Genitourinary Surgery

MOSBY'S PERIOPERATIVE NURSING SERIES

Genitourinary Surgery

Gratia M. Nagle, RN, BA, CNOR, CRNFA, CURN

Nursing Director
Paoli Surgery Center
RN First Assistant/Clinical Urology Nurse
Adult and Pediatric Urology/Infertility
Great Valley Erectile Dysfunction Clinic
Paoli, Pennsylvania

*Chapter 3 authored by and select sections
co-authored by:*

James R. Bollinger, MD, FACS

Adult and Pediatric Urology/Infertility
Great Valley Erectile Dysfunction Clinic
Chairman, Department of Urology
Paoli Memorial Hospital
Paoli, Pennsylvania

with 778 illustrations

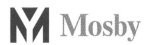 Mosby

St. Louis Baltimore Boston Carlsbad Chicago Naples New York Philadelphia Portland
London Madrid Mexico City Singapore Sydney Tokyo Toronto Wiesbaden

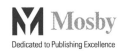 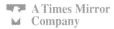

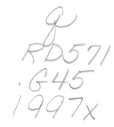

Vice President and Publisher: Nancy L. Coon
Editor: Michael Ledbetter
Developmental Editor: Nancy O'Brien
Project Manager: Dana Peick
Senior Production Editor: Stavra Demetrulias
Manuscript Editor: Carl Masthay
Senior Composition Specialist: Joan Herron
Designer: Amy Buxton
Manufacturing Manager: Betty Muellar
Cover Art: Stacey Lanier/AKA Design
Cover Photo: Catherine Nagle
Photography: Gratia M. Nagle
Illustrator: Cindy Bollinger

Printed in the United States of America
Composition by Mosby Electronic Production
Lithography/color film by Arthur Morgan Co.
Printing/binding by Von Hoffmann

Mosby–Year Book, Inc.
11830 Westline Industrial Drive
St. Louis, Missouri 63146

ISBN 0-8151-7029-7

97 98 99 00 01 / 9 8 7 6 5 4 3 2 1

Consultants

Emmie J. Amerine, RN, BS, CURN
Clinical Urology/Radiology Nurse
Adult and Pediatric Urology/Infertility
Great Valley Erectile Dysfunction Clinic
Paoli, Pennsylvania

Sharon Anderson, PhD
Reproductive Endocrinology
Main Line Reproductive Science Center
Wayne, Pennsylvania

Nancy Arnold
Laser Peripherals
Minnetonka, Minnesota

Norma L. Baer, RN, BSN
District Clinical Manager
Heraeus Surgical
Milipitas, California

Phil Bilello, MD
Departments of Anesthesia
Paoli Memorial Hospital and
   Paoli Surgery Center
Paoli, Pennsylvania

James R. Bollinger, MD, FACS
Adult and Pediatric Urology/
   Infertility/Erectile Dysfunction
Chairman, Departments of Urology
Paoli Memorial Hospital and
   Paoli Surgery Center
Paoli, Pennsylvania

Marcia L. Collymore, RN, MHS
Facility Manager
Paoli Surgery Center
Paoli, Pennsylvania

Thomas J. Connor
Regional Manager
Cook Urological, Inc.
Spencer, Indiana

Larry Davis
Southeast Regional Sales Manager
Heraeus Surgical
Milipitas, California

Dennis Daye, PA-C
Adult and Pediatric Urology/Infertility
Great Valley Erectile Dysfunction Clinic
Paoli, Pennsylvania

Jill Dooling
Certified Stapling Technician
Auto Suture Co.
Norwalk, Connecticut

Brian Dye
Sales Consultant/
   Field Sales Trainer
Bard Urological Division
CR Bard, Inc.
Covington, Georgia

Joseph Ferroni, MD, FACOG
Chairman, Department of
   Obstetrics/Gynecology
Paoli Memorial Hospital and
   Paoli Surgery Center
Paoli, Pennsylvania

Rick Flynn
Technical/Sales Consultant
Erbe USA
Marietta, Georgia

Eileen Gehn
Valley Laboratory
Boulder, Colorado

Mary R. Gosline
Technical/Sales Consultant
Opto-Systems, Inc.
Newtown, Pennsylvania

Thomas Hakala
Director of Operations
Laser Peripherals
Minnetonka, Minnesota

Evan W. Hauck, PhD
Professor of Languages
Great Valley School District
Malvern, Pennsylvania

Jane A. Hibbler, RN, BS, CPTC
Transplant Coordinator
Delaware Valley Transplant Program
Philadelphia, Pennsylvania

Benjamin Jacobs, MD
Anodyne Associates
Chairman, Departments of Anesthesia
Paoli Memorial Hospital and
   Paoli Surgery Center
Paoli, Pennsylvania

Mark W. McClure, MD, DABU
Central Carolina Urology Associates PA
Raleigh, North Carolina

Earl E. Sands, MD, FACOG
Gynecology, Obstetrics, and Infertility
Pottstown, Pennsylvania

Virginia Schuster
Implant Consultant
American Medical Systems
Minnetonka, Minnesota

Gregory Thompson, MS, MD
Adult and Pediatric Urology
Paoli, Pennsylvania

Richard Yelovich, MD
Radiation Oncology
Paoli Cancer Center
Paoli Memorial Hospital
Paoli, Pennsylvania

J. Clifford Vestal, MD
Adult and Pediatric Urology
Phoenixville, Pennsylvania

Reviewers

Ellen Carson, PhD, RNCS
Associate Professor
Pittsburg State University
Pittsburg, Kansas

Wanda L. Dunkel, BAN, RN, CNOR
Clinical Nurse III
Laser and Microscope Coordinator
Operating Room
Memorial Medical Center
Springfield, Illinois

Brigitte Gerbert, RN
Clinical Urology Nurse
Fetze-Claire Urology Association
Allentown, Pennsylvania

Susan Musser, BSN, CNOR
Operating Room Manager
Lancaster Surgery Center
Lancaster, Pennsylvania

For Jane, Jim, and Rich

Preface

"The real essence of nursing, as of any fine art, lies not in the mechanical details of execution, nor yet in the dexterity of the performer, but in the creative imagination, the sensitive spirit, and the intelligent understanding lying back of these techniques and skills. Without these, nursing may become a highly skilled trade, but it cannot be a profession or a fine art. All the rituals and ceremonials which our modern worship of efficiency may devise, and all our elaborate scientific equipment will not save us if the intellectual and spiritual elements in our art are subordinated to the mechanical, and if the means come to be regarded as more important than ends."

Stewart, 1929

The genitourinary patient is vulnerable, and entrusts him or herself to our care. The perioperative nurse has the opportunity and responsibility to function as the advocate of each patient. Care of the genitourinary patient requires critical thinking and creativity.

To date, too little information has been available to the genitourinary perioperative nurse. The intent of this book is to provide a resource for perioperative nurses specializing in genitourinary surgery. This book expands the perioperative role beyond the confines of the operating room walls to encompass preoperative and postoperative teaching and care. It is meant to be a guide for those in practice and those entering practice, and should be adapted to the situation of each reader.

The focus is the adult genitourinary patient: to emphasize the unique needs of each patient, and to identify the perioperative considerations and interventions that form the basis of professional genitourinary practice. It is intended to be a comprehensive coverage of perioperative genitourinary nursing. Medical/surgical nursing, critical care nursing, and rehabilitation are extensively addressed in other texts, and only briefly mentioned here. Space constraints necessitate concentrating on the more common procedures. Renal transplant is detailed from the aspect of the donor harvest only, the transplant itself belonging to the realm of dedicated institutions. Pediatrics is mentioned as a point of reference, but it is beyond the scope of this writing to deal with the subject in any detail. That must be the topic of a separate book.

Part I, Foundations of Genitourinary Surgical Nursing, begins with the history of genitourinary surgery (Chapter 1) and provides a perspective from which to gain an understanding of the roots of urologic intervention. The anatomy and physiology of the genitourinary system (Chapter 2); surgical pathophysiology (Chapter 3); the diagnostic techniques essential in determining surgical care (Chapter 4); the genitourinary team and the elements of perioperative nursing standards, process, and care (Chapter 5); and the equipment and instruments required for implementing that care (Chapter 6) are detailed.

Part II details the surgical interventions that will be encountered most frequently. Endoscopic and laser interventions are discussed in Chapter 7; laparoscopic procedures are covered in Chapter 8; classic open procedures are addressed in Chapters 9, 10, and 11; microscopic approaches are reviewed in Chapter 12; and more advanced technology, such as ESWL and cryotherapy, are detailed in Chapter 13.

The methods and supplies are intended to be generic, for each practice setting will differ in terms of surgical theory, training, and technique. Much of the information provided is left open to discussion for precisely this reason. There are no hard and fast rules, only recommendations based on the experience and expertise of those in practice. That is what makes perioperative genitourinary nursing so exciting—it is constantly growing, bringing change and improvement with that growth.

Some of the unique features of Genitourinary Surgery *are:*

- Surgery through the ages, showing how little, as well as how much, has changed.
- The components essential to an interdisciplinary approach to patient care.
- A review of anatomy and physiology from the urologic perspective.
- The pathophysiology that brings the genitourinary patient to the surgical arena.
- Diagnostic methods that determine the course chosen for the genitourinary patient.
- Comments regarding nursing and surgery from those long past, those who helped form the foundations of our present practices.
- The holistic nursing process and its adaptation to a specialized focus.

- In depth approaches, with illustrations, to positioning.
- A sample care plan and critical pathway to use as a guide for all genitourinary procedures.
- Considerations for the RN First Assistant related to genitourinary surgery.

- A step-by-step description of the procedures with accompanying rationale, alternatives, creative innovations, complications, and expected sequealae.
- Colored photographs of surgery in process to augment the procedural descriptions.

"We need to realize and affirm anew that nursing is one of the most difficult of arts. Compassion may provide the motive, but knowledge is our only working power. Perhaps, too, we need to remember that growth in our work must be preceded by ideas, and that any conditions which suppress thought, must retard growth. Surely we will not be satisfied in perpetuating methods and traditions. Surely we shall wish to be more and more occupied with creating them."

M. Adelaide Nutting, 1925

Acknowledgements

"In the beginning, God created nursing. He (or She) said, I will take a solid, simple, significant system of education and an adequate, applicable base of clinical research, and On these rocks, will I build My greatest gift to Mankind—nursing practice. On the seventh day, He—threw up His hands. And has left it up to us."

MM Styles

This text would not have been possible without the assistance of my colleagues in nursing and medicine. Their ready support enabled me to turn an idea into a reality.

First and foremost, I thank my Facility Manager, Marcia Collymore, RN, MHS, for her continual support, critiques, and encouragement. Many thanks to my staff at the Paoli Surgery Center, especially, Michelle, Debbie, Jeanne, Judy, BJ, Karla, Char, and Steve; and to my Regional Vice-President, Shelvy Frank, RN, MS. Sincere thanks also to Dottie Moser, RN, MHA, Operating Room Nurse Manager at Paoli Memorial Hospital, and members of her operating room staff: Norma, Janice, Helen, Desmond, Ken, Tim, Joann, Debbie, Jeff, Patti, JoAnne, Kathy, Betty, Beth, and Kay.

Thanks also to Pottstown Memorial Hospital, Sandi at Chester County Hospital, and Barbara and Margie at Phoenixville Hospital and their operating room nurses. I appreciate being allowed to intrude and sometimes interrupt your flow.

To my friends in the various anesthesia departments: Phil, Ben, John, Elaine, Mary Ann, Pat, Vince, Barb, Betty, and Terry —thank you!

Many thanks to the surgeons who have believed in me and taught me over the years. It would take a chapter to name all of you, but you each know who you are. My growth as a perioperative nurse is in large part due to your influence. Surgeons were also instrumental to the outcome of this text by providing me key operative moments to capture on film. Sincere gratitude to James Bollinger, MD; Francis Fanfera, MD; Earl Sands, MD; Clifford Vestal, MD; Joseph Conti, MD; and Mary Diephaus, MD. And to those willing subjects, otherwise known as the surgical patient, I won't name you, but I certainly thank you for participating.

Special thanks to Cook Urological for their financial assistance, providing the opportunity to attend a seminar critical to the development of this project. I am truly grateful.

Company representatives provided material crucial to creating this book. I thank Steven Lambert from Circon, Mark Goodwin from Innerdyne, Ginny Schuster from AMS, Brian Dye from CR Bard Urological, Jill Dooling from Auto Suture, Tom Connor from Cook Urological, and Mary Gosline from Opto-Systems.

No photographer could achieve a product without help. Thank you Dennis; Jim; Michelle at PSC; and Debbie, Norma, and Janice at PMH for snapping shots when I couldn't be there. In addition to photographs, illustrations were a necessity. Thank you, Cindy, for your wonderful drawings.

To my Mosby family, thank you for your belief in me by offering this opportunity and guiding me through the process. Many thanks to the unsung members of the production staff. Michael, Teri, Julie, and Nancy: you were terrific! I could not have done it without your support.

Thank you to my family, for putting up with me. It has been a long year.

Contents

Genitourinary Surgery

Foundations of GENITOURINARY SURGICAL NURSING

1

The History of Genitourinary Surgery

I will not use knife, not even on sufferers from stone, but will withdraw in favor of such men as are engaged in this work.

Hippocrates

For centuries urology has held an ambivalent position, at best, in the practice of medicine. Despite being the only specialty specifically mentioned in the Hippocratic oath, the men engaged in the specialty were considered in a lower class, both socially and professionally.

George Livermore in his 1933 presidential address to the American Urological Association expressed the situation in the following manner: "Urology was born in filth and degradation, nourished in ignorance and superstition; espoused by quacks and charlatans, in whose vicious clutches it reached its zenith in avariciousness and cupidity...."[4]

It cannot hinder, but rather assist, the genitourinary perioperative nurse to survey the evolution of urology through the ages. An overview of how the specialty began and progressed will provide insight to present day methods and mind-set.

PRERENAISSANCE PERIOD

Humankind has been beset by dysfunction of the genitourinary system since the dawn of time. In ancient China surgery was limited to the castration of men and boys seeking advancement at court. Originally, castration was exercised as a form of severe punishment, but eventually total removal of the penis and testicles came to be a pledge of absolute allegiance to the monarchy.

Ancient Babylonian writings, dating to 2300 BC, contain descriptions of venereal disease and attest that Abraham performed circumcisions. An illustration in the Hebraic Bible, dated 1299, displays ceremonial sacrificial vessels and circumcision knives used by the ancients. Physicians of ancient Greece based what was known of human anatomy in rational thought, giving the bladder, rectum, buttocks, and pelvic bones precise topographic relationships to each other.

Urinary infections, as well as renal and bladder calculi, have been identified in the mummies of early Egypt. A link between the functioning of the outside world and internal human function may have prompted the Egyptians to view man's physiology as a system of channels *(metus)* similar to the irrigation canals throughout the country. They believed that air was ingested

through the nose and ears and entered these channels; it was then delivered to the heart and from there to all parts of the body. These channels were also thought to carry urine, sperm, blood, tears, and feces. Information from the patient and complex physical examination that included the study of body emanations such as urine formed the basis for diagnostic methods. References were made to bloody urine, possibly indicating cystitis, infection, or calculi. Egyptian scrolls from approximately 2000 BC, as well as the Old Testament (the Books of Chronicles, Exodus, Leviticus, Kings, and Proverbs), describe the rite of circumcision and promote strict rules regarding prophylaxis against contagion through sexual relations.

Of the ancient cultures, India displayed the most skill at surgical intervention. Written discussions describe tumor excisions, amputations, hernia and harelip repairs, cesarean sections, and removal of bladder stones. More than 125 surgical instruments are depicted, including trocars and catheters, as well as instructions for handwashing and the bandaging of wounds. The Vedas, Holy Sanskrit books written in 1600 BC, comprise four volumes. One volume, the Atharva Veda, contains innumerable incantations and charms for the practice of magic; disease, injuries, sanity, health, and fertility are mentioned. Although methods of diagnosis included magical approaches, the patient was also scrutinized carefully, especially their body fluids such as urine. Diabetes was detected by the sweet taste of a patient's urine. Medical and surgical theoretical instruction incorporated memorization and recitation of the Vedas. Practical training included performing surgical procedures on the bladders of animal carcasses.

The advent of Hippocratic methods in 400 BC placed the focus on the patient rather than the condition. Great emphasis was placed on the observation and evaluation of physical findings. Hippocratic writings from ancient Greece promulgate directions for giving large amounts of fluid for kidney cases.

According to Galen (130 to 200 AD), considered the last of the great minds of Greece, elaborate diagnoses were based on symptomatology, with virtually every symptom a disease.

1

Twelve diseases of the bladder were established with emphasis on the condition rather than the patient. Much of Galen's knowledge of anatomy stemmed from animal dissection, accounting for some of his errors. The frontispiece from a 1565 collection of his works depicts him dissecting the internal organs, including the kidneys and bladder, from a pig.

Of the great minds in history, mention should be made of Celsus (130 to 200 AD). Although not regarded as a true medical practitioner by many scholars (partly because he wrote in Latin rather than Greek), his perceptive and detailed descriptions of anatomy and surgical interventions are appreciated by modern day surgeons. These writings, found in the *De Medicina*, covered a wide range of topics including thorough instructions for hernia repair, with mention made of the scrotal cavity, tunica, and plastic restoration of the penile prepuce.

Much Greek and Roman theory and methodology owes its preservation to the seventh century influence of Islam. Arabic physicians used essentially the same methods as their Greek and Roman counterparts. Because of the emphasis placed on uroscopy (examination of urine), the half-filled urine flask became the symbol for the physician. The color, consistency, sediment, smell, and taste of urine helped in determining what was wrong with a patient, thus aiding prognosis and guiding treatment (Fig. 1-1).

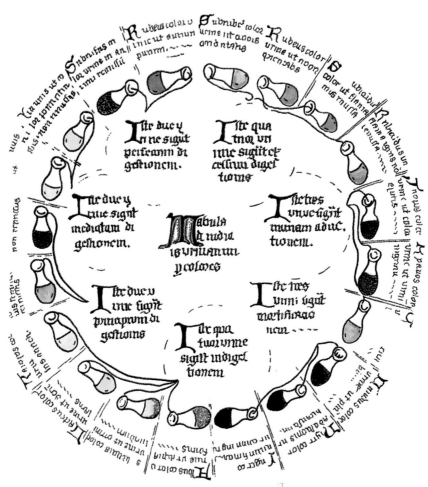

Fig. 1-1 Medieval uroscopy chart illustrating the study of urology. Written in the commonly spoken Latin, vulgar Latin, the table addresses the quality of urine by its color and the clinical ramifications associated with each color ranging from clear to black. Translation: The chart title is in the center, revolving in a counter-clockwise direction and setting forth the symptoms of worst digestion to better digestion. It makes its observations in comparative groups of 2, 3, and 4 examples. In addition to several levels of digestion, deadly indications and burning urine are mentioned. The outermost border denotes the colors that present with the symptomatic findings. Black/gray accompanies very grave circumstances; red/blue shades are synonymous with burning. The most healthful indications are associated with clear urine. Milky urine is indicative of indigestion. *(Illustration courtesy Bodleian Library, Oxford, England. Artwork by Cindy J. Bollinger. Translated by Evan W. Hauck, Language Dept., Great Valley School District, Malvern, Penn.)*

THE DARK AGES

During the late Middle Ages (500 to 1500), an extensive specu-
lative system was erected on weak foundations. Data was based
on the study of astrology, urine, and herbal and pulse lore. This
was in part a result of the ban placed by Pope Boniface VIII on
the dissection of human corpses, which brought medical and
surgical advancements to a halt.

Chaucer, in his *Canterbury Tales,* relates a story of a fourteenth century pilgrimage. Among the travelers was a physician,
depicted in a drawing performing uroscopy on a flask of urine.
The fourteenth century Greek manuscript *Antidotarium* pic-
tures a physician in a pharmacy examining urine.

While many outstanding practitioners performed surgery
and continued to document their experiences, lithotomy
(removal of urinary bladder stones) was condemned, no doubt
because of the poor results. The fourteenth century Roman
manuscript *Rolandus Parmensis Chirurgia* depicts an operation
for removing bladder stones, a procedure with very poor outcome at that time.

Girolamo Fracastoro of Verona acquired medical fame in
1530 through his celebrated poem *Syphilis Sive Morbus Gallicus,*
which recognized the venereal cause of what was termed the
"French disease," renaming it syphilis. The poem epitomized
contemporary knowledge of the condition, its suspected mode
of transmission, and a treatment remedy. In 1539 Diaz da Isla of
Barcelona wrote of the previously unknown, unseen, and unde-
scribed disease that appeared in 1493 after the voyage of
Columbus, which by all accounts was obviously syphilis.
During this same period, Paracelsus began referring to the mal-
ady as "French gonorrhea," causing confusion lasting until the
nineteenth century.

RENAISSANCE PERIOD

An illustration from the fifteenth century *Epistle of Othea,* by
Christine de Pisan of France, depicts a physician examining a
patient's urine that was carried to him by messenger. This typ-
ifies the reliance on uroscopy for diagnosis that existed in virtually every culture. Other depictions may be found in the seventeenth century French paintings "The Village Doctor" by
David Teniers the Younger and "The Dropsical Woman" by
Gerard Dou.

The fifteenth century brought with it outstanding advances
resulting from a revolt against the authority of the church and
the restrictions initiated in 1300 by Pope Boniface VIII. A foundation of accurate knowledge regarding the function and structure of the human body was built through the dissection of
human cadavers. The text *Fasciculus Medicinae,* written in 1491
by Johannes de Ketham of Italy, contains 10 woodcuts depicting
contemporary medical practice, including didactic lectures and
human anatomic dissection.

The invention of the printing press allowed for greater dissemination of new knowledge and led to an increase in vernac-
ular texts. In 1543, Andreas Versalius published *De Humani
Corporis Fabrica,* which was based on direct observation and
thus removed Galenic errors, marking the beginning of modern
anatomy. Ambroise Pare, known as the father of modern
surgery, elevated the practice to a more dignified position in
1564 through his treatise *Ten Books of Surgery* (Fig. 1-2).

One of earliest examples of pelvic surgery dates to 1561
when Pierre Franco of Lausanne reported the removal of a large
bladder calculus through a suprapubic cystotomy. During this
time the first surgical procedure on the prostate was also
reported. In Valetta in 1575 the Knights of Malta erected one of
the first hospitals. The institution was specifically intended for
cases of hemorrhage, lithotomy, and insanity.

During the 1603 syphilis epidemic in London a change in
social attitude regarding promiscuity developed as a result of
the newly acquired knowledge of sexual transmission. Secrecy
began to surround such activity, resulting in the foregoing of
treatment and consequent spread of the disease. Barber surgeons treated the lesions with painful salves of mercury.

THE SCIENTIFIC REVOLUTION

The seventeenth century brought many advances in medicine.
De Motu Cordis was published in 1628 by William Harvey,
establishing him as the founder of modern physiology. In 1651
Exercitationes de Generatione Animalium, his contribrution to
embryology, was published.

A renowned clinician, Thomas Willis, performed many
human autopsies in order to relate clinical symptoms to pathology. He was one of the first to emphasize the sweetness of urine
in diabetes mellitus, differentiating it from the unrelated condition diabetes insipidus.

An engraving in *Specimen Medicinae Sinicae,* written in
1682, depicts acupuncture with points marked for kidney treatment. The invention of the microscope by Anton von
Leeuwenhook in Holland brought diagnostics to a new level.
Through the implementation of his invention he became the
first to describe spermatozoa.

During this time theories concerning alkalosis and acidosis
were postulated as causes of chemical imbalance, and quantitative discoveries of capillary circulation and metabolism became
medical landmarks. Anatomists of this time still have their

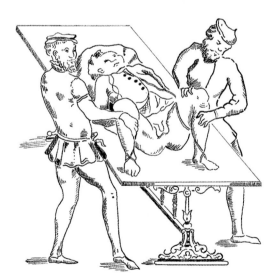

Fig. 1-2 Patient properly positioned for bladder stone
removal, from the *Ten Books of Surgery* by Ambroise Paré,
1564. *(Illustration courtesy The New York Academy of Medicine,
New York, N.Y. Artwork by Cindy J. Bollinger.)*

names attached to the structures they were responsible for discovering. One such example is Cowper's gland in the male . This century also brought the first appearance of medical journals. Although strides were made in virtually every nation, Italy was the leader in science and medicine.

AGE OF ENLIGHTENMENT

Eighteenth century medicine began an era of accelerated discovery, such as the masterful research in transplantation by John Hunter of Scotland. He transformed surgery into a rational science. The approach to lithotomy (cutting into the peritoneum to remove urinary bladder calculi) was improved when Jacques de Beaulieu, a French friar, used a lateral incision. An English contemporary, Richard Wiseman, published numerous case histories on similar attempts in the 1700s. Later, William Cheselden, also of England, gained recognition for lithotomy. Considered an expert when speed in any surgical procedure was essential, Cheselden reportedly performed the technique in less than one minute. Unfortunately, progress in medical science was often hampered by the perpetuation of elaborate hoaxes. One particularly significant hoax was accomplished by Joanna Stephens of England, who milked the gullible of thousands of pounds and convinced even Cheselden that she had discovered a remedy for dissolving urinary stones.

The first recorded lithotomy in America occurred circa 1760. John Jones of New York was reported to have successfully performed the technique in 3 minutes or less. The father of American surgery, Philip Syng Physick, afflicted by kidney stones himself, had an avid interest in urology. After beginning his surgical practice in 1792, he developed his own bougies of linen and beeswax to treat urinary obstruction and vesical stones. He tapped hydroceles with trocars and irrigated the cavity with wine. In 1795, Physick designed a lancet-cannula for internal urethrotomy and a gorget with interchangeable blades for bladder neck incisions.

MODERN MEDICINE

The nineteenth century continued to offer advancement in medicine as it elevated nursing to a new level of expertise. Bacteriology and immunology developed as separate disciplines. Precision instruments for diagnosis and treatment began to be introduced.

The 1800s heralded the first attempts to incorporate bowel segments into the urinary tract. Jean Civale of France invented a lithotrite for crushing urinary bladder stones. American Benjamin W. Dudley, in practice from 1806 to 1839, was a surgical mainstay of the Medical School of Transylvania in Kentucky. His most common and successful operative intervention was lithotomy performed through a lateral approach. Dudley devised urologic instrumentation including a silver catheter, retractors, a urethrotome, calculus extractors for dislodging urethral stones and bladder stone fragments, a flexible silver catheter, and a urethral dilator, as well as a gorget modified from one invented by Henry Cline of London. Attempts were made in 1830 to dilate the prostatic urethra with a gold beater's balloon (Fig. 1-3).

In 1827, in addition to the discovery of antiseptics by Lister, Amussat of France removed a hazelnut-sized tumor protruding

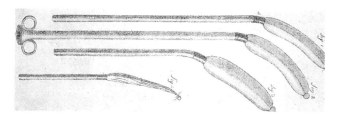

Fig. 1-3 Circa 1830 balloon dilatation device. *(From Kirby RS et al:* Benign prostatic hyperplasia, *London, 1993, Mosby-Wolfe.)*

from the bladder neck in a patient with bladder outlet obstruction. Another French contributor during this era was Charles Edouard Brown-Sequard. Often spoken of as the founder of endocrinology, his lectures taught that the adrenals, kidneys, thyroid, spleen, pancreas, and liver all had secretions, which are now called hormones, that enter the bloodstream and are useful in treatment. He also believed that injections of extracts from the testis would produce rejuvenation. As a result, patients are now being treated with injections of testosterone for loss of libido resulting in sexual dysfunction.

Germany produced leaders in pathologic anatomy and physiology, among them Karl von Rokitansky and Rudolf Virchow, the founder of cellular pathology. Virchow's text, *Cellular Pathology Based on Physiological and Pathological Histology,* has been called one of the three greatest medical books since Hippocrates. Friedrich Wohler broke the barrier between inorganic and organic chemistry in 1828 when he successfully synthesized urea from ammonia and carbon dioxide.

In 1831 John Marshall, Chief Justice of the Supreme Court, put himself in Physick's hands. He was successfully diagnosed and treated for multiple bladder calculi that had been causing dysuria and obstructive symptoms for 2 to 3 years.

In the 1840s Philippe Ricord of France demonstrated the character of syphilis, dividing it into three distinct stages and differentiating it from gonorrhea.

J.M. Sims of the United States quite inadvertently discovered a patient positioning technique (knee-chest followed by dorsal lithotomy) that allowed for repair of vesicovaginal fistula in 1845. During this same period, masterful reports by Richard Bright of London on the pathologic and clinical nature of diseases of the kidneys led to the name *Bright's Disease* for chronic nephritis. A colleague of Bright, Thomas Addison, performed such thorough examinations with perceptive analyses that he successfully isolated pernicious anemia and adrenal insufficiency. Both are still referred to as Addison's anemia and Addison's disease of the adrenals.

The year 1851 saw the first urologic publication in America. Written by Samuel D. Gross, *A Practical Treatise on the Diseases, Injuries and Malformations of the Urinary Bladder* was 3 years in the making. The text became widely used, resulting in subsequent extended editions. In the same year as Gross's treatise, Willard Parker described the first cystotomy for inflammation and rupture of the bladder.

More difficult urologic interventions began to be attempted. Joseph Pancoast of Philadelphia performed the first successful surgery for exstropy of the bladder in 1858. The first successful excision of a diseased human kidney occurred in 1861 in Milwaukee under the hands of Erastus W. Wolcott.

Nursing gained recognition when Preston described the ideal nurse as an artist and in 1863 developed a 6-month course of nursing instruction. The training covered surgery, medicine, obstetrics, poultice and plaster preparation, diet principles, and cooking methods.

Edward Keyes of Bellevue opened the first hospital ward in America for genitourinary patients in 1875. Urology as a specialty was finally given its first academic recognition in 1877 by the Bellevue Hospital Medical College with the appointment of William H. Van Buren as Professor of Diseases of the Genitourinary System and Clinical Surgery. A text he wrote in collaboration with Keyes, *Diseases of the Genito-urinary Organs, with Syphilis,* was a common medical school book for more than 50 years. In 1878 Henry Bigelow made one of the most important contributions to urology with his invention of the lithotrite and successful development of the first litholapaxy procedure. Samuel Alexander became a partner of Keyes in 1887 and is considered one of the first true urologists in the specialized sense. His lengthy article on prostate disease, *The Technique of Median Prostatectomy,* was published in 1911.

In 1879 Neisser discovered gonococcus, and in 1882 Koch reported discovery of the tubercle bacillus. Also in 1879, Nitze and Leiter of Germany invented the first practical cystoscope. The light source consisted of an exposed platinum wire lit by electric current. It took until the 1920s, however, to devise a feasible technique to adequately visualize the urinary tract.

The application of local anesthesia in urology came about in 1884 when Fessenden Nott Otis tried a 4% concentration of cocaine hydrochlorate to numb a strictured urethra before litholapaxy. The 10-minute procedure was performed following administration of the agent and the patient felt no pain. In addition to this achievement, Otis designed the Otis urethrometer and the dilating urethrotome. The latter is still in use today.

The first transvesical, or suprapubic, prostatectomy to completely remove obstructing prostate tissue was performed by von Dittel in 1885. The patient died of sepsis on the sixth postoperative day. William Belfield of Chicago performed the first successful suprapubic (transvesical) prostatectomy in 1887, followed closely by McGill. Belfield won an international reputation with his book, *Diseases of the Prostate,* published in 1893. He was the first to identify the tubercle bacillus and gonococcus by microscopic smears.

The year 1893 ushered in many advances in urology. James Brown, chief of the Genitourinary Dispensary at John Hopkins Hospital, performed the first ureteral catheterization of a male patient. He accomplished this with his own modification of the Nitze-Leiter cystoscope and a soft, pliable catheter. George Edebohls reported on his treatment of movable kidney with nephropexy. In 1899 he performed the first procedure to relieve chronic nephritis and in 1901 introduced renal decortication for Bright's disease. Howard Kelly successfully distended a female patient's bladder with air and effectively visualized and catheterized the ureteral orifices under direct vision. In 1894 Kelly developed a technique of uretero-ureteral anastomosis utilizing a catheter as a temporary splint. Kelly, in collaboration with Dumm, introduced the Kelly plication for incontinence in women in 1914.

Eugene Fuller of New York performed the first complete enucleation of a prostatic adenoma in 1894, and in 1895 stressed the importance of complete enucleation. The discoveries of x-rays by Wilhelm Konrad Roentgen in 1895, of radioactivity by Antonio Henri Becquerel in 1896, and of radium by Marie and Pierre Cure in 1898 initiated a new realm for science. Around this same time, in 1897, Tuffier placed a rigid metal stylet into a ureteral catheter outlining the ureter on an abdominal radiograph, thereby initiating the development of urographic contrast material. Roentgen's discovery enabled him to show that abdominal radiographs could also demonstrate radiopaque urinary calculi. Soon the radiographic location of the ureters and kidneys was accomplished by the retrograde placement of radiopaque ureteral catheters. By the first decade retrograde pyelogram was being performed by Voelcker and von Lichtenberg, but the colloidal silver contrast material was found to cause kidney injury.

Internationally, twentieth century medicine continued to expand at a rapid pace. Ether and chloroform proved to be effective anesthetic agents. The role of the nurse anesthetist became integral with the increased sophistication of surgery. The fields of surgery and urology did not, however, attract many female practitioners. This possibly was due to the presumption that a woman would not be accepted by patients of either sex, as well as long-standing professional resistance.

Treatment for incontinence in women began to be approached in earnest during the 1900s. The Goebell-Frangenheim-Stoeckel technique utilizing a rectus fascia strip that remained attached to the midline was proposed by these German gynecologists. Modifications of this technique are achieving successful results today.

In 1901 Jokichi Takamine isolated epinephrine from the adrenal medulla and Peter Freyer of London achieved continued success with suprapubic prostatectomies. Albarran made the first endoscopic diagnosis of an upper urinary tract tumor in 1902. Lewis allowed successful stone passage in 1905 by dilating the ureter on a patient with ureterovesical junction obstruction. That same year Albarren described RPF (retroperitoneal fibrosis, a dense desmoplastic process that may involve any or all structures within the peritoneum). Also in 1905 the spirochete of syphilis was identified through darkfield microscopy by Fritz Schaudinn and Erich Hoffmann in Berlin. In 1906 serodiagnostics for syphilis were introduced by August von Wasserman.

O'Coner credits van Stockum for the first retropubic prostatectomy for benign prostatic hyperplasia (BPH) in 1908. In 1909 Franz Torek reported on his technique for orchiopexy and established the pattern for numerous operations. Rowntree and Geraghty developed the phenolsulfonphthalein kidney-function test, called the Hopkin's test, resulting in another giant step in diagnostics. In 1909 Leo Buerger introduced the first indirect irrigating observation and double catheterizing cystoscope, by adding modifications to the instrument pioneered by F. Tilden Brown. It was aptly called the Brown-Buerger cystoscope (Fig. 1-4).

Hugh Hampton Young, the father of modern American urology, performed the first rigid ureteroscopy in 1912 but the procedure did not become routine until Goodman and Lyon in 1977. Young, of John Hopkins Hospital and University, created the first

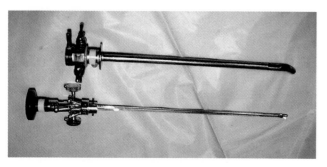

Fig. 1-4   Brown-Buerger cystoscope.

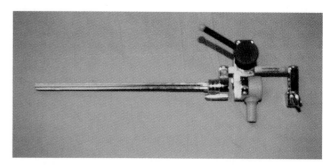

Fig. 1-5   McCarthy resectoscope working element.

official residency program in urology in 1916. The program was based at the James Buchanan Brady Urological Institute on the Hopkins campus, a donation from his friend and patient "Diamond" Jim Brady. Other achievements to Young's credit are the development of the Young prostatic tractor and the prostatic punch. In 1917 the first issue of the *Journal of Urology* was published with Young as editor-in-chief. Known for his sense of humor, Edward Keyes is reported to have said "The prostate makes most men old, but it made Hugh Young."

With the dawn of the 1920s transmission of light through glass fibers became known. Walter B. Cannon of Harvard coined the phrase *homeostasis* to describe the dynamic equilibrium regulating human physiology. John Caulk used infiltration anesthesia on the internal vesical orifice for the removal of minor obstructions, utilizing a cautery punch of his own design. Bumpus discussed the distribution of lymph node metastasis from prostate adenocarcinoma in 1921, stating that if the iliac glands could be examined satisfactorily, their early involvement would undoubtedly be proven. Also in 1921 the operating microscope was introduced by Nylen, but it did not enter the realm of urology or gynecology until the 1970s. Osbourne and Rowntree performed the first intravenous urography at the Mayo Clinic in 1923, but the contrast material consisted of inorganic iodide salts that led to poor opacification and a high incidence of adverse reactions.

The advancements in visualizing the urinary tract led to the invention of specialty instrumentation. The first of these tools was the observation and operating cystourethroscope invented by Joseph McCarthy in 1923, followed by the metal-cone-tipped–dilator set created by Lyons in 1924 for the treatment of incontinence in women. Later McCarthy became known for his foroblique panendoscope and resectoscope (Fig. 1-5). The first successful dye was discovered in Berlin by Binz and Swick. They developed Selectan-neutral pyridine compound that opaqued the kidneys, and later Uroselectan (Iopax). The technique of intravenous injection for urinary tract radiography developed by Swick in 1929 was the forerunner of later, more sophisticated angiography. Hugh Hampton Young first visualized a child's ureter and renal pelvis with a rigid pediatric cystoscope in 1929. He passed the instrument into the renal pelvis of a 2-week-old patient with massively dilated upper collecting systems secondary to posterior urethral valves, and visualized the interior of the ureters, renal pelves, and calyces.

In the 1930s outstanding hospitals and universities still combined urology and general surgery, and much urologic inter-vention was performed by general practitioners and surgeons. Retropubic prostatectomy was popularized through the efforts of Jacobs and Casper in the United States in 1933 and Hybbinnette in Sweden in 1935. Edwin Beer perfected the first practical pediatric cystoscope in 1935. The problem of impotency also began to be addressed, and in 1936 Bogoras created a prosthesis for penile rigidity from a patient's rib. The year 1938 saw a published compilation of the current tenets of penile lymph anatomy by Rouviere of France.

During the 1930s a 12-month internship in urology became a universal component of American medical education. Nurses began assisting in the operating room, delivery room, and outpatient units as the trend to specialized care evolved into expanded and extended roles during the 1940s.

In 1941 W.J. Kolff put kidney dialysis on a functioning basis with his artificial kidney and the discovery of a suitable filtering material. Aldridge perfected his version of the Goebell-Frangenheim-Stoeckel fascial sling for incontinence in women in 1942. Corrective techniques for impotency were still being attempted. In 1944 penile implants constructed from resected rib were placed bilaterally, in the dorsal corporal canals, by Frumkin. In 1945 retropubic prostatectomy for BPH was reintroduced and popularized by Terrance Millin of Ireland. He showed that his technique offered excellent visualization of the bladder neck and allowed for improved hemostasis. Metalcone–shaped dilators with interchangeable tips, for placement into the ureteral orifice under direct vision, were introduced by Dourmashkin in 1945. Marshall, Marchetti, and Krantz began intervention for incontinence in women in 1949. Their procedure involved a retropubic suspension of the vagina and urethral wall to the symphysis pubis, or retropubic urethropexy, with the patient in dorsal lithotomy position.

In 1950 Wallingford synthesized "urokon," a triiodinated benzoic acid derivative (sodium acetrizoate), for visualizing the urinary tract radiographically. Bricker initiated the ileal conduit for urinary diversion (a cutaneous urinary diversion) in 1950. Also in 1950 Richard Lawlor initiated a major contribution to urology when his team transplanted a cadaver kidney. Using an end-to-end anastomosis, Lawlor and his team afforded a woman with bilateral polycystic disease 5 extra years of life.

The 1950 Nobel Prize for medicine was awarded to E.C. Kendall and P.S. Hench of the United States and Tadeus Reichstein of Switzerland for describing the structure and biologic effects of suprarenal cortex hormones.

It was 1954 before advanced endoscopic technology was introduced by Hopkins, Kapany, and Van Heel. In 1955 Goodwin and associates performed the first percutaneous nephrostomy to decompress an obstructed kidney.

Advances in surgical treatment for cancer developed as a result of the 1959 Flocks and Whitmore reports. A significant incidence of clinically unsuspected metastasis to the obturator, hypogastric, and external iliac nodes was found in separate studies of patients with clinically localized adenocarcinoma of the prostate. This same year a needle bladder neck suspension for stress incontinence in women was promoted by Pereyra. A special cannula for a blind suprapubic stab through the retropubic space and paraurethral tissues was the primary instrumentation for this technique (Fig. 1-6).

The 1960s brought the development of flexible instrumentation by Bush and associates and the invention of the current rod lens system for rigid endoscopy by Harold H. Hopkins. Hopkins revolutionized light transmission with his rigid rod lens system that enhanced endoscopic illumination, and he developed the fiberoptic technology that led to flexible endoscopes. Inserting the endoscope cystoscopically like a ureteral catheter, he visualized the upper urinary tract. Forced diuresis provided irrigation as accessories were manipulated alongside the endoscope. In 1961 Burch devised a retropubic suspension of the perivaginal fascia to Cooper's ligament for the treatment of stress incontinence. This was accomplished by elevating the vaginal fascia lateral to the urethra and entering the retropubic space.

Quackels performed the first successful cavernospongiosum shunt for priapism in 1963, and in 1964 Grayhack devised the saphenocavernosum shunt, also for priapism. Successful utilization of a 3 mm fiberscope (or ureteroscope) transurethrally through a 26 Fr cystoscope into the distal ureter to visualize a stone at 9 cm was accomplished by Marshall in 1964. There was no method to change the angle of the tip or irrigate and distend the ureter but visualization remained excellent.

Harer and Genther modified the Pereyra bladder neck suspension in 1965 with a vaginal incision to mobilize the urethra and absorbable sutures to approximate the paraurethral tissues across the midline. In 1966 Smith described the pathology and attempted to define the cause of penile scarring (Peyronie's disease) as a vascular inflammatory process beginning in the space between the tunica and the erectile tissue of the penis. It was felt an association with Dupuytren's contracture existed. Also in 1966 Beheri performed an intracorporeal placement of a penile prosthesis constructed of polyethylene rods.

Takagi developed and successfully utilized a narrow flexible fiberscope, 2.7 mm in diameter and 70 cm long, through a ureterotomy in 1966. Another major step took place in this same year when Victor Marshall successfully carried out a renal autotransplantation. In 1967 Pereyra and Lebherz modified the original bladder suspension technique by entering the retropubic space under finger control and opening the lateral paraurethral tissues. In the same year, Taubner and Wapler further modified this method by employing the cystoscope to place the suspension sutures under direct visual control. Also in 1967 Pearman placed a silicon single rod penile prosthesis between the dorsal aspect of Buck's fascia and the tunica albuginea.

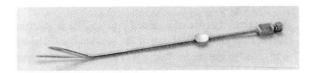

Fig. 1-6 Pereyra needle. *(Courtesy Pilling Co., Fort Washington, Penn.)*

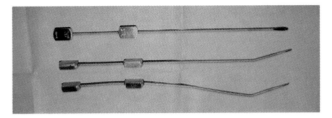

Fig. 1-7 Stamey needles, 0, 15, and 30 degrees.

In 1969 Almen proposed the use of radiographic nonionic compounds with the same opacity as the benzoates but less osmolality. These contrast solutions became known as iopamidol (Isovue) and iohexol (Omnipaque).

Stamey modified the needle suspension for stress incontinence in 1973 by placing dacron buttresses under cystoscopic control and creating a set of three needles angulated at 0, 15, and 30 degrees for suture placement (Fig. 1-7). The cystoscope, along with elevation of the suspension sutures and bolsters for additional bladder neck support, allowed accurate placement at the bladder neck and visualization of the bladder neck closure. In 1973 advances in the manufacture of penile prosthetics also took place. Scott introduced the inflatable AMS 700 CX system, Mentor promoted their hybrid polyurethane copolymer device known as the Bioflex, and the team of Small and Carrion invented a pair of silicone semirigid rod implants. A further modification of the Pereyra bladder neck suspension that eliminated a vaginal incision was developed by Winter in 1976.

Lasers began to be utilized during urologic intervention and in 1976 Staehler revealed a full thickness bladder burn with the argon-beam laser. Advances since have enabled clinical applications of the Nd: YAG, holmium: YAG, CO_2, KTP, and pulse-dyed lasers as well. Progress with penile prosthetics continued with the introduction of the 1977 Finney-Flexirod developed by Finney. A modification of the cavernosa-glans shunt for priapism was described by Al-Ghorab in 1978, and Cobb and Ragde presented a double prong needle with a barrel knot for bladder neck suspension. This needle allowed for a sufficiently supportive fascial bridge with the nylon knot supporting the paraurethral tissues. This was their alternative to the dacron buttress.

Raz further modified the needle suspension in 1981 by creating an inverted U incision, mobilizing the urethra, and placing helical sutures. AMS presented the AMS 600 semirigid, semimalleable paired tapered silcone rod penile implants in 1983, and in 1985 produced the hydroflex implant. In 1986 the Flexi-Flate penile implant by Surgitek-Finney hit the market. In

1987 Gittes and Loughlin began to use the Stamey needles instead of the Pereyra and developed an incisionless technique. Around this same time Eddehoj performed the first corpora-glans shunt for priapism.

RECOGNITION AS A SPECIALTY

Specialty organizations were established over the passing years. In 1886 the American Association of Genito-Urinary Surgeons was formed. Around the same time, Belfield of Chicago started the Chicago Urological Society. The American Urological Association came into being in 1902 with Ramon Guiteras as the first president. This organization is presently the primary association for urologists nationwide, with chapters throughout the country. The (AMA) *American Medical Association* established the Section on Genito-Urinary Diseases in 1910, which has since been renamed the Section on Urology. The addition of the subspecialty of pediatric urology marks the growth still occurring within the specialty. The restructuring of the American Board of Urology in the 1970s placed the specialty in perspective and has led to improved education, research, and practice.

Nursing organizations have also been formed to gather those specializing in the practice of genitourinary nursing. Registered nurses, licensed practical nurses, surgical technologists, physician assistants, physicians, surgeons, and other allied health care workers from all practice settings are welcomed. The American Urological Association Allied, Inc. (AUAA), formed in the 1970s, was the official genitourinary nursing branch of the American Urological Association (AUA). Restructured in 1995, the Society of Urologic Nurses and Associates (SUNA) is now the official genitourinary nurses organization and a separate entity from the AUA. Another less widely known organization is the International Urologic Society (IUS) which functions on a similar premise. Certification in the specialty of urology may be attained through Certification Board for Urologic Nurses and Associates (CBUNA) in Pitman, New Jersey.

The past few decades have seen urology blossom into a full-grown and accepted specialty. Urologic specialists have collaborated with specialists in other disciplines to coordinate treatment efforts. New methods of treating old problems, old methods revitalized and enhanced, and new problems to be addressed are here. The individualized and group specialty goal remains the same as in the beginning: improved patient care.

Bibliography

1. Davidson AJ, Hartman DS: *Radiology of the kidney and urinary tract,* Philadelphia, 1994, WB Saunders.
2. Donahue MP: *Nursing: the finest art,* St. Louis, 1985, Mosby.
3. Droller MJ: *Surgical management of urologic disease,* St. Louis, 1992, Mosby.
4. Eaton Laboratories: *A bicentennial history of the practice of urology in the United States,* Northfield, 1976, Medical Communications, Inc.
5. Emmett JL, Witten DM: *Clinical urography,* vol 2, Philadelphia, 1971, WB Saunders.
6. Huffman JL, Bagley DH, Lyon ES: *Ureteroscopy,* Philadelphia, 1988, WB Saunders.
7. Kirby RS, Christmas TJ: *Benign prostatic hyperplasia,* London, 1993, Gower.
8. Lilly: *200 years of surgery: milestones in American medicine,* Indianapolis, 1976, Eli Lilly and Co.
9. Lyons AS, Petrucelli RJ: *Medicine: an illustrated history,* New York, 1978, Harry N. Abrams.
10. Rogers FB: *A syllabus of medical history,* Boston, 1962, Little, Brown.
11. Rogers FB: *Medical education in the United States,* Hagerstown, 1974, HarperCollins.
12. Smith V: *Fifty glorious years: mid-atlantic section American Urological Association, 1941-1991,* Richmond, 1992, Wm. Byrd Press.

2

Genitourinary System

Remember that anatomy which is learned by memory is easily forgotten and is often useless, but anatomy which you have grasped by your reason and understanding will last forever...Let me therefore caution you again—do not depend on anatomy which you have committed to memory, but learn anatomy by using your sense of understanding and of reason, as well as the sense of seeing and feeling. Learn to understand the structures of the body, on which depends your ability to do surgery, by studying its development from the egg stage to completion. Your knowledge of anatomy and of physiology must not depend upon what you read in books; it must be founded on observations made by yourself by the use of your senses and the use of instruments of precision. You can have no scientific knowledge as long as you depend upon the authority of books and lectures. Science abhors authority. It requires demonstration of facts, it believes nothing upon anyone's authority.

Augustus Charles Bernays

Knowledge of the anatomic structures and an understanding of renal physiology is necessary to appropriately facilitate safe patient positioning and proper instrumentation. The urologist's plan of care should be coordinated with perioperative nursing care in preparing the genitourinary patient for surgery.

The normal genitourinary system includes two kidneys, two ureters, the urinary bladder, the urethra, and the prostate gland in the male. Also considered essential to the genitourinary system are the adrenal glands, male reproductive organs, and the female urogynecologic system. As technology expands and new procedures are developed, genitourinary surgery finds itself crossing paths with other specialties.

The normal physiology of the urinary tract is discussed in this chapter with pertinent clinical concepts to provide the novice student with a memory mechanism. The subject is addressed in more detail in Chapter 3, which describes pathophysiologic disorders.

ANATOMY AND PHYSIOLOGY
Adrenal Glands
Anatomy
The adrenal glands cap the medial aspects of the superior pole of each kidney and lie retroperitoneally beneath the diaphragm (Fig. 2-1). Triangular in shape, the right adrenal is adjacent to the inferior vena cava. The rounded, crescent-shaped gland on the left lies posterior to the stomach and pancreas. Each adrenal gland is composed of a cortex that secretes steroids (cortisol) and hormones (aldosterone), and a medulla that secretes norepinephrine and adrenaline (epinephrine). Pituitary gland activity stimulates these secretions. Branches from the aorta and the inferior phrenic and renal arteries provide a liberal arterial blood supply. On the right, venous blood drains into the inferior vena cava, while on the left it exits through the left renal vein. The lymphatics accompany the suprarenal vein and empty into the lumbar lymph nodes.

Physiology
The adrenal glands function as two distinct organs. The adrenal cortex and medulla each have specific physiologic functions.

The cortex produces the steroids that maintain metabolic homeostasis, regulate salt retention, and modulate sexual activity. These steroids are derived from cholesterol and pregnenolone (the basic steroid structure). The zona glomerulosa, the outer zone of the adrenal cortex, produces aldosterone and is the only source of this mineralocorticoid. The other zones, the fasciculata and reticularis, produce cortisol, the androgens (male hormones), dehydroepiandrosterone, dehydroepiandrosterone sulfate, and androstenedione.

Aldosterone serves to maintain sodium and potassium balance with active sites in the kidneys, intestines, salivary glands, and sweat glands. In all locations its effect is to increase sodium absorption and potassium secretion (see Chapter 3).

Metabolic blockade in the pathway of cortisol production may lead to adrenal cortical hyperplasia because of overstimulation by adrenocorticotropic hormone (ACTH) produced by the pituitary gland (see Chapter 3). Cortisol is essential for life. Its effects include the accumulation of glycogen (carbohydrate) in the liver and muscle, enhancement of the cellular production of glucose (gluconeogenesis), impairment of peripheral glucose utilization, and interactions with other hormones.

Production of cortisol from cholesterol requires that enzymes be present. These may be congenitally absent. A deficiency of one or more enzymes may lead to overproduction of steroid hormones, the intermediates in the production of cortisol, and may have variable clinical effects that are dependent on the steroid effect.

Adrenal androgens are only weakly active compared with androgens of testicular origin unless a pathologic state exists, such as congenital adrenal hyperplasia, where masculinization may occur (an increase in male secondary sexual characteristics such as body habitus and hair distribution).

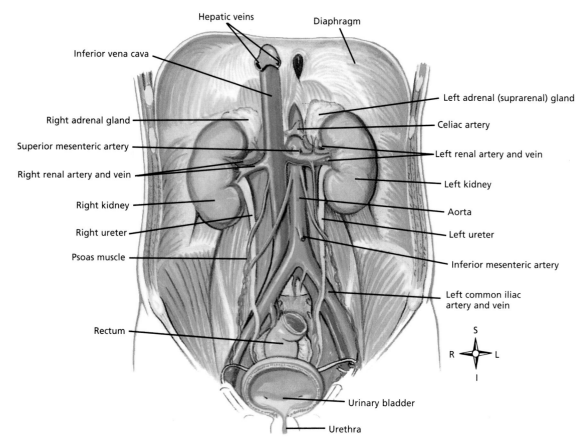

Hepatic veins

Diaphragm

Inferior vena cava

Left adrenal (suprarenal) gland

Right adrenal gland

Celiac artery

Superior mesenteric artery

Left renal artery and vein

Right renal artery and vein

Left kidney

Right kidney

Aorta

Right ureter

Left ureter

Psoas muscle

Inferior mesenteric artery

Left common iliac artery and vein

Rectum

Urinary bladder

Urethra

Fig. 2-1 Location of the urinary system organs. Anterior view of urinary organs with peritoneum and visceral organs removed. *(Courtesy Ernest W. Beck. From Thibodeau GA, Patton KT:* Anatomy and physiology, *ed 3, St. Louis, 1996, Mosby.)*

The adrenal medulla produces 14% of the body's epinephrine, 13% of its dopamine, and 73% of its norepinephrine. These hormones are known as catecholamines. The medulla of the adrenal gland is bathed in the blood from the adrenal cortex and contains high levels of glucocorticoids. The glucocorticoids in this blood are necessary for the activation of the enzyme phenylethenolomine-N-methyltransferase for the biosynthesis of epinephrine.

Catecholamines cause varied clinical effects by stimulating different receptor sites (protein binding sites). The actions of epinephrine and norepinephrine are not independent but rather dose dependent. Receptor sites are classified as alpha and beta depending on the effect produced when stimulation occurs. For example, the alpha-1 effect on smooth muscle, blood vessels, and the prostate is contraction; the alpha-2 effects include constriction of large veins and relaxation of the intestines. Beta actions include the beta-1 effects of increased heart rate and efficiency; and the beta-2 effects of airway (bronchioles) dilatation and relaxation of the intestine and uterus. Dopaminergic reactions include vasodilation and inhibition of norepinephrine release.

The metabolism of catecholamines includes degradation by the enzymes catecholamine-O-methyl transferase and monoamine oxidase. In addition, the catecholamines may be taken up by the neurons swhere they were released initially. They are removed from the circulation rapidly, with a half life of only 20 seconds. The metabolic product of their degradation is vanilmandelic acid (VMA), with metanephrine and normetanephrine contributing. These are excreted in the urine and are assayed during evaluation for pheochromocytoma (see Chapter 3).

Kidneys

Anatomy

The kidneys lie along the lateral borders of the psoas muscle in the retroperitoneal space. One is located on each side of the vertebral column at the level of the twelfth thoracic vertebra to the third lumbar vertebra. The liver rests above and anterior to the right kidney, causing its location to be several centimeters below the left kidney. The adult kidney weighs from 115 to 175 grams, is approximately 11 cm long from the upper pole to the lower pole, averages 5 to 7 cm in width, and is up to 3.5 cm in thickness. Generally the kidney in a female is smaller.

Loose, fatty areolar tissue known as perirenal fat surrounds each kidney. A capsule of fascia renalis, or Gerota's fascia, encloses the renal space (Fig. 2-2). These structures help to maintain the kidneys in their normal anatomic position as well as to serve as protective cushions in an otherwise lean body mass area. Figure 2-3 shows the anterior and posterior relationships of the kidneys.

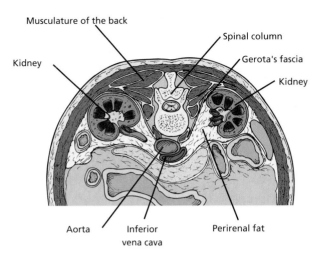

Fig. 2-2 Protective covering of kidneys. *(From Gray M: Genitourinary disorders, St. Louis, 1992, Mosby.)*

The renal vessels (artery and vein) and the ureter enter and leave through a concave area known as the *hilum* on the medial side of each kidney. The renal pelvis is a funnel-shaped structure, lying posterior to the renal vascular pedicle, that divides into several branches (calyces) within the kidney (Fig. 2-4). The renal parenchyma is composed of the medulla and the cortex. The medulla consists primarily of pyramids (triangular wedges) with bases that face the cortex laterally and narrow papillae that face the hilum. Each papilla protrudes into a calyx where the urine leaving the papilla is collected for transport from the kidney. The cortex surrounds the medulla and dips in between the pyramids, forming columns and lobules.

Blood supply to the kidney is conveyed through the renal artery, a large branch of the aorta, and leaves through the renal vein, making it a highly vascular organ (Fig. 2-5). Upon entering the kidney the renal artery divides into anterior and posterior sections. These sections divide further into interlobular arteries from which smaller afferent branches (arterioles) thread to the glomeruli. Efferent arterioles in the glomeruli then pass to the tubules of the nephron. At any one time the kidneys process approximately one fifth of the body's entire blood volume.

The renal lymphatic supply, originating beneath the capsule of the kidney, empties into the lumbar lymph nodes at the renal vascular pedicle-aortal junction. The nerves of the involuntary (autonomic) nervous system originate from the lumbar sympathetic trunk and the vagus nerve. The pedicle of the kidney consists of a renal artery, renal vein, nerves, and lymphatics. Renal function is not impaired by destruction of the nerve pathways.

Physiology

Renal physiology includes developmental anatomy, microanatomy, renal blood flow, renal metabolism of electrolytes, concentration mechanism, acid-base balance, excretion of organic solutes, and the effect of hormones on renal function.

The kidneys receive one fifth of the cardiac output, constitute less than 1% of the total body mass, and filter 180 L of fluid out of the blood each day at a rate of 1 L of blood per minute to produce approximately 1 ml of urine per minute. Total renal blood flow is 1200 ml per minute per 1.73 squares meters (m^2)

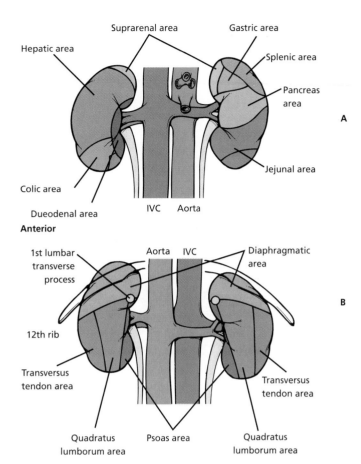

Fig. 2-3 Anterior, **A**, and posterior, **B**, relationship of kidneys and ureters to organs in peritoneal cavity, to vertebral column posteriorly, and to main arteries and veins. *(From Meeker MH et al: Alexander's care of the patient in surgery, St. Louis, 1995, Mosby.)*

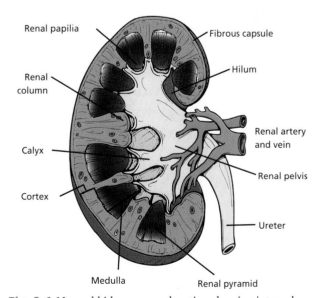

Fig. 2-4 Normal kidney, coronal section showing internal structures. *(From Thibodeau GA, Patton KT: Anatomy and physiology, ed 3, St. Louis, 1996, Mosby.)*

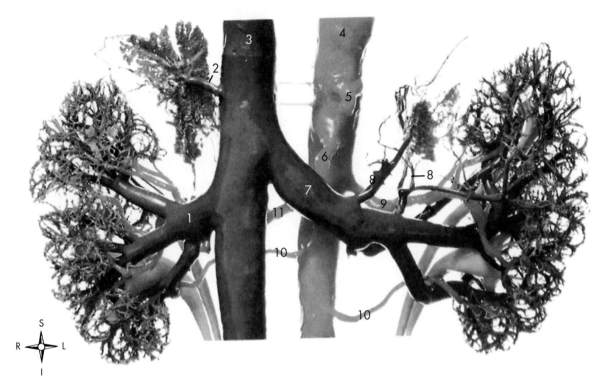

Fig. 2-5 Renal blood supply, anterior view. *1,* Right renal vein; *2,* Right suprarenal vein; *3,* Inferior vena cava; *4,* Aorta; *5,* Celiac trunk; *6,* Superior mesenteric artery; *7,* Left renal vein; *8,* Left suprarenal vein; *9,* Left renal artery; *10,* Accessory renal arteries; *11,* Right renal artery. *(From Thibodeau GA, Patton KT: Anatomy and physiology, ed 3, St. Louis, 1996, Mosby.)*

of body surface. Ninety percent of the blood flow is distributed to the renal cortex and the remainder to the medulla, or inner portion of the kidney tissue.

The functional unit of the kidney is the nephron, which is composed of the glomerulus, proximal convoluted tubule, loop of Henle, distal convoluted tubule, and collecting duct (Fig. 2-6). Production of urine begins with the filtration of blood passing through the afferent arteriole of the glomerulus. The filtrate passes into Bowman's space (capsule) and the lumen of the tubule of the nephron at the level of the glomerulus. The filtered blood passes out via the efferent arteriole. Following a set path, the filtrate then passes through the proximal convoluted tubule, the loop of Henle, and the distal convoluted tubule into the collecting duct, the renal pelvis, and down the ureter. The filtrate is modified along its path by the reabsorption of certain components as well as the secretion of others. Still other components are excreted without secretion or reabsorption.

Clearance is a quantitative description of the rate of excretion of substances compared with their concentration in the bloodstream. A substance that is neither reabsorbed nor secreted has a clearance equal to the glomerular filtration rate (GFR) and is used in clinical situations as a measure of renal function. A carbohydrate polymer of fructose, inulin, has a clearance equal to GFR because it is neither reabsorbed nor secreted. Endogenous creatinine is used to estimate GFR because of the difficulty in performing inulin clearances clinically. Creatinine clearance is calculated by multiplying the concentration of creatinine in urine by the total urinary volume over 24 hours; the result is divided by the concentration of creatinine in the plasma multi-

plied by 1440 minutes. At lower clearance rates creatinine is secreted and clearance determination overestimates renal function. Kidney function and weight vary with body surface area. In calculating GFR it is sometimes appropriate to describe it in terms of the standard body surface area (1.73 m^2). Without collecting urine over 24 hours the GFR may be estimated using the following formula:

Male patient

$$\frac{(140 - \text{age}) \ (\text{Kg of weight})}{(72) \ (\text{serum creatinine})} = \text{creatinine clearance mL/min}$$

Female patient

$$\frac{(140 - \text{age}) \ (\text{kg of weight})}{(72) \ (\text{serum creatinine})} \ (0.85) = \text{creatinine clearance mL/min}$$

This is particularly helpful when calculating GFR to determine the appropriate dose of a potentially nephrotoxic medication such as one of the aminoglycosides (e.g., gentamicin).

Glomerular filtration is driven primarily by the hydrostatic pressure in the glomerular capillary, and the afferent and efferent arterioles. In addition the colloid osmotic (oncotic) pressure in Bowman's space, the tubules of the nephron, and the interstitial tissues just outside the nephron, moderate the effect of the head of pressure exerted in the glomerular capillary. The autoregulation of glomerular filtration pressure by the kidney serves as a protective mechanism for the nephron. Normally, at blood pressures between 80 and 180 mm Hg, there is only a 10% variation in renal plasma flow and glomerular filtration rate. Only at arterial pressures below 80 mm Hg is there an

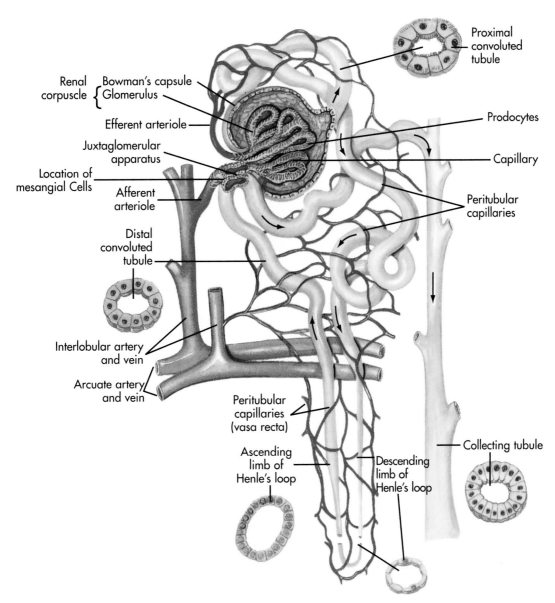

Fig. 2-6 Nephron, the basic functional unit of the kidney, showing the surrounding peritubular blood vessels. *(From Thibodeau GA, Patton KT:* Anatomy and physiology, *ed 3, St. Louis, 1996, Mosby.)*

increase in resistance to blood flow in the efferent arteriole, thereby maintaining GFR at the nephron level.

The autoregulatory mechanism for blood flow is not clearly understood, but may be due to the rate, or osmolality, of filtrate flowing through the distal tubule (the distal tubuloglomerular feedback mechanism), the muscle tone in the afferent arteriole related to systemic pressure changes (myogenic theory), or the presence of vasodilatory metabolites such as prostaglandins (metabolic theory). At arterial pressures below 80 mm Hg, GFR drops with a corresponding decrease in urinary output, as seen in cardiogenic or hypovolemic shock (prerenal oliguria).

The fluid entering Bowman's space is almost free of albumin. Filtration is restricted by the selective permeability of the glomerulus, which is due to pore size and electrical charge. Neutral dextran, which is the same size as albumin but has no net negative charge, is filtered 100 times more easily than albumin. Filtration of molecules greater than 14 angstroms (Å) in radius is progressively restricted so that those of 40 Å cannot filter through into Bowman's space.

Regulation of sodium and water, sodium excretion, and urinary dilution and concentration are a result of selective absorption of components of the filtrate through the proximal and distal tubules, the loop of Henle, and the collecting duct as they pass through the kidney from the cortex toward the medulla. The ducts of the nephron pass through a milieu (environment) that has progressively more oncotic pressure around them to facilitate absorption of components of the filtrate. This is known as the countercurrent multiplier mechanism.

To maintain acid-base balance the kidney reabsorbs 80% of the filtered bicarbonate (HCO_3^-), a base, in the proximal convoluted tubule. In addition the kidney manufactures additional bicarbonate by secreting hydrogen (H^+). The collecting tubule provides the final mechanism for excretion of acid with titration of ammonia, phosphate, and other titratable buffers (compounds that bind hydrogen ions without allowing dissociation at the pH of the filtrate). Carbonic anhydrase is an enzyme that catalyzes the hydration of carbon dioxide to form carbonic acid, which dissociates into bicarbonate and H^+. This enzyme is present in the cells of the tubules and the luminal surface (brush border) so that net absorption of bicarbonate and secretion of acid is accomplished. Factors that affect proximal tubular reabsorption of bicarbonate include hydration (decrease in hydration facilitates absorption of bicarbonate) and increased CO_2 in respiratory insufficiency (increases absorption as does potassium depletion). Parathyroid hormone and phosphate depletion inhibit reabsorption.

Most net acid excretion occurs in the collecting duct, where it is secreted by metabolic pumps (systems requiring the expenditure of energy) that are also dependent on intracellular carbonic anhydrase. The net rate of acid excretion may be modified by a change in the electrical gradient between the collecting tubule cells and the lumen, primarily by changes in the amount of sodium delivered to the distal tubule. Increases in sodium in the distal tubule increase the secretion of acid because the sodium is reabsorbed. Acid is secreted to maintain electrical neutrality in the lumen of the tubule. Mineralocorticoids, such as aldosterone, can directly stimulate the capacity of the pump secreting acid. Alterations in the availability of titratable buffer, such as ammonia, may change the net rate of acid excretion.

Defects in the ability of the kidney to excrete acid may occur because of defects in the secretory mechanisms in the proximal or distal tubules. Proximal renal tubular acidosis (Type 2) is caused by a lowered threshold for reabsorption of bicarbonate. Normally, 80% of filtered bicarbonate is reabsorbed in the proximal tubule. In this disorder excretion of calcium and potassium is increased but formation of renal calcifications is rare. Clinically, children affected by this disorder may have osteomalacia, rickets, abnormal intestinal calcium absorption, and decreased phosphorus levels and vitamin D metabolism.

Distal renal tubular acidosis (Type 1) may be complete or incomplete. The clinical features include nephrocalcinosis and acidosis in the complete form, and an inability to secrete a urine with a level below pH 5.4 with an acid load in the incomplete form.

Most of serum potassium (90%) undergoes filtration, the majority absorbed in the proximal tubule. Potassium excretion is augmented by increased tubular flow, as occurs after diuretic administration, with increased sodium load, or from the effect of aldosterone.

Plasma calcium that is not bound to plasma proteins is filtered by the glomerulus. There is a subsequent 98% tubular reabsorption in the proximal tubule and the ascending loop of Henle. Calcium reabsorption follows sodium and is excreted in increased amounts after administration of the diuretic agent furosemide (Lasix). Chlorthiazide, also a diuretic, inhibits sodium transport and increases reabsorption of calcium. This is the therapeutic effect often sought for some patients with the tendency to form urinary stones.

Urea is the major metabolic end product of protein breakdown and is freely filtered by the glomerulus. The rate of urea reabsorption is inversely related to the rate of flow through the tubules. This accounts for the disproportionate increase in blood urea nitrogen (BUN) levels compared with serum creatinine levels during dehydration (prerenal azotemia).

Glucose is also freely filtered at the glomerulus and is completely reabsorbed in the early portion of the tubule. With increasing amounts of glucose in the filtrate, a tubular maximum glucose tolerance is reached beyond which it begins to pass into the urine.

Citrate apparently helps prevent the formation of urinary calcium lithiasis (stones) by binding calcium. It is metabolized into CO_2 and water inside the cell, and its excretion is dependent on the presence of acidosis or alkalosis.

The kidney has important endocrine functions, at times interacting with its excretory function. Important endocrine functions include renin-angiotensin, prostaglandin, kallikrein-kinin, erythropoietin, and vitamin D metabolism.

The renin-angiotensin-aldosterone system is one of the most important renal hormone mechanisms regulating systemic blood pressure, sodium and potassium levels, and blood flow. This system plays an integral role in the development of renovascular hypertension. Renin is secreted in response to influences that reduce arterial blood pressure, such as heart failure, sodium depletion, and hemorrhagic shock. The system responds by generating elevated levels of angiotensin II, a potent vasoconstrictor. In addition, angiotensin II stimulates the adrenal zona glomerulosa to increase production of aldosterone, which elevates the reabsorption of sodium (Fig. 2-7). The renin-angiotensin-aldosterone system plays a major role in protecting against sodium depletion, despite a rising systemic blood pressure resulting from vasoconstriction and decreased organ perfusion. In the kidney, angiotensin II acts directly on the renal vasculature by causing constriction. The basis for prehydration of surgical patients with saline solutions is to minimize the risk of postoperative renal failure (acute tubular necrosis) which may occur as a result of constriction of the renal vasculature secondary to increased circulating levels of angiotensin II.

Atrial natriuretic peptide, produced in the atrium of the heart, regulates both sodium metabolism and systemic blood pressure. In the kidney it acts to increase GFR and renal plasma flow and to decrease tubular reabsorption of sodium leading to diuresis. It has a dilatory effect on vascular smooth muscle and inhibits aldosterone secretion from the adrenal gland.

Insulin receptors are present in the kidney and when stimulated cause decreased excretion of sodium and phosphate. The action of glucagon appears to be opposite, leading to increased excretion of sodium and phosphate.

Catecholamines such as adrenaline appear to have activities in the kidney affecting renal blood flow and distribution, GFR, renin secretion, and tubular fluid reabsorption. The actions appear to be mediated through alpha- and beta-adrenergic receptor sites.

The kidney is the major site of conversion of vitamin D to its active form. The site of action of both vitamin D and parathyroid hormone appears to be the distal nephron.

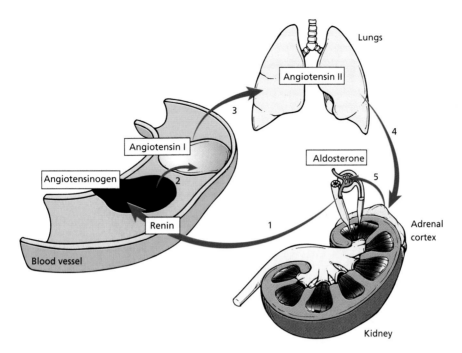

Fig. 2-7 Renin-angiotensin mechanism for regulating aldosterone secretion.
1. The juxtaglomerular apparatus secretes renin into the blood when incoming blood pressure drops below a certain level.
2. Renin, an enzyme, facilitates conversion of angiotensinogen to angiotensin I.
3. Angiotensin I is converted to angiotensin II in the lungs, by enzymes in the capillaries.
4. Angiotensin II stimulates secretion of aldosterone in the adrenal cortex.
5. Aldosterone causes increased reabsorption of sodium, resulting in increased water retention, which leads to increased blood volume. Increased blood volume elevates the blood pressure and causes the renin-angiotensin mechanism to stop.

(Courtesy Joan M. Beck. From Thibodeau GA, Patton KT: Anatomy and physiology, *ed 3, St. Louis, 1996, Mosby.)*

Erythropoietin is the most important hormone involved in the regulation and maintenance of normal circulating levels of red blood cells (erythrocytes). This hormone is derived primarily from the kidney in the adult (and the liver in the infant). Under normal conditions the production of red blood cells is controlled by the level of oxygen in the bloodstream. In anemic patients with normal kidney function an increase in the production of erythropoietin by the kidneys stimulates the production of red blood cells in the bone marrow. Chronic renal failure leads to a decrease in the production of erythropoietin, resulting in the anemia seen in this condition. Patients on chronic renal dialysis who are treated with erythropoietin experience an increased level of exercise tolerance associated with their increased red blood cell count.

Eicosanoids are fatty acids that are synthesized in the renal cortex and medulla. These may have vasoconstrictor as well as vasodilatory activity. They are known as prostaglandins, prostacyclins, and thromboxanes.

Prostaglandins play a limited role during normal physiologic activity, but during general anesthesia production increases and maintains normal renal blood flow. Drugs that decrease the production of prostaglandins include the nonsteroidal antiinflammatory drugs (NSAIDs) such as aspirin, naproxen, ibuprofen, and indocin.

Hormones metabolized in the kidney include insulin, parathyroid hormone, calcitonin, glucagon, angiotensin, growth hormone, vasopressin, erythropoietin, thyroid-stimulating hormone (TSH), luteinizing hormone (LH), follicle-stimulating hormone (FSH), and human chorionic gonadotropin (hCG). Nephrectomy (removal of a kidney) prolongs the time required for the release of hormones from the circulation into the urine. Successful renal transplantation will facilitate metabolism and excretion.

In a similar way excretion of drugs from the urinary tract may be delayed in patients with renal insufficiency. This is particularly important when the drug may be nephrotoxic, as with the aminoglycoside class of antibiotics (gentamicin, tobramycin, amikacin).

Ureters

Anatomy

The ureter is a continuation of the renal pelvis, extending in a smooth **S** curve to the base of the bladder. Relative to the position of the kidneys, the left ureter is slightly longer than the right. A fibromuscular cylindrical tube composed of three layers, the adult ureter averages 25 to 30 cm long and 4 to 5 mm in diameter with a lumen that varies from 0.2 to 1 cm in diameter. A fibrous outer protective sheath gives way to smooth muscle, which overlies the submucosal lamina propria of vessels and nerves. The interior is lined by transitional-cell epithelial mucosa (urothelium) that is resistant to the secretion or reabsorption of components in the urine.

Lying on the psoas muscle, the ureter passes medially to the sacroiliac joint and lateral to the ischial spine. Curving backward toward the base of the bladder, the ureter inserts into the trigone muscle. Three areas in the ureter are more susceptible to obstruction from calculi because of normal anatomic narrowing: the ureteropelvic junction (UPJ), the point where it crosses the external iliac vessels, and the ureterovesical junction (UVJ).

The renal pelvis and ureter form a continuous tube that extends from the hilum of the kidney to the base of the bladder. The UPJ is where the pelvis of the kidney tapers into the ureter. The UVJ is composed of the lower ureter, the trigone muscle, and the bladder wall. The lower ureter enters near the ureterovesical outlet at the lateral aspect of the trigone. A portion of the ureter, the intravesical ureter, enters through the bladder wall and is unique from the upper ureter. Approximately 1.5 cm long, it is composed of the intramural segment surrounded by detrusor muscle and the submucosal segment, which travels under the mucosa. The smooth muscle bundles of the upper ureter form a complex network while the intravesical ureteral bundles are arranged longitudinally to promote closure of the lumen. Terminating as the ureterovesical valve, the intravesical ureter opens into the bladder. The muscle bundles fan out and terminate in the trigone at the base of the bladder (Fig. 2-8).

An adventitia of dense connective tissue anchors the lower ureter to the bladder. The superficial layer is an extension of the bladder wall's connective tissue and the inner layer is an extension of the ureteral adventitia. A plane of loose connective tissue, Waldeyer's sheath, lies between these layers. This tissue affords mobility to the intravesical ureter, allowing it to accommodate to structural changes that occur in the bladder as it fills with urine.

Ureteral arterial blood supply varies. The upper ureter may receive blood from the branches of the renal, adrenal, or gonadal arteries. The lower ureter may receive blood from branches of the obturator artery, the uterine artery in females, or the deferential artery in males. A venous plexus allows drainage of venous blood into vessels that parallel the arterial supply. Paraaortic or renal node chains and the common or external iliac node chains provide for lymphatic drainage.

Physiology

Urine is transported from the kidney through a process called efflux. Slight distention occurs in the renal pelvis as urine accumulates, approximately 15 to 20 ml, initiating a propulsive wave of muscular contractions extending along the ureter. Urine is propelled down the ureter and into the urinary bladder through this peristaltic action. Neural, endocrine, and pharmacologic influences also affect the smooth muscle contractions of the ureter. If alpha-adrenergic receptors in the ureteral wall are stimulated, the strength and number of contractions is increased. If beta-adrenergic receptors are stimulated, relaxation results. When cholinergic receptors are stimulated, the release of catecholamines appears to cause more vigorous contractions. Peristalsis is enhanced with the administration of epinephrine or catecholamines.

Urinary Bladder
Anatomy

The urinary bladder is a hollow viscus organ, composed of detrusor muscle fibers, that acts as a reservoir for the storage of urine until micturition (voiding) occurs. It is lined by an inner urothelial layer, a vascular submucosa, and an outer adventitial layer. The urothelium consists of transitional epithelial cells and the submucosa is composed of arteries, veins, connective tissue, lymphatic channels, and nerves. Formed of connective tissue, the adventitia is loosely connected to the peritoneal fascia and anchored to the abdominal wall by the urachus. The base of the bladder is formed by the trigone, a small triangular area. The trigone consists of superficial and deep muscle. The deep, tightly bound smooth muscle is a continuation of Waldeyer's sheath and terminates at the bladder neck in a circular layer of smooth muscle fibers that contribute to continence. The superficial muscle is an extension of the muscle fibers of the intravesical ureter and extends into the bladder neck in females and the proximal urethra in males.

The three corners of the trigone correspond to the openings (orifices) of the ureters and the bladder neck (opening of the urethra) (Fig. 2-9). The ureteral orifices lie on the proximal trigone at the interureteric ridge and are approximately 2.5 cm apart. Converging detrusor muscle fibers of the bladder wall form the bladder neck (internal sphincter), help secure the intravesical ureter at its point of entry, and pass distally to become the smooth musculature of the urethra. As the bladder fills with urine it expands into the abdominal cavity.

The main arterial supply of the bladder includes the superior and inferior vesical arteries and the vesiculodeferential, or uterine, artery. These vessels arise from the internal iliac (hypogastric), the internal pudendal, and the inferior gluteal arteries. The superior vescial artery supplies the dome and the posterior aspect of the bladder, while the vesiculodeferential artery feeds the fundus of the uterus and the terminal ureter. The inferior vesical artery supplies the bladder base, the proximal urethra, and the prostate. The obturator artery and vaginal artery in the female also contribute to the blood supply. The rich venous supply of the bladder drains into the lateral plexi around the ureter and the prostatovesical plexus (pudendal plexus, Santorini's plexus). The veins empty into the internal iliac vein from these plexi. The vesical, the external and internal iliac, and the common iliac lymph nodes supply the lymphatic system.

The bladder's size, position, and proximity to the bowel, rectum, and reproductive organs are in direct relation to the amount of bladder distention. The vagina lies dorsal to the base of the bladder and parallel to the urethra (Fig. 2-10). The prostate gland is interposed between the bladder neck and the urethra (see Fig. 2-9). These anatomic correlations serve as valuable landmarks during pelvic surgery and often influence the symptoms that the patient may experience.

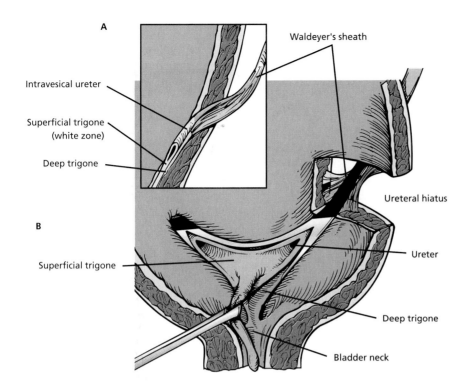

A

Waldeyer's sheath

Intravesical ureter

Superficial trigone
(white zone)

Deep trigone

B

Superficial trigone

Ureteral hiatus

Ureter

Deep trigone

Bladder neck

Fig. 2-8 Normal ureterovesical complex. **A,** Side view of Waldeyer's sheath surrounding intravesical ureter and continuing downward as the deep trigone, extending to the bladder neck. **B,** Waldeyer's sheath connected by a few fibers to the detrusor muscle in the ureteral hiatus. This sheath, inferior to the ureteral orifice, becomes the deep trigone. Ureteral musculature continues downward as the superficial trigone. *(From Tanagho EA: Anatomy of the lower urinary tract. In Walsh PC: Campbell's urology, ed 5, Philadelphia, 1986, WB Saunders.)*

Physiology

Bladder evacuation is initiated by nerve cells from the sacral division of the autonomic nervous system. These reflex centers are controlled by the higher voluntary centers in the brain. The contraction of bladder muscles and the relaxation of bladder outlet sphincters are controlled by stimulation to these sacral centers. Closure of the sphincters is managed by the muscles inside and adjacent to the urethral wall, and by the pelvic floor, enabling continence.

The UVJ allows the passage of urine without reflux (regurgitation in a retrograde fashion). Pressure produced by peristaltic waves propels urine through the UVJ. Active and passive adaptation of the UVJ prevents reflux when intravesical pressure rises during micturition. Muscles of the intravesical ureter and trigone contract immediately before contraction of the detrusor muscle, preventing urine from moving through the junction. The contraction of the detrusor muscle also closes the UVJ, a mechanism that protects the bladder from reflux during exercise or stress. Tone is maintained for approximately 20 seconds following micturition, after which relaxation allows efflux to resume and the bladder to refill.

A stretching mechanism increases the surface area of the urothelium as the bladder fills, allowing the bladder to accommodate the rising urine volume. This process is a result of changes in the configuration of protein structures in the urothelium and the smoothing of redundant wrinkles. The urothelium is impermeable to the excretion or reabsorption of water and solutes, thus preventing the accumulation of urinary waste products before micturition.

Urethra/Urethrovesical Unit

Anatomy

In men the urethra is normally 25 to 30 cm long and extends from the bladder neck to the tip of the penis with a diameter that varies from 7 to 10 mm. It is divided into two portions: the sphincteric (proximal) urethra and the anterior (distal or conduit) urethra, both of which undergo further division. The proximal urethra is commonly referred to as the posterior urethra at the point where it is elevated by the verumontanum, extending from the bladder neck through the prostate and the membranous portions. It is called the membranous urethra at the point where it exits the prostate and crosses the pelvic (urogenital) diaphragm. The distal, or anterior, urethra is subdivided into the bulbar, pendulous (penile), and glandular urethras (Fig. 2-11). Approximately 15 cm long, the distal urethra extends from the membranous urethra to the base of the penis. The areas most prone to strictures in males are the membranous and the bulbar urethras.

The widest portion of the male urethra is the proximal urethra, which is usually about 3 cm long. The verumontanum lies on the floor of the proximal urethra and contains the openings for the ejaculatory ducts. The shortest portion of the urethra is the membranous portion, measuring approximately 2.5 cm. It extends from the external sphincter to the apex of the prostate. The pendulous urethra lies within the corpus spongiosum. The urothelium of the urethra is continuous with that of the bladder.

The periurethral muscles lie immediately adjacent to the membranous urethra in males. Intrinsic urethral skeletal muscle (rhabdosphincter) in the proximal urethra provides pro-

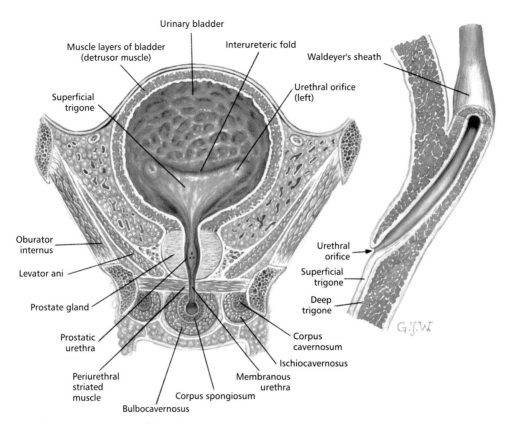

Fig. 2-9 Ureterovesical junction. *(From Gray M:* Genitourinary disorders, *St. Louis, 1992, Mosby.)*

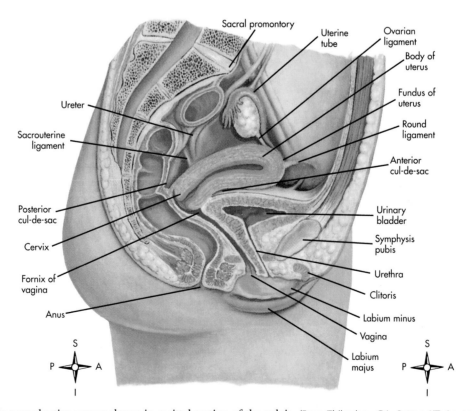

Fig. 2-10 Female reproductive organs shown in sagittal section of the pelvis. *(From Thibodeau GA, Patton KT:* Anatomy and physiology, *ed 3, St. Louis, 1996, Mosby.)*

longed tension to prevent urinary leakage (see Fig. 2-9). The male urethra is composed of an inner urothelium lined by transitional epithelium and numerous secretory cells. Below this is a submucosal layer containing lymphatic channels, vessels, and nerves. Branches of the internal pudendal artery provide the arterial blood supply. The deep penile vein and pudendal plexus are the sites of venous drainage. The subinguinal node chain accepts the lymphatic drainage.

The pelvic floor muscles include groups of slow twitch fibers that support the pelvic viscera and rapid twitch fibers that respond to the sudden pressure changes occurring with coughing, sneezing, and exercising (Fig. 2-12). Extending from the anterior to the posterior aspects of the pelvis, these muscles are divided into superior and inferior segments and form a supportive sling for the rectum, reproductive organs, and the urethrovesical unit. The superior division forms part of the rectal sphincter and the periurethral muscles that aid the urethral sphincter mechanism. The inferior portion contributes to the rectal fossa in men but adds little to urethrovesical function in women.

In women the urethra is a narrow, membranous tube approximately 3 to 5 cm long and 6 to 8 mm in diameter. It is slightly curved and lies behind the symphysis pubis, anterior to the vagina. It passes through the internal and external sphincters and the urogenital diaphragm. The distal urethra is fused to the anterior vaginal wall. The proximal urethra is composed primarily of smooth muscle fibers. Skeletal muscle fibers in the middle third form the rhabdosphincter. The female urethra is also characterized by an inner urothelium consisting of transitional epithelium with numerous mucus-producing cells. Lymphatic chains, a rich vasculature, and nerves are found in the submucosal layer. Opening on the floor of the urethra just inside the meatus are the periurethral glands of Skene. These are the homologues to the prostate in males. The muscles of the pelvic floor form the periurethral musculature near the distal urethra and contribute to the urethral sphincter mechanism (Fig. 2-13). A low percentage of urethral strictures appear in women.

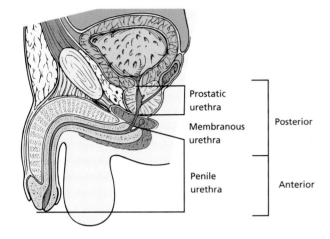

Fig. 2-11 Male urethra. *(From Thompson JM: Mosby's clinical nursing, ed 3, St. Louis, 1993, Mosby.)*

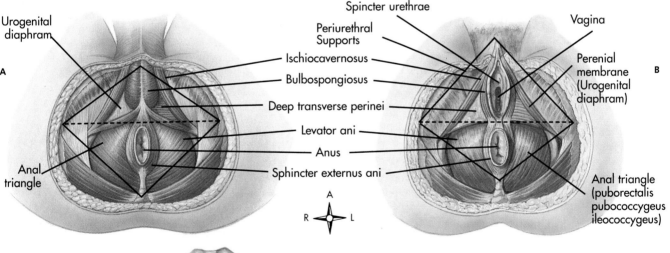

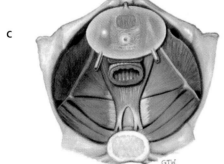

Fig. 2-12 Muscles of the pelvic floor. **A,** Male, inferior view. **B,** Female, inferior view. *(From Thibodeau GA: Anatomy and physiology, ed 3, St. Louis, 1996, Mosby.)* **C,** Abdominal view of pelvic floor muscles in relation to the bladder. *(From Gray M: Genitourinary disorders, St. Louis, 1989, Mosby.)*

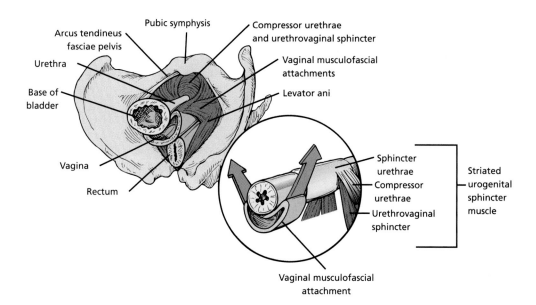

Fig. 2-13 Component parts of urethral support and sphincteric mechanism. Proximal urethra and bladder neck are supported by the anterior vaginal wall and its musculofascial attachments to the pelvic diaphragm. *Inset*, Contraction of the levator ani elevates the anterior vagina, bladder neck, and proximal urethra, aiding bladder neck closure. The sphincter urethrae, urethrovaginal sphincter, and compressor urethrae are part of the striated urogenital diaphragm (triangle or sphincter muscle). *(From Walters MD:* Clinical urogynecology, *St. Louis, 1993, Mosby.)*

Physiology

Any alteration in the structural integrity of the urethrovesical unit will affect the transport, storage, and expulsion of urine and cause incontinence. Neural centers in the brain, spinal cord, and peripheral system also modulate urinary continence. Bladder function may be influenced by the cerebral cortex, thalamus, hypothalamus, basal ganglia, or limbic system. The brainstem also controls the detrusor reflex, with two centers in the pons directly influencing urinary control. One center initiates the detrusor response while the other coordinates bladder contraction and relaxation of the pelvic floor.

The sympathetic nerve chain sends messages from the T10 to L2 spinal levels to the bladder and sphincter mechanism, which promote filling and storage of urine through detrusor relaxation and sphincter closure. The parasympathetic system promotes micturition by causing the detrusor to contract and the sphincter to open. Somatic and peripheral nerves regulate the pelvic floor muscles.

The hypogastric plexus transmits sympathetic input to the bladder, and beta-adrenergic nerve endings respond by relaxing the detrusor muscle, in turn allowing the filling and storage of urine. Alpha-adrenergics at the bladder neck, proximal urethra, and rhabdosphincter react by increasing sphincter closure tension, which also promotes filling and storage. The pelvic plexus sends parasympathetic signals to the detrusor muscles and cholinergic receptors in the bladder wall contract the muscle and aid micturition. Cholinergic receptors in the rhabdosphincter may also promote relaxation of the sphincter mechanism. The pudendal nerve aids the function of the skeletal and periurethral muscles in the pelvic floor by providing tone for bladder contraction and relaxation.

Prostate Gland

Anatomy

The prostate gland, an accessory reproductive gland, is located at the base of the bladder neck and the triangular ligament. It is a fibromuscular organ that completely surrounds the urethra in a "donut" configuration. Measuring 4 cm at its base and about 2 cm in depth, it weighs approximately 20 g (Fig. 2-14).

The prostate gland consists of four glandular regions: two major regions, the peripheral and central zones, and two minor regions, the transitional and periurethral zones. Some clinicians still divide the prostate into the intraurethral lobes (right and left lateral), and the extraurethral lobes (posterior and median). The posterior lobe is easily palpable during a digital rectal examination (DRE).

A fibrous sheath separating the prostate gland and the seminal vesicles from the rectum, located behind the prostatic capsule, is known as the true prostatic capsule. When perineal prostatectomy is considered, this fascia is an important landmark.

A highly alkaline fluid is secreted from the prostate gland, diluting the testicular secretions as they are released from the ejaculatory ducts. These secretions are believed to be essential to the life and passage of spermatozoa. Arterial blood supply to the prostate gland originates from the pudendal, inferior vesical, and hemorrhoidal arteries.

Physiology

The prostate gland is a male accessory sex gland that contributes unique secretions to the ejaculate to facilitate insemination and probably helps to protect the lower urinary tract from infection. The development of the prostate is under hor-

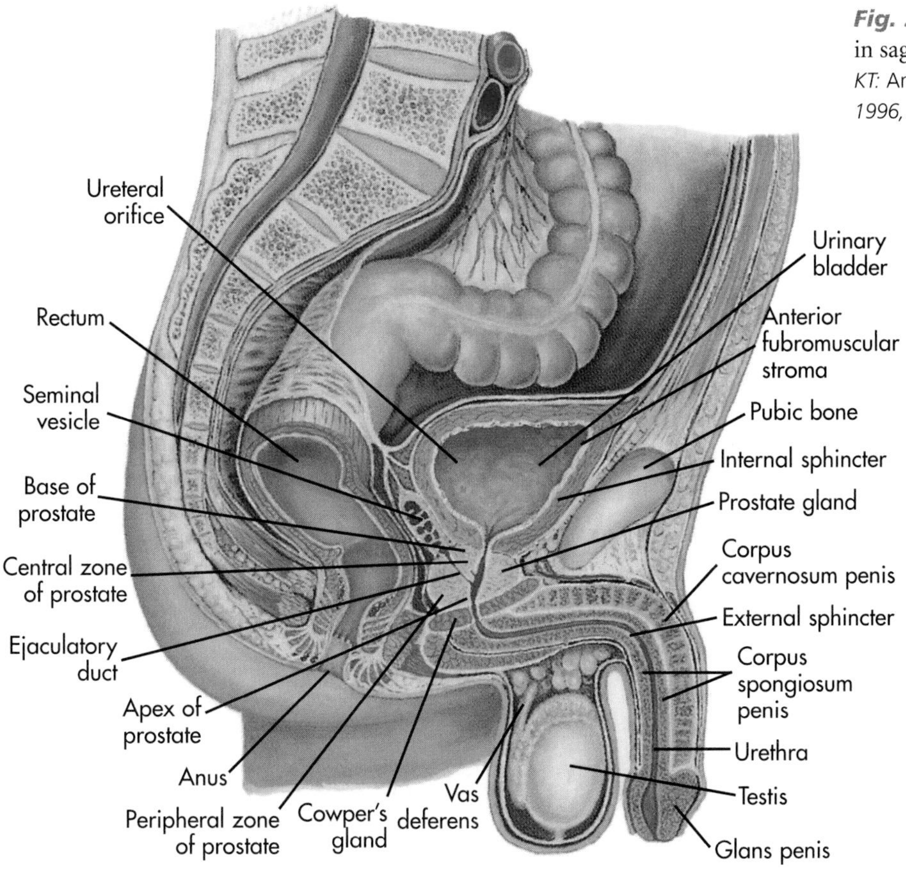
Ureteral orifice
Urinary bladder
Anterior fubromuscular stroma
Rectum
Seminal vesicle
Pubic bone
Internal sphincter
Base of prostate
Prostate gland
Central zone of prostate
Corpus cavernosum penis
External sphincter
Ejaculatory duct
Corpus spongiosum penis
Apex of prostate
Urethra
Anus
Testis
Vas deferens
Peripheral zone of prostate
Cowper's gland
Glans penis

Fig. 2-14 Male reproductive organs shown in sagittal section. *(From Thibodeau GA. Patton KT: Anatomy and physiology, ed 3, St. Louis, 1996, Mosby.)*

monal control, with demonstrated histologic changes occurring at birth, puberty, and later life.

The prostate contributes 15% of the ejaculatory volume and is the primary source of zinc, calcium, magnesium, and citrate in the ejaculate. The majority of the ejaculatory volume is a product of the seminal vesicles. The presence of fructose in the ejaculate stems from the seminal vesicles and may be a differential point in diagnosing congenital absence of the seminal vesicles and obstruction of the vas deferens. Zinc may have important antibacterial activity in the prostate, but the role of citrate, a binder of metal ions, is unclear.

Nitrogenous compounds, phosphorylcholine, and the polyamines spermine and spermidine are secreted in prostatic fluid. Enzymatic degradation of spermine generates aldehydes, which give semen its characteristic odor and may be antibacterial.

Prostate specific antigen (PSA) and prostatic acid phosphatase (PAP) are compounds measurable in the serum. Produced in increased amounts by malignant prostatic cells, they are used to assess the presence or progress of cancer.

The male sex hormone testosterone is necessary for the prostate to develop. The primary sources of testosterone are the Leydig's cells of the testes. The testes also produce estrogens, which may be responsible for the development of benign prostatic hypertrophy. Benign enlargement of the prostate ultimately occurs in approximately 75% of men and may require medical or surgical intervention depending on its severity (see Chapter 3).

Male Reproductive Organs

Anatomy

Several paired structures compose the male reproductive system. These structures are the testes, epididymides, seminal ducts (vas deferens), seminal vesicles, ejaculatory ducts, and bulbourethral glands. Other organs vital to the reproductive system are the penis, urethra, and prostate gland.

The **scrotum,** located behind and below the base of the penis and in front of the anus, is divided into two sections by an internal median raphe (septum). Two cavities, or sacs, lined with smooth, glistening tissue (tunica vaginalis) are contained within the scrotum. Normally a small amount of clear fluid is found within each sac. One testis, epididymis, and a section of the spermatic cord are supported within each loose sac (see Fig. 2-14).

The **testes,** responsible for the manufacture of spermatozoa, also contain specialized Leydig's cells that produce the male hormone testosterone. The sperm are formed in numerous small tubules surrounded by dense capsules of connective tissue within the testes. Adjacent to the epididymis, these tubules coalesce and continue into the epididymis, where the sperm mature and are stored (Fig. 2-15). The appendix testis, found at the upper pole of each testis, is a small, rounded body that may be stalked or pedunculated (flat).

The **epididymis,** a long, convoluted duct along the posterolateral surface of the testis, is closely attached to the testicle by fibrous tissue. Seminal fluid, which provides a liquid, migratory medium for the sperm, is excreted from the epididymis. The vas deferens (ductus deferens or seminal duct) is a distal continuation of the epididymis as it enters the prostate gland and transports sperm to the seminal vesicles (see Fig. 2-15).

The **spermatic cord,** located in the inguinal area, contains the vas deferens along with veins, arteries, lymphatics, nerves, and surrounding connective tissue (cremaster muscle). These structures provide testicular support. The ejaculatory duct is the terminal portion of the vas deferens. It passes between the prostatic lobes and opens into the posterior urethra.

The seminal vesicles, prostate gland, and bulbourethral gland are the accessory reproductive glands. The seminal vesicles are located behind the bladder and unite with the vas deferens to produce protein and fructose for the nutrition of the sperm cells. At ejaculation both sperm and prostatic fluid are released.

The **bulbourethral glands** (Cowper's glands) are located along each side of the urethra at the juncture of the membranous and bulbar urethras (see Fig. 2-14). Mucous secretions are emptied into the urethra from each gland through its ductal system. These are the homologues to Bartholin's glands in females.

The **suspensory ligaments** are the fibrous attachments that suspend the penis from the pubic symphysis. Three distinct, vascular, spongelike bodies within the penis surround the urethra: two outer bodies, the right and left corpus cavernosum, and an inner body, the corpus spongiosum urethra (Fig. 2-16). A network of vascular channels within these tissues fill with blood during erection (Fig. 2-17). The skin at the distal end of the penis is doubly folded to form a prepuce (foreskin), which serves as a covering for the glans penis. The urethral orifice (meatus) is located in the glans penis.

Physiology

The testes, epididymides, vas deferentia, seminal vesicles, ejaculatory ducts, and prostate gland function as a unit to produce viable sperm, contained in the semen and designed for

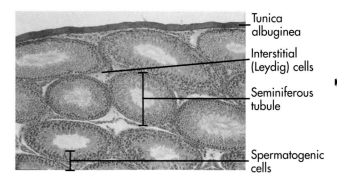

Fig. 2-15 A, Tubules of the testis and epididymis. *(Courtesy Ernest W. Beck.)* **B,** Testis, macrophotograph showing seminiferous tubules within testis. *(From Thibodeau GA, Patton KT: Anatomy and physiology, ed 3, St. Louis, 1996, Mosby.)*

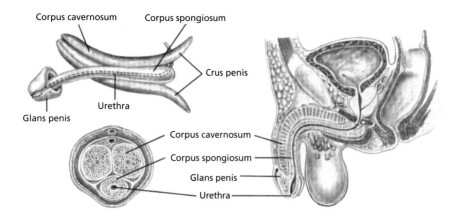

Fig. 2-16 Penile anatomy. *(From Seidel HM: Mosby's guide to physical examination, ed 3, St. Louis, 1995, Mosby.)*

reproduction. The vas deferens, seminal vesicle, and ejaculatory duct assist reproduction by transporting mature sperm cells. The prostate and vas deferens add needed nutrients to the fluid that accompanies the sperm during ejaculation.

The reproductive system is regulated by hormonal influences and ejaculation is controlled by neuromuscular activity modified by endocrine actions. Luteinizing-hormone–releasing hormone (LHRH) is released in the hypothalamus and travels to the pituitary gland to cause production of LH and FSH. Both LH and FSH act in the testes to stimulate production of male androgens, in particular testosterone and dihydrotestosterone. These hormones encourage spermatogenesis.

Gonadal androgens are essential to the production of viable, mature sperm cells. Spermatogenesis takes place in three distinct stages. Primary spermatocytes, with 92 chromosomes, are formed by mitotic division in the seminiferous tubule. Four secondary spermatogenia are formed through two meiotic divisions, yielding 23 chromosomes. Spermatids mature into spermatozoa capable of independent movement and fertilization finally occurs.

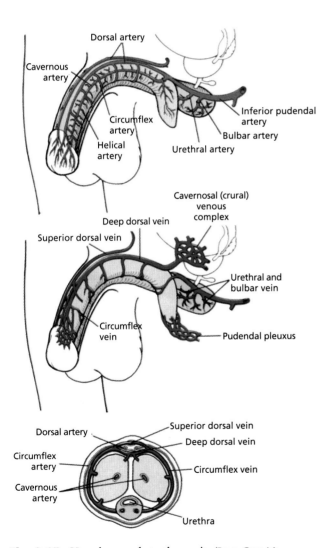

Fig. 2-17 Vascular supply to the penis. *(From Gray M: Genitourinary disorders, St. Louis, 1989, Mosby.)*

Erectile function is under neurovascular and hormonal control. Tumescence begins with smooth muscle relaxation at the capillary level, increasing blood flow to the corporal bodies. As the sinus spaces in the corporal bodies fill, the increased volume initially increases the length and volume of the penis. The corporal bodies of the penis once engorged with blood develop an erection rigid enough for vaginal entry. Venous occlusion maintains this engorgement, possibly because of increased muscle tone that occludes drainage, valves in the vein that prevent drainage, or mechanical compression of the penile veins from the increased pressure against the tunica albuginea.

Female Urogynecologic System
Anatomy and physiology

Historically, care of women with conditions involving pelvic floor dysfunction has been managed by gynecologists. Only in recent years has there been a significant trend toward specialized genitourinary care and treatment. The female urogynecologic system consists of the vaginal vault and the supporting fascial and ligamentous attachments that link the vagina to the bladder neck and the rectal wall.

The female **urethra**, configured in an elongated **S** shape, is closely related to the pubic bones and arch. Component parts of the endopelvic fascia, or suspensory mechanism, maintain the anatomic positioning. The suspensory attachments include the anterior pubourethral ligament, the posterior pubourethral ligaments, and the intermediate (connecting) ligament. The anterior and posterior ligaments are formed by the inferior and superior fascial layers of the perineal membrane (formerly called the urogenital diaphragm) and fix the distal urethra to the pubic bone. The proximal urethra and bladder base are supported in a slinglike manner by the anterior vaginal wall, which attaches bilaterally to the levator ani muscles and the arcus tendineus fasciae pelvis (pelvic diaphragm). The levator ani muscle is divided into three parts: the puborectalis, the pubococcygeus, and the ileococcygeus (see Fig. 2-12). These muscles form a sphincter for the urethra, vagina, and rectum.

The urethral musculature is an extension of the vesical musculature. The urethral smooth muscle and mucosa coapt (fuse) together to form the extrinsic sphincter mechanism. It is composed of an inner striated component, lying within and adjacent to the urethral wall, and an outer component of skeletal muscle fibers of the pelvic diaphragm. The inner mechanism consists of the sphincter urethrae, which surrounds the proximal two thirds of the urethra. The outer mechanism, known as the deep transverse perineus muscle (compressor urethrae and urethrovaginal sphincter), arches over the ventral surface of the distal one third of the urethra (see Fig. 2-13). When functioning as a single unit, these three muscles are termed the *striated urogenital sphincter muscle*. Primarily consisting of slow twitch fibers, it exerts tone on the urethral lumen over prolonged periods. It may also assist voluntary interruption of the urinary stream as well as urethral closure with stress by a reflex muscle contraction. The striated periurethral sphincter is a superior extension of the perineal membrane and is innervated by branches of the pudendal nerve. Pudendal nerve function is needed for tonic and reflex sphincteric closure.

The **anterior pubourethral ligament** is a deep extension of the suspensory ligament of the clitoris and attaches near the external urethral meatus. The posterior pubourethral ligaments run a course from the pubic bone to the urethra. They are firmly attached near the midline and just proximal to the subpubic arch. The ligaments attach broadly to the paraurethral tissues at the junction of the upper one third and the distal two thirds of the urethra, approximately 10 to 15 mm from the subpubic arch. A broad fascial sheath originating from this attachment runs across the levator ani fascia and fuses at variable distances from the urethra. The investing fascia of the bladder is fused to a second fascial extension that passes downward along the superior surface of the urethra. The last extension meets and fuses with the anterior pubourethral ligament and is termed the *intermediate ligament*. It is believed that this point of attachment is the site of continence control in females. Anatomic defects in the pubourethral ligaments are thought to be a contributing factor to urinary incontinence in women.

The **vagina** is suspended in a hammock fashion between the pubis and cervix, with loose lateral attachments to connective tissues and the pelvic diaphragm. The anterior vaginal wall is contiguous with the bladder base and the urethra. The terminal ureters pass closely to the lateral vaginal vault. The fibers of the pelvic diaphragm form a U-shaped muscle layer, the urogenital hiatus, which permits opening of the pelvic viscera to the perineum and is instrumental in vaginal support. The perineal membrane lies below the urogenital hiatus and attaches laterally to the pubococcygeus muscle at the UVJ. The vagina and urethra pass through the perineal membrane and are supported by it. Together the pelvic diaphragm and perineal membrane compose the pelvic floor. Anterolaterally the vagina is supported by the endopelvic fascia (Fig. 2-18). The upper endopelvic fascia is identified surgically as the cardinal and uterosacral ligament complex.

Both the bladder and urethra depend on the vaginal wall for support. There are three levels of vaginal support: the perineal membrane, the paravaginal supports (see Fig. 2-12), and the intraperitoneal cardinal and ureterosacral ligaments. Anterior vaginal wall support to the pelvic diaphragm provides a stable base on which the bladder neck and proximal urethra are compressed with increased abdominal pressure. These paravaginal supports enable posterior movement of the vesical neck, as seen with micturition, and elevation of the pelvic floor when the urinary stream is halted. Defects in the paravaginal supports probably result in urethral hypermobility, with resulting loss of the posterior urethrovesical angle, which may lead to incontinence.

GLOSSARY

Acid Derived by partial exchange of replaceable hydrogen; water-soluble compound capable of reacting with a base to form a salt; hydrogen-containing molecules able to give up a proton to a base; able to accept an unshared pair of electrons from a base.

Acid-base balance State of equilibrium between proton donors and proton acceptors in the buffering system

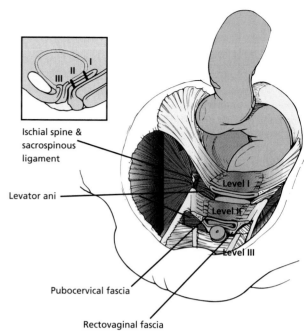

Ischial spine & sacrospinous ligament

Levator ani

Level I

Level II

Level III

Pubocervical fascia

Rectovaginal fascia

Fig. 2-18 Levels of support of the upper and mid-vagina. In Level I the endopelvic fascia suspends the vagina from the lateral pelvic walls; fibers extend vertically and posteriorly toward sacrum. In Level II the vagina is attached to the arcus tendineus fascia pelvis and superior fascia of the levator ani muscles. *(From DeLancey JO: Am J Obstet Gynecol 166:1717, 1992. In Walters MD et al: Clinical urogynecology, St. Louis, 1993, Mosby.)*

of the blood, maintained at an approximate pH of 7.35 to 7.45 in arterial blood under normal conditions.

Acidosis An elevated level of acid in the bloodstream.

Adrenaline Epinephrine

Adrenergic Activated by adrenaline; resembling adrenaline in physiologic action.

Adrenocorticotropic hormone (ACTH) Hormone that stimulates the adrenal cortex.

Adventitia Outer layer that makes up a tubular organ, composed of collagenous and elastic fibers, not covered by peritoneum.

Afferent To conduct inward or toward.

Albumin Simple heat coagulable, water-soluble protein in blood plasma or serum and muscle.

Aldehyde Any of a variety of highly reactive compounds characterized by the carbohydrate (CHO) group.

Alkalosis Abnormal condition of increased alkalinity in tissues and blood.

Aminoglycoside A group of antibiotics that inhibit bacterial protein synthesis and are active against gram-negative bacteria; streptomycin, neomycin.

Androgen Male sex hormone.

Androstenedione Steroid sex hormone secreted by the testes, ovary, and adrenal cortex; acts more strongly in production of male characteristics than testosterone.

Angiotensin Any of two forms of a kinin, one with severe vasoconstrictive activity; Angiotensin I is the physiologically inactive form composed of 10 amino-acid residues, a precursor to Angiotensin II; Angiotensin II is the physiologically active form, a protein with vasoconstrictive activity composed of eight amino-acid residues.

Angstrom (Å) Unit of length equal to one ten-billionth of a meter.

Arteriole Any of small terminal twigs of an artery that end in capillaries.

Atrial natriuretic peptide Hormone secreted by atrium that regulates blood pressure and stimulates diuresis and natriuresis.

Autonomic Occurring involuntarily; having an effect on tissue supplied by autonomic nervous system.

Base Alkaline; water-soluble compound capable of reacting with an acid to form a salt; molecules or ions able to take up a proton from an acid; able to give up an unshared pair of electrons to an acid.

Biosynthesis Production of a chemical compound by a living organism.

Buffer Substance or mixture of substances, such as bicarbonates and some proteins in biologic fluids, that in solution stabilize the hydrogen ion concentration by neutralizing both acids and bases.

Bulb Of the penis—proximal extended part of the corpus cavernosum of the male urethra; of the vestibule—structure in the female vulva homologous to the bulb of the penis; consists of elongated mass of erectile tissue on each side of the vaginal opening united anteriorly to the contralateral mass by a narrow median band passing along the lower surface of the clitoris.

Bulbocavernous Located near the bulb of the penis.

Bulbourethral Of or relating to the bulb of the penis and the urethra; Cowper's gland.

Calcitonin Polypeptide hormone from the thyroid gland that tends to lower the calcium level in blood plasma.

Carbonic anhydrase Zinc-containing enzyme in red blood cells that aids carbon dioxide transport from the tissues and its release from the blood in the lungs by catalyzing the reversible hydration of carbon dioxide to carbonic acid.

Catecholamine Various substances that function as hormones or neurotransmitters or both; epinephrine, norepinephrine, dopamine.

Cavernous Composed largely of vascular sinuses and capable of dilating with blood to bring about the erection of a body part.

Chorionic gonadotropin A hormone produced by the chorion, a portion of the placenta.

Clitoris Small erectile organ at the anterior or ventral part of the vulva homologous to the penis.

Coalesce To grow together.

Coapt Cause to adhere, close, fuse, or fasten together.

Colloid A substance in a state of division, preventing passage through a semipermeable membrane; gelatinous or mucinous substance in diseased tissues or normally as in the thyroid.

Corpus main part of a bodily structure or organ.

Cortisol hydrocortisone.

Cremaster thin muscle consisting of loops of fibers derived from the internal oblique muscle and descending on the spermatic cord to surround and suspend the testicle.

Dehydroepiandrosterone androgenic ketosteroid found in urine and adrenal cortex; thought to be an intermediary in the biosynthesis of testosterone.

Detrusor outer, largely longitudinally arranged musculature of the bladder wall.

Dextran polysaccharide that yields only glucose on hydrolysis but otherwise differs from starch and glycogen; used in physiologic saline as a plasma substitute.

Diuresis increased excretion of urine.

Dopamine a monoamine that occurs as a neurotransmitter in the brain and serves as an intermediary in the biosynthesis of epinephrine.

Dopaminergic activated by the neurotransmitter activity of dopamine; nerve pathway.

Efferent conducting outward from a part or organ; conveying nervous impulses to an effector.

Eicosanoid compounds derived from polyunsaturated fatty acids and involved in cellular activity; prostaglandins, thromboxanes.

Endogenous growing from or on the inside; caused by factors within the body; arising from an internal structure; produced by metabolic synthesis in the body.

Enzyme complex protein produced by living cells, catalyzing specific biochemical reactions at body temperature.

Epinephrine a sympathomimetic hormone that is the principal blood pressure raising hormone secreted by the adrenal medulla; used medicinally as a heart stimulant, as a vasoconstrictor to control hemorrhage of the skin and prolong the action of local anesthetics, and as muscle relaxant for bronchial asthma.

Epithelium membranous cellular tissue covering a free surface or lining a tube or cavity to enclose or protect the other parts of the body; produces secretions and excretions and functions in assimilation.

Erythropoietin a hormone produced in the kidney and responsible for formation of red blood cells.

Fasciculata fibroaerolar tissue and fat around the kidney forming a sheath for the organ.

Follicle stimulating hormone, FSH hormone from anterior lobe of pituitary gland that stimulates the growth of ovum-containing follicles in the ovary and activates sperm-forming cells; follitropin.

Glucagon protein hormone produced by pancreatic islets of Langerhans that promotes an increase in the blood sugar level by increasing the rate of breakdown of glycogen in the liver.

Glucocorticoid Group of corticoids involved in carbohydrate, protein, and fat metabolism; tend to increase liver glycogen and blood sugar by increasing glyconeogenesis; antiinflammatory and immunosuppressive; hydrocortisone, dexamethasone.

Gluconeogenesis Formation of glucose by the liver from fats and proteins; glyconeogenesis.

Glycogen Polysaccharide that is the principal form in which carbohydrates are stored in tissues; occurs especially in liver and muscle.

Hapten Small part of an antigen that reacts with an antibody but cannot stimulate antibody production without a carrier protein molecule.

Homeostasis Maintenance of relatively stable internal physiologic conditions (such as body temperature or pH of blood) under fluctuating conditions.

Hydrostatic Relating to fluids at rest or to the pressure they exert or transmit.

Hyperplasia Abnormal or unusual increase in the elements of a part (tissue cells).

Hypovolemic Decreased volume of circulating blood.

Interlobular Lying between, connecting, or transporting the secretions of lobules (ducts).

Kallikrein Hypotensive proteinase that liberates kinins from blood plasma proteins that are used therapeutically for vasodilatation.

Kinin Polypeptide hormones formed locally in the tissues; primary effect is on smooth muscle.

Lamina propria Highly vascular layer of connective tissue under the membrane lining a layer of epithelium.

Levator Muscle used to raise a body part.

Leydig's cell Interstitial cell of testis; considered the primary source of testicular androgens.

Luteinizing hormone, LH Hormone of protein-carbohydrate composition, obtained from anterior lobe of pituitary gland; in females stimulates development of corpus lutea and with FSH the secretion of progesterone; in males stimulates development of interstitial tissue in the testis and the secretion of testosterone.

Meatus A natural body passage; canal, duct.

Medulla Medullary portion of a gland, such as in the adrenal gland.

Meiotic Cellular process resulting in a 50% reduction in the number of chromosomes in gamete-producing cells; involving a reduction division where one of each pair of homologous chromosomes passes to a daughter cell and a mitotic division.

Mineralocorticoid Corticosteroid that chiefly affects the fluid and electrolyte balance; aldsoterone.

Metanephrine A catabolite of epinephrine found in the urine and some tissues.

Micturition Urination.

Milieu; environment; "milieu interieur" The body fluids regarded as an internal environment in which cells of the body are nourished and maintained in a state of equilibrium.

Mitotic series of steps resulting in the formation of two new nuclei, each with the same number of chromosomes as the parent nucleus; takes place in the nucleus of a dividing cell.

Monoamine oxidase enzyme that functions in the nervous system by breaking down monoamine neurotransmitters.

Myogenic originating in muscle; functions in rhythmic fashion by reason of the inherent properties of cardiac muscle rather than from a specific neural stimuli; heartbeat.

Natriuresis excess loss of cations, especially sodium in the urine.

Nephrocalcinosis calcification of the tubules of the kidney.

Nitrogenase an iron-containing enzyme that catalyzes the reduction of molecular nitrogen to ammonia.

Nitrogenous a compound containing nitrogen in its combined form; nitrates, proteins.

Norepinephrine a catecholamine that is the chemical means of transmission across synapses of the postganglionic neurons of the sympathetic nervous system and parts of the central nervous system; vasopressor hormone of the adrenal medulla and precursor of epinephrine; also called noradrenalin (Levophed).

Normetanephrine metabolite of norepinephrine found in the urine.

Oliguria reduced excretion of urine.

Oncotic pressure exerted by plasma proteins on the capillary wall.

Osmolality concentration of an osmotic solution measured in osmols per liter.

Osmotic pressure produced with osmosis, dependent on molar concentration and absolute temperature; maximum pressure that develops in a solution separated by a membrane permeable to a solvent; pressure necessary to prevent osmosis.

Parathyroid hormone, PTH parathormone.

Peristalsis successive waves of involuntary contraction passing along the walls of hollow muscular structures and forcing contents outward.

Periurethral tissues surrounding the urethra; occurring in the tissues surrounding urethra.

Pheochromocytoma tumor derived from chromaffin cells and associated with paroxysmal or sustained hypertension.

Phosphorylcholine a hapten used in the form of its chloride to treat hepatobiliary dysfunction.

Polyamine compound with more than one amino group.

Pregnenolone unsaturated hydroxy-steroid ketone that is formed by the oxidation of steroids like cholesterol and yields progesterone on dehydrogenation.

Prepuce foreskin; similar fold invests clitoris.

Prostacyclin Prostaglandin that inhibits aggregation of platelets and dilates blood vessels.

Prostaglandin An oxygenated unsaturated cyclic fatty acid with hormonelike actions such as controlling blood pressure or smooth muscle contraction.

Psoas Either of two internal loin (flank) muscles.

Pudendal In the region of the external genital organs.

Raphe Seamlike union of two lateral halves of an organ with external ridge or furrow and internal fibrous connective septum.

Renin An enzyme produced and secreted by the juxtaglomerular cells of the kidney.

Reticularis Network of cells; formed of certain structures within cells; formed of connective tissue fibers between cells; catalyzes norepinephrine and epinephrine.

Retroperitoneal Occupying the space behind the peritoneum.

Seminal Consisting of seed or semen.

Seminiferous Producing or bearing seed or semen, such as epithelium of testes.

Spermatid One of the cells formed by division of secondary spermatocytes that differentiate into spermatozoa.

Spermatogenesis Process of male gamete formation including meiosis and transformation of four spermatids into spermatozoa; spermiogenesis.

Spermidine A crystalline amine found in semen.

Spermine A crystalline tetramine found in semen in combination with phosphoric acid.

Subpubic Just below the pubic bone (symphysis).

Suprapubic Above the pubis.

Thromboxane Potent regulator of cellular function formed from endoperoxides; first found in thrombocytes.

Titration Process of determining the concentration of dissolved substances in terms of the smallest amount of a reagent of a known concentration required to bring about a given effect in reaction with a known volume.

Thyroid-stimulating hormone TSH, thyrotropin.

Transferase Enzyme that promotes transfer from one molecule to another.

Trigone Smooth triangular area on the inner surface of bladder, limited by the apertures of urethra and ureters.

Tunica Enveloping membrane or layer of body tissue; (albuginea) white, fibrous capsule of the testis; (vaginalis) pouch of serous membrane derived from the peritoneum and covering the testis.

Urea Soluble nitrogenous compound that is the chief component of urine and an end product of protein decomposition; used intravenously as a diuretic drug; carbamide.

Urogenital The organs of or functions of excretion and reproduction.

Vanilmandelic acid, VMA A principal catecholamine metabolite whose presence in excess in the urine is used as a test for pheochromocytoma; vanillylmandelic.

Vasopressin Polypeptide hormone secreted with oxytocin by the posterior lobe of the pituitary gland; increases blood pressure and has antidiuretic effect.

Verumontanum Elevation in the floor of prostatic portion of the urethra where the seminal ducts enter.

Vesical Relating to the urinary bladder.

Vesicle Membranous and usually fluid-filled pouch.

Viscus Internal organ of the body located in the large cavity of the trunk.

Zona glomerulosa Outermost of the three cortical adrenal layers, consisting of round masses of epithelial cells.

Bibliography

1. Bernays AC: *Golden rules of surgery*, St. Louis, 1906, Mosby.
2. Brundage DJ: *Renal disorders*, St. Louis, 1992, Mosby.
3. Campbell JB, Campbell JM: *Mosby's survival guide to medical abbreviations and acronyms*, St. Louis, 1995, Mosby.
4. Doughty DB: *Urinary and fecal incontinence: nursing management*, St. Louis, 1991, Mosby.
5. Drach, GW: *Common problems in infections and stones*, St Louis, 1992, Mosby.
6. Emmett JM, Witten DM: *Clinical urography*, vol 2, Philadelphia, 1971, WB Saunders.
7. Gershenson DM, DeCherney AH, Curry SL: *Operative gynecology*, Philadelphia, 1993, WB Saunders.
8. Gillenwater JY et al: *Adult and pediatric urology*, ed 3, St. Louis, 1996, Mosby.
9. Glenn JE: *Urologic surgery*, Philadelphia, 1991, Lippincott.
10. Gray H: *Anatomy: descriptive and surgical*, St. Louis, 1991, Mosby.
11. Gray M: *Genitourinary disorders*, St. Louis, 1992, Mosby.
12. Grunfeld JP et al: *Advances in nephrology*, vol 24, St. Louis, 1995. Mosby.
13. Hampton BG, Bryant RA: *Ostomies and continent diversions: nursing management*, St. Louis, 1992, Mosby.
14. Hashmat AI, Das S: *The penis*, Philadelphia, 1993, Lea & Febiger.
15. Hinman F: *Atlas of urosurgical anatomy*, Philadelphia, 1993, WB Saunders.
16. Horne MM, Swearingen PL: *Pocket guide to fluid, electrolyte, and acid-base balance*, St. Louis, 1993, Mosby.
17. Kirby R, Christmas T: *Benign prostatic hyperplasia*, London, 1993, Gower.
18. Lloyd-Davies W et al: *Color atlas of urology*, London, 1994, Mosby-Wolfe.
19. Meeker MH, Rothrock JC: *Alexander's care of the patient in surgery*, St. Louis, 1995, Mosby.
20. Pagana KD, Pagana TJ: *Diagnostic and laboratory test reference*, St. Louis, 1992, Mosby.
21. Resnick MI, Kursh ED: *Current therapy in genitourinary surgery*, St. Louis, 1992, Mosby.
22. Resnick MI, Novick AC: *Urology secrets*, St. Louis, 1995, Mosby.
23. Tanagho EA, McAninch JW: *Smith's general urology*, Norwalk, Conn, 1995, Appleton & Lange.
24. Thibodeau GA, Patton KT: *Anatomy and physiology*, ed 3, St. Louis, 1996, Mosby.
25. Walsh PC, Retrick ST: *Campbell's urology*, ed 6, Philadelphia, 1992, WB Saunders.
26. Walters MD, Karram MM: *Clinical urogynecology*, St. Louis, 1993, Mosby.
27. Zacharin RF: The anatomic supports of the female urethra, *Obstetrics and gynecology* 32:6, 1968.

3

Genitourinary Pathophysiology

James R. Bollinger

I do not pretend to teach her how, I ask her to teach herself, and for this purpose I venture to give her some hints.

Florence Nightingale

The organs of the urinary tract are the adrenal glands, kidneys, ureters, urinary bladder, prostate gland, male genital system, and female vagina and urethra, where current urologic intervention applies.

An overview of the pathologically altered physiologic characteristics of the organs of the urinary tract and the conditions that most commonly lead the patient to the operative theater are described in detail in this chapter to provide an understanding of surgical treatment. Additional and less common conditions are covered in less detail and are the subjects of other texts.

ADRENAL GLAND

Aldosterone acts at the level of the renal tubules to maintain sodium levels in the bloodstream. Cortisol bears the responsibility of maintaining the blood glucose level and producing sex hormones. Norepinephrine has a direct stimulatory effect on the heart and blood vessels. Cushing's syndrome, pheochromocytoma, neuroblastoma and adrenocortical carcinoma, as well as primary aldosteronism, are conditions that affect the adrenal gland and may prompt its removal surgically.

Cushing's Syndrome and Disease

The production of excessive adrenocorticotropic hormone (ACTH) by the pituitary gland will result in bilateral adrenal hyperplasia known as Cushing's disease. The hormones that are produced by the adrenal gland by a primary adrenal tumor, or where the adrenal cortex is being stimulated by an extraadrenal ACTH-producing tumor, cause a symptom complex known as Cushing's syndrome (Fig. 3-1).

The clinical presentation of Cushing's syndrome (caused by overproduction of adrenocortical hormones) includes pronounced weakness, centripetal obesity or a moon-shaped face, fat pads over the area of the clavicles and the seventh cervical vertebra (buffalo hump), red striae over the abdomen and thighs (Fig. 3-2), irritability, insomnia, hypertension, osteoporosis, possible psychotic behavior, and an abnormal diabetic glucose tolerance test with an elevated fasting plasma glucose level. The fundamental abnormality in Cushing's syndrome caused by an adrenocortical tumor is the overproduction of adrenocortical hormones. The differentiation of the cause of the hormone overproduction is made by laboratory measure-

ments of ACTH and cortisol levels, as well as 24-hour urinary 17-hydroxycorticosteroids and 17-ketosteroids levels, and by suppression of production of these hormones using varying doses of dexamethasone. At times, total bilateral adrenalectomy is indicated when the source of ACTH cannot be removed surgically. However, if the source of ACTH is found in the pituitary, it may be treated by neurosurgical resection (transphenoidal hypophysectomy). In the presence of an adrenocortical carcinoma, usually diagnosed by computed tomography (CT) scan, adrenal resection is indicated.

Aldosteronism

Primary aldosteronism, or an excessive production of aldosterone, leads to a combination of hypertension that is usually persistent, diminished serum potassium levels, and symptoms that may include increased nocturia, polyuria, diabetes insipidus, alkalosis, and tetany. Muscular weakness and orthostatic hypotension may be exhibited because of the patient's hypokalemic state. An adenoma of the adrenal gland is the usual finding in female patients. However, bilateral nodular adrenal hyperplasia occurs predominantly in young men. Laboratory findings include a slightly elevated serum sodium level with a very low potassium level of less than 3 mEq. Masses of the adrenal glands in this setting may be from l to 2 cm in diameter and may be localized with CT scan or radionuclide investigation. In bilateral nodular hyperplasia, medical treatment is recommended. Adrenalectomy is the treatment of choice in the presence of an aldosterone-producing tumor. Two thirds of aldosteronomas present on the left side.

Pheochromocytoma

Pheochromocytoma, a benign or malignant tumor, derived from the adrenal medulla is responsible for an increased production of catecholamines. These hormones have a stimulatory effect on the cardiovascular system and include norepinephrine, epinephrine, metanephrine, and vanilmandelic acid (VMA). Systolic and diastolic hypertension may be sustained or paroxysmal and often is followed by a feeling of profound weakness. Symptoms are commensurate with the severity of the hypertension and may include increased sweating, nausea and vomiting, a feeling of flushing or blanching, tachycardia and

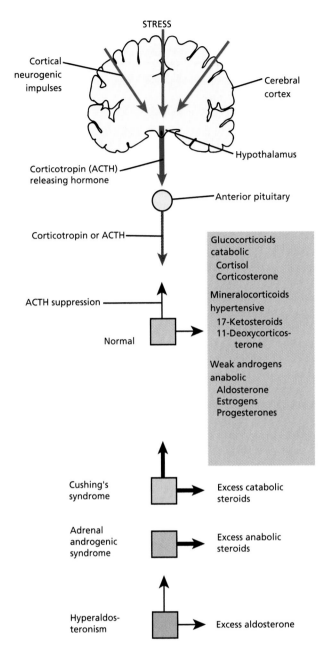

Fig. 3-1 The hypothalamic-pituitary-adrenocortical relationships in various syndromes. *(Modified from Tanagho EA, McAninch JW, Smith's general urology, ed 14, Norwalk, Conn., 1995, Appleton & Lange.)*

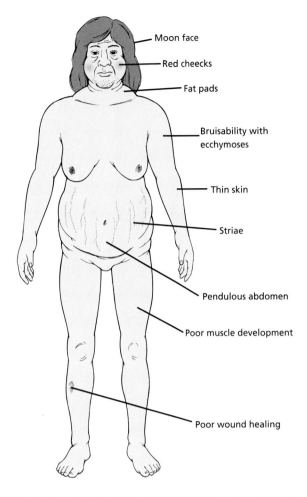

Fig. 3-2 Cushing's syndrome symptoms displaying principal clinical features. *(Modified from Forsham PH: William's textbook of endocrinology, ed 4, Philadelphia, 1968, WB Saunders.)*

palpitation, orthostatic hypotension, headache, and weight loss that results from anorexia. Diagnosis is considered when patients present with the above symptoms and 24-hour urine collections that exhibit elevated normetanephrine, metanephrine, and VMA (breakdown products of epinephrine and norepinephrine).

Pheochromocytomas may be extraadrenal and located in the retroperitoneum, between the adrenal gland and the bladder, and at the organ of Zuckerkandl (adrenal tissue in an ectopic location, usually anterior to the aortic bifurcation). Surgical excision accompanied by careful alpha-blocker anesthetic prepa-ration with early ligation of the adrenal vein is indicated. Care must be taken to avoid handling the tumor before its resection.

Neuroblastoma

Neuroblastoma may develop from any portion of the sympathetic chain in the retroperitoneum (45% involve the adrenal gland). These tumors offer the poorest prognosis, with most presenting in the first $2^{1}/_{2}$ years of life. Those discovered as late as the sixth decade are apparently less aggressive.

An abdominal or flank mass may be the first finding noted by the patient's physician or parents. Symptoms in the child include fever, malaise, failure to thrive, and constipation or diarrhea. Fifty percent of these tumors contain small areas of calcification. The plain abdominal film will demonstrate displacement of adjacent gas in the intestinal tract, but the diagnosis is typically made by CT scanning. Treatment is followed by surgical excision and preoperative radiation therapy. If the tumor is believed to be unresectable, chemotherapy has also been found to be effective.

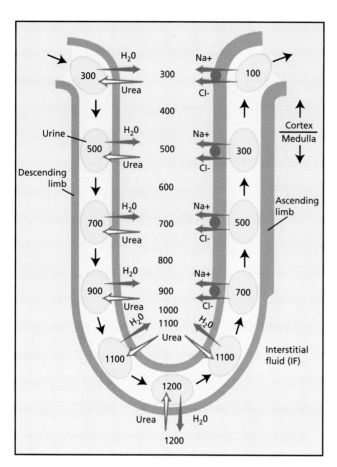

Fig. 3-3 The countercurrent multiplier system in the loop of Henle. Na+ and Cl- are pumped from the ascending limb and moved into the interstitial fluid (IF) to maintain a high osmolality there. Because the salt content of the medullary IF increases, this is called a "multiplier" mechanism. Because ion pumping also lowers the tubule fluid's osmolality by 200 mOsm, fluid leaving the loop of Henle is only 100 mOsm (hypotonic), compared to 300 mOsm (isotonic) when it entered the loop. Numbers in the diagram are expressed in milliosmoles (mOsm). (*From Thibodeau GA, Patton KT:* Anatomy and physiology, *ed 3, St. Louis, 1996, Mosby.*)

KIDNEYS

Renal Parenchymal Disease

The function of the kidneys includes regulation of body fluid, osmolality and volume, electrolyte and acid-base balance, excretion of metabolites and foreign products, and the production and secretion of hormones.

The nephron, glomerular complex, and countercurrent balance system are responsible for the filtration and concentration of components to be reabsorbed and excreted from the blood (Fig. 3-3). Renal parenchymal disorders such as glomerulonephritis may lead the patient to renal biopsy. This may be necessary to establish an accurate diagnosis, differentiate proportionate causes, determine probability of reversibility, choose the correct therapy, follow the progress of a chronic renal process, to prognosticate, and for investigative purposes. The anatomic characteristics of the kidney displaying the relative

position and size of the nephron, the basic functional unit of the kidney, can be seen in Fig. 2-6. Many disease processes may affect any portion of the nephron and may require biopsy of the renal parenchyma. One example is systemic lupus erythematosus (SLE) for which the World Health Organization has developed a system of classification depending on the severity of the involvement. This classification demonstrates the advantages of utilizing light microscopy, immunofluorescence, and electron microscopy to classify each biopsy. By utilizing these three techniques, it is possible to assign the biopsy to one of the five classes of SLE nephritis. Class I renal biopsy specimens demonstrate normal histologic findings, are rare, and are seen only in the beginning of the systemic disease. Class II is also known as the mesangial lesion. An important component of the glomerulus, the mesangium, is the supporting structure for the glomerular capillaries (see Fig. 2-6). It secretes the extracellular matrix, exhibits phagocytic activity, and secretes prostaglandins. The glomerulus is the capillary tuft and, because of its position relative to the capillaries, is responsible for filtering the blood directly to the kidneys. The mesangial cells may affect the ability of the kidneys at the level of the glomerulus to perform this function. In SRE, patients involved with this form of nephritis do not usually require specific treatment.

In class III, focal tubular (proximal and distal convoluted tubules) and interstitial (outside the tubules) changes are present. Urinary sediment reflects the presence of nephritis with the demonstration of red blood cells, red blood cell casts, and a variable amount of protein. Approximately one fourth of patients with a class III lesion excrete at least 3.5 g of protein in the urine per 24 hours (nephrotic syndrome, i.e., generalized edema).

Class III and class IV are really a continuum, with all the histologic changes demonstrated in class III as a focal lesion being present universally in class IV biopsy specimens. Patients with a class IV lesion have a dramatically thickened form of lesion known as a wire-loop lesion, demonstrate an abundant deposit of material in the subendothelial space on electron microscopy, and excrete red cells and red casts and at least 3.5 g of protein in the urine per 24 hours. A high proportion of these patients progress to renal failure. In class V, membranous glomerulonephritis, the patient population is generally older, with proteinuria significant enough to cause generalized edema. Some of these patients present with a set of symptoms known as nephrotic syndrome, the result of significant protein loss caused by the disease. This classification has a more indolent course but can progress to renal failure over time. Renal vein thrombosis may be a feature of this classification of lupus nephritis.

Acute Renal Failure

Acute renal failure indicates that renal function is not sufficient to maintain the body's metabolic balance. This may result from insufficient perfusion of the kidneys and may be prerenal, caused by hypovolemia or diminished cardiac function; renal, secondary to intrinsic kidney failure; or postrenal, caused by an obstructive process involving both ureters or the bladder. Intrinsic renal failure may be caused by injury to any of the components of the nephrons including vascular (afferent and efferent arterioles), glomerular, tubular, or interstitial. Pathologically, acute renal failure associated with histologic evidence of epithelial cell death may be attributed to ischemia from diminished cardiac output or shock, or may be nephrotic and known as acute tubular necrosis. Acute tubular necrosis generally occurs in a hospitalized patient, and the causes, though generally apparent, may be multifactorial. In acute tubular necrosis, kidney function, or specifically glomerular filtration rate, declines to zero. This decline has four contributing factors: decreased blood flow to the kidneys from constriction of the afferent arteriole leading to the glomerulus; tubular obstruction with secondary increased hydrostatic pressure in the tubules; passive backleak of glomerular filtrate across the injured tubular epithelial barrier; and mesangial contraction leading to a decreased glomerular surface area. The diagnosis of acute tubular necrosis is generally possible biochemically. Renal tissue may also be available by virtue of an associated surgical procedure or by biopsy.

Renal dialysis either by continuous arteriovenous hemofiltration or by peritoneal access may be necessary to control fluid and electrolyte imbalance and maintain blood urea nitrogen (BUN) levels below l00 mg/dl. Studies have failed to show, however, an improved mortality, making the role of this treatment modality as yet unclear. Care must be taken to avoid hypotension and fluid volume depletion, which may occur during dialysis and potentially prolong renal ischemia and recovery from acute tubular necrosis.

Chronic Renal Failure

Chronic renal failure is a common problem, with an estimated l70,000 patients currently receiving hemodialysis. The number of patients with chronic renal insufficiency, however, is much larger. This insufficiency may occur because of any insult, but it is generally believed that glomerular hypertension and hyperperfusion of surviving glomeruli after an initial insult eventually lead to destruction of the glomerulus. Serum BUN and creatinine will remain within the normal range until the glomerular filtration rate is reduced below half, and serum electrolyte and acid-base balance are usually maintained until the glomerular filtration rate (GFR) falls below l0% of normal. Complications of chronic renal insufficiency may include anemia because of a decreased production of erythropoietin, suppression of bone marrow production of red blood cells by uremic toxins, and decreased red blood cell survival. Hypertension must be controlled to prevent cerebrovascular and cardiac injury as well as to protect renal function. Angiotensin and angiotensin-converting enzyme (ACE) inhibitors both decrease loss of protein in the urine and prevent the progression of glomerular disease. However, these may be associated with a decreased GFR, causing a worsening of anemia and hyperkalemia in patients with advanced renal insufficiency, and they must be used with caution. Platelet dysfunction may be treated temporarily and normalized with administration of desmopressin (DDAVP, which exerts an antidiuretic effect), or for longer periods of time with estrogen therapy. Renal osteodystrophy occurs before dialysis is necessary, and treatment involves restriction of dietary phosphorus with supplementary dietary calcium. In chronic renal insufficiency the combination of increased parathyroid hormone levels and diminished vitamin D levels decrease intestinal calcium absorption and increase bone resorption.

Diabetic Glomerulopathy

Diabetic glomerulopathy is a disease entity that involves one fourth of patients with diabetes mellitus. The greatest proportion of patients with diabetes mellitus are non–insulin-dependent, or Type II, diabetics. Renal involvement in these patients is less common than in the insulin-dependent, or Type I, diabetics. There is, however, a higher prevalence of non–insulin-dependent diabetics, resulting in overall comparable numbers of patients with renal involvement with Type I or Type II diabetes mellitus.

Diabetic glomerulopathy, the most common form of diabetic renal disease, develops when mesangial cells become thickened and eventually destroy the glomerulus. Protein deposits known as hyalin also form throughout the kidney and are similar to the changes that occur in and account for diabetic retinopathy and coronary artery disease.

The finding of hyalinosis and narrowing of glomerular efferent arterioles along with Bowman's capsular drop formation (replacement with hyalin) is pathognomonic for diabetic glomerulopathy. Clinically the disease may be silent, be present with small amounts of albumin in the urine, or be a gross nephrotic syndrome. The development of nephrotic-range proteinuria, the loss of up to l2 to l5 g of protein in the urine in a 24-hour period, is associated with a rapid decline of the glomerular filtration rate. The loss of larger amounts of protein in the urine prompt the search for an alternative cause for the patient's glomerular disease. Other clinical manifestations of diabetes mellitus with renal involvement include hyperkalemia and hyperchloremic acidosis disproportionate to the decrease in renal function. This is caused by decreased production of aldosterone by the juxtaglomerular apparatus and the deposition of hyalin in the arterioles at this location. Atherosclerosis involving the renal circulation tends to be increased in diabetic patients as it is in other organs. This presents as narrowing of the proximal opening of the renal artery by atheromatous plaque and may be the cause of renal failure. A patient who is diabetic and presents with worsening hypertension requiring increasing doses of antihypertensives and perhaps the presence of an abdominal bruit, suggests the diagnosis. Screening tests including captopril renal nuclear scan and ultimately renal arteriography, the gold standard for diagnosis, may be necessary to confirm suspicions. Be wary of the increased risk of acute renal failure after administering radiocontrast material to diabetic patients and provide adequate volume expansion.

Patients who are diabetic are at increased risk for chronic urinary retention by virtue of autonomic neuropathy, which affects the urinary bladder. In addition, these patients are more prone to urinary tract infection and its complications, such as papillary necrosis, pyelonephritis with gas-producing organisms, perinephric abscess, and xanthogranulomatous pyelonephritis. Diabetic patients are more susceptible to acute renal insult such as exposure to intravenous iodinated contrast material and volume depletion.

The life expectancy of a diabetic patient entering dialysis is less than 4 years. The statistic can be improved upon only by a successful transplant from a donor fully matched for human lymphocyte antigen.

Renovascular Hypertension

Renovascular hypertension is another entity for which surgical intervention may be necessary to correct uncontrolled hypertension and its associated problems. The basis for the development of this is the formation of atheromatous plaque in the proximal 2 cm of the renal artery (distal arterial or branch involvement is uncommon). Fibrous dysplasia accounts for approximately 40% of all renovascular disorders and is classified according to the portion of the artery involved. Medial fibroplasia is the most common of the fibrous lesions, accounting for 75% to 80% of the total. It generally occurs in 25- to 50-year-old women, often involves both renal arteries, and may involve the carotid, mesenteric, iliac, and other vessels. Renovascular disease may be treated with percutaneous angioplasty or renal artery bypass if conservative therapy has failed.

The development of renovascular hypertension should be considered when there is deteriorating renal function, loss of renal parenchyma, a combination of these, or accelerating hypertension despite conservative management. Diagnosis may be established by performing captopril radioiostope renography and renovascular angiography (Fig. 3-4). The physiologic basis for the development of renovascular hypertension is the production of renin by the juxtaglomerular apparatus. Renin facilitates the conversion of angiotensinogen to angiotensin I (see Fig. 2-7). Captopril must be used with caution. It blocks the effect of renin, depriving the affected kidney of the increased head of pressure necessary for perfusion, and may temporarily elevate the patient's BUN and creatinine. The administration of this drug with simultaneous administration of radioisotope will demonstrate findings suggestive of a renovascular lesion, indicating the need for investigation with arteriography (Fig. 3-5).

Congenital Renal Anomalies

Congenital anomalies of the kidneys occur more frequently than in any other organ and may be associated with gross deformity of an external ear, maldevelopment of facial bones on the same side, lateral displacement of the nipples, and congenital scoliosis and kyphosis. Congenital anomalies include agenesis, hypoplasia, supernumerary kidneys, dysplastic and multicystic kidneys, polycystsic kidneys, solitary simple renal cysts, anomalies of fusion, ectopic kidneys, kidneys in abnormal rotation, and abnormalities of the renal vessels in addition to medullary sponge kidney disease.

Renal agenesis

Unilateral renal agenesis has an occurrence of 1 in 5000, is seen more on the left side, and is more common in males. This abnormality most likely occurs because the ureter fails to develop and does not reach the tissue that will ultimately become the fully formed kidney. Without an intact drainage system, the tissue that should ultimately become the functioning kidney never develops. This is associated with no symptoms but may be associated with other congenital anomalies including abnormalities of the heart or vertebral column, anal anomalies, and congenital abnormalities of the long bones, hands, and genitalia. The ureter may drain into an abnormal, ectopic location in the urethra, seminal vesicle, or vagina. Bilateral renal agenesis is uniformly fatal. A list of associated anomalies can be found in Box 3-1.

Hypoplastic kidneys

Renal hypoplasia implies a small but fully formed kidney and may be congenital (Fig. 3-6). A congenitally small kidney is of normal configuration but may not have a full complement of calyces and nephrons. Dysplasia indicates the presence of distortion of the renal architecture. Causes of acquired dysplasia include vesicoureteral reflux, chronic pyelonephritis, chronic glomerulonephritis, and diminished renal blood flow with ischemia. Supernumerary kidneys, or the presence of additional fully formed kidneys without duplication or triplication, are rare anomalies.

Dysplastic kidneys

Dysplastic kidneys, or renal dysplasia, implies malformation of renal tissue, which may clinically present as a multicystic kid-

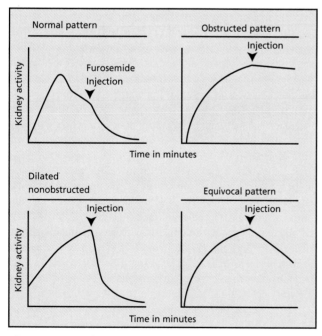

Fig. 3-4 Normal standard dynamic renal scan and renogram using ^{123}I-hippuran. Divided function: L/L + R = 62%. (*From Gillenwater JY et al, editors:* Adult and pediatric urology, *ed 3, St. Louis, 1996, Mosby.*)

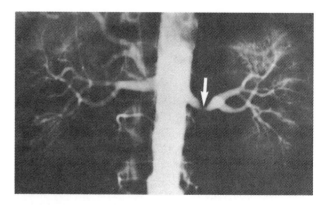

Fig. 3-5 Bilateral arterial disease is present and more pronounced on the left than on the right. (*From Gillenwater JY et al, editors:* Adult and pediatric urology, *ed 3, St. Louis, 1996, Mosby.*)

ney in the newborn or adult (Fig. 3-7). This is almost always unilateral and is characterized by an irregular lobulation of cysts with a ureter that is absent or atretic. The underlying cause of the various forms of multicystic kidneys in the infant appears to be obstruction in utero and may be seen in cases of ureteral duplication where a congenital ureterocele obstructs the upper pole. In instances where posterior urethral valves obstruct the bladder and kidney, the presence of bilaterally dysplastic or multicystic kidneys may also be seen.

Multicystic kidneys

Adult complications of multicystic kidney disease may include tumor (with only six documented cases), infection, hypertension, and flank pain. At one time it was believed that dysplastic or multicystic kidneys should be removed surgically within the first year of life. This has been shown to be unnecessary, though there still are strong proponents of this procedure. Associated abnormalities with renal dysplasia are listed in Box 3-2.

Polycystic kidneys

Polycystic kidney disease is hereditary and almost always a bilateral disease. The congenitally dominant form of polycystic kidney disease is generally diagnosed in adulthood. However, the recessive form is diagnosed in infancy and is associated with a short life expectancy. Polycystic kidney dis-

ease is believed to occur because of blind secretory tubules connected to functioning glomeruli that become cystic (Fig. 3-8). These units develop progressive functional impairment. Medullary sponge kidney disease may be part of the condition but in a milder form. The kidneys are often palpable on physical examination. Hypertension is found in 60% to 70% of these patients, who develop a gradually deteriorating renal function. Polycystic kidney disease may be associated with Lindau's disease, cerebellar cysts, vascular malformations of the retina, tumors or cysts of the pancreas, multiple bilateral cysts, or adenocarcinomas of both kidneys. In tuberous sclerosis (epiloia), a condition associated with polycystic kidney disease, mental retardation, and convulsive seizures, lesions known as hamartomas may develop in the skin, brain, retinas, bones, liver, and heart, as well as the kidneys.

Treatment of these individuals is usually conservative and supportive. Flank pain, fever and chills, infection, hemorrhage

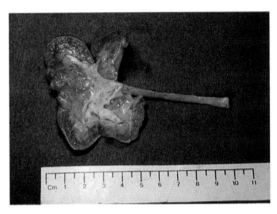

Fig. 3-6 Hypoplastic kidney. Cross section shows thin cortex and very little functioning renal tissue. It was discovered on routine examination for essential hypertension. *(From Lloyd-Davies W et al: Color atlas of urology, ed 2, London, 1994, Mosby-Wolfe.)*

Box 3-1 **Anomalies Associated with Unilateral Renal Agenesis**

Albright's syndrome
Arnold-Chiari syndrome
Cardiac septal defects
Imperforate anus
Myelomeningocele
Poland's syndrome
Pulmonary anomalies
Sacral agenesis or hypoplasia
Sirenomelia or monomelia
Spina bifida
Tracheoesophageal fistula
Urethral diverticula
VATER syndrome (vertebral defects, imperforate anus, tracheoesophageal fistula, and radial and renal dysplasia)

FEMALES
Ovarian ectopia
Tube and ligament abnormalities
Turner's syndrome
Uterine anomalies
Vaginal atresia

MALES
Absent vas deferens, seminal vesicles, ejaculatory ducts
Epididymal abnormality
Hypospadias
Testicular agenesis
Undescended testes

Modified from Seidman EJ, Hanno PM: *Current urologic therapy,* ed 3, Philadelphia, 1994, WB Saunders.

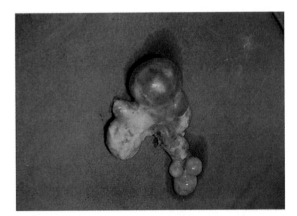

Fig. 3-7 Dysplastic kidney. This kidney is an example of the group of disorders in which abnormal metanephric differentiation is seen, frequently associated with cyst formation. The abnormal structures are recognized histologically. Most cases described as aplastic or multicystic kidney are really variants of this disorder. *(From Lloyd-Davies W et al: Color atlas of urology, ed 2, London, 1994, Mosby-Wolfe.)*

into the cysts, and the development of gross total hematuria may, however, prompt surgical intervention. Percutaneous aspiration or surgical unroofing of multiple renal cysts may be necessary to relieve flank pain in these patients.

Simple renal cysts

Simple renal cystic disease is a very common finding on urologic investigation of the upper urinary tracts with ultrasound examination or CT scan. Differentiation of simple renal cystic disease from polycystic disease is usually easily accomplished. Difficulty may occur when the cyst is multiple and septated, or bilateral, though they are commonly unilateral involving only the lower pole.

It is unclear whether simple renal cystic disease is congenital or acquired. Its origin may be similar to polycystic disease, where the functioning renal unit (the nephron) is unable to drain properly. Simple cysts have been produced in animals by causing tubular obstruction and local ischemia.

Because of their size, cysts may sometimes compress the ureter, causing obstruction or infection. In polycystic kidney disease, enlargement of cysts and compression of adjacent renal tissue rarely cause a significant loss of functioning kidney tissue (Fig. 3-9).

The most important differentiation is between renal cystic disease and renal malignancy. The usual presentation of a renal cyst is as an incidental finding on evaluation of the upper urinary tracts with ultrasound, CT scan, or intravenous pyelography (IVP), with or without tomography. The characteristics of a benign simple cyst are (1) the demonstration of a thin wall and smooth contour, (2) the absence of multiple chambers in the cyst, (3) no calcification present in the cyst or its wall, and (4) a CT density (measured in Hounsfield units) that is close to 0. Margination of the lesion when compared with functioning adjacent kidney tissue is based on the absence of the uptake of contrast media in the cyst wall or its contents.

Box 3-2 **Abnormalities Associated with renal dysplasia**

Beckwith-Wiedemann syndrome (Wilm's tumor)
Dandy-Walker syndrome
Familial renal dysplasia
Jeune's syndrome (asphyxiating thoracic dystrophy)
Meckel-Gruber syndrome (microcephaly, cleft palate, hepatic dysgenesis)
Cerebral dysgenesis
Multicystic kidney
Posterior urethral valves
Prune-belly syndrome
Renal retinal dysplasia
Hydrocephalus
Trisomy D
Ureteral orifice ectopia
Ureterocele
Vesicoureteral reflux
Zellweger syndrome

Modified from Seidman EJ, Hanno PM: *Current urologic therapy*, ed 3, Philadelphia, 1994, WB Saunders.

The classification proposed by Bosniak is helpful in the evaluation and follow-up treatment of benign and complicated simple renal cysts. Class I is a benign simple cyst that fulfills the criteria as above. Class II is a minimally complicated cyst by virtue of multiple septations, minimal calcification, and no increase in density on CT evaluation. These lesions may be followed with repeat evaluation at periodic intervals. Class III is a moderately complicated cyst with some findings seen in malignant lesions that cannot be clearly differentiated from them. Some of these will be found to be benign. A surgical approach to these lesions may be that of simple enucleation or partial nephrectomy. It is at times difficult for the pathologist to rule out the presence of a malignancy on either microscopic or gross examination. Elderly patients may be more appropriately followed with repeat radiographic evaluation by CT scan or ultrasonography until the diagnosis becomes clear. Class IV, cystic carcinoma, can usually be readily diagnosed. If the carcinoma is not metastatic, treatment should be radical nephrectomy.

Fusion anomalies

Anomalies of renal fusion occur in about 1 in 1000 individuals, with the most common being horseshoe kidney in which

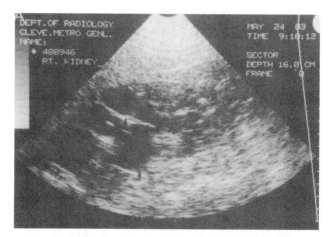

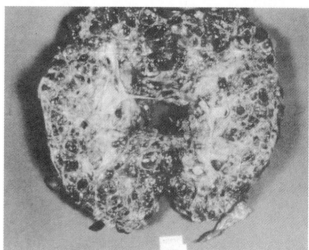

Fig. 3-8 **A,** Ultrasonography of polycystic kidneys. **B,** Adult polycystic kidney. *(From Gillenwater JY et al, editors:* Adult and pediatric urology, *ed 3, St. Louis, 1996, Mosby.)*

the lower poles of the kidney fuse across the midline. There are two ureters that open normally into the urinary bladder. Extraurologic anomalies occur in 78% of the patients, and 65% will exhibit other genitourinary defects (Fig. 3-10). The tissue that will become functioning kidney tissue in later life apparently fuses early in embryonic life. Under these circumstances the kidney lies lower than normal in the retroperitoneal space and derives its blood supply from adjacent arteries such as the aorta and iliac. Since the ureters must pass over the fused portion of the kidney tissue, or the isthmus, they tend to become dilated above this area, increasing the incidence of stone disease, infection, and tumors.

Renal ectopia (ectopic kidneys)

An ectopic kidney is located in an abnormal position and usually manifests as a kidney that did not rise to its normal position in the renal fossa under the liver on the right, or just below the spleen on the left. This usually presents in a position over the pelvic brim, in the pelvis, and, rarely, in an ectopic position in the chest. As in horseshoe kidney, these kidneys take

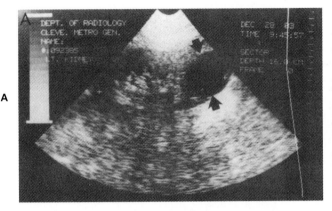
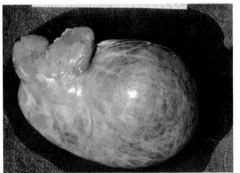

Fig. 3-9 A, Ultrasonography of longitudinal section of kidney shows a lower-pole smooth-walled cyst with complete absence of any echoes. *(From Gillenwater JY et al, editors: Adult and pediatric urology, ed 3, St. Louis, 1996, Mosby.)* **B,** Macroscopic view of typical renal cyst showing the classic blue-domed appearance. *(From Lloyd-Davies W et al: Color atlas of urology, ed 2, London, 1994, Mosby-Wolfe.)*

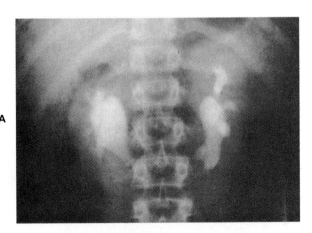
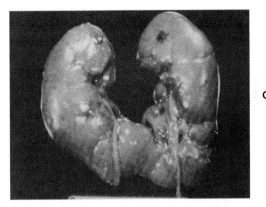
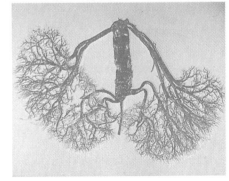

Fig. 3-10 A, The horseshoe kidney is the most common variety of renal fusion. **B,** Blood supply of horseshoe kidney. The arteries to the apical upper middle posterior segments on either side of the aorta are of the same pattern as those of normal kidneys. Not only have the right lower segmental arteries arisen from a common trunk, but also the posterior branches have arisen earlier than the anterior branches and almost directly from the aorta. **C,** Horseshoe kidney cross section showing the lower poles fused across the midline with the ureters passing down anteriorly *(A and C from Gillenwater JY et al, editors: Adult and pediatric urology, ed 3, St. Louis, 1996, Mosby; B from Lloyd-Davies W et al: Color atlas of urology, ed 2, London, 1994, Mosby-Wolfe.)*

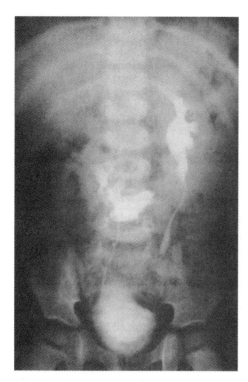

Fig. 3-11 Crossed ectopia of one kidney fused with the other kidney and both having only one pelvicalyceal system. *(From Gillenwater JY et al, editors: Adult and pediatric urology, ed 3, St. Louis, 1996, Mosby.)*

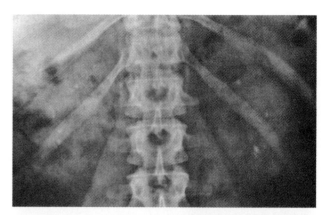

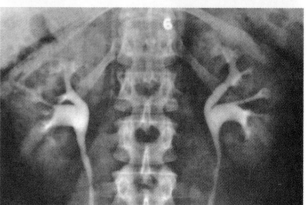

Fig. 3-12 A, IVU of medullary sponge kidney. **B,** Advanced medullary sponge kidney with calcification. *(From Gillenwater JY et al, editors: Adult and pediatric urology, ed 3, St. Louis, 1996, Mosby.)*

their blood supply from adjacent arteries, and it is important to remember this congenital entity when one encounters a pelvic mass on abdominal or pelvic examination. Ectopic kidneys are most often asymptomatic unless associated infections, stone disease, or obstruction intervene. Ectopic kidneys may be crossed with or without fusion (Fig. 3-11).

Anomalous renal arteries are not uncommon, as opposed to a single renal artery. Three or four arteries may be seen on renal angiography and, because of their location relative to the ureteropelvic junction (UPJ), one in particular may cause obstruction, requiring surgical correction. Anomalous arteries do not represent a significant problem unless surgical intervention is required because the patient is a kidney donor.

The "nutcracker phenomenon" presents as gross, usually painless, hematuria because of increased pressure in the venous circulation of the left kidney, caused by an anomalous position of the duplicated left renal vein, underneath the inferior mesenteric artery. This may be treated with irrigation of the collecting system with a dilute solution of silver nitrate but, if the patient requires transfusion, may necessitate surgery to correct the anomalous venous drainage.

Medullary sponge kidney

Medullary sponge kidney disease is a congenital recessive defect. The collecting tubules represented in the earlier figure of the nephron are dilated, predisposing the patient to infection and calculus formation. It is related to polycystic kidney disease and occasionally associated with hemihypertrophy of the body.

There is generally no surgical intervention necessary except to treat the occasional complications of the disease, infection and stone formation (Fig. 3-12).

Renal Trauma

Blunt injury

The treatment of renal trauma may depend on the mechanism of injury, the number and severity of associated intraabdominal injuries, the age of the patient, and the clinical and radiographic presentation of the patient. Renal trauma may be classified as blunt, penetrating, or renal pedicle injuries. Blunt renal injuries are contusions that result in superficial cortical lacerations; 70% to 80% manifest without significant bleeding or urinary extravasation. These may be managed with conservative treatment (Fig. 3-13). The remainder of blunt renal injuries are associated with significant bleeding (requiring repeat transfusion) with or without urinary extravasation and will ultimately lead to infection, obstruction, or hypertension. The need for operative intervention becomes apparent (Fig. 3-14). A small proportion of blunt renal injuries are associated with significant injury to adjacent organs, mandating laparotomy to salvage as much of the organ system as possible and the patient's life.

Several caveats apply to the evaluation and treatment of renal trauma patients. First, in the absence of gross hematuria,

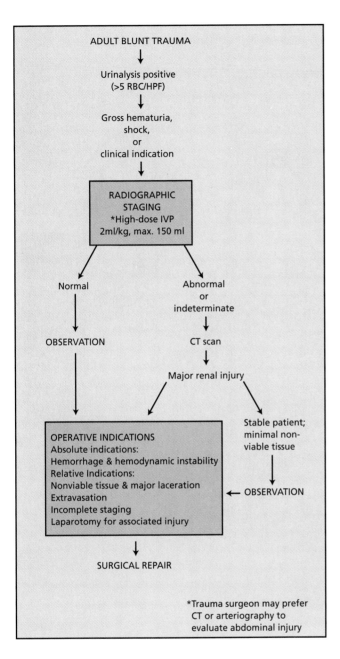

ADULT BLUNT TRAUMA

↓

Urinalysis positive
(>5 RBC/HPF)

↓

Gross hematuria,
shock,
or
clinical indication

↓

RADIOGRAPHIC
STAGING
*High-dose IVP
2ml/kg, max. 150 ml

Normal / Abnormal or indeterminate

OBSERVATION / CT scan

↓

Major renal injury

OPERATIVE INDICATIONS
Absolute indications:
Hemorrhage & hemodynamic instability
Relative Indications:
Nonviable tissue & major laceration
Extravasation
Incomplete staging
Laparotomy for associated injury

Stable patient;
minimal non-
viable tissue

↓

← OBSERVATION

↓

SURGICAL REPAIR

*Trauma surgeon may prefer
CT or arteriography to
evaluate abdominal injury

Fig. 3-13 Management protocol for adult with suspected blunt renal trauma. *(From Resnick MI: Current therapy in genitourinary surgery, ed 2, St. Louis, 1992, Mosby.)*

radiographic evaluation may not be necessary. However, one must be aware of the mechanism of injury. If a disruption of the UPJ or pedicle is believed to be consistent with the patient's injury, radiographic evaluation is imperative to make this diagnosis early on. The incidence of renal artery thrombosis is more common in the pediatric age group because of the relative lack of protection afforded the kidneys in the pediatric retroperitoneum, as compared with the adult. Further, if the patient's clinical condition changes after the initial evaluation, signifying possibly more serious internal injury, radiographic evaluation of the urinary tract is imperative.

The traditional approach to radiographic evaluation is the administration of 2 ml/ kg of intravenous contrast for an IVP—diagnostic for 80% of significant upper urinary tract injuries. CT scan has the advantage of providing imaging of adjacent organs and is the most commonly used single study to evaluate trauma victims. Evaluation using color Doppler ultrasonography of the renal pedicle may be helpful in selected cases but requires a skillful operator to localize the renal artery and measure its blood flow.

Blunt injury to the renal vascular structures occurs in fewer than 5% of cases of renal trauma, 90% of it in the pediatric or young-adult age group. The renal artery is stretched during the contusion leading to tearing of the arterial intima with subsequent subintimal dissection and thrombosis. The mortality for renovascular injuries is as high as 40%, primarily as a result of extensive associated injury. In addition, significant symptoms associated with renal pedicle injury may be absent, and so a high index of suspicion must be maintained. Since the kidney can tolerate only 30 minutes of warm ischemic time without significant loss of function and after 2 hours there is some degree of irreversible loss of renal function, the presence of a renal pedicle injury requires immediate operative intervention (Fig. 3-15).

Penetrating injury

Penetrating renal injuries account for approximately l5% to 20% of all renal injuries, and the kidneys are involved in l0% of all abdominal penetrating wounds. There is a trend toward conservative management of these injuries, but it must be decided early whether the injury was from a high- or low-velocity missile. A high-velocity missile (over 2000 feet/sec) generates significant associated injury because of the shock impact to surrounding tissue, and abdominal exploration and débridement is required. Approximately 70% of patients who have suffered penetrating injury will present with gross hematuria. However, any patient with more than five red blood cells per high-powered field should undergo radiographic evaluation. In the case of a stab wound, the size of the entrance wound has little correlation to the degree of injury sustained below this level. However, up to 90% of patients with stab wounds may be managed nonoperatively.

Renal Tumor

Renal cell carcinoma

Approximately 80% of malignancies of the kidney are renal cell carcinomas. In the United States in l993 there were just under 30,000 new cases representing 2% of new cancers. The origin of renal cell carcinoma is unclear but appears to be associated with a known genetic abnormality.

Renal cell carcinoma usually involves only one pole of the kidney and is generally discovered when ultrasonography or IVP is performed for the evaluation of hematuria. A flank mass or flank pain may be the presenting symptom. Computerized tomography is most often the first-line diagnostic study to stage and diagnose this lesion. Surgical extirpation (excision) is the gold standard for curative therapy in these individuals but may not be possible once the tumor has penetrated through the renal capsule into Gerota's fascia or adjacent structures.

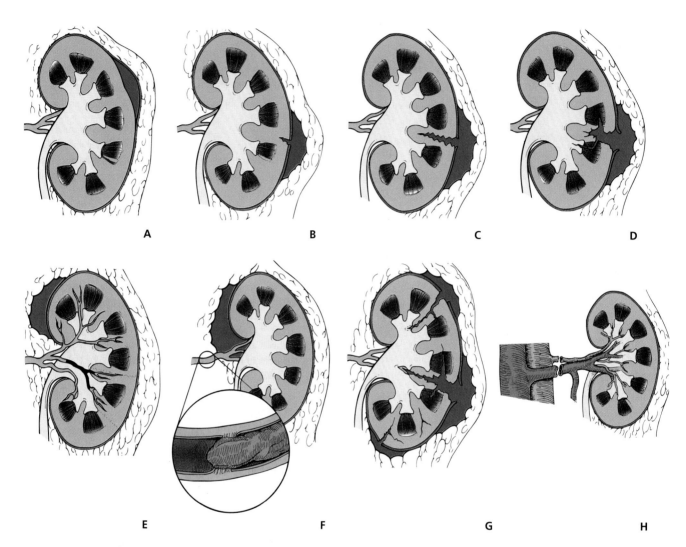

Fig. 3-14 Classification of renal injuries. Grades I and II are minor; grades III, IV, and V are major. **A,** *Grade I:* microscopic or gross hematuria, normal findings on radiologic studies, contusion or contained subcapsular hematoma without parenchymal laceration. **B,** *Grade II:* nonexpanding, confined perirenal hematoma or cortical laceration less than 1 cm deep without urinary extravasation. **C,** *Grade III:* parenchymal laceration extending more than 1 cm into the cortex without urinary extravasation. **D,** *Grade IV:* parenchymal laceration extending through the corticomedullary junction and into the collecting system; a laceration at a segmental vessel may also be present. **E,** *Grade IV:* thrombosis of a segmental renal artery without a parenchymal laceration but with corresponding parenchymal ischemia. **F,** *Grade V:* thrombosis of main renal artery with intimal tear and distal thrombosis displayed in *inset.* **G,** *Grade V:* multiple major lacerations resulting in a "shattered" kidney. **H,** *Grade V:* avulsion of main renal artery or vein, or both. (*From Resnick MI:* Current therapy in genitourinary surgery, *ed 2, St. Louis, 1992, Mosby.*)

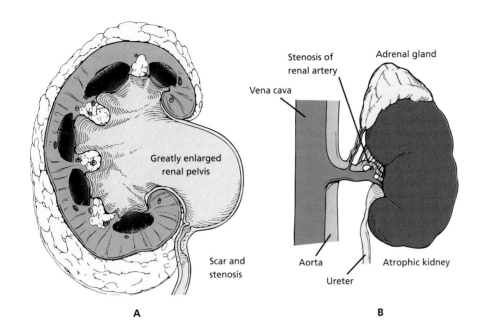

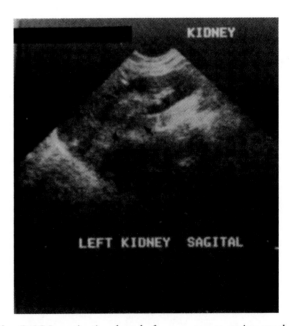

Fig. 3-15 Late pathologic findings in renal trauma. **A,** Ureteropelvic stenosis with hydronephrosis secondary to fibrosis from extravasation of blood and urine. **B,** Atrophy of kidney caused by stenosis from injury to arterial blood supply. *(Modified From Tanagho EA, McAninch JW:* Smith's general urology, *ed 14, Norwalk, Conn., 1995, Appleton & Lange.)*

Additional studies necessary to stage the disease include a chest radiograph to rule out pulmonary metastatic disease, a CT scan of the brain to rule out cerebral metastatic disease, and a chemistry survey to rule out elevated alkaline phosphatase and potential skeletal involvement. Alkaline phosphatase is important to the metabolic production and destruction of bone. Although elevation of this enzyme may be attributed to other causes, it is always elevated in the presence of bony metastatic disease and may prompt a bone scan to confirm the diagnosis. Since the complete removal of all malignant tissue is the only way to be assured of a cure, undiagnosed renal masses ultimately require surgical examination. A complete metastatic work-up should be performed before nephrectomy to establish the absence of distant disease. The presence of enlarged lymph nodes in the retroperitoneum, adjacent to a solid renal mass on CT scan, does not contraindicate surgical extirpation. The appearance of enlarged lymph nodes does not guarantee the presence of metastatic disease in the lymphatic chain. Fine-needle aspiration is sometimes helpful, though the presence of a normal needle aspirate does not guarantee the absence of microscopic malignant extension. The performance of a retroperitoneal lymph node dissection in cases of renal cell carcinoma remains controversial. However, obtaining staging information from a retroperitoneal lymph node dissection is gaining importance as new biologic therapies are included in postoperative adjuvant trials. In the presence of extensive retroperitoneal disease, nephrectomy is generally not indicated unless the patient suffers from significant pain secondary to mass effect, significant bleeding, or requires nephrectomy as part of a plan for postoperative protocol therapy. Direct extension into an adjacent organ, however, should not deter the surgeon from removing all disease, provided that it can be completely excised (Fig. 3-16).

Because of improved surgical technique, or partial nephrectomy, nephron-sparing surgery is being considered in selected

Fig. 3-16 Investigational study for a space-occupying renal lesion. Transverse view on ultrasound showing distortion of the renal outline by a superficial echogenic mass suggestive of a solid renal tumor. The presence or absence of echoes indicates if a lesion is solid or cystic. *(From Gillenwater JY et al, editors:* Adult and pediatric urology, *ed 3, St. Louis, 1996, Mosby.)*

individuals. This may be used in patients in whom radical nephrectomy would result in the need for permanent dialysis. In the absence of this condition, radical nephrectomy is the standard of care for excision of renal cell carcinoma.

Renal cell carcinoma may be approached through a standard flank incision if the lesion is not particularly large and involves the upper or lower pole, or with an anterior or thoracoabdominal approach to gain access for renal vessel ligation before disturbing the tumor for dissection and removal. The selection of incision is generally tailored to the patient's anatomy and the size of the lesion as determined by preoperative computerized tomography. The diagnosis of renal vein involvement with tumor should be considered preoperatively and investigated with CT scan, magnetic resonance imaging (MRI), or vena cavography in order to plan the surgical approach (Fig. 3-17). The prognosis for renal cell carcinoma patients treated with nephrectomy depends on the grade of tumor and the size and extensiveness of the disease. When the tumor is located within the kidney and is surrounded by normal renal tissue without lymphatic extension, the 5-year survival rate is approximately 70%. Extension through the capsule decreases the 5-year survival rate to 50%. Involvement of the renal vein or vena cava decreases the 5-year survival another l0%, and extension to the lymph nodes further decreases survival expectancy to 0 or up to 30%. Involvement of contiguous organs implies a maximum 5-year survival rate of only l0%.

Treating patients with metastatic disease with high-dose interleukin-2 (IL-2) may result in less than a 10% complete response rate in high-performance patients. Additional information indicates that optimum immune therapy used to treat patients with metastatic renal cell carcinoma may be curative. At the University of California, Los Angeles, 28 patients treated

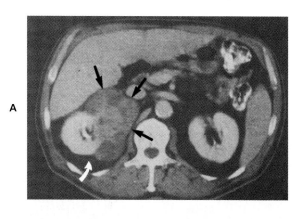

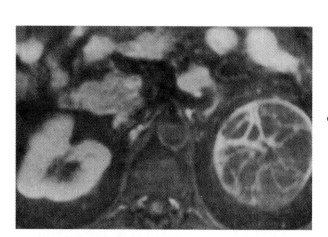

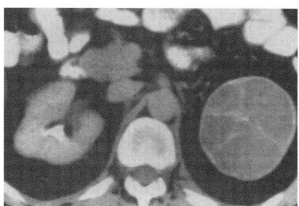

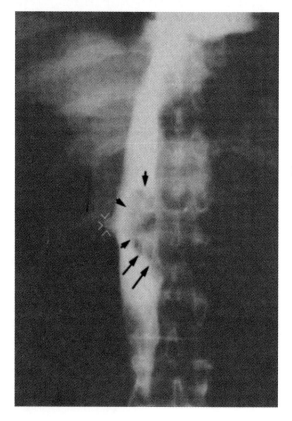

Fig. 3-17 CT scan showing the variation of density exhibited by the renal tumor on transverse abdominal cuts. CT scan with contrast is the first-line approach to investigation of renal cortical carcinomas. **A,** CT scan of large renal tumor appearing as partly solid mass with classical areas of necrosis. **B,** CT scan showing possible liver involvement by the renal tumor. MRI is used for problem cases and the detection of other organ involvement. **C,** MRI of same tumor occupying the entire upper pole of the right kidney, suggesting other organ involvement by virtue of its size. **D,** Cavography of vascular invasion of the main renal vein with visible tumor. *(From Gillenwater JY et al, editors:* Adult and pediatric urology, *ed 3, St. Louis, 1996, Mosby.)*

with tumor-infiltrating lymphocyte cells from nephrectomy specimens and a low dose IL-2 regimen achieved complete response ranging from 4 to 28 months in 25% of the 28 patients undergoing treatment.

Transitional cell carcinoma

Approximately 80% of tumors arising from the collecting system and pelvis of the kidney and ureter are transitional cell carcinomas that have a similar appearance, both grossly and histologically, to tumors that arise in the urinary bladder. Fifteen percent of these are squamous cell carcinomas, occurring more commonly in women. Adenocarcinomas and sarcomas are rare.

URETERS

Congenital ureteral anomalies, a common finding on IVP, may be associated with stasis of urine and therefore hydronephrosis and the development of infection or calculus disease. Duplication abnormality is apparently caused by a dominant gene that has incomplete expression (penetrance) as shown in

Fig. 3-18. Most cases occur in female patients, for reasons that are unclear, and the development of the ureter may be incomplete. In this case, the tissue that will ultimately become the kidney formed a hypoplastic, or multicystic, kidney (Fig. 3-19).

Congenital Ureteral Anomalies

The usual presentation of ureteral duplication is that of the Y configuration (Fig. 3-20). When ureteral duplication is complete, the ureter that drains the upper pole of the kidney has its opening closest to the neck of the bladder. The ureter that drains the lower pole of the kidney opens into the bladder farther up and away from the neck of the bladder and has a drooping lily presentation on x-ray. The ureter draining the lower pole of the kidney therefore enters the bladder with a more direct passage across the bladder wall and is predisposed to reflux of urine with its associated difficulties (infection and scarring of the kidney). The ureter that enters closest to the bladder neck and drains the upper pole of the kidney is the one that results in ureterocele formation (Fig. 3-21). The junction of

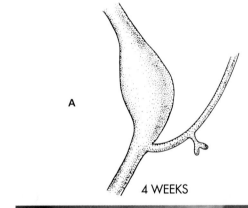

A

4 WEEKS

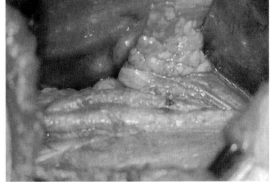

C

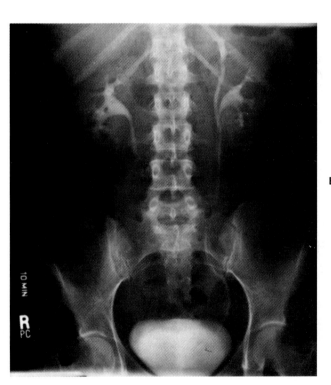

B

Fig. 3-18 **A,** Diagram of embryo at 4 weeks showing two ureteric buds. Ureteric anomalies account for about 30% of all congenital abnormalities in the urinary tract. Approximately 10% of patients have some ureteric abnormality. Ureteral duplication is caused by early branching of the ascending ureter; its extent depends on when it branches or by the second ureteric bud arising from the mesonephric duct. The diagram shows two ureteric buds causing the duplication in the urinary tract. **B,** Bifid kidney. The division, caused by late branching of the ureteric ampulla, is in the upper third of the ureter. This can give rise to abnormal peristalsis in the ureter leading to the "yo-yo" flow of urine from one portion to the other. **C,** Duplex system, indicative of late branching, starts at the upper third of the ureter. (**A** *from Gillenwater JY et al editors:* Adult and pediatric urology, *ed 3, St. Louis, 1996, Mosby;* **B,** *from Walters MD:* Clinical urogynecology, *St. Louis, 1993, Mosby;* **C** *from Lloyd-Davies W:* Color atlas of urology, *ed 2, London, 1994, Mosby-Wolfe.)*

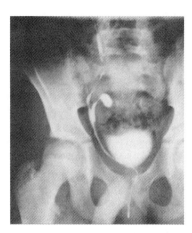

Fig. 3-19 Retrograde pyelogram of lower third ureteric duplication. One ureter opens into an ectopic hypoplastic kidney as a result of the failure of one of the duplicated ureters to develop. *(From Lloyd-Davies W et al: Color atlas of urology, ed 2, London, 1994, Mosby-Wolfe.)*

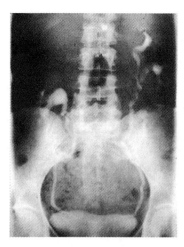

Fig. 3-20 Upper third duplex system with drooping-lily appearance of the opposite side. *(From Lloyd-Davies W et al: Color atlas of urology, ed 2, London, 1994, Mosby-Wolfe.)*

the ureter with the lumen of the urinary bladder never opens completely and drains through a pinpoint orifice, causing dilation of the ureter at the level of its entrance into the urinary bladder (ureterocele). This may cause obstruction in the upper pole of the kidney and its attached ureter and may actually be ectopic (opening in an abnormal location). This condition has been exhibited in the labia or vagina in females and in the seminal vesicle in males. Treatment of a ureterocele, segmental hydronephrosis of the kidney, or problems caused by an ectopic ureter (such as incontinence), is determined by the results of a complete urinary tract evaluation. If damage to a dilated upper pole segment is severe, leaving little functioning kidney tissue remaining, removal of this portion of the kidney by means of partial nephrectomy may be appropriate. If significant function remains and if the attachment of the ureter to the urinary bladder is not in an abnormal location, it may be possible to attach the normal ureter to the dilated portion through a ureteroureterostomy at the level of the kidney. Reflux can be treated with reimplantation of the refluxing segment. It may also be possible to achieve improvement in ureteral drainage by merely incising the ureterocele endoscopically, though reflux at this level may occur, necessitating more definitive treatment.

Retrocaval ureter

Another ureteral anomaly that occurs rarely is that of retrocaval ureter (Fig. 3-22). This may lead to ureteral obstruction with associated destruction of the kidney, stone formation, and infection accompanied by flank pain. This is diagnosed by IVP or retrograde pyelography (RGP). The occurrence of an ectopic ureteral opening can result in continuous leakage of urine, which should prompt the clinician to suspect its presence. This anomaly may occur as a separate entity without a duplication anomaly of the upper urinary tract. Under normal circumstances the ducts that drain the primitive kidney will in later life become the genital ductwork. The tubules for the primitive and mature kidney drainage systems separate as development pro-

gresses, so that normal differentiation will occur. When the ductwork that is attached to the primitive kidney does not separate, an ectopic ureter develops. The ureter from the mature upper urinary tact will drain into a duct that was a portion of the primitive kidney.

Ureteropelvic and ureterovesical narrowing

Congenital narrowing of the ureter may occur either at the UPJ, adjacent to the kidney, or just proximal to the entrance of the ureter into the urinary bladder (Fig. 3-23). Both cause hydronephrosis with its associated complications of infection, stone formation, and destruction of the kidney (Fig. 3-24). Clinically these may manifest as the onset of flank pain after drinking fluid that has a diuretic effect, such as alcoholic or caffeinated beverages, and is known as "beer-drinker's kidney."

Acquired Ureteral Anomalies

Ureteral stricture

Acquired ureteral stricture may be caused by any inflammatory process that occurs around the ureter. This may be attributable to extensive abdominal or pelvic surgery, radiation therapy, scar formation as a result of periureteral bleeding or surgical repairs, compression of the ureters by lymph nodes or malignancies, and intrinsic ureteral scarring caused by ischemia related to prolonged obstruction with ureteral calculi or infection. The ureter may become stenotic because of uterine prolapse or retroperitoneal fibrosis secondary to chronic analgesic use. Retroperitoneal fibrosis may also be associated with chronic use of ergot derivatives (e.g., Cafergot; Sansert for migraine headache; Methergine to promote uterine contractions) as a discrete entity or may be contributed to by granulomatous bowel disease such as Crohn's disease. Ureteral integrity can also be compromised by infections such as tuberculosis or bilharzial infection (schistosomal infestation) or affected by aortic or iliac artery aneurysms. UPJ stenosis may also be associated with the inflammatory influence of vesicoureteral reflux.

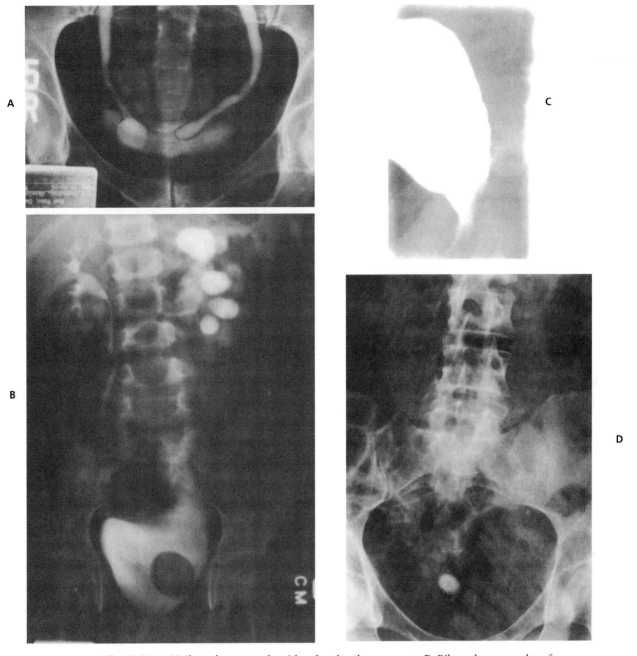

Fig. 3-21 **A,** Unilateral ureterocele with cobra-head appearance. **B,** Bilateral ureteroceles of differing size, a large right ureterocele and a small left cobra-head ureterocele. **C,** Prolapsing ureterocele, the most common cause of urinary retention in women. **D,** Kidney and upper bladder x-ray view of ureterocele with midsized calculus. *(**A** and **B** from Gillenwater JY et al, editors: Adult and pediatric urology, ed 3, St. Louis, 1996, Mosby; **C** from Lloyd-Davies W et al: Color atlas of urology, ed 2, London, 1994, Mosby-Wolfe; **D** from Tanagho EA, McAninch JW: Smith's general urology, ed 14, Norwalk, Conn., 1995, Appleton & Lange.)*

Malignancies of the lower urinary tract such as bladder carcinoma or carcinoma of the prostate may stenose the UVJ, or it may be compromised by elevation of the trigone related to benign enlargement of the prostate. Chronic constipation can contribute to lower ureteral dilatation. Endometriosis can invest the ureter as well as the bladder, resulting in obstruction.

Ureteral Tumors

Transitional cell carcinoma

Malignant tumors of the ureter and renal pelvis are primarily transitional cell carcinomas similar to those found in the urinary bladder. They are predisposed to by the excretion of metabolites of tryptophan as found in cigarette smoke. Renal pelvic tumors may be solid or papillary. Solid tumors are pri-

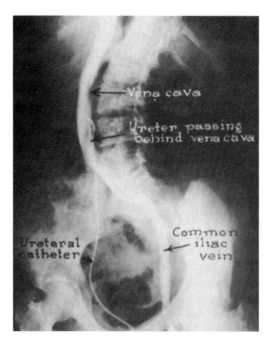

Fig. 3-22 Retrocaval ureter clearly showing the characteristic curve of the ureter. Retrocaval ureter is caused by persistence of the precursor of the vena cava remaining anterior to the ureter. *(Modified from Tanagho EA, McAninch JW: Smith's general urology, ed 14, Norwalk, Conn., 1995, Appleton & Lange.)*

marily squamous cell carcinomas and are found more commonly in women because of the increased incidence of infection. These may be difficult to differentiate from tissue associated with inflammation. These tumors may primarily invade the kidney tissue, rather than causing hypertrophic growth into the pelvis of the kidney, making diagnosis difficult.

The incidence of renal pelvic tumors appears to be increasing. Earlier in the century the ratio between renal and parenchymal tumors was 1 to 18, whereas the present ratio seems to be closer to 1 to 4. This may be secondary to carcinogens in the environment, in particular the use of tobacco and the use of certain analgesics (APCs).

The diagnosis of a ureteral or renal pelvic tumor may be suspected when the patient presents with painless hematuria that on cystoscopic examination of the urinary bladder appears to be emanating from one side, or with hematuria associated with flank pain on the involved side. IVP or RGP findings often are virtually diagnostic. CT scan with intravenous contrast material may be beneficial in establishing the diagnosis and may help to rule out the presence of adjacent involved lymph nodes or metastatic disease in the lung or liver. Normal urinary cytologic features do not exclude a malignancy of significant potential in the ureter or renal pelvis. The primary management of renal, pelvic, and ureteral tumors is excision of the associated kidney with the ureter and a cuff of urinary bladder. Malignant cells may seed portions of the ureter below the tumor, increasing the chance of tumor forming dis-

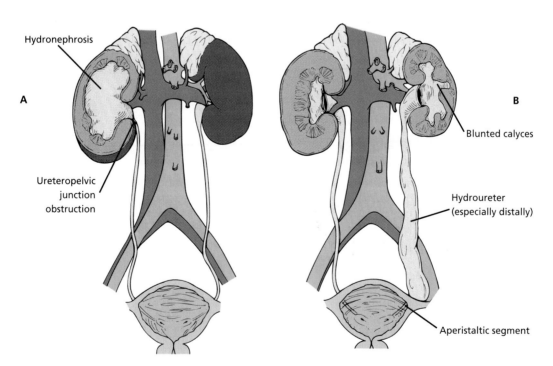

Fig. 3-23 Congenital ureteral obstruction. **A,** Right UPJ obstruction with hydronephrosis. **B,** Left UVJ obstruction (obstructed megaureter) with hydronephrosis. *(Modified from Tanagho EA, McAninch JW: Smith's general urology, ed 14, Norwalk, Conn., 1995, Appleton & Lange.)*

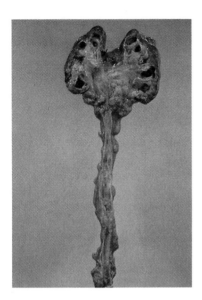

Fig. 3-24 Hydronephrotic kidney caused by combined pelvic and ureteric tumors. *(From Lloyd-Davies W et al: Color atlas of urology, ed 2, London, 1994, Mosby-Wolfe.)*

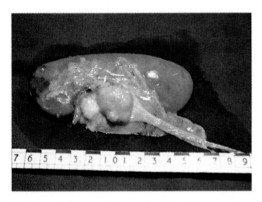

Fig. 3-25 Rounded tumor in renal pelvis. Cross section shows papillary differentiated transitional cell carcinoma of renal pelvis growing in the lumen of the renal pelvis. *(From Lloyd-Davies W et al: Color atlas of urology, ed 2, London, 1994, Mosby-Wolfe.)*

tal to the primary lesion (Fig. 3-25), with the significant likelihood of an associated bladder lesion. In certain instances, endoscopic treatment with resection or laser ablation may be feasible by virtue of a tumor's small size and location and the patient's overall condition. In more recent years laparoscopic nephroureterectomy has been performed with less morbidity than that associated with the traditional open technique. Nephroureterectomy must be contemplated only in the presence of a normal-appearing opposite kidney and ureter. In selected cases instillations of bacille Calmette-Guérin (BCG) may be used to treat superficial and recurring ureteral or renal transitional cell carcinomas. Radiotherapy may be used for inoperable patients or those with poor prognosis. Chemotherapy utilizing a platinum-based regimen has also shown significant promise. The ureter may be the site of metastatic tumors arising from the breast, colon, prostate, stomach, kidney, and lymphoma.

It may be acceptable to perform only a simple nephrectomy where palliation, because of the local extent of the tumor, is the goal of therapy, where the tumor is a squamous lesion with rare ureteric involvement, or if the patient is a poor surgical risk. Five-year survival statistics from the Memorial Sloan-Kettering series was 77% for noninvasive lesions, 57% for superficially invasive lesions, and 5% for lesions extending beyond the kidney. Patients with transitional cell carcinomas, treated with simple nephrectomy, have a 65% recurrence in the ureteral stump. This may be amenable to treatment with resection or endoscopic fulgeration, with or without laser ablation, at a later time.

Ureteral Obstruction
Ureteral calculi
Renal colic is the term applied to the sudden onset of flank pain experienced when a renal calculus passes from the kidney into the ureter. Approximately two thirds of the calculi are composed of calcium and oxalate, or mixtures of calcium oxalate with calcium phosphate. Magnesium ammonium phosphate (struvite) stones account for 15% of all calculi and occur in a clinical setting where a urea-splitting bacteria, such as *Proteus mirabilis*, elevates the urinary pH and predisposes the patient to the precipitation of calculus material. Uric acid and cystine stones account for 10% of urinary calculi. In addition, there are other miscellaneous causes of stone formation such as xanthine, silicates, or matrix calculi, as well as metabolites of certain drugs, such as the earlier forms of the sulfonamides or triamterene. Calculus formation may occur where crystals ("Randall's plaques") serve as the center (nidus) for calculus crystallization and enlargement. These may enlarge until they can no longer be held in their position at the renal papillae. Another cause of calculus formation may be dehydration (as occurs in hot climates or with excessive perspiration) vomiting, or diarrhea. Structural anomalies of the urinary tract as seen with medullary sponge kidney disease may lay the groundwork for the formation of urinary calculi. As previously indicated, the presence of urea-splitting organisms may increase the urinary pH and predispose the patient to the formation of magnesium ammonium phosphate calculi. Excessive ingestion of dietary or medicinal calcium may lead to calcium stone formation because the excessive ingestion of food high in certain amino acids, such as purines, may cultivate the formation of uric acid calculi. Cabbage, rhubarb, spinach, tomatoes, celery, black tea, and cocoa may set up the basis for the formation of oxalate stones, as small bowel disease does with hyperabsorption of dietary oxalate.

Calculi consisting of calcium oxalate account for 80% of all urinary calculi, 60% of which occur because of absorptive hypercalciuria. This is caused by increased sensitivity of the intestinal tract to vitamin D leading to the increased absorption of calcium. When the dietary calcium level is restricted to 150 mg/day, the increased levels of calcium in the urine revert to normal. Increased levels of water intake may aid in reducing stone production. A decrease in sodium intake to 100 mEq/day will lead to further absorption of calcium from the blood filtered by the glomerulus and therefore diminish the amounts of calcium excreted daily. A decrease in calcium absorption must be achieved by intake of cellulose phosphate, which increases the binding of calcium in the intestinal tract, to prevent its absorption. Calculus formation from diminished citrate excretion in the urine may occur and can be tested with orally administered potassium citrate time-released tablets. Orthophosphates, on the other hand, curb the formation of calculi by increasing the excretion of the urinary inhibitors pyrophosphate and citrate.

Another cause of urinary calculus formation, renal hypercalciuria, occurs when the kidney is incapable of reabsorbing normal amounts of calcium from the urinary filtrate. Thiazide diuretics increase the reabsorption of calcium from the distal convoluted tubule and thereby lower the daily excretion of calcium in the urine.

The diagnosis of urinary tract calculus is directly related to its degree of density under x-ray (radiopacity) (Table 3-1). The initial investigation in a patient who presents with renal colic, dull aching flank pain (which is less acute), or recurrent urinary tract infection (leading one to suspect urinary calculus) is the plain abdominal film of the kidneys, ureters, and urinary bladder (KUB). Further evaluation with IVP or intravenous urogram (IVU) may be necessary to assess the degree of obstruction and to rule out the presence of a nonopaque or partially opaque calculus (such as uric acid calculus), which may be causing obstruction but not be apparent on x-ray film. After the initial episode of renal colic has been treated and relieved with analgesics (intravenously or intramuscularly administered morphine, ketorolac [Toradol], or a similar antiinflammatory agent), subsequent treatment will depend on the size and position of the

ureteral calculus and whether or not the patient has associated complications that would precipitate intervention. The majority of patients who present with renal colic secondary to a ureteral calculus can be managed through periodic office visits. The indications for hospitalization, ancillary therapy, or surgical intervention include urinary tract infection associated with fever, a calculus that is greater than 6 mm in diameter and is unlikely to pass without mechanical assistance, the presence of symptoms that are too severe for ambulatory (home care) management, and calculi in both ureters (or in one ureter when the patient has a solitary kidney). The typical plan for management of a patient with ureteral calculus and renal colic is outlined in Table 3-2.

The majority of calculi less than 5 mm in width will pass spontaneously within a month after the onset of symptoms. Almost all stones greater than 8 mm in diameter and 65% of stones greater than 6 mm will be in the ureter after 1 year. Obstruction that is untreated for more than 4 to 6 weeks can cause irreversible renal damage. Patients with calculi greater than 5 mm should be treated after 4 weeks if the calculus does not appear to be traveling distally in the ureter (Fig. 3-26).

Hübner in Vienna followed 63 patients with asymptomatic calyceal calculi for up to 7 1/2 years. In 52% of the patients the calculi migrated into the ureter and almost always became symptomatic. Only 16% of these calculi were spontaneously passed, usually with renal colic. Of the remaining patients, 45% had calculi that grew in size, and 40% of these patients eventually required some type of surgical intervention. In 6 patients, obstruction and infection had damaged the kidneys severely enough to mandate nephrectomy.

Currently available alternatives for the treatment of ureteral and renal calculi include extracorporeal shock-wave lithotripsy (ESWL), ureteroscopic removal using electrohydraulic lithotripsy (EHL), or laser lithotripsy. In certain cases of percutaneous stone removal ultrasonic lithotripsy may be desirable. The equipment incorporates an ultrasound probe that fragments the calculus and an aspiration apparatus that removes the small calculus particles as they are created. During the last 10 years the development of extracorporeal shock-wave lithotriptors and the current availability of small-diameter, flexible, and rigid ureteroscopes have revolutionized the treatment of urinary tract calculi.

Table 3-1 **Stone Density Related to Opacity**

CONSISTENCY	DENSITY	RADIOPACITY
Calcium phosphate	22	Very opaque
Calcium oxalate	10.8	Opaque
Magnesium ammonium phosphate	4.1	Moderately opaque
Cystine	3.7	Slightly opaque
Uric acid	1.4	Nonopaque
Xanthine	1.4	Nonopaque

Modified from Tanagho EA, McAninch JW: *Smith's general urology,* ed 14, Norwalk, Conn, 1995, Appleton & Lange.

Table 3-2 **Treatment for Ureteral Calculi**

CHARACTERISTICS	LOCATION	TREATMENT
Stones <6 mm	Upper and middle of ureter	Wait 4 weeks
Stones <6 mm	Upper and middle of ureter	Proximal dislodgment Extracorporeal shock-wave lithotripsy (ESWL) *or* In situ ESWL with stent *and then* Ureteroscopic retrieval
	Distal portion of ureter	Ureteroscopic extraction
Stones with associated pathologic condition	Any ureteral site	Ureteroscopic retrieval *and then* Open ureterolithotomy

Modified from Resnick MI, Kursh E: *Current therapy in genitourinary surgery,* ed 2, St. Louis, 1992, Mosby.

Treatment is predicated on the calculus being symptomatic a dull aching pain in the flank, as seen in the case of calyceal calculi; renal colic; recurrent urinary tract infection; and an avenue for egress of the fragments in the associated urinary tract. Some believe that the treatment of asymptomatic calyceal calculi may be acceptable to prevent the complications associated with their passage. Treatment of the patient thereafter with some type of conservative therapy aimed at prevention of additional calculus formation is recommended (Table 3-3).

ESWL is most successful in cases where the calculus is less than 2 cm in diameter. In these cases the 3-month stone-free

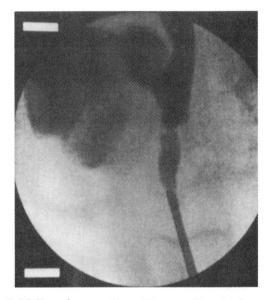

Fig. 3-26 Ureteric stone. *(From Gillenwater JY et al, editors:* Adult and pediatric urology, *ed 3, St. Louis, 1996, Mosby.)*

rate is approximately 75% to 90%. Results of treatment in the upper ureter and kidney have a higher success rate, one approaching 90%, whereas in the middle and lower parts of the ureter, ESWL may achieve only 40% to 75% success. Contraindications to ESWL include a bleeding diathesis (abnormal tendency) that is uncorrected, associated obstruction below the calculus, and pregnancy. The presence of a cardiac pacemaker requires attention to the timing of the ESWL, taking into consideration the patient's pacemaker rate, to prevent complicating cardiac arrhythmias.

Some patients (10% to 25%) may require an additional procedure to aid in the passage of calculus fragments, such as the placement of a ureteral stent. The accumulation of distal ureteral calculi in the ureteral lumen creates an x-ray appearance known as *Steinstrasse* (street of stones) (Fig. 3-27). Recent studies have demonstrated the absence of significant hypertension after ESWL. The final determination of this complication awaits the report of a prospective multicenter clinical trial.

With the development of narrow flexible and rigid ureteroscopes, it has become possible to remove calculi from the urinary tract endoscopically. With the use of small-diameter EHL probes it may be possible to remove 90% of the urinary tract calculi encountered. A distinct advantage in the use of an endoscopic approach in the treatment of ureteral calculi is that the entire calculus can be removed with no time interval required for the passage of fragments, as may be seen with ESWL. However, the use of ureteroscopic techniques are associated with an 8% to 10% complication rate, primarily in the form of localized perforation. The symptoms resolve with ureteral stenting in the majoriy of cases. The use of a 7 Fr rigid ureteroscope further decreases the incidence of perforation in the distal third of the ureter, but instrumentation and possible stenting is still required.

Table 3-3 **Specific Medical Treatments**

CONDITION	FIRST CHOICE	SECOND CHOICE
Absorptive hypercalciuria		
Type I, severe	Sodium cellulose phosphate	Thiazide + K$_3$Cit
Type I, mild-moderate	Thiazide + potassium citrate (K$_3$Cit)	Orthophosphate
Thiazide resistant	Sodiium cellulose phosphate Orthophosphate	
Type II	Dietary calcium restriction	Thiazide
Hypophosphatemic (Type III)	Orthophosphate	Thiazide
Renal hypercalciuria	Thiazide + K$_3$Cit	
Hyperuricosuric calcium nephrolithiasis		
Severe	Allopurinol	K$_3$Cit
Mild-moderate	K$_3$Cit	Allopurinol
Distal renal tubular acidosis	K$_3$Cit	
Chronic diarrheal syndrome	K$_3$Cit	
Thiazide-induced hypocitraturia	K$_3$Cit	
Idiopathic hypocitraturia	K$_3$Cit	
Gouty diathesis	K$_3$Cit	
With hyperuricemia	K$_3$Cit + allopurinol	

Modified from Resnick MI, Kursh E: *Current therapy in genitourinary surgery,* ed 2, St. Louis, 1992, Mosby.

The treatment of ureteral calculi with ureterolithotomy (stone removal through a surgical incision), once the standard of care for trapped calculi greater than 5 mm, is virtually no longer used. An exception to this is the presence of an associated ureteral disorder such as obstruction, tumor, massive reflux, or unsuccessful endourologic stone removal or ESWL. A calculus lodged in the upper portion of the ureter is generally treated with a dorsal lumbotomy or subcostal flank incision, whereas calculi in the midureter portion are approached through a right abdominal muscle-splitting incision, and those in the lower portion of the ureter are approached through a curved lower quadrant incision, also by muscle-splitting technique. In each situation, the ureter is incised longitudinally, after the stone is trapped in its location, and the ureter is then repaired with absorbable suture material, with or without stenting.

Ureteropelvic junction obstruction

Primary UPJ obstruction is a congenital lesion that causes obstruction of the kidney at the junction of the renal pelvis and the ureter (Fig. 3-28). This may be attributed to an intrinsic ureteral stricture at the UPJ (Fig. 3-29) but may also be present at the uterovesical junction (UVJ). UPJ obstruction may also be secondary to tortuosity with kinking of the proximal ureter, a tapering stenosis just below the UPJ, extrinsic bands that compress the ureter, compression of the ureter between an artery and vein that pass through the lower pole of the kidney, a congenitally high insertion on the renal pelvis, or any combination of these (Fig. 3-30).

As one of the three narrowest areas in the lumen of the ureter, UPJ obstruction may also be secondary to vesicoureteral reflux. The others are at the pelvic inlet (where the ureter

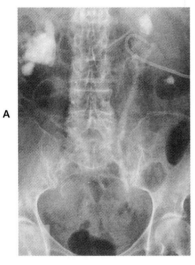

A

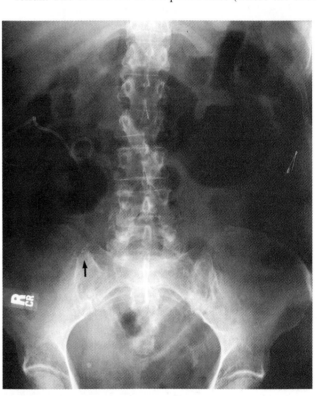

B

Fig. 3-27 A, Bilateral staghorn calculi with extensive *stein-strasse* and nephrostomy tube in place after ESWL. **B,** Large volume *steinstrasse* on right. (**A** *from Lloyd-Davies W et al: Color atlas of urology, ed 2, London, 1994, Mosby-Wolfe.*)

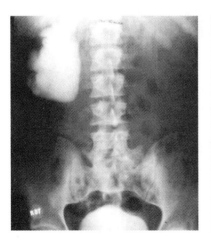

A

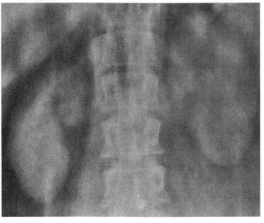

B

Fig. 3-28 A, IVU of hydronephrotic right kidney with no function on left. **B,** Tomogram of large left kidney. (**A** *from Lloyd-Davies W et al: Color atlas of urology, ed 2, London, 1994, Mosby-Wolfe;* **B** *from Gillenwater JY et al, editors: Adult and pediatric urology, ed 3, St. Louis, 1996, Mosby.*)

crosses the external iliac vessels) and at the UVJ (where the ureter passes through the wall of the urinary bladder). UPJ obstruction has been associated with congenital renal abnormality on the opposite side, such as a multicystic kidney.

UPJ obstruction may be present in a newborn. One in 800 fetuses have dilatation of the collecting system of the kidney, and approximately half of these persist. Renal ultrasonography demonstrating a dilated pelviocalyceal system in an infant with a one-sided abdominal mass confirms the diagnosis.

Later in life, UPJ obstruction may be suggested by the pain after oral ingestion of fluids that produce a diuretic effect, elicited from the inability of the kidney to excrete the urine produced. An IVP that demonstrates a dilated pelviocalyceal system with a normal upper ureter again points to UPJ obstruction. If the kidney's collecting system has the characteristic appearance, dilated calyces with an apparent compromising renal mass, RGP is performed to rule out associated lower ureteral abnormalities and to determine the length of the narrowed area. When the diagnosis is unequivocal, radioisotope diuretic renography may be beneficial. This study is performed in the nuclear medicine department by injection of a radioactive tracer and a diuretic. Under normal circumstances, the clearance of radioactive tracer from the two kidneys should be approximately equal, assuming that their function is equal. In a situation where there is an obstruction, the radioactive tracer will linger in the collecting system because the narrowed area in the ureter does not allow kidney clearance in a normal time interval (Fig. 3-31). The ultimate diagnosis of UPJ obstruction may be made by combining the patient's clinical history (incidence of pain or associated infection) with a more definitive study, the Whitaker test. This is done by infusing saline or contrast material through a catheter that is placed percutaneously into the kidney. At the same time, measurements are taken from the lower portion of the ureter. Differential pressure measurements can then be made above and below the area under suspicion (Fig. 3-32).

There are three approaches to the treatment of UPJ obstruction. The traditional approach, the dismembered pyeloplasty, is an open removal of the obstructing portion of the ureter at the UPJ with a reconnection of the ureter to the pelvis of the kidney. A nephrostomy tube is placed to control urinary drainage during the postoperative period.

An endopyelotomy may be performed in the absence of constricting fibrous bands or arterial compression of the UPJ. After gaining access to the dilated collecting system of the kidney, through either an antegrade or a retrograde approach, the UPJ is incised and an endopyelotomy stent placed, along with a nephrostomy tube, to control urinary drainage in the postoperative period. The stent is allowed to remain in place for several weeks, during which time the ureteral wall will advance around the newly placed stent to create a normal-sized ureteral lumen at the location of the previously narrowed area (Fig. 3-33).

The third operative procedure is performed in the retrograde direction by gaining access to the upper portion of the ureter with an operating ureteroscope and incising the narrowed area transurethrally. A variation of this is the use of a dilating balloon that incorporates a surgical wire electrode along the long access of the balloon. The balloon is inflated under fluoroscopic guidance at the level of the UPJ and electrocautery is applied to the cutting electrode to incise the area of narrowing. Subsequent to this a stent is placed and left in situ for several weeks to allow healing of the incised portion of the ureter.

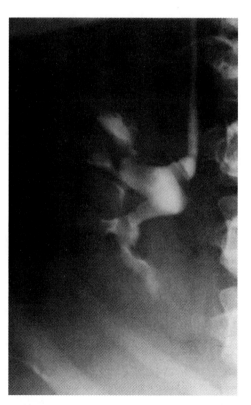

Fig. 3-30 UPJ obstruction caused by a vessel crossing the ureter, causing the pelvis to fall over the ureter, which becomes acutely kinked, resulting in progressive hydronephrosis. *(From Droller MJ: Surgical management of urologic disease, St. Louis, 1992, Mosby.)*

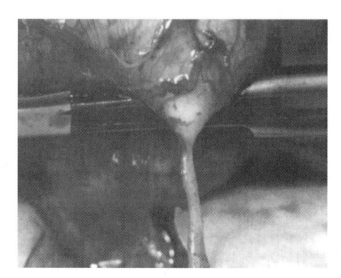

Fig. 3-29 UPJ obstruction showing interior close-up of the UPJ with the dilated pelvicalyceal system above. *(From Gillenwater JY et al, editors: Adult and pediatric urology, ed 3, St. Louis, 1996, Mosby.)*

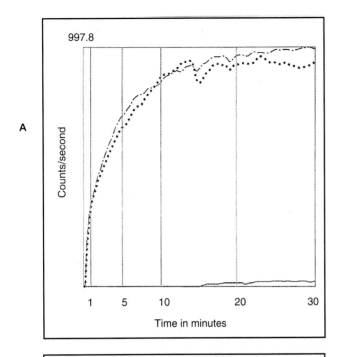

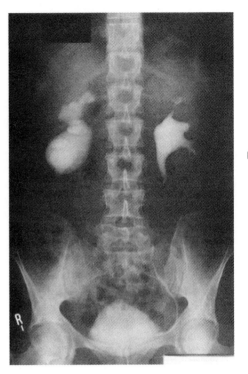

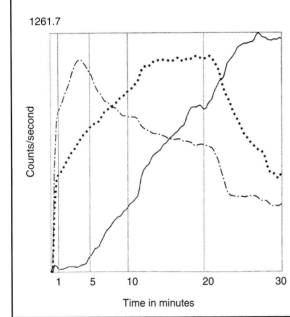

Fig. 3-31 **A,** Renogram of a patient with bilateral UPJ obstruction. Tracer is retained despite administration of furosemide at 20 minutes. Left renogram*, —— • ——; right renogram*, —— • ——; bladder activity,—— • ——. Relative function: left, 50%; right, 50%. Urinary flow rate, 1.14 ml/min; volume voided, 40 ml. **B,** IVU of patient with bilateral hydronephrosis. A renogram is needed to show if obstruction is present. **C,** Renogram showing prompt washout of tracer on the left side before administration of furosemide, indicating a nonobstructed left kidney. Tracer is retained for up to 20 minutes on the right side, but after furosemide there is prompt washout, indicating a nonobstructed right kidney. Left renogram*,—— • ——; right renogram*, —— • ——; bladder activity, —— • ——. Relative function: left, 64%; right, 36%. Urinary flow rate, 14 ml/min; volume voided, 550 ml. *Curves are not normalized and are background subtracted. *(From Lloyd-Davies W et al: Color atlas of urology, ed 2, London, 1994, Mosby-Wolfe.)*

Repair of UPJ obstruction can also be performed laparoscopically using the same technique as the open approach. Although long-term results on this procedure are not yet available, the decreased morbidity of laparoscopic surgery in this disease entity is attractive.

The ureter passes from the kidney, adjacent to the aorta on the left and the vena cava on the right, and is a delicate fibromuscular structure that because of its length, is prone to injury during operative procedures in the abdomen and pelvis. Some of the more common causes of ureteral stricture that result from these injuries are listed in Table 3-4. The treatment of these injuries may be by an endoscopic or an open approach as listed in Tables 3-5 and 3-6.

Vesicovaginal and ureterovaginal fistulae

A ureterovaginal fistula should be suspected when there is vaginal drainage of urine in the immediate postoperative period after a procedure that violated the vagina and possibly the ureter. In cases of vesicovaginal fistula, correcting the fistula between the bladder and the vagina will not correct the patient's incontinence or the ureteral obstruction on the injured side. Diagnosis is accomplished with a combination of IVP and RGP. Several open techniques for the correction of ureteral stricture include the Davis intubated ureterotomy, transureteroureterostomy, psoas hitch procedure, and the Boari flap procedure (Figs. 3-34 to 3-37). Primary anastomosis of the normal portions of the ureter, after excising the stricture, is also an option.

Text continues on p. 54

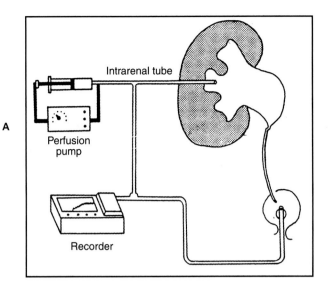

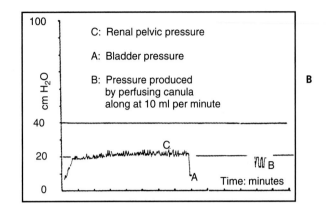

Fig. 3-32 The Whitaker test measures the pressure drop between the renal pelvis and the bladder and is another method of differentiating between an obstructive and a nonobstructive lesion in the urinary tract. A pressure drop of less than 10 cm H_2O at an injection rate of 10 ml/min indicates no obstruction. **A,** Diagram of the apparatus for investigating a pelviureteric obstruction. Pressure is measured in the pelvis and the bladder at a perfusion of 10 ml/min. **B,** Normal recording of Whitaker test. *(From Lloyd-Davies W at al:* Color atlas of urology, *ed 2, London, 1994, Mosby-Wolfe.)*

Table 3-4 **Common Causes of Ureteral Stricture**

Category	%	Examples	Cause
Urologic surgery	44	Ureteroileal anastomosis	Ischemia
		Ureterolithotomy	Recurrent malignancy
		Ureteroneocystotomy	
		Ureteroureterostomy	
General or vascular surgery	4	Aortobifemoral bypass	Surgical ligation, transection, clamping
		Abdominoperineal resection	Ischemia
		Colon resection	Periureteral inflammation
		Appendectomy	
		Transplant ureter	
Gynecologic surgery	6.8	Hysterectomy	Surgical ligation, transection, clamping
		Cesarean section	
		Ovarian cystectomy	Ischemia
Endoscopic urologic procedure	20	Ureteroscopy	Ureteral perforation or resection
		Ureteral stone retrieval	Ischemia, scarring
		Percutaneous stone manipulation	
		Ureteral catheterization	
		Intraureteral lithotripsy	
		Electrocautery or laser ablation	
Passage of calculus	13.2		Ischemia
Miscellaneous	9	Retroperitoneal fibrosis	Infection
		Chronic urinary tract infection	Periureteral inflammation
		Pelvic radiation	
		Genitourinary tuberculosis	
		Recurrent pelvic carcinoma	
Unknown	3	No apparent cause	

Modified from Resnick MI, Kursh E: *Current therapy in genitourinary surgery,* ed 2, St. Louis, 1992, Mosby.

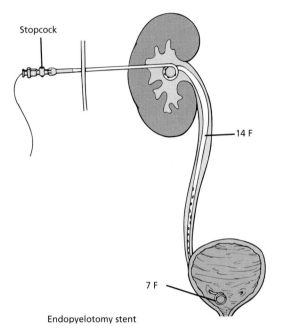

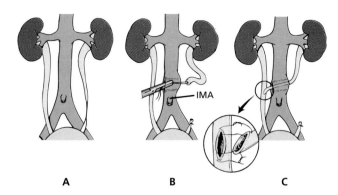

Fig. 3-35 **A,** Transureteroureterostomy. There is a long stricture in the left ureter that cannot be managed with ureteroureterostomy. **B,** Division of the ureter and retroperitoneal tunneling of the ureter in front of the aorta, above the level of the inferior mesenteric artery to the contralateral side. **C,** End-to-side watertight anastomosis of the left ureter to the right ureter. *(From Resnick MI:* Current therapy in genitourinary surgery, *ed 2, St. Louis, 1992, Mosby.)*

Fig. 3-33 Endopyelotomy stent postoperatively. Diameter changes from 14 Fr gauge at the site of the endopyelotomy to 7 Fr at the bladder. *(From Resnik MI:* Current therapy in genitourinary surgery, *ed 2, St. Louis, 1992, Mosby.)*

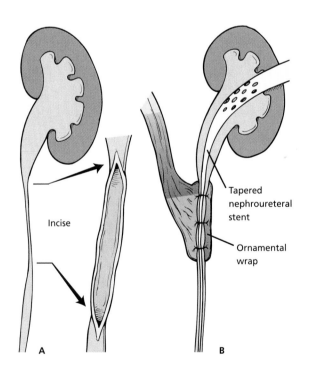

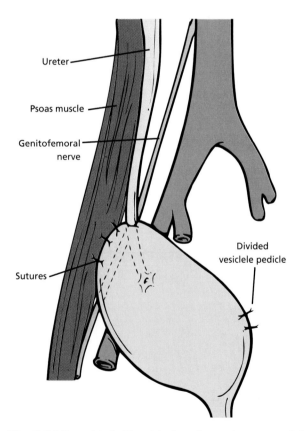

Fig. 3-34 **A,** Davis intubated ureterotomy. The stenotic area is incised until the proximal and distal point of the incision show a wide lumen. **B,** A nephrostomy and a ureteral stent, or a combination nephroureteral stent, is used. The edges of incised ureter are partially reapproximated over the stent. A piece of omentum can be mobilized and wrapped around this segment to provide good blood supply for viability and ureteral regeneration. *(From Resnick MI:* Current therapy in genitourinary surgery, *ed 2, St. Louis, 1992, Mosby.)*

Fig. 3-36 Psoas hitch. The right lateral superior aspect of the bladder is sutured to the psoas muscle. The contralateral vesical pedicle may need to be divided to achieve this degree of mobilization. The reimplantation of the ureter is performed after the bladder is fixed to the psoas muscle. *(From Resnick MI:* Current therapy in genitourinary surgery, *ed 2, St. Louis, 1992, Mosby.)*

Table 3-5 **Surgical Treatment of Ureteral Stricture**

TREATMENT	AUTHOR	NUMBER OF PATIENTS	SUCCESS (%)	COMMENTS
Stenosis from UPJ to iliac vessels				
Ureteroureterostomy with renal mobilization	Carlton (1971)	25	92	Watertight anastomosis
Davis intubated ureterotomy	Davis (1951)	N/A	90	Wrapped incision with fat to prevent adhesions
Boari flap	Thompson (1974)	23	100	100% had reflux, 87% with sterile urine; no restenosis
Ileal replacement	Boxer (1978)	89	81	Contraindicated with serum creatinine >2.0
Renal autotransplantation	Bodie (1986)	23	87	Two kidneys removed postoperatively because of hemorrhage
Pelvic ureteral stenosis				
Ureteroneocystostomy with psoas hitch	Ehrlich (1975)	52	95-100	Two cases reflux; no restenosis
Boari flap	Flynn (1979)	41	95-100	
Transureteroureterostomy	Udall (1973)	42	98	One failure led to nephrectomy
All stenoses				
Ureterolysis with omental wrap	Baker (1988)	54	25-100	Success greater with functioning kidney and postoperative corticosteroids
Urinary diversion (cutaneous ureterostomy)	Faminella (1971)	70	Varied	1. Flush stoma; 95% restenosis 2. Protruding stoma; 45%-64% restenosis
Nephrostomy drainage				Temporary decompression in septic patient; diagnostic for stricture
Nephrectomy				Definitive in completely obstructed kidney; 10% total renal function on scan

Modified from Resnick MI, Kursh E: *Current therapy in genitourinary surgery,* ed 2, St. Louis, 1992, Mosby.
N/A, Not applicable.

Table 3-6 **Endourologic Management of Ureteral Stenosis**

TREATMENT	AUTHOR	DILATION EXTENT	NUMBER OF STRICTURES	STRICTURE TYPE	SUCCESS (%)	COMMENTS
Mechanical dilatation						
Ureteral catheterization	Witherington (1980)	8 Fr	4	Postsurgical, short	100	50% had multiple dilatations before resolved
Bougie dilatation	Vliestra (1953)	To 20 Fr	37	N/A	N/A	
Balloon dilatation, antegrade	Banner (1984)	12 Fr	44	Varied	48	Fair success
Balloon dilatation, retrgrade	Eshghi (1988)	to 18 Fr	25	Varied	74	Best success with short membranous stricture
Endoscopic incision						
Cold-knife	Eshghi (1988)	Varied	61	Varied	98	Failure with one long stricture, treated with ureteroureterotomy successfully
Hot-knife	Thomas (1988)	To 24 Fr with full-thickness incision	14	N/A	64	Strictures >1.5 cm failed

Modified from Resnick MI, Kursh E: *Current therapy in genitourinary surgery,* ed 2, St. Louis, 1992, Mosby.
Fr, French gauge; *N/A,* not applicable

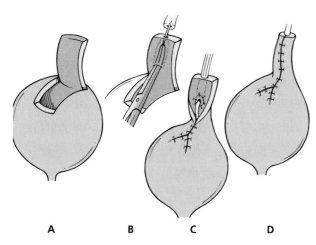

A   **B**   **C**   **D**

Fig. 3-37 Boari flap with ureteral reimplantation. **A,** Flap is developed from the anteroposterior aspect of the bladder. **B,** The submucosal tunnel is created, and the ureter is advanced. **C,** The ureter is fixed to the completed submucosal tunnel. **D,** The flap is closed in a cylindrical manner. *(From Resnick MI: Current therapy in genitourinary surgery, ed 2, St. Louis, 1992, Mosby.)*

A stricture may be incised ureteroscopically to achieve adequate drainage. The location of the incision is important to avoid damage to the residual blood supply to the ureter. In cases of injury this supply may be tenuous at best. Recommended sites for incision of ureteral strictures are depicted in Fig. 3-38.

The interposition of a segment of small intestine, in cases where large portions of the ureter have been damaged, is also an option. Additionally, in selected cases, renal autotransplantation can be performed. The kidney may be detached from its artery and vein and moved into the anatomic pelvis, in the site for a renal transplant, and reanastomosed to the vessels there with implantation of the normal residual ureter into the urinary bladder. In selected cases nephrectomy may be a last resort.

URINARY BLADDER
Congenital Anomalies

Congenital conditions of the urinary bladder include bladder exstrophy, bladder diverticula, urachal cysts, and associated anomalies. Urinary bladder exstrophy is a congenital condition that affects 1 in 330,000. It is a severe malformation that is part of an abnormality in the formation of the lower urinary tract. The bladder is not incorporated into the pelvis and exists as an open structure on the lower part of the anterior abdominal wall. This entity may also involve portions of the cloaca, an early embryologic compartment, which receives both solid waste from the alimentary canal and liquid waste from the urinary tract. There is an associated divided symphysis pubis in approximately 10% of the cases. The upper urinary tracts are almost always normal and the babies are healthy, with other anomalies of genitourinary and musculoskeletal organs appearing rarely. Undescended and retractile testes and inguinal hernias are not uncommon, however. In the female patient, the clitoris may be bifid and the vagina short, stenotic, and anteriorly displaced.

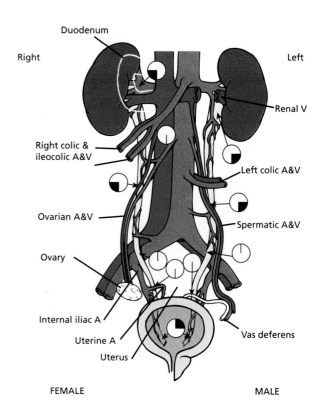

Fig. 3-38 Anatomic sites for stricture incision, based on the surface anatomy of the ureter and paraureteral structures. Utilizing these recommended sites will preserve the blood supply of the ureter while avoiding vital structures. *(From Resnick MI: Current therapy in genitourinary surgery, ed 2, St. Louis, 1992, Mosby.)*

The surgical challenge in reconstruction of exstrophy epispadias (Fig. 3-39) is considerable but its discussion is beyond the scope of this text. The goal of therapy is to create cosmetically acceptable and functional genitalia. This usually requires multiple procedures (on average, three) for reconstruction of the lower urinary tract as an internal organ, in addition to reconstruction of the external genitalia and fusion of the bony pelvis.

Bladder diverticula

Urinary bladder diverticula may be congenital or acquired. Generally, congenital bladder diverticula exhibit themselves during childhood. Variable amounts of muscle cover the mucosal lining of the urinary bladder, which protrudes laterally beyond the bladder wall. These may be associated with reflux of urine into the kidneys through the ureteral openings in the bladder, causing a propensity toward recurrent urinary tract infection and subsequent kidney damage. Congenital diverticula may require surgery if they are greater than 2 cm in diameter, drain poorly, or are in a location and of a size that incorporates the ureteral orifice. The presence of multiple diverticula suggests the presence of a secondary problem such as neurogenic bladder disorder (without normal neurologic innervation). Congenital diverticula are excised surgically when indicated. This is most commonly performed through a low Pfannenstiel incision with muscle-splitting technique.

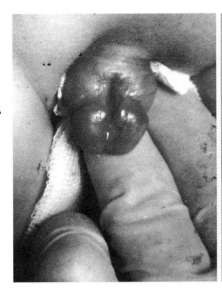
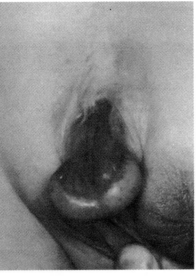

A

B

Fig. 3-39 **A,** Glandular epispadias. The patient is usually continent, and the glans is flattened with a dorsal split.
B, Penopubic or subsymphyseal epispadias. Severe form with the urethral opening at the penopubic junction, accompanied by incontinence. The distal urinary sphincter is deficient, and the verumontanum is visible within the urethral opening. The pubic bones are widely separated. *(From McGuire EJ et al:* Advances in urology, *vol 8, St. Louis, 1995, Mosby.)*

Acquired Diverticula

Acquired bladder diverticula occur in the adult and are generally believed to be caused by bladder outlet obstruction as a result of benign prostatic enlargement, carcinoma of the prostate, or altered coordination between contraction of the bladder and relaxation of the sphincter to void (detrusor sphincter dyssynergia) as seen in neurogenic bladders. Complications of bladder diverticula include recurrent urinary tract infection. During voiding the diverticula become filled with urine and do not empty completely. Patients with bladder diverticula are prone to stone formation because of urinary stasis in approximately 16% of the cases and to tumor formation in 2.9% to 6.7% of the cases. Less frequent complications include an inflammatory process around the diverticulum (peridiverticulitis), spontaneous rupture, and upper urinary tract obstruction because of compromised ureteral drainage. Urinary retention caused by bladder neck compression is a rare condition.

Bladder diverticula can be treated endoscopically by fulguration that destroys the lining of each bladder diverticulum, incision in the neck of the diverticulum to facilitate drainage, resection of the neck, or a combination of these techniques. Most often, the diverticulum is excised through a low Pfannenstiel, extraperitoneal incision but has been removed laparoscopically as well.

The development of bladder tumor inside a diverticulum has propensity for early dissemination, since the bladder diverticulum does not have a muscular wall preventing penetration of tumor cells. Therefore one should be certain to visualize the entire lining of the diverticulum (Fig. 3-40).

Urachal Anomalies

The urachus is a fibrous cord that in embryonic life carries waste from the primitive urinary tract to the outside of the body through the umbilical cord. By the time of birth, it has deteriorated into a fibrous cord and should no longer be patent. When the urachus or portions of its tubular structure remain open, four variations of patent urachal anomalies can present (Figs. 3-41 and 3-42)

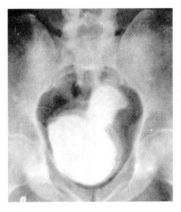

Fig. 3-40 A filling defect and irregular external tumor wall of a diverticulum caused by an extensive tumor. These may often be visualized through an endoscope introduced through the mouth of the diverticulum. Ultrasonography may help delineate the tumor. *(From Lloyd-Davies W et al:* Color atlas of urology, *ed 2, London, 1994, Mosby-Wolfe.)*

- A *patent urachus*, which, in the adult, may drain foul-smelling fluid from the umbilicus (40%)
- A *urachal sinus*, an opening at the umbilicus that does not connect to the urinary bladder (18%)
- A *urachal diverticulum*, a diverticular structure located on the anterior wall of the urinary bladder that does not connect with the umbilicus (3%)
- A *urachal cyst*, a bladder diverticulum that emanates from the anterior wall and has a narrow connecting neck from the cyst to the urinary bladder (31%)

Several clinical problems may occur as a result of urachal anomalies. One of these, drainage of foul-smelling fluid from the umbilicus, prompts the adult patient to seek urologic help. The urachal cyst may harbor urine that has become infected and will lead to stone formation. This will manifest itself as a recurrent urinary tract infection (UTI). In infancy, a patent urachus may present in cases where lower urinary tract obstruction

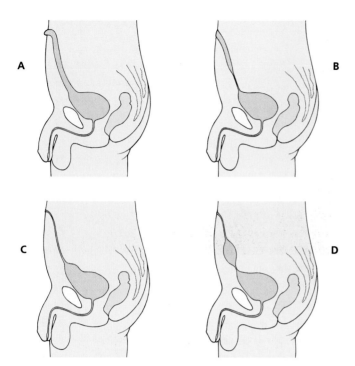

Fig. 3-41 Four urachal anomalies. **A,** Patent urachus. **B,** Urachal sinus. **C,** Urachal diverticulum. **D,** Urachal cyst. *(Modified from Bauer SB, Retik AB:* Urol Clin North Am 5:195, 1978.)

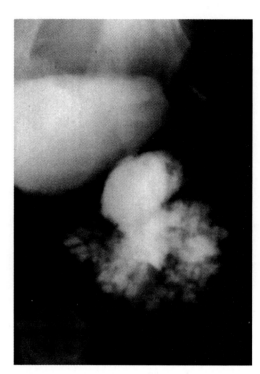

Fig. 3-42 Infected urachal cyst visualized on percutaneous sinogram with concomitant cystogram. *(From Resnick MI:* Current therapy in genitourinary surgery, *ed 2, St. Louis, 1992, Mosby.)*

is present, as in cases of posterior urethral valves. Additional congenital anomalies of the urinary tract should be suspected when urachal anomalies are present. The urachus has been, on rare instances, known to perforate into the peritoneal cavity in pediatric patients. One of the most significant sequelae of a urachal remnant is a malignant tumor in that remnant, usually presenting as an adenocarcinoma of the urinary bladder. These are located on the anterior wall of the urinary bladder and tend to be aggressive lesions requiring total cystectomy to achieve a cure. In the absence of a malignancy, three surgical options are available: incision and drainage of the urachal cyst, first-stage excision or incision and drainage of the infected material, and second-stage excision of the remnant at a later time. Drainage alone has a recurrence rate of approximately 30% and represents inadequate therapy.

Excision of the urachal remnant should involve excision of the umbilicus and the urachal remnant, the extraperitoneal fascial attachments down to and including the urinary bladder, and a cuff of urinary bladder at the attachment point.

Urachal anomalies may be associated with prune-belly syndrome or Eagle-Barrett syndrome, a rare syndrome of unknown cause. Its features include the absence of abdominal wall muscles, gross dilatation of the urinary tracts, bilateral intraabdominal testes, and bilateral inguinal hernias (Fig. 3-43).

Bladder Tumors

Bladder tumors are the second most common urologic malignancy. Three-fourths are found in men and one-fourth in women. The average age at diagnosis is 65 years. Neoplasms of the urinary bladder are transitional cell carcinoma (90%), squamous cell carcinoma (8%), adenocarcinoma (2%) as seen in malignant deterioration of the urachal remnant, and rhabdomyosarcoma (less than 1%).

Papillary transitional cell carcinoma is associated with the increased excretion of metabolites of tryptophan. This is seen in higher concentrations in the urine of smokers and patients with transitional cell carcinoma of the urinary bladder. Fundamentally, transitional cell carcinoma may be divided into those that are superficial and those that are invasive. A transitional cell malignancy that exists and grows on the wall of the urethelium, does not tend to become papillary, and extends into the lumen of the urinary bladder is termed *carcinoma in situ* (CIS). This condition tends to be insidious unless there is an associated significant inflammatory reaction in the urinary bladder, for it is not easily visualized endoscopically (Figs. 3-44 to 3-47).

Bladder tumors may initially present as microscopic hematuria. More typically the patient demonstrates gross, painless hematuria accompanied by the passage of clots. The diagnosis is made on investigative endoscopic examination of the urinary bladder. Employment in occupations likely to have increased exposure to toxins may be associated with the formation of bladder tumors.

Superficial tumors

Superficial bladder tumors generally lend themselves well to treatment with transurethral resection. Since transitional cell carcinoma is a disease of the entire transitional cell lining of the

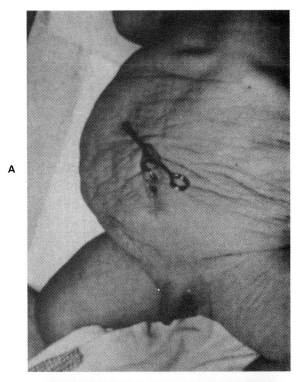

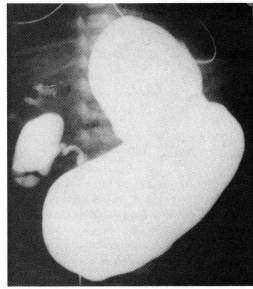

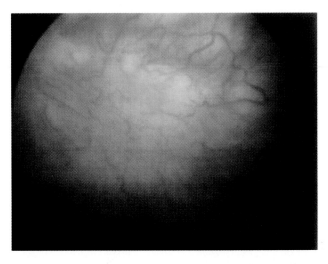

Fig. 3-44 Discrete small papillary T1 tumor with normal surrounding bladder mucosa and fronded appearance.

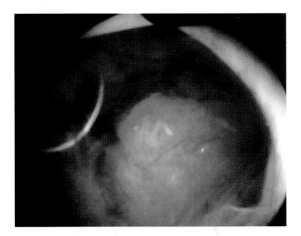

Fig. 3-45 Sessile T2 tumor on the base of the bladder.

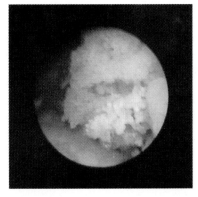

Fig. 3-43 Prune-belly syndrome. **A,** Prune-like appearance of abdomen with empty scrotum. **B,** Cystogram of prune-belly syndrome. Urethral irregularity without obstruction is common. Bladder has characteristic hourglass shape with horizontal configuration and a persistent, possibly patent, urachal remnant. *(From Gillenwater JY et al, editors:* Adult and pediatric urology, *ed 3, St. Louis, 1996, Mosby.)*

urinary tract, recurrences are not uncommon in sites other than the location of the initial presentation. After transurethral resection, rates for recurrence of papillary tumors may be as high as 90%, most occurring within the first year. Approximately 10% to 15% of patients with superficial tumors will subsequently develop invasive tumors. To accurately deter-

Fig. 3-46 Infiltrating T3a papillary tumor with superficial hemorrhage and necrosis. T3a tumors are irregular and single and may have surface slough. Presenting symptoms are hemorrhage, dysuria, frequency, and occasional straining caused by superimposed secondary infection. *(From Lloyd-Davies W et al:* Color atlas of urology, *ed 2, London, 1994, Mosby-Wolfe.)*

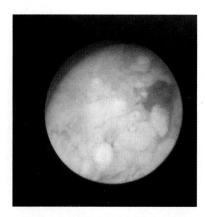

Fig. 3-47 Nodular infiltrating T3b tumor with early ulceration *(From Lloyd-Davies W et al: Color atlas of urology, ed 2, London, 1994, Mosby-Wolfe.)*

mine the grade and extent of the malignant involvement, patients must be staged with a complete history concerning prior urethelial tumors and with a cystoscopy and biopsy of existing lesions. Random biopsies to identify other possible sites and bimanual examination (under anesthetic) to evaluate the depth of bladder infiltration, the presence of a mass, or fixation of the bladder to the pelvic sidewall are justified. Because ultrasonography does not provide a physiologic evaluation of the urinary tract from a radiologic standpoint, IVP to detect other possible urinary tract lesions or intramural ureteral obstruction is necessary. Biopsy of the prostatic urethra is necessary when extension is suspected and a urinary diversion procedure is being contemplated.

After the initial transurethral resection and staging, some form of intravesical chemotherapy may be administered should a recurrence develop. It may be instilled as prophylactic therapy after a complete transurethral resection of a bladder tumor. In addition, intravesical chemotherapy should be given in cases of carcinoma in situ, since poor endoscopic presentation makes progress difficult to assess. A urinary cytologic examination should be performed at periodic intervals to assess for a complete response to chemotherapy.

The most common intravesical chemotherapeutic agents include thiotepa, which eliminates existing disease 35% of the time but eradicates carcinoma in situ in only 15% of the cases; doxorubicin (Adriamycin), which averages a 30% elimination of existing disease and a 25% eradication of carcinoma in situ; and mitomycin (Mutamycin-C), which shows a 50% elimination of existing disease and a 40% eradication of carcinoma in situ. Bacille-Calmette-Guérin (BCG) carries the highest rate of eradication of carcinoma in situ. Used as a prophylactic agent intravesically, BCG has demonstrated complete response rates ranging from 63% to 100% after 1 year posttreatment. Rates of recurrence for patients receiving thiotepa, doxorubicin, mitomycin, and BCG are 45%, 40%, 30%, and 20% respectively.

Adverse reactions to BCG therapy, bladder irritation and fever, generally subside with cessation of therapy. However, in certain cases, administration of antituberculin agents is necessary. Failure to eradicate carcinoma in situ leads to considera-

tion of other alternatives including radical cystectomy with urinary diversion as a definitive form of treatment. Solitary invasive bladder tumors may be treated aggressively with transurethral resection along with laser therapy. The laser treatment is capable of extending the margin of electrocautery dissection for a distance of 0.5 cm, decreasing the likelihood that residual invasive cancer cells have been left behind. Laser light energy can be delivered quite easily through a flexible fiber, through either a rigid or a flexible cystoscope, and, for cases of transitional cell carcinoma of the upper urinary tract, through one of the newer flexible, narrow-gauge ureteroscopes.

Invasive tumors

Invasive carcinoma of the urinary bladder is most often transitional cell carcinoma. Less often is the origin of the malignancy an adenocarcinoma (usually seen in cases of a urachal remnant), or a squamous cell carcinoma (more often seen in a dysfunctional bladder or with infestation of the urinary tract with tropical parasites known as *Schistosomas*). Only one third of patients who originally have a superficial transitional cell carcinoma ultimately develop an invasive lesion.

The definitive treatment for an early invasive malignancy of the urinary bladder is total removal of the urinary bladder with adjacent lymph nodes. This requires the formation of an alternative mechanism for handling the patient's urine. Traditionally, this has been the ileal conduit, which is a segment of small intestine that has been isolated from the intestinal tract (except for its blood supply). One end is closed, and the other end is opened to the outer abdominal wall to drain into an external collection device. The internal end of the ileal conduit is attached to the ureters. More recently, additional types of urinary diversion using the small and large intestine have been developed where a catheterizable stoma may be formed. This is brought out on the abdominal wall, or the new bladder (neobladder) is attached to the urethra (orthotopic diversion) after frozen-section biopsy results of the urethra are negative for tumor extension. With improvements in surgical techniques, the development of urinary diversions that do not require an external drainage device, and improvements in anesthetics and methods of preoperative and postoperative care, the concept of total removal of the urinary bladder with urinary diversion is less of a psychologic obstacle for surgical candidates. In addition, with the development of penile prosthetic devices and the artificial urinary sphincter the patient can look forward to regaining sexual activity and continence during the postoperative period.

At the time of radical cystectomy, pelvic lymph nodes are removed for tumor staging purposes. Additionally, it is the standard of care to also remove the prostate gland or uterus. It may be possible to spare the neurovascular bundle on at least one side. This nerve and vessel complex supplies the erectile mechanism. The patient may be able to reestablish sexual activity without artificial assistance. Vaginal reconstruction is also possible when bowel segments are used. Sexual activity is now possible for the female patient with an invasive carcinoma of the urinary bladder that mandates sacrificing the vagina.

In cases where the bladder is involved by numerous areas of carcinoma in situ or the prostate is involved with tumor, urethral recurrence will develop in approximately 9% of the cases by 5 years and in 17% of the cases by 10 years. It is not considered safe to leave the patient's urethra unresected. In these cases it is possible to use a short length of the terminal ileum to create a narrow catheterizable stoma that may be brought out through the abdominal wall on the right side, either the upper or the lower quadrant, or through the umbilicus (catheterizable continent urinary diversion).

For patients undergoing radical cystectomy and urinary diversion, multiple alternatives must be in place before surgery. The involvement of a wound-ostomy-continence nurse (WOCN) before surgery is therefore desirable to aid in counseling the patient regarding potential needs: external collection devices, instruction in intermittent catheterization, dealing with possible urinary incontinence in the early or extended postoperative period, and coping with the psycho-social ramifications that may occur because of the alterations in body image and lifestyle.

Candidates for radical cystectomy with urinary diversion include patients with a muscle-invading tumor regardless of the grade, patients with high-grade superficially invasive tumors with lymphatic invasion, patients with diffuse CIS, or patients with recurrent superficial carcinoma that intravesical therapy could not control.

A determination of candidates for continent urinary diversion depends on the patient's concept of his or her own body, the willingness to accept an external collection device, the patient's overall medical condition, and the condition of the patient's intestinal tract, particularly the portion needed to form the neobladder.

Bladder Trauma

Trauma to the urinary bladder may result in either an extraperitoneal or intraperitoneal rupture. In the former, there is a rupture of the urinary bladder, caused by blunt trauma, that results in leakage of urine outside the urinary bladder but confined to the space outside the peritoneal cavity. A cystogram with the urinary bladder filled to a range of 350 to 500 ml is the most reliable test to rule out the presence of a ruptured urinary bladder. However, a properly performed CT scan of the bladder will also demonstrate bladder rupture. In the presence of a pelvic fracture as demonstrated by KUB, a bladder injury will be present approximately 15% of the time.

Extraperitoneal injury

Extraperitoneal rupture of the urinary bladder may be treated without surgical intervention by Foley catheter drainage for 7 to 10 days. If on subsequent cystography the rupture has not healed or there are attendant complications because of the rupture, such as sepsis, surgical intervention may be necessary (Fig. 3-48).

Intraperitoneal injury

Intraperitoneal rupture indicates that the rupture of the urinary bladder has occurred across the peritoneal covering over the bladder dome, allowing urine to drain into the peritoneal cavity (Fig. 3-49). This is a condition that requires surgical repair through a laparotomy incision (Fig. 3-50). Additional injuries should be determined by intraabdominal exploration

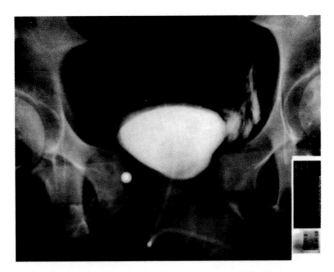

Fig. 3-48 Cystogram showing extraperitoneal bladder rupture. *(From Resnick MI:* Current therapy in genitourinary surgery, *ed 2, St. Louis, 1992, Mosby.)*

and palpation and then repaired. A suprapubic catheter should be left in place for approximately 7 to 10 days.

Urinary Incontinence

Stress urinary incontinence has been recognized as an important public health concern as evidenced by the National Institutes of Health conference on the topic in 1988. With the increasing number of middle-aged and elderly people in our population at large, this problem promises to be of growing concern.

Urinary incontinence may be of several types. Urinary urge incontinence connotes the loss of urine that cannot be controlled during bladder contraction. This generally occurs when a patient appreciates the urge to urinate but is unable to reach the bathroom in time. This usually implies some type of neurologic deficit involving the sphincter mechanism such as that seen after an extensive pelvic operation, carcinoma of the colon, or cerebrovascular accident (CVA).

Urinary overflow incontinence implies the loss of small amounts of urine, frequently after the bladder has reached capacity and can contain no more. At this point the bladder will contract briefly, and the patient may be unable to withhold the small amount of urine that is voided "off the top" of the large residual volume. This may be seen in patients with diabetes mellitus who have an autonomic neuropathy and the inability to void to completion.

Incontinence in the female patient

Urinary stress incontinence in the female patient may be divided into an anatomic incontinence or intrinsic sphincter dysfunction (ISD). The first of these is secondary to the loss of anatomic support with an otherwise functional urethral sphincter mechanism. A typical history is a complaint of involuntary loss of urine during coughing, sneezing, laughing, or varied aerobic activities (e.g., tennis, jogging, dancing, exercising).

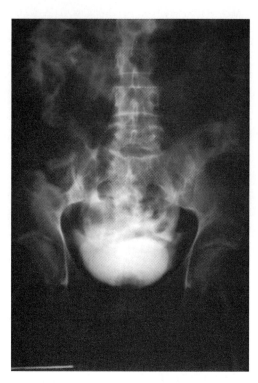

Fig. 3-49 Cystogram showing intraperitoneal bladder rupture and loops of bowel outlined by contrast medium. *(From Resnick MI: Current therapy in genitourinary surgery, ed 2, St. Louis, 1992, Mosby.)*

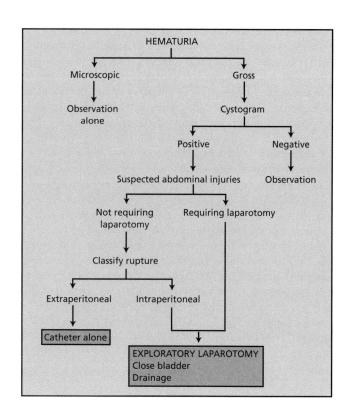

Fig. 3-50 Algorithm for suspected bladder rupture. *(From Resnick MI: Current therapy in genitourinary surgery, ed 2, St. Louis, 1992, Mosby.)*

ISD implies the lack of a normally functioning sphincter mechanism that may manifest clinically as loss of urine upon minimal provocation, such as when standing from a seated position or walking. ISD may also coexist with other anatomic changes that contribute to incontinence.

It is not uncommon for a degree of vaginal prolapse to be present with either anatomic incontinence or ISD. These patients must be assessed for urinary urgency and urge incontinence, since this component may not be improved by correction of the anatomic or intrinsic deficit. The patient may also have other medical conditions that preclude certain types of therapy, such as significant coronary artery disease, diabetes mellitus, or neurologic dysfunction. The impact of incontinence on the patient's lifestyle must be evaluated to determine what importance the patient places on urinary leakage, if her social activities have been affected, or if she is content to wear pads routinely. The patient's wishes and goals are important to assess when considering alternative options. A patient who refuses surgery may be willing to perform pelvic floor (muscle-strengthening) exercises, with or without biofeedback techniques. This has been shown in the majority of cases to improve or cure urinary stress incontinence. On the other hand, the patient who has incontinence during sexual activity and wishes to maintain her present level of sexual participation, but has failed pelvic muscle exercises previously, may seek a more permanent solution.

Aside from pelvic floor exercises, the conservative forms of therapy include alpha-adrenergic receptor agents such as ephedrine or phenylpropanolamine (Entex), since these have been shown to be effective in increasing the tone of the sphincter mechanism, in some cases decreasing the tendency toward urinary incontinence. These agents must be continued in order to remain effective but tend to exacerbate underlying hypertension.

Pelvic floor exercises were originally advocated by Arnold Kegel, a California gynecologist who popularized these exercises along with monitoring the strength of the contraction with a "perineometer." He was able to demonstrate that patients who were faithful to the exercise regimen were able to achieve an 84% success rate. More recently, vaginal cones have been substituted as a biofeedback device. Patients may use them at home and are successful in achieving improved continence the majority of the time. Pelvic exercises, with or without biofeedback, need to be performed consistently to maintain the strength of the continence mechanism.

Estrogen therapy has been used to increase the blood supply and pliability of the vaginal tissues and improve the coaptation of the urethral lining. The possible increased risk of endometrial and mammary carcinomas with the use of estrogens must be explained to the patient. On the other hand, estrogen therapy helps decrease the incidence of osteoporosis.

Tricyclic antidepressants may be used as a conservative approach, since they exhibit both anticholinergic and alpha-adrenergic activity. The difficulty with tricyclics, such as thorazine, is that they may not be well tolerated, especially in the geriatric population, and must be carefully monitored. There are surgical alternatives for intrinsic sphincter dysfunction or stress urinary incontinence. The determination of the appropriate course of surgical therapy depends on the results of the patient's history and physical examination and urodynamic testing.

By examining the patient in the lithotomy position, vaginal prolapse may be diagnosed. A cotton applicator (Q-Tip) inserted into the urethral meatus may be seen to bend toward the ceiling during straining, reflecting urethral hypermobility, compatible with urinary stress incontinence. Cystoscopic evaluation may demonstrate hypermobility of the proximal portion of the urethra and the opening of the bladder neck during abdominal straining with a partially filled urinary bladder. Additionally, an endoscopic examination may demonstrate an occasional bladder tumor or inflammatory changes, which may contribute to urinary urgency. This is frequently alleviated with a course of antibiotic therapy and the removal of any small lesions that are present.

Examination of the patient in the erect position with a filled bladder is a vital part of the physical evaluation for urinary incontinence. Abdominal straining in the erect position will demonstrate the degree to which the patient has vaginal prolapse and the degree to which incontinence occurs during abdominal straining. Loss of bladder content in the erect position without straining implies the presence of ISD. A more precise definition is obtained by urodynamics. The loss of bladder content occurs with intraabdominal pressures of less than 30 cm of water and has been defined as intrinsic sphincter dysfunction (low leak point pressure). Another important feature of the physical examination for planning the surgical therapy is the determination of the presence or absence of rectocele and enterocele. This should be done by digital examination of the posterior and anterior portions of the patient's vagina while she is in the supine position.

Videourodynamic (VUD) studies can be performed to more precisely differentiate anatomic causes from primary intrinsic sphincteric dysfunction. This study combines the fluoroscopic appearance of the bladder neck and the proximal portion of the urethra, with and without abdominal straining, with time measurements of intraabdominal and intravesical pressures. The results of this study can then be reviewed by the physician and patient. Properly selected patients for correction of anatomic incontinence can be treated with open bladder neck suspension utilizing a Marshall-Marchetti-Krantz (MMK) or Burch procedure, or with a needle suspension technique such as the modified Raz, Stamey, and Pereyra procedures. Because of the small incision required, with limited dissection necessary, needle suspensions are preferable over the traditional open approaches unless other intraabdominal procedures will be performed. The objective of these procedures is to recreate the normal anatomy of the pelvis so that the bladder neck and urethra are suspended. The incontinence caused by descent of the bladder neck during straining is thereby eliminated. The success rate should be more than 90% when patients are properly selected.

For cases of ISD the success of the standard approach to bladder neck suspension is at best 70%. Pubovaginal sling procedures, however, place a strip of fascia or synthetic mesh behind the bladder neck. This supports the bladder neck so that the incontinence is alleviated. Overall success rates are 90% to 95%, but the rate of urinary retention ranges from 5% to 20%. The presence of prior neurologic problems, chronic obstruction, or bladder augmentation predict a higher rate of permanent urinary retention. Rate of detrusor instability after sling procedures is approximately 15%, though in the majority of cases this can be addressed with anticholinergic therapy. Instability presents as urinary urgency to the point of incontinence. Behavioral therapy, pelvic floor exercises, and electrical stimulation have also been used to treat urge incontinence and instability postoperatively. Anatomic incontinence is treated with bladder neck suspension and repair of associated vaginal prolapse. Intrinsic sphincter dysfunction (also called deficiency), associated with bladder neck instability, is treated with the pubovaginal sling procedure. When ISD is not associated with prolapse of the bladder neck and urethra, the proximal part of the urethra can be injected with heterologous collagen (Contigen) or autologous fat to serve as a bulking agent to maintain the bladder neck in a closed position during filling.

Incontinence in the male patient

Urinary incontinence in the male patient is more common than originally believed. Only 5% of incontinent men, however, seek help. Between 15 and 64 years of age, 2% experience some type of incontinence. After 64 years, the incidence increases to 17%. In institutionalized males, up to 55% are incontinent.

The causes of incontinence may be neurologic, idiopathic, and secondary to prostatectomy or trauma. Neurologic factors most commonly associated with incontinence are multiple sclerosis (MS), CVA, or myelodysplasia (abnormal development of the lower spinal cord). Additionally, radiation therapy or surgical injury to the pelvic nerves may result in incontinence.

Prostatectomy is the urologic procedure that most often contributes to incontinence. Transurethral resection may be associated with incontinence 1% of the time. Radical retropubic prostatectomy, performed for removal of malignant prostate glands, may result in continued incontinence 1 year postoperatively approximately 11% of the time. The rate of postoperative incontinence after perineal prostatectomy is 3%, in the same time.

The usual factor precipitating urge incontinence is detrusor (bladder muscle) instability, though local irritation such as a urinary tract infection may also prompt this condition. In cases where a known neurologic disease exists, bladder urgency is said to be attributable to detrusor hyperreflexia. Conservative efforts at controlling male incontinence are generally unsuccessful except for the use of anticholinergic medication to alleviate urge incontinence. A common example of this type of medication is oxybutynin chloride (Ditropan).

Alternatives for postprostatectomy incontinence include bladder neck reconstruction, injection of urethral bulking agents such as collagen, or insertion of an artificial urinary sphincter. The most successful of these choices has been the artificial urinary sphincter. This device may be implanted after 1 postoperative year of persistent incontinence. The prosthesis is placed through two incisions, perineal and small inguinal. Patient satisfaction ranges at about 95%. The injection of collagen or fat has been successful in only a few select cases. Bladder neck reconstruction is uncommon in view of the implant results.

PROSTATE GLAND

Neoplasms of the prostate gland, benign or malignant, constitute a large portion of urologic practice and surgical procedures. The internal anatomy of the prostate gland has become standardized by virtue of our appreciation of the prostate on transrectal ultrasonography (Fig. 3-51). The zonal anatomic features of the prostate detected by transrectal ultrasonography are illustrated as depicted by McNeill in the early 1970s (Fig. 3-52).

Benign Prostatic Hyperplasia

The natural history of benign prostatic hyperplasia (BPH) is that of a gradual onset of obstructive symptoms spanning several years. The development of rapidly progressive symptoms of obstruction should raise suspicions of prostatitis or prostatic carcinoma associated with prostatic enlargement. The histologic changes of BPH begin in the early thirties. It is estimated that a 50-year-old man has a 20% to 25% chance of requiring some type of surgical intervention for BPH during his lifetime. It is estimated that up to one third of patients who present initially with obstructive symptoms will have stabilization in the progression of their symptoms or, in some cases regression, making intervention unnecessary. The symptoms are generally progressive in the remainder of patients. Presently the timing of intervention allows for a stepwise program of therapeutic options that include the use of alpha-adrenergic receptor blockers and ultimately transurethral incision or resection of the prostate.

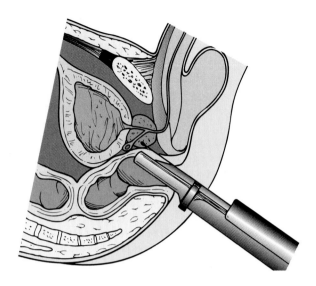

Fig. 3-51 Ultrasound imaging of prostate provides a full ultrasound map of the whole prostate and demonstrates the prostatic capsule at all levels. The seminal vesicles and bladder base are differentiated from surrounding tissues, allowing measurement of prostatic dimensions. An ultrasound probe with rotating transducer is inserted into the anal canal to enter the lower rectum. The probe tip is surrounded by conductive gel inside a condomlike probe cover. The linear array 7 MHz transducer provides a 135-degree scan of the prostate in all directions. Ultrasonograms of the prostate from the bladder base and seminal vesicles to the prostatic apex are obtained by withdrawal of the probe at 0.5 cm intervals and needle biopsy specimens taken from any abnormal or suspicious areas. *(From Gillenwater JY et al, editors:* Adult and pediatric urology, *ed 3, St. Louis, 1996, Mosby.)*

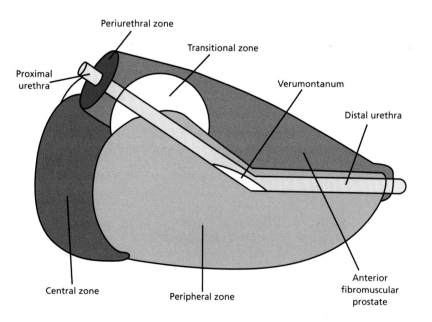

Fig. 3-52 Three-dimensional representation of the prostate showing anatomic relationships of the zones. *(From Kirby RS, Christmas T:* Benign prostatic hyperplasia, *London, 1993, Gower.)*

BPH occurs in the upper two thirds of the prostate gland in the transition zone near the periurethral zone because of enlargement of the transition zone. This compresses the urethra and causes obstruction of the bladder neck. Obstructive symptoms include hesitancy, an intermittent stream, terminal dribbling, diminished size and force of the urinary stream, a sensation of incomplete emptying, increased nocturia, increased daytime urinary frequency, and urgency with burning (dysuria) on urination. Evaluation of the patient should include a digital rectal examination to assess the gland for size (normal is approximately walnut size) and for areas of hardening (nodules) indicative of carcinoma. In the absence of associated hematuria, cystoscopy does not necessarily need to be performed. An ultrasonographic examination to check for residual urine and dilatation of the upper urinary tract caused by prostatic enlargement, or an IVP, is typically performed to assess the overall urinary tract.

Appropriate investigation in the treatment of the symptoms potentially caused by BPH is warranted. Treatment of a patient for BPH when symptoms are caused by some other process will not necessarily improve the patient's condition. Among the pitfalls are the patient with previous CVA, neurovesical dysfunction secondary to spinal disease, or peripheral neuropathy as seen in diabetes mellitus, alcoholism, or Parkinson's disease. Patients with multiple sclerosis may have detrusor sphincter dyssynergia, a functional obstruction displayed by contraction of the sphincter mechanism when the patient attempts voiding, causing obstruction of the bladder outlet. The presence of a small prostate gland with symptoms that indicate the presence of bladder outlet obstruction (BOO) should lead to more than just a rudimentary investigation. Urethral stricture disease is not uncommon and may cause symptoms of outlet obstruction.

A urinary flow study may be done to document a diminished peak and average urinary flow rate. If the diagnosis is somewhat equivocal, a voiding pressure study may be performed where the intravesical pressure determination may be combined with a flow study to demonstrate diminished urinary flow rate with simultaneous increased intravesical pressure, indicating obstruction. Cystoscopy would rule out the presence of urethral stricture associated with bladder calculi, or tumors

in the case of hematuria (Fig. 3-53). A VUD study with voiding and differential pressure studies may be performed to combine with the results of the urinary flow, the urethral pressure just below the prostate, the fluoroscopic image of the bladder neck, and the visualization of the urethra and bladder, to further document outlet obstruction (Fig. 3-54).

Endoscopic findings include trabeculation of the urinary bladder (Fig. 3-55), saccule formation (Fig. 3-56) and diverticula, bladder wall thickening, and distortion of the trigone and ureters caused by cephalad enlargement of the prostate that raises the trigone toward the abdomen (Fig. 3-57). This last finding may be seen on IVP and is known as fish-hook deformity of the ureters (Fig. 3-58).

When the symptoms are early and mild, the patient may be treated with alpha-adrenergic blocking agents. These drugs block alpha$_1$-receptor sites, in the prostatic urethra and bladder neck. When stimulated, these increase the muscle tone of the sphincteric fibers in the apex of the prostate and the bladder neck. After taking an alpha-blocker, the patient generally notes a mild to moderate but significant diminution in his obstructive symptoms if the tissue composition of his prostate gland is primarily fibromuscular. The effect of an alpha-adrenergic receptor blocking agent in treating patients with bladder outlet obstruction secondary to prostatism is generally immediate. If the patient's symptoms are mild and he has not yet developed any complications of bladder outlet obstruction secondary to prostatism and he has not responded to an alpha-blocker, another drug called *finasteride* (Proscar) may be used. This is a 5-alpha-reductase inhibitor that blocks the conversion of testosterone to its active form in the prostate. The drug must be taken routinely for a period of 6 to 12 months to allow time for the glandular component of prostatic enlargement to reduce in size, creating a more normal voiding pattern. If the patient's symptoms have not responded to conservative management and infection has been eliminated as a possible source of irritative symptoms, transurethral resection or incision of the prostate (TURP, TUIP) may be considered.

TURP has been the gold standard for the treatment of bladder outlet obstruction secondary to prostatism and continues to achieve the highest results in terms of relieving bladder outlet obstruction secondary to prostatic enlargement. Before performing a TURP, the associated disease entities in patients regarded as viable candidates should be considered and evaluated. The more commonly encountered conditions and rates of occurrence are cardiac myopathy (25%), pulmonary disease (14.5%), gastrointestinal disorders (13.2%), and renal disease (9.8%).

With the use of the Nd:YAG laser, KTP laser, and the new resectoscope roller-ball probe, TURP may be achieved with as little as a 23-hour hospital stay or as an outpatient. Investigators have reported equivalent results to standard transurethral resection.

TUIP may be performed in patients who have a relatively small obstructing gland. The advantages of transurethral incision include a lower rate of retrograde ejaculation and postoperative stricture. TUIP has a practically equivalent result in terms of eradicating obstruction when compared with standard transurethral resection of the prostate.

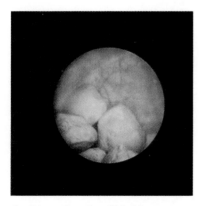

Fig. 3-53 Calculi in trabeculated bladder. *(From Lloyd-Davies W et al: Color atlas of urology, ed 2, London, 1994, Mosby-Wolfe.)*

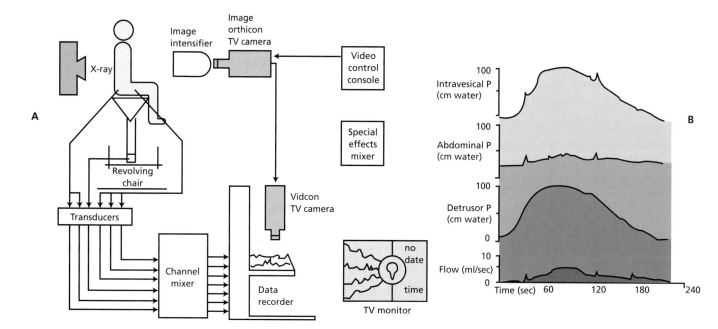

Fig. 3-54 A, Urethral pressure profile equipment. A catheter with a closed end and a rosette of subterminal openings is placed into the bladder. Fluid is infused slowly with a constant low rate pump, and the catheter is mechanically withdrawn at a constant rate. The pressure within the catheter is recorded, and a profile of the static pressure conditions along the length of the urethra is obtained. The patient may be asked to contract the external sphincter to observe alterations in the profile. **B,** Pressure-flow study of normal micturition. In the normal bladder, filling results in a small pressure rise to the point of fullness. Micturition is under voluntary control and accomplished by a smooth increase in intravesical pressure. Because detrusor fibers are present in the proximal portion of the urethra, the bladder neck is open. The external sphincter relaxes coincidentally. *P,* Pressure. **(A,** *Modified from Tanagho EA, McAninch JW: Smith's general urology, ed 14, Norwalk, Conn., 1995, Appleton & Lange;* **B** *from: Gillenwater JY et el, editors:* Adult and pediatric urology, *ed 3, St. Louis, 1996, Mosby.)*

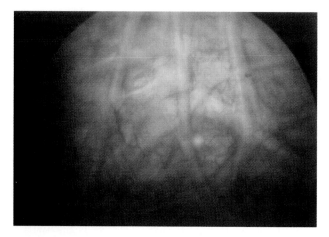

Fig. 3-55 Trabeculation of bladder. Classic ribbing of the thickened bladder muscle occurs when the bladder responds to outflow obstruction with hypertrophy.

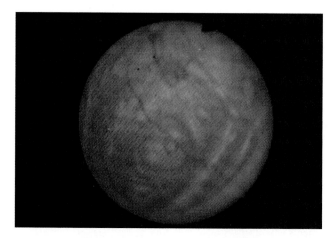

Fig. 3-56 Trabeculation with early sacculation may advance to diverticulum formation.

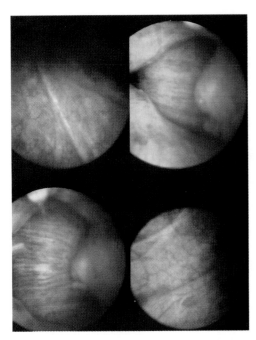

Fig. 3-57 Very large middle prostatic lobe.

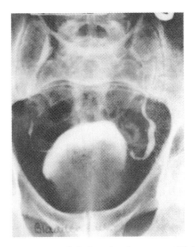

Fig. 3-58 Lower ureteral deformity, known as "fishhooking," caused by middle lobe enlargement of prostate. *(From Lloyd-Davies W et al: Color atlas of urology, ed 2, London, 1994, Mosby-Wolfe.)*

Prostatic Carcinoma

Carcinoma of the prostate is the most prevalent malignancy in American men, with approximately 200,000 new cases annually and 38,000 deaths each year. Autopsy series indicate that 30% of 50-year-old men and 75% of 75-year-old men have carcinoma of the prostate. Approximately 5% to 10% of the population over 50 years of age will develop clinically significant cancers that have a volume of more than 0.5 cc. These lesions have variable growth rates (potential for slower rate in men greater than 70 years old) and may be associated with a propensity toward metastatic disease and death.

The cause of carcinoma of the prostate includes a strong genetic propensity to develop this disease. In addition, the male hormones influence the prostate toward malignant deterioration. Environmental influences such as herbicides and insecticides and the increased fat content in the average diet may also play a role. Regional and racial differences in the incidence of carcinoma of the prostate are well known. Among African Americans the incidence of carcinoma of the prostate is 50% higher than in white Americans. Infectious agents have not been demonstrated to be conclusively implicated in the development of carcinoma of the prostate. Prostate cancers are adenocarcinomas and arise from the prostate acinar (gland) cells. It is believed that malignant deterioration occurs in atrophic gland cells that begin to form around the fifth to seventh decades of life.

Experience with transrectal ultrasonography and mapped prostate biopsies has demonstrated the anatomic position of prostatic carcinoma within the prostatic internal anatomy. Approximately 70% of tumors occur in the peripheral zone of the gland, 15% to 20% arise in the central zone, and 10% to 15% in the transitional zone. Additionally, prediction of stage and aggressiveness of the disease can be made by the numbers of prostate biopsy specimens that contain malignancy and the relative proportion of each biopsy taken that contains a malignancy. A larger proportion of involvement in each biopsy specimen and

The use of open prostatectomy for elimination of benign obstructing adenoma is limited to less than 10% of the cases. The alternative choice is a standard TURP. The resectionist, however, must decide, based on the results of digital rectal examination, x-ray studies, ultrasonographic findings, and the cystoscopic appearance of the gland, whether TURP is feasible. This depends in part on the rate at which obstructing tissue can be removed compared with the stability of the patient and the likelihood of significant blood loss and hyponatremia during a lengthy transurethral resection. Suprapubic prostatectomy is carried out through a low Pfannenstiel or low vertical midline incision. A suprapubic catheter is generally left in place in addition to a urethral Foley catheter. Although operative times are shorter than TURP for a large obstructing prostate, the hospital stay is more prolonged because of the need for an incision and extended recovery.

Balloon dilatation of the prostatic urethra (transcystoscopic urethroplasty) had been popularized during the last 5 years. It has however, fallen to the wayside, since results of a series of patients treated in this manner indicate that the relief of obstruction is no better than when a simple cystoscopy is performed.

Additional new forms of therapy for BPH are on the horizon. One of these is hyperthermia, where the prostatic tissue is heated to achieve involution (shrinkage) with the passage of time and the performance of additional therapy sessions. In addition, the insertion of a metal prostatic stent in poor-risk patients whose survival is limited holds some promise of alleviating obstruction for the short-term. This is a metal tubularized mesh that is inserted into the prostatic urethra to hold the lobes of the prostate apart and achieve more normal voiding.

the numbers of biopsy specimens containing malignant growth imply a larger-volume tumor. This raises the likelihood that the tumor has already penetrated through the capsule of the gland and may have already metastasized either locally or distantly.

The Gleason grading system, the most widely accepted method of histologic grading, is used by pathologists to describe the growth potential of prostatic malignancies. The Gleason grading system utilizes the appearance of the malignancy in the primary and secondary growth pattern (the largest area involved with malignancy on biopsy and the second largest involved with malignancy). These two areas are graded on a scale from 1 to 5, and the Gleason score is obtained by adding the two numbers, resulting in a sum that is on a scale from 2 to 10. The higher the Gleason score, the more likely the tumor will be aggressive, metastasizing early. The largest proportion of tumors are moderately differentiated, or Gleason grade 5 to grade 7. The most commonly used staging system, designating the extent of the malignancy, is the TNM system (Table 3-7).

Prostate specific antigen (PSA) is a screening blood test that may be done, in addition to the digital rectal examination (DRE), to aid in initially detecting the presence of prostatic carcinoma. Top normal range for PSA is 4 ng/dl. Between 4 and 10 ng/dl there is a 20% probability that a suspicious-looking area on transrectal ultrasonography will be malignant on biopsy, even if there is no suspicion of carcinoma on the DRE. With a suspicious area on digital rectal examination, this is raised to 25%. With a PSA of 20 ng/dl there is at least a 5% chance of pelvic lymph node involvement. Less than 5% of prostate cancers will be detectable with PSAs that are less than 4 ng/dl. Large benign glands and glands involved with prostatitis may also cause an elevation of the PSA and must be differentiated from carcinoma. Transrectal ultrasonography is an ultrasound

examination of the prostate performed by placing a transducer (probe) inside the rectum to look at the prostate gland. The characteristic appearance of malignancy on transrectal ultrasonography is a dark (hypoechoic) area in the peripheral zone. Biopsies of the prostate can be guided under transrectal ultrasonography to gain access to the areas most suspect for malignancy. Color Doppler imaging of the prostate with transrectal ultrasound (representation of blood flow in the prostate in color, usually red and blue) may help in localizing small cancerous lesions that have a normal echo appearance, since malignancies usually occur in the regions of increased blood flow.

CT scan and MRI are helpful in assessing the lymph node–bearing areas for cancerous lymphatic involvement with an accuracy that ranges between 83% and 89% and a sensitivity that ranges between 88% and 90%. These two modalities, however, do not rule out the presence of microscopic extension through the capsule or seminal vesicle.

Traditional pelvic lymphadenectomy is a surgical procedure that is done through a low anterior abdominal incision outside of the peritoneal cavity to remove lymph nodes from the vascular structures in the pelvis in order to rule out the presence of microscopic nodal extension. As an alternative and less invasive technique, this same procedure can be performed intraperitoneally or extraperitoneally with the laparoscope. This procedure is done by inserting three to four trocars in the lower abdomen to remove nodal chains in a similar manner as the open technique. It is generally considered appropriate to perform radical prostatectomy in the face of lymph nodes that do not contain microscopic involvement with metastatic disease.

Bone scanning uses a radioactive labeled molecule to assess the skeleton for metastasis from the prostate. It has been shown that the likelihood of finding bone metastasis with the patient's PSA less than 10 ng/dl is below 5%. The exception is in instances where the Gleason score is 8 to 10 ng/dl, indicating the likelihood of aggressive malignancies.

It is generally accepted that patients who have at least a 10-year life expectancy are candidates for radical removal of the prostate gland, either by radical retropubic prostatectomy or radical perineal prostatectomy. In the case of the perineal approach, the lymph nodes are retrieved through a separate incision, or laparoscopically. The prostate is removed through an incision between the rectum and the scrotum. Its advantages include a shorter hospital confinement, less blood loss, an earlier return of urinary continence, and diminished postoperative pain. Radical retropubic prostatectomy incorporates pelvic lymphadenectomy.

The neurovascular bundles (nerve-vessel complex supplying the erectile bodies) may be spared by either surgical approach, offering the patient a chance to maintain potency in the postoperative period. Continence rates 1 year postoperatively for perineal prostatectomy are approximately 97% and between 89% to 99% for radical retropubic prostatectomy. Complications include intraoperative hemorrhage; injury to the obturator nerve, ureter, or rectum; deep venous thrombosis (DVT); pulmonary embolism; symptomatic pelvic lymphocele; and wound or urinary tract infection. The incidence for these complications remains less than 3% if appropriate precautions are taken.

Table 3-7 **Clinical Staging for Carcinoma of Prostate**

DESCRIPTION	AJC (TNM)
Localized	
Clinically unsuspected	T1
Focal, low grade	T1a
Intragland lump (diffuse/high grade)	T1b
Clinically suspected	T2
<1.5 cm, confined to one lobe	T2a
>1.5 cm, confined to one lobe	T2a
Bilateral lobes	T2b
Disseminated	
Periprostatic	T3, T4
Base seminal vesicle/lateral sulcus	
Base seminal vesicle/other structures	T4
Distant	
Pelvic lymph node	T1-4/N1
Bones, lung, etc.	T1-4/NO-3
Elevated PAP only	T1-4/N3

Modified from Alexander: *Care of the patient in surgery,* ed 10, St Louis, 1996, Mosby.

AJC, American Joint Committee on Cancer Staging; *PAP,* prostatic acid phosphate; *TNM* refers to tumors, nodes, metastases, the counterpart staging system to the Jewett, Marshall, Strong system of tumor staging.

As an alternative to surgical extirpation, radiation therapy in the form of external beam therapy or interstitial therapy may be administered. External-beam radiation therapy carries survival statistics that are equal to surgery at 10 years but diminished thereafter. External-beam radiation therapy is generally delivered over a 6-week period. Interstitial radiation therapy utilizes iodine or palladium isotopes and is delivered percutaneously into the prostate by means of needles containing 5 mm isotope seeds under transrectal ultrasonographic guidance.

The advantage of interstitial radiation is the delivery of a higher total dose of radiation therapy in the range of 10,000 to 17,000 rads to the prostate (as compared with 6800 to 7000 rads with an external beam) without damaging surrounding structures such as the rectum and bladder neck. The overall results are comparable. Interstitial radiation implantation is generally carried out on an outpatient or 24-hour inpatient-stay basis and may be combined with pelvic lymphadenectomy.

A recent, innovative form of therapy, cryoablation, circulates liquid nitrogen through five probes, placed in the prostate under ultrasonographic guidance, to freeze the prostate to temperatures of $-180°$ C. Preliminary results are encouraging; however, long-term results are needed before this can be offered as a standard form of therapy.

An additional form of surgical therapy may be bilateral orchiectomy. This may be offered to patients to remove the source of male sex hormones and diminish the symptoms of metastatic disease as well as produce involution of the prostate gland. This form of therapy has to a large degree been replaced by other medical forms of androgen ablation.

The use of traditional cytotoxic agents for the treatment of metastatic prostate cancer has been disappointing so far and is used only in selected cases as a last alternative.

URETHRA

Stricture Disease

Urethral stricture disease in its acquired form is a common problem in urologic practice. It is generally caused by previous infection or instrumentation and presents with symptoms of a diminished stream, postvoid dribbling with or without chronic prostatitis, and urinary tract infection. Peak and average urinary flow rates will be less than 10 ml and 5 ml/sec respectively, and diagnosis may be made by urethroscopy or retrograde urethrography (RUG).

Urethral strictures are fibrous constrictions of the urethra that occur because of infection (venereal disease) or instrumentation (Fig. 3-59). Not uncommonly the urologist is called upon to insert a catheter in a situation where hospital personnel have been unable to relieve a patient's bladder obstruction. Initially the well-anesthetized (with topical anesthetic) urethra should be dilated with filiforms and followers. Urethral dilatation should be carried out to 22 Fr and a l6 Fr catheter inserted. A Council, coude, or Foley catheter may be used, depending on the position of the bladder neck and the ease of dilatation. This does not cure the stricture but allows for monitoring urinary output and temporary relief of obstruction. Periodic dilatations at lengthening intervals may provide for a cure, as determined by assessment at 1 year. Van Buren sounds may be used to dilate a strictured urethra if anatomic knowledge of the urethra is available as demonstrated by RUG. If dilation is not possible with the above, direct visualization cystoscopically and dilatation over a guidewire passed into the bladder may be necessary.

Optical internal urethrotomy (incision of the stricture under direct vision) is usually done on an outpatient basis under topical anesthesia with sedation. In the short term, success rates are 70% to 80% and are easily repeated, and the procedure holds few complications. If the stricture is not amenable to permanent dilation with these techniques, some type of urethroplasty is in order. If the stricture is short enough, primary excision and anastomosis of the normal portions of the urethra can be accomplished after spatulating the opposite walls. The patient is placed in lithotomy or exaggerated lithotomy position to facilitate exposure. If necessary, more complex forms of urethroplasty can be performed with advancement flaps and split-thickness or full-thickness grafts.

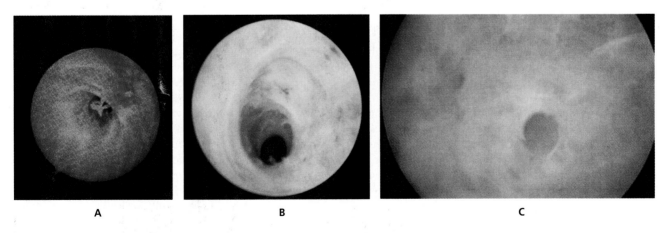

A   **B**   **C**

Fig. 3-59 **A,** Inflamed urethral mucosa with stricture. **B,** Scarred, fibrotic, long-standing urethral stricture. *(From Lloyd-Davies W et al: Color atlas of urology, ed 2, London, 1994, Mosby-Wolfe.)* **C,** Tight urethral stricture.

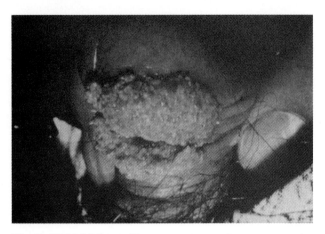

Fig. 3-60 Multiple papillary warts. *(From Gillenwater JY et al editors:* Adult and pediatric urology, *ed 3, St. Louis, 1996, Mosby.)*

Condylomas

Urethral condylomas (warts) are found just inside the meatus of the male urethra and may be associated with irritative symptoms or scant bloody discharge. The fleshy lesions may be found endoscopically anywhere along the male urethra and are generally sexually transmitted. They have been implicated in the development of female cervical dysplasia. Treatment must include evaluation of the sexual partner. Meatal lesions may be removed, using local anesthesia, through fulguration of the site of attachment. Those that present farther up the canal may be treated with endoscopic resection and laser ablation. For lesions involving the penile shaft (Fig. 3-60), local excision, CO_2 laser ablation, electrofulgeration, or regular applications of podophyllin may be effectively utilized. Follow-up evaluation is indicated because of the high recurrence rate no matter what form of therapy is employed. Condylomas may also occur as a large lesion known as Buschke-Löwenstein tumor.

MALE REPRODUCTIVE SYSTEM
Testis

Testicular tumor occurs in 2 to 3 of 100,000 males in the United States. Germ cell tumors constitute 90% to 95% of these. The remainder are non–germinal cell neoplasms such as Leydig's cell, Sertoli's cell, and gonadoblastoma cell tumors. The highest incidence of testicular tumor is in adult males from the late teens to approximately 30 years of age. Cryptorchidism (nondescent of the testis) is associated with a higher incidence of testicular tumor on either side, with occurrence ranging from 7% to 10%. The highest risk of developing testicular malignancy occurs in testes that are intraabdominal. An inguinal testis has a significantly lower risk at 1 to 80 compared with 1 to 20 for the abdominal testis. Placement of the testis in the scrotum facilitates examination for the detection of tumor, though probably if done after 3 years of age it does not significantly increase the fertility on that side. Causal relationships between trauma and infection in the testis afflicted with carcinoma have been associated but no definitive answer has been established. However, the use of exogenous estrogens by the mother during pregnancy

is associated with an increased incidence of testicular carcinoma to up to five times over the expected incidence.

The classification of testicular tumor depends on the location at which the abnormal cell travels down an abnormal pathway of development. The original germ cells that are present in the embryo (totipotential germ cells) can travel along different pathways in the formation of the tumor cell type that they will ultimately have. The most common of these is seminoma, which accounts for 35% of testicular carcinoma. This represents the development of the germ cell into a mature type of testicular cell that has become malignant. Embryonal cell carcinoma accounts for 20% of testicular carcinomas and is a malignancy in which the original precursor germ cell develops into a malignant cell, representing an abnormal growth of the embryo. Teratomas may be seen in children and adults and represent 5% of testicular carcinomas. Mixed germ cell types account for 40% and are a combination of teratoma and embryonal cell carcinomas. Choriocarcinoma accounts for less than 1% and is rare in its pure form. These are particularly aggressive lesions that demonstrate early bloodborne spread with paradoxically small intratesticular lesions associated with widespread metastatic disease.

The entity of carcinoma in situ of the testis is still not completely understood. This lesion appears to be a premalignant entity, but the ideal treatment is unclear. A testicular carcinoma on one side with biopsy findings consistent with carcinoma in situ on the second side certainly indicates cautious follow-up care.

Clinical staging for testicular carcinoma is aimed at detecting metastatic disease in the retroperitoneum and the lungs. A chest x-ray study and CT scan of the abdomen are the primary forms of radiographic investigation. Laboratory determination of tumor markers such as alpha-fetoprotein (α-FP; elevated in embryonal carcinoma and teratocarcinoma), LDH (lactate dihydrogenase; its elevation correlates with tumor burden in nonseminomatous germ cell tumors), and human chorionic gonadotropin (elevated in all nonseminomatous tumors and to a lesser extent in seminoma).

The most important clinical finding is the development of a painless hard mass in the testis (Fig. 3-61). The delay of diagnosis correlates with the onset of metastatic disease and can be as long as 3 to 6 months. An incorrect diagnosis is established in approximately 25% of patients with testicular tumors. A history of epididymitis or testicular trauma is commonly a deceptive feature masking underlying testicular tumor diagnosis. Hydrocele (collection of excess fluid around the testis) may mask the underlying testicular tumor as well. Testicular ultrasonography is a noninvasive diagnostic study that can be performed relatively easily in patients who are in an age group at risk for the development of testis tumors.

The treatment of testicular tumor is determined by the type of cells present in the lesion, the tumor markers present, and the results of CT and chest x-ray examinations. Seminoma is exquisitely sensitive to radiotherapy, and a relatively low dose of retroperitoneal irradiation yields an average 5-year survival rate of 87%. Patients who relapse may be treated with salvage chemotherapy as are patients with high-stage seminomas. Low-stage nonseminomatous germ cell tumors may be treated after

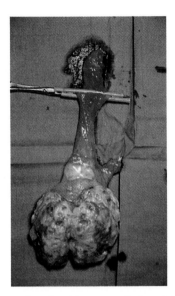

Fig. 3-61 Bisected testis with tumor displayed. *(From Lloyd-Davies W et al: Color atlas of urology, ed 2, London, 1994, Mosby-Wolfe.)*

inguinal orchiectomy by surveillance. This involves a series of CT scans and chest x-ray films initially performed at 8-week intervals and continued at lengthening periods of time for 3 or more years.

As an alternative, the classic approach has been to perform retroperitoneal lymph node dissections on patients with non-seminomatous tumors. However, 75% of node dissections result in negative biopsy results. Retroperitoneal lymph node dissection removes the lymph nodes both in the renal hilum and around the aorta and vena cava to the level of the bifurcation of the iliac artery on the affected side. Modifications of the areas dissected in retroperitoneal lymphadenectomy have been responsible for the preservation of seminal emission in patients where disruption of the sympathetic chain was the causative agent in the classic surgical approach. High-stage nonseminomatous tumors are treated with a primary platinum-based combination chemotherapy after inguinal orchiectomy. Residual tumor mass seen on CT scan after chemotherapy will contain a tumor 20% of the time, teratoma 40% of the time, and fibrosis 40% of the time. Residual tumor masses in the retroperitoneum after chemotherapy may be resected and additional cycles of chemotherapy administered.

Fertility among patients with testicular tumors is generally suboptimal. However, a discussion of sperm cell banking before orchiectomy and further treatment is in order so that this issue is addressed.

Hydrocele

Hydrocele is a collection of straw-colored fluid within the tunica vaginalis and may be congenital or acquired. The congenital type is found in childhood where a patent opening between the abdominal cavity and the tunica vaginalis exists (the processus vaginalis). This tends to fill with fluid during the day and drain at night. It may close spontaneously before 1 year of age, but if it contains bowel it should be surgically corrected.

In children a communicating hydrocele should be explored with an inguinal incision, since it really represents a potential inguinal hernia that should be closed by ligation of the opening into the peritoneal cavity. Chronic hydrocele usually occurs in men after 40 years of age, and its cause is not entirely clear. It may be caused by increased production of fluid that accumulates inside the tunica vaginalis because the lymphatic channels that absorb the fluid may not be functioning normally as a result of inflammation. It is important to rule out associated inguinal hernia and to diagnose hydrocele by transilluminating the scrotum with a flashlight. In a darkened room, a flashlight held against the bottom of the scrotum will transilluminate light through the fluid to the skin on the superior surface of the scrotum. If, on the other hand, there is a testicular mass or bowel in the scrotum, transillumination will not occur. Ultrasonography will confirm the diagnosis.

Hydroceles should be repaired if they are uncomfortable because of their size or if they represent a cosmetic problem for the patient. The anterior area of the scrotum is generally incised, the tunica vaginalis exposed and incised on its anterior surface, the fluid drained, and excess hydrocele sac excised. The cut edges that remain are brought to the posterior surface of the testis and sutured in place, and the testis is returned to the scrotum. The Lord procedure, which suture plicates the walls of the hydrocele sac upon themselves, is an alternative form of treatment. Hydroceles tend to recur approximately 15% of the time.

Varicocele

A varicocele is a varicosity of the scrotum that may interfere with fertility by increasing the temperature of the testis. A varicocele may cause a dull aching pain that is alleviated by lying down. Onset may occur after adulthood if a retroperitoneal process develops and interferes with normal venous drainage from the testes (Figs. 3-62 and 3-63).

Varicocele may be treated surgically by ligation at the level of the external inguinal ring, at the level of the internal inguinal ring through an inguinal incision, or laparoscopically between the bifurcation of the aorta and the internal inguinal ring. The more invasive retroperitoneal approach generally is not commonly performed.

Spermatocele

A spermatocele is a painless cystic mass containing sperm cells and lies just above and posterior to the testis but is separate from the testis and attached to the epididymis. It is different from hydrocele in that it contains testicular fluid and sperm cells and probably arises from tubules that connect the testis to the epididymis. It is a benign lesion that can be transilluminated normally but contains cloudy fluid and should be repaired if it is annoying to the patient.

Testis torsion

Torsion of the spermatic cord is an extremely painful condition that usually affects adolescent males. It may be partial or complete, and in complete cases the testis will turn 720 degrees on the spermatic cord. If the torsion is not corrected within 4 to 6 hours, infarction usually occurs resulting in death of the testicle (Fig. 3-64). Torsion causes the left testis to rotate counter-

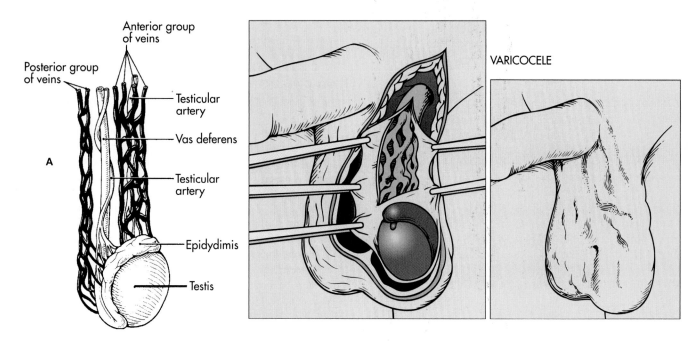

Fig. 3-62 **A,** Vascular anatomy of spermatic cord. **B,** Stage I varicocele where cremasteric veins are not involved. *(From Droller M: Surgical management of urologic disease, St. Louis, 1992, Mosby.)*

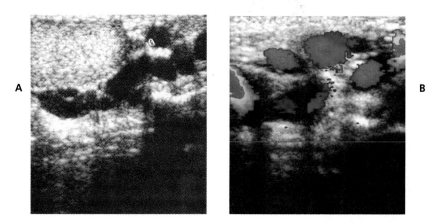

Fig. 3-63 Ultrasonograms of varicocele. **A,** High-resolution ultrasonogram of varicocele with structures surrounding the lower pole. **B,** Increasing venous pressure by means of a Valsalva maneuver seen as increased blood flow on color Doppler ultrasonography, indicating a significant varicocele. *(From Lloyd-Davies W et al: Color atlas of urology, ed 2, London, 1994, Mosby-Wolfe.)*

clockwise and the right testis to rotate clockwise. Manual detorsion may be attempted if the torsion is discovered within the first 1 or 2 hours of its occurrence, turning the testis in the respective opposite direction in which torsion has occurred. This can be accomplished by infiltrating the spermatic cord with a local anesthetic. If manual detorsion fails, immediate surgical exploration and detorsion must be carried out, accompanied by fixation of the opposite testis to prevent the same condition on that side.

Torsion of the testis is sometimes suspected in cases of torsion of the appendix of the testis and epididymis (small vestigial structures attached to the testis or epididymis). With careful physical examination one may see a "blue dot sign" moving underneath the testicular coverings. As an alternative, color Doppler imaging may be used to differentiate testicular torsion from a torsed appendix, testis, or epididymis. In the latter case (Fig. 3-65), pain will gradually subside over 5 to 7 days, and unless the diagnosis is unclear surgical exploration is unnecessary.

Penis

Peyronie's disease

Peyronie's disease is a condition that presents as a curvature of the penile shaft, or extreme pain, when erection occurs. In

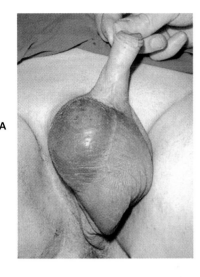

A

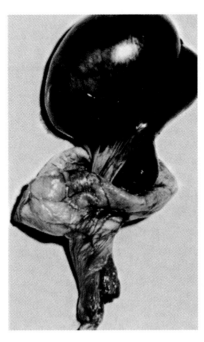

B

Fig. 3-64 A, Torsion of testicle. Torsion leads to a true urologic emergency. In the infant, the entire cord may twist resulting in testicular infarction. In the adolescent, torsion of the body of the testis or epididymis occurs within the tunica vaginalis, and the testis may lie horizontally ("bell-clapper" testis). Onset may not be dramatic, and the initial pain not severe, making the diagnosis difficult. The condition may be easily confused with epididymo-orchitis. If torsion is suspected, treatment must occur within 4 to 6 hours of onset to avoid irreversible infarction. **B,** Resected infarcted testis. (**A** *from Lloyd-Davies W et al:* Color atlas of urology, *ed 2, London, 1994, Mosby-Wolfe;* **B** *from Resnick MI:* Current therapy in genitourinary surgery, *ed 2, St. Louis, 1992, Mosby.)*

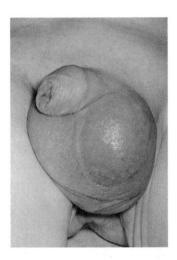

Fig. 3-65 Epididymitis. An enlarged inflamed epididymis and testicular body associated with scrotal erythema and a complication of urinary tract infection. Torsion may produce a similar clinical picture complicating the diagnosis. *(From Lloyd-Davies W et al:* Color atlas of urology, *ed 2, London, 1994, Mosby-Wolfe.)*

more advanced cases erection may not be possible. Diagnosis is made when examination of the penis reveals a dense thickening of the coverings over the erectile bodies (tunica albuginea). At times these may be calcified and visible on radiographic examination of the penis.

The cause of Peyronie's disease is unclear, but trauma and congenital predisposition are likely. Other areas of abnormal fibrous accumulation in the hands, spine, ears, and feet may also be evident. In some cases the fibrous plaques may spontaneously resolve after 18 to 24 months. Initial treatment is conservative with oral vitamin E supplements, or Potaba (potassium *para* aminobenzoic acid).

Surgical correction of curvature may be performed if adequate erections are possible. Excision of fibrous plaque and dermal grafting is preferable in some instances. Ultimately, implantation of a penile prosthesis accompanied by a straightening procedure may be required.

Priapism

Priapism is a prolonged, painful, and unwanted erection that may result in impotence if left untreated longer than a few hours. The cause is unknown in at least half the cases, but it has been associated with leukemia, sickle cell disease, pelvic tumors or inflammations, spinal cord trauma, and the use of certain medications. The most frequent cause is the injection of intercavernosal pharmacologic agents used for the treatment of erectile dysfunction.

If conservative efforts to reduce the priapism are unsuccessful, it may be necessary to perform a shunt (opening for the passage of blood) between the erectile bodies and the glans penis. If the priapism persists for a long enough time, scarring of the entire interior of the erectile body (corpus cavernosum) occurs, requiring a penile prosthetic implantation to regain sexual activity.

Carcinoma

Carcinoma of the penis occurs in 1% to 2% of 100,000 men per year in western societies and may be located on the penile shaft, glans, or foreskin. It is believed to be associated with the accumulation of smegma (secretions from cutaneous glands) under the foreskin because of inadequate cleansing. Giant condyloma may be difficult to distinguish from low-grade squamous cell carcinoma, but a viral cause for carcinoma of the penis has not been proven. Other penile lesions such as leukoplakia (a white plaque often seen in diabetics) and balanitis xerotica obliterans (a white lesion associated with meatal stricture) may also be related to carcinoma. Carcinoma in situ (local, noninvasive growth) is known as Bowen's disease, or erythroplasia of Queyrat.

Circumcision may be adequate for lesions localized to the foreskin, but partial or total penectomy is indicated for lesions of the penile shaft or glans penis.

Proper staging of the disease may necessitate lymph node dissection of the groin and pelvis in addition to CT and bone scans, and chest x-ray films. Ulceration and a significant inflammatory reaction may accompany inguinal lymph node involvement. Distant metastasis is apparent less than 10% of the time. Five-year survivals are 90% for node-negative cases, 50% in inguinal node–positive conditions, 20% with iliac (pelvic) node involvement, and none in instances of distant metastasis. Chemotherapy offers limited usefulness, but radiation therapy may afford some alleviation of pain.

Phimosis

Phimosis is the inability to retract the foreskin in the uncircumcised male (Fig. 3-66). It results in irritation under the foreskin because of an accumulation of smegma that has become infected. The incidence of infection appears to be lower in those males who are able to retract the foreskin for proper cleansing.

Circumcision, the operative procedure to remove the foreskin from the penis, is most commonly performed just after birth by the obstetrician, pediatrician, or urologist for traditional and social reasons. Phimosis may also be treated by performing a dorsal slit procedure. This technique incises the foreskin on the anterior area of the glans penis, from the opening in the foreskin at the penile tip to its attachment to the penile shaft, just behind the glans. Circumcision may be accomplished by application of a Gomco clamp, which crushes the skin at its attachment, or by incision of the tissue with a scalpel.

Paraphimosis

Paraphimosis results when the foreskin has been retracted above the glans and cannot be repositioned (reduced) to cover the glans. This results in an emergency situation, for if left untreated, the constriction created will cause the glans to lose venous blood supply followed by the loss of arterial blood flow.

Balanoposthitis

Balanoposthitis (balanitis) presents with inflammation and cracking of the foreskin in the uncircumcised male. When an adult develops this condition, the possibility of adult onset diabetes should be considered because this is often one of the first symptoms (Fig. 3-67).

ERECTILE DYSFUNCTION

Male sexual dysfunction may be secondary to arterial or venous insufficiency of the erectile bodies, neurologic deficit, or hormonal deficit or may be psychologic in origin. Psychologic causes of erectile dysfunction are generally quickly suspected, and appropriate referral is made. Hormonal deficit can be suspected if the patient complains of a diminished libido and can be ameliorated by appropriate hormonal replacement.

Neurologic deficit is generally suspected if the patient complains of associated neurologic deficit such as peripheral neuropathy as in diabetics, or patients with known multiple sclerosis. Arterial and venous insufficiency is suspected in the presence of associated disease processes, such as hypertension and cardiovascular disease, and is associated with hypercholesterolemia and tobacco use. Alcoholism is another significant cause of erectile dysfunction and in approximately 50% of the cases may not improve with the cessation of drinking.

Many medications may interfere with the ability of the male patient to achieve a satisfactory erection, and a list of these medications with an appropriate discussion is available in several references specific to erectile dysfunction.

Color Doppler ultrasonography of the erectile bodies may be used, along with pharmacologic injections of the cavernous bodies, to screen for arterial and venous insufficiency. Pharmacologic injections or the use of vacuum devices are alternative forms of treatment in patients who respond to the vasodilators used to stimulate the onset of erection, such as papaverine and prostaglandin-E. Vacuum erectile devices may be used by patients who are willing to use such external devices. A vacuum is applied to the lubricated penis during foreplay to

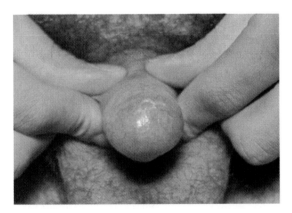

Fig. 3-66 Phimosis. *(From Lloyd-Davies W et al: Color atlas of urology, ed 2, London, 1994, Mosby-Wolfe.)*

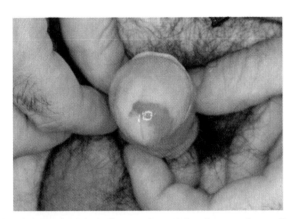

Fig. 3-67 Balanitis. Inflammation of the glans penis usually occurs with an associated phimosis. The inflamed glans is seen with the prepuce retracted. *(From Lloyd-Davies W et al: Color atlas of urology, ed 2, London, 1994, Mosby-Wolfe.)*

establish an erectilelike state. A constriction ring is placed at the penile base after it has become engorged with blood.

Venous insufficiency may be suspected by continued blood flow between cardiac cycles, duplex Doppler ultrasonography, and significant blood flow in the more superficial venous channels of the penis. This abnormality can be confirmed by dynamic infusion cavernosography and cavernosometry (DICC). Refer to Chapter 4 for a more complete description of this procedure.

In very select patients, with a large discrete venous leak, ligation of the abnormal venous channels may improve sexual function. Excision of the deep dorsal vein of the penis with emissary vein ligation has fallen into disuse because of the limited 50% success achieved at 2 years.

For patients who are unable to perform and find the use of injection therapy or vacuum devices unacceptable and in whom sexual activity plays an important part in their lifestyle, the insertion of a penile prosthesis is an attractive alternative. The overall success rate and patient acceptance is in the range of 95%.

Penile prosthetics are of several different types. Prosthetics may be of the inflatable type with a separate reservoir pump and cylinders that are implanted into the erectile bodies. As an alternative, self-contained inflatable devices may be implanted, but these generally produce a less cosmetically desirable erection and flaccid state than the three-piece device. A malleable prosthesis involves the implantation of a silicone-covered malleable wire, one of which is placed in each erectile body, producing enough rigidity for penetration but malleable so that the penis may be bent down and concealed.

Penile prosthetics are generally inserted either through an incision just below the pubis or between the scrotum and the penis. This procedure can be performed on an outpatient or short-hospital-stay basis. Penile prosthetic patients are generally comfortable enough to use the prosthesis after 4 to 6 weeks.

Surgical intervention and treatment of male infertility may occur in cases where testicular biopsy is required to differentiate between vasal or epididymal obstruction and primary testicular failure, ligation of varicocele, correction of vasal obstruction secondary to previous vasectomy, or microscopic epididymal sperm aspiration (MESA) for assisted reproductive techniques, such as intracytoplasmic injection of sperm cells (ICSI) into the female partner's egg.

GLOSSARY

Ablation Removal, especially by cutting.

Acetylcholine Neurotransmitter released at the autonomic synapses and neuromuscular junctions; active in the transmission of nerve impulses and formed enzymatically in the tissues from choline.

Acinar Relating to an acinus, or gland cell.

Agenesis Absence of development.

Albright's syndrome Polyostotic fibrous dysplasia, patchy dermal pigmentation, and endocrine dysfunction; also called Albright's disease and McCune-Albright syndrome.

Alkaline phosphatase A phosphate, such as the phosphomonoesterase from blood plasma or milk, active in an alkaline medium; enzyme active in bony metabolism splitting compounds for production and destruction of bone; elevated in children and in metastasis to the bone.

Alpha-blocker Agent that blocks alpha-adrenergic receptor sites such as the cardiovascular and respiratory systems and the bladder outlet.

Alpha-fetoprotein Fetal blood protein present abnormally in adults with some forms of cancer.

Angiomatosis Multiple angiomas, hemangiomas, lymphangiomas composed of blood vessels or lymphatic vessels.

Angiotensinogen Serum globulin formed by the liver and cleaved by renin to produce angiotensin I; hypertensinogen.

Anomalous Deviated from normal, as in development of body parts or organs.

Anticholinergic Group of drugs having activity that blocks or opposes acetylcholine and the transmission of nerve impulses; reaction similar to atropine, causing dry mouth, blurred vision, decreased contractility of the bladder and gastrointestinal tract, and tachycardia.

APC Abbreviation for medicinal tablet composed of aspirin, phenacetin, and caffeine.

Aplastic Never developed, no tissue present; tendency to form cysts in place of organ, as with kidney.

Arnold-Chiari syndrome Congenital anomaly in which the cerebellum and the medulla oblongata, which is elongated and flattened, protrude into the spinal canal through the foramen magnum; may be associated with many other defects, including spina bifida occulta and meningomyelocele; also called Arnold-Chiari deformity.

Atretic Pertaining to atresia, absence or closure of an anatomic part or natural passage.

Atrophic Shrunken, as atrophic testis caused by testis torsion.

Autologous Derived from the same individual.

Bacille Calmette-Guérin Derivative of the tubercle bacillus, used therapeutically in the treatment of bladder tumors.

Balanitis xerotica obliterans Condition involving the glans penis with scarring, depigmentation, and narrowing of the urethral meatus.

Bifid Divided into two lobes or parts.

Bilharzial Schistosomal, named after Bilharz, a German anatomist who described the parasite responsible for schistosomiasis.

Boari flap Flap of bladder wall used to anastomose to the ureter where a portion of the ureter has been destroyed or removed.

Captopril Drug that is an angiotensin inhibitor, used therapeutically, or with radionuclide testing to aid in the diagnosis of renovascular hypertension.

Choriocarcinoma Malignant tumor developing in the uterus from a trophoblast and rarely in the testes from a neoplasm.

Cloaca Common chamber into which the intestinal, urinary, and generative canals discharge; terminal part of the embryonic hindgut.

Cortex Cortical area surrounding the periphery of a gland, as in the adrenal.

Countercurrent balance Balance in the flow of materials in opposite directions; kidney system.

Cystine Amino acid containing sulfur, a component of nonopaque urinary calculi.

Cytotoxin Substance having a toxic effect on cells.

Dandy-Walker syndrome Congenital hydrocephalus caused by obstruction of the foramina of Magendie and Luschka; also called Dandy-Walker deformity.

Davis intubated ureterotomy Technique of relieving the obstruction in a long narrowed ureteral segment.

DDAVP Trade name for desmopressin acetate (1-deamino-8-D-arginine vasopressin acetate), a drug used to treat enuresis (bed wetting) and with antidiuretic (water-conserving) effect on the kidneys.

Dexamethasone Synthetic glucocorticoid used as an antiinflammatory and antiallergen.

Diathesis Predisposition.

Dysplasia Developed abnormally.

Dyssynergia Altered coordination during contraction of the bladder and sphincter because bladder and sphincter probably contract simultaneously during voiding.

Ectopic Positioned in an abnormal location.

Electrical stimulation Form of therapy used for the treatment of urinary incontinence whereby the muscles of the pelvic floor are passively exercised and strengthened.

Embryonal cell Type of testis tumor with components similar to those found in the embryo but with malignant alteration.

Enterocele Herniation of small intestine into the vagina from its apex or uppermost part.

Ephedrine Drug that is similar in action to epinephrine (adrenaline) and stimulates the sphincter mechanism to maintain continence.

Epiloia Dominant genetic trait characterized by mental deficiency and multiple tumor formation of the skin and brain; maintained by a high mutation rate; tuberous sclerosis.

Epispadias Congenital defect in which the urethra opens upon the upper surface of the penis.

Ergot Any of a group of alkaloids used medicinally for their contractile effect on smooth muscle; derived from the fungi of infected rye.

Exstrophy Eversion of a part or organ; congenital malformation of the bladder where the normally internal mucosa is exposed on the abdominal wall because of failure of union between the halves of the pubic symphysis and the adjacent halves of the abdominal wall.

Extracellular matrix Tissue located outside the glomerulus and produced by the juxtaglomerular cells.

Extravasation Leakage into adjacent tissues, as extravasation of urine.

Fibroplasia Process of forming fibrous tissue as in wound healing.

Fibrous Composed of fibrous connective tissue.

Gerota's fascia Fibrofatty layer surrounding and protecting the kidneys and investing the adrenal glands.

Hamartoma Mass resembling a tumor that represents anomalous development of tissue natural to a part or organ rather than a true tumor.

Heterologous Derived from a different species.

Hounsfield unit Unit of measurement of density in computerized tomography.

Hyalinosis Condition characterized by hyalin degeneration as exhibited by scar tissue resulting from an accumulation of protein, especially in the kidney.

Hydronephrosis Abnormal dilatation of the kidney, usually caused by obstruction.

Hyperchloremic Elevated level of chloride in the bloodstream.

Hypercholesterolemia Elevated serum cholesterol.

Hyperkalemia Elevated serum potassium level.

Hypermobility As in urethral hypermobility, which predisposes to urinary stress incontinence caused by loss of normal anatomic support.

Hypernatremia Elevated serum sodium level.

Hyperreflexia Inappropriate contractions, as in inappropriate bladder contractions, where a known neurotic diagnosis exists.

Hypoechoic Decreased reflectivity of ultrasound imaging.

Hypophysectomy Surgical removal of the pituitary gland.

Hypoplastic Underdeveloped, partially developed, incomplete.

Immunofluorescence Labeling of antibodies or antigens with fluorescent dyes for the purpose of demonstrating the presence of a particular antigen or antibody in a tissue preparation of a smear.

Interleukin-2 Chemotherapeutic agent used to treat metastatic renal cell carcinoma.

Intima Lining as the tunica intima of an artery.

Intracytoplasmic Inside the cytoplasm of the cell.

Isthmus Narrow connection, as the isthmus of horseshoe kidneys.

Juxtaglomerular Group of cells, known as the juxtaglomerular apparatus, that have important regulatory functions relating to the glomerulus and the regulation of blood pressure.

Kyphosis Abnormal backward curvature of the spine.

Leukoplakia Condition considered precancerous; thickened white patches of epithelium occurring on mucous membranes of mouth, vulva, and kidney pelvis.

Lindau's disease Rare genetic disease characterized by angiomatosis of the retina and cerebellum and by cysts of the liver, pancreas, and kidneys.

Lord procedure Procedure to surgically correct scrotal hydrocele by suturing the hydrocele walls onto themselves.

Lymphocele Abnormal collection of lymphatic fluid, such as that occurring after lymph node dissection or renal transplantation.

Lymphoma Malignant tumor of the lymphatic system.

Matrix calculus Calculus composed of protein without crystallization, serving as the center for potential stone formation.

Nocturia Voiding that occurs at night.

Obturator nerve Nerve extending from the bifurcation of the iliac artery through the obturator fossa to supply the adductor muscles of the thigh.

Ortho-paraphosphate Any one of a number of compounds in this group used to treat a propensity toward urinary stone formation by increasing the binding of calcium in the intestinal tract or increasing the excretion of paraphosphate, which inhibits stone formation in the urinary tract.

Orthostatic hypotension Decrease in blood pressure when one assumes an erect position; also sometimes called postural hypotension.

Osteodystrophy Defective formation of bone usually associated with abnormalities of calcium and phosphorus metabolism.

Papillary necrosis Condition usually found in diabetics, where the renal papillae are destroyed by infection.

Parenchyma Essential and instinctive tissue of an organ or an abnormal growth as distinguished from its supportive framework.

Perinephric Perirenal, circumrenal, surrounding the kidney.

Peripheral neuropathy Pathologic condition that affects the peripheral nervous system, as in diabetic peripheral neuropathy.

Periureteral Outside the ureter, as in periureteral fibrosis.

Pfannenstiel Low curved transverse abdominal incision, usually used with muscle splitting.

Phagocytic Functioning as a phagocyte by engulfing foreign material and consuming debris and foreign bodies.

Podophyllin Resin obtained from the podophyllum (or rhizome and rootlet of mayapple, *Podophyllum peltatum*) used as a caustic.

Posterior valve Obstructing flap of tissue in the prostatic urethra of male infants affected with this diagnosis.

Postural hypotension *see* orthostatic hypotension.

Prognosticate Make a prognosis about a probable outcome.

Psoas hitch Technique to attach the bladder to a shortened ureter by suturing the bladder dome to the psoas muscle.

Pyelonephritis Urinary tract infection involving the kidneys associated with identifiable microscopic inflammatory changes and associated with fever, chills, and flank pain clinically.

Radiopacity Density under x-ray beam and appearing white on film; opaque to radiation.

Randall's plaque Submucosal calcification in the renal collecting system.

Recessive Expressed only when the determining gene is in the homozygous condition.

Rectocele Herniation of the rectum forward into the vagina.

Reflux Passage of urine in the opposite direction of its normal passage.

Renal papillae Apices of a renal pyramid that project into the lumen of a calyx of the kidney and through which collecting tubules discharge urine.

Retrograde ejaculation Passage of seminal fluid into the bladder during ejaculation instead of the normal (antegrade) direction.

Rhabdomyosarcoma Malignant tumor composed of striated muscle cells.

Saccule Depression in the lining of the urinary bladder between trabeculae where a diverticulum (protrusion through the bladder wall) may form.

Schistosome Parasite transmitted to freshwater swimmers in areas of Asia, causing urinary tract disease known as schistosomiasis, or bilharziasis.

Septated Divided by septa, or multiple separations.

Sireno-monomelia Related to or affecting only one limb.

SLE nephritis Systemic lupus erythematosus nephritis; involvement of the kidneys by this disease, with varying severity.

Struvite Urinary calculus associated with urinary tract infection with a urea-splitting organism such as one of the *Proteus* species.

Supernumerary Extra, as in supernumerary kidneys.

Teratoma Tumor derived from more than one embryonic layer and made up of a heterogeneous mixture of tissues (bone, muscle, cartilage).

Thiazide Group of diuretics used orally to treat hypertension; also one used to treat renal calculus disease by its action of increasing absorption of calcium from the urine.

Trabeculation Formation or presence of bundles of fibers, as in trabeculation of the bladder.

Transsphenoidal Surgical approach across the sphenoid sinus to the pituitary gland.

Transureteroureterostomy Technique of anastomosing a ureter to the ureter on the opposing side by passing it retroperitoneally.

Tricyclic antidepressant Group of antidepressants (imipramine) that increase the action of epinephrine (adrenaline) and have an inhibitory effect on the bladder

Trisomy The presence of an extra chromosome of one type in an otherwise diploid cell.

Trytophane By-product of cigarette smoke associated with the development of bladder tumors; tryptophan.

Tuberous sclerosis Genetic trait in man characterized by mental deficiency and multiple tumor formations of the skin and brain.

Turner's syndrome A disorder of gonadal differentiation, marked by short stature, undifferentiated (streak) gonads, and other abnormalities that may include webbing of the neck, low posterior hair line, increased carrying angle of the elbow, cubitus valgus, and cardiac defects.

Ureterocele Dilated ureteral opening into the bladder.

Ureteroureterostomy Reanastomosis of transected ureter.

Uric acid calculus Calculus composed of uric acid; uric acid is also the component of gouty arthritic tophi.

VATER syndrome Vertebral defects, imperforate anus, tracheoesophageal fistula, and radial and renal dysplasia.

Xanthine Basic compound that occurs especially in animals or plant tissue, is derived from guanine and hypoxanthine, and yields uric acid on oxidation; also any of various derivatives of this.

Xanthogranulomatous Unusual severe, chronic inflammatory condition of the kidney, usually seen in the elderly, and usually in women.

Zuckerkandl's organs Small masses of chromaffin cells (like in adrenal medulla) in close relation to sympathetic ganglia, aortic paraganglia; also called Zuckerkandl's bodies.

Bibliography

1. Agency Health Care Policy and Research (AHCPR): Urinary Incontinence Guideline Panel: *Urinary incontinence in adults*, *Clinical Practice Guidelines*, 92-1038, Rockville, Md, 1992, Department of Health and Human Services.
2. Aronson S et al: Cystic renal masses: usefulness of the Bosniak classification, *Urol Radiol* 13:83, 1991; comments in 13:91, 1991.
3. Bosniak MA: The current radiographic approach to renal cysts, *Radiology* 158:1, 1986.
4. Gillenwater JY et al, editors: *Adult and pediatric urology*, ed 3, St. Louis, 1996, Mosby.
5. Fisher-Rasmussen W: Treatment of SUI, *Ann Med*, 22:455, 1990.
6. Horstman WG et al: Comparison of computed tomography and conventions cystography for detection of traumatic bladder rupture, *Urol Radiol* 12:188, 1991.
7. Jeter JF: Pelvic floor exercises with and without biofeedback for treatment of urinary incontinence problem, *Urology* 5:72, 1991.
8. Kilalis RP et al: Observation of renal extopia and fusion in children, *J Urol* 110:558, 1973.
9. Kirby R, Christmas T: *Benign prostatic hyperplasia*, London, 1993, Gower.
10. Koeppen BM, Stanton BA: *Renal physiology*, ed 2, St. Louis, 1992, Mosby.
11. Lloyd-Davies W et al: *Color atlas of urology*, London, 1994, Mosby-Wolfe.
12. Meeker MR, Rothrock JC: *Alexander's care of the patient in surgery*, ed 10, St. Louis, 1995, Mosby.
13. Nightingale F: *Notes on nursing*, London, 1859, Harrison & Sons.
14. Novick AC: Surgical correction of renovascular hypertension, *Surg Clin of North Am* 68:1007, 1988.
15. Resnick MI, Kursh E: *Current therapy in genitourinary surgery*, ed 2, St. Louis, 1992, Mosby.
16. Seidmon EJ, Hanno PM: *Current urologic therapy three*, Philadelphia, 1994, WB Saunders.
17. Strause MB, Welt L: *Disease of the kidney*, Boston, 1971, Little, Brown.
18. Tanagho EA, McAninch JW: *Smith's general urology*, ed 14, Norwalk, Conn, 1995, Appleton & Lange.
19. U.S. Department of Health and Human Services: *Current urologic therapy*, 1992.
20. Walsh PC, Retrick ST: *Campbell's urology*, ed 6, Philadelphia, 1992, WB Saunders.

4

Diagnostic Interventions

Before surgical intervention on a patient, extensive examination and diagnostic testing takes place. In order to provide optimal care for the patient, the genitourinary nurse should have an understanding of these preparatory investigative work-ups. One or several diagnostic procedures may have been performed before the decision was made that surgery is indicated.

INVASIVE DIAGNOSTIC PROCEDURES

Before surgical intervention several invasive diagnostic examinations are available to the genitourinary surgeon. Preoperative testing may include intravenous pyelograms (IVP) or intravenous urograms (IVU), retrograde pyelograms (RGP), retrograde urethrograms (RUG), renal arteriogram, renal venogram, video urodynamic study (VUD), urethrocystogram (UCG), nephrogram and nephrotomogram, duplex Doppler, dynamic infusion cavernosometry and cavernosography (DICC), and transrectal ultrasound biopsy of the prostate (TRUS Bx). Which tests are performed depend on the patient's complaint and the anticipated procedure.

IVU is a series of radiographic studies that are enhanced by an ionic or nonionic contrast medium (dye). Through the detailed information provided, the overall function of the entire urinary tract may be evaluated, as well as the ability of the kidney to concentrate and excrete urine (Fig. 4-1). After intravenous injection of the contrast material, sequential x-rays of the abdomen and pelvis are taken, enabling evaluation of the transport of urine from the renal pelvis to the bladder. The patient's ability to empty the bladder is reviewed on an x-ray taken after voiding.

Common indications for IVU are urinary calculi, recurrent urinary tract infections, pain from the urinary tract, hematuria, renal mass or tumor, urinary system tumor, trauma, obstruction, and congenital anomalies. Assessment of the bony structures and renal calcifications, and evaluation of hydronephrosis, filling defects, and malposition are possible through this examination.

The study holds a risk for an untoward reaction in patients with a history of allergies or asthma, and a risk for renal toxicity in patients with diabetes mellitus, hyperuricosuria, amyloidosis, preexisting renal insufficiency or failure, or heart disease. It is contraindicated in patients with multiple myeloma. Some of the underlying heart conditions that pose an increased threat include myocardial, atherosclerotic, or valvular disease, and existing conduction disturbances.

If there is a known contraindicating disease or allergy to iodine-based contrast material, shellfish, or cutaneous iodine-based cleansing solutions, the procedure should be omitted in favor of an RGP. Allergic reactions are apparent immediately after the injection of the contrast material, and are potentially severe. The caregiver needs to be observant for the early signs of hypersensitivity, which include transient nausea, urticaria, itching, and respiratory distress that can rapidly turn into respiratory failure and death.

Contrast material can induce cardiac arrhythmias, conduction abnormalities, and myocardial ischemia. The most commonly seen arrhythmia is premature ventricular contraction; the most severe reaction noted is ventricular tachycardia and fibrillation; less common is atrioventricular block. An increase in cardiac rate is believed to lead to an increased requirement for oxygen and is the likely cause for symptoms of ischemia. The exact cause of contrast-induced cardiotoxicity is uncertain. Suggested causative factors are the sudden introduction of a hypertonic volume load, direct toxicity to the myocardium, and stimulation of the neural reflex pathways.

RGP provides a detailed series of x-rays that display anatomic views of the ureter, ureteropelvic junction (UPJ), renal pelvis, and calyces (Fig. 4-2). Endoscopic visualization of the ureterovesical junction (UVJ) is necessary. A ureteral catheter is placed in the lower ureteral tract and the contrast medium is infused by gravity or injected into the upper urinary tract. The only significant precaution is a known allergy to cutaneous iodine-based cleansing solutions, requiring discretion in the selection of the surgical preparation.

Potential risks include pyelonephritis related to instrumentation and injection of material into a sterile body cavity, or overdistention of the renal collecting system resulting in extravasation of contrast material. Patients undergoing RGP should be observed for flank pain, dysuria, chills, and fever for 24 to 48 hours after the procedure. Adequate postoperative fluid intake is an important point to stress during the preoperative teaching session. Fluids should include fruit juices because overhydrating with water alone will deplete the body of needed potassium.

Retrograde urethrograms (RUG) necessitate the installation of a small volume of iodine-based contrast material into the urethra from a retrograde direction (Fig. 4-3). This may be achieved through a catheter-tipped syringe, through a Foley catheter snugged in the fossa navicularis and balloon-inflated with 1 ml of fluid, or through a special holder. Oblique x-rays of the urethra are taken after installation of 15 to 30 ml of contrast material. This procedure may be used to determine the presence of urethral stricture, urethral fistula, urethral trauma, urethral diverticulum, or urethral tumor.

Renal arteriograms allow evaluation of the arterial blood supply to the kidneys by means of a series of x-rays (see Chapter 3, Fig. 3-5). A radiopaque catheter is threaded through the femoral or axillary artery into the abdominal aorta and renal artery, under fluoroscopy, in the radiology suite. Contrast material is injected intraarterially. Several images are obtained in the first 2 to 4 seconds after injection of the dye. This affords visualization of the renal arterial system. Opacification of the contrast material in the renal parenchyma marks the nephric phase and lasts for 15 to 20 seconds (Fig. 4-4). The venous phase that follows has limited diagnostic value because of extensive renal extraction and concentration of the contrast medium.

Common indications for renal arteriogram are renal trauma, renal mass or tumor, renal vascular hypertension, hematuria, or preoperative planning for removal of large renal, adrenal, retroperitoneal, or pelvic masses, and for investigation before nephron-sparing renal surgery or renal transplantation. An allergy to iodine-based contrast material is the primary contraindication.

Potential complications after the examination include bleeding from the puncture site and allergic reactions. Pressure needs to be applied to the puncture site and the area observed for frank bleeding for 48 hours after the procedure. Observation of pedal pulses, capillary filling of the nailbeds, (shortness of breath, wheezing, and rhonchi are indicative of an allergic response) and respiratory exchange should be vigilant during and after the procedure.

Renal venograms are radiographic assessments of the kidney's venous system. The right femoral vein is cannulized with a radiopaque catheter that is advanced to the left renal vein. Contrast material is injected and the catheter is angled upward into the contralateral renal vein and the procedure repeated. Injection of epinephrine into the renal artery approximately 10 seconds after venography often enhances the imaging.

This procedure should be avoided in patients with allergy to iodine-based contrast material. Common indications for renal venograms are renovascular hypertension, to obtain renal vein

renin samples, renal mass or tumor, congenital urinary system anomalies, renal vein thrombosis, and renal tumor thrombus (renal cell carcinoma). The same potential complications apply as with renal arteriogram.

Video urodynamic studies (VUD) are the gold standard for evaluation of lower urinary tract dysfunction during the filling, storage, and voiding phases (Fig. 4-5). Multichannel urodynamic parameters are combined with video imaging and fluoroscopy of the lower urinary tract to assess the physiology and morphology of the lower urinary tract (Fig. 4-6). Indications may include urinary incontinence, voiding dysfunction without incontinence, neuropathic bladder dysfunction, bladder outlet obstruction, urinary retention of unknown cause, and suspected urethral obstruction. If a urinary tract infection or an illness limiting mobility is present, the test may be contraindicated.

Uroflowmetry is a urinary flow study that evaluates the urinary flow rate (Fig. 4-7). The patient urinates into a funnel that is connected to a flow rate metering apparatus that produces

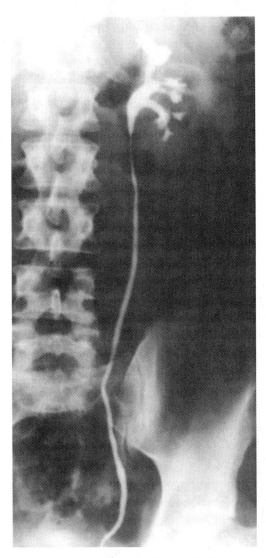

Fig. 4-2 Retrograde pyelography, fine detail of pelviocalyceal system. *(From Tanagho EA, McAninch JW: Smith's general urology, ed 14, Norwalk, Conn., 1995, Appleton & Lange.)*

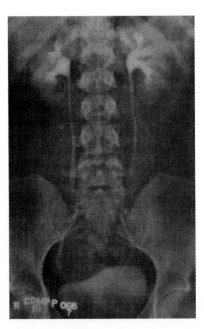

Fig. 4-1 Normal IVU, full length film. *(From Gillenwater et al: Adult and pediatric urology, ed 3, St. Louis, 1996, Mosby.)*

analog or computer-generated graphic results. It is a valuable screening measure that detects abnormal flow patterns often indicative of outlet obstruction or deficient detrusor contractility. It is also a useful quality control measure before a pressure-flow study, providing a "normal" flow pattern for each patient, before the invasive instrumentation used with more detailed testing.

Cystometrogram (CMG) is a bladder filling test, combined with radiography, that compares volume with intravesical pressure through an analog or computer-generated graph (Fig. 4-8).

With the patient supine, one or more catheters are introduced through urethral or suprapubic access into the bladder. The bladder is filled with water or saline and a CMG is obtained in both supine and upright positions. A voiding pressure study generally follows, providing flow data to combine with the

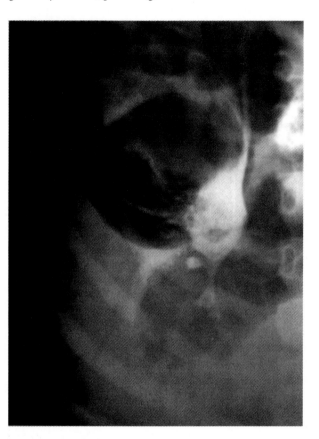

Fig. 4-4 Nephrographic phase shows dense rim around avascular mass. *(From Drach GW:* Common problems in infections and stones, *St. Louis, 1992, Mosby.)*

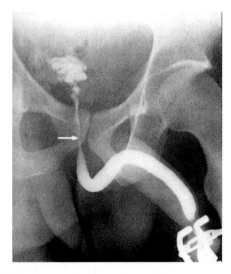

Fig. 4-3 Urethrography, normal ascending urethrogram. The urethra is smooth and narrows normally in the region of the external sphincter. The verumontanum is shown as a filing defect in the prostatic urethra. *(From Lloyd-Davies W:* Color atlas of urology, *ed 2, London, 1994, Mosby-Wolfe.)*

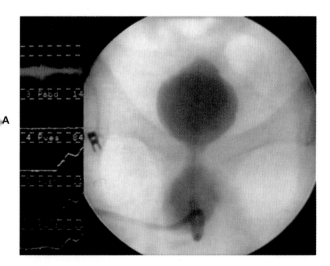

A

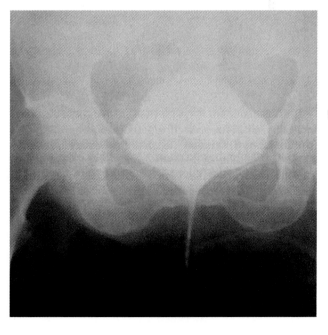

B

Fig. 4-5 A, Video urodynamic (VUD) image. *(From Gray M* Genitourinary disorders, *St. Louis, 1992, Mosby.)* **B,** X-ray taken during VUD.

CMG. Two-catheter technique avoids the tendency toward artifact found with the single-catheter method and offers the advantage of removing the filling catheter, enhancing the pressure-flow study.

Additionally, an abdominal pressure catheter may be employed to detect artifact produced by abdominal pressure changes caused by movement or straining. This consists of a fluid-filled balloon catheter that may be inserted rectally or vaginally. Connection to a pressure transducer records values on a polygraph or computer (Fig. 4-9). The detrusor pressure, an approximate representation of the smooth muscle bladder wall's contribution to filling and micturition pressures, is

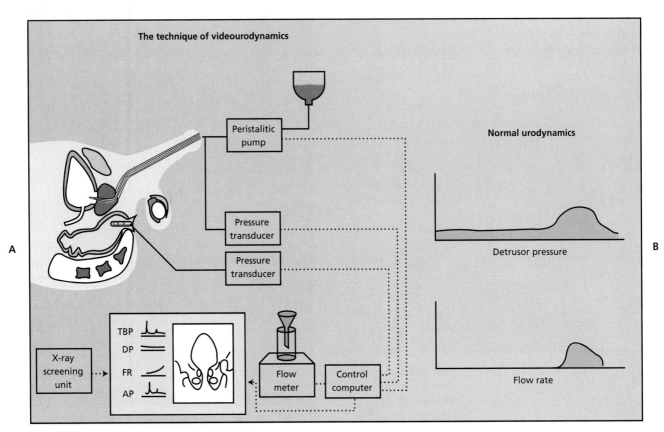

Fig. 4-6 **A,** Schematic diagram showing technique of VUD. **B,** Normal VUD graph.
(From Kirby RS: Benign prostatic hypertrophy, *London, 1993, Gower.)*

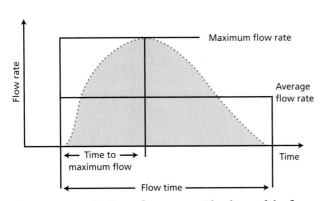

Fig. 4-7 Normal urinary flow pattern. The shape of the flow pattern is significant and when it becomes flattened, prolonged and intermittent, it indicates outflow obstruction. Maximum flows under 20 ml/sec are abnormal. This noninvasive test helps monitor progress following many treatment regimens. *(From Gillenwater et al:* Adult and pediatric urology, *ed 3, St. Louis, 1996, Mosby.)*

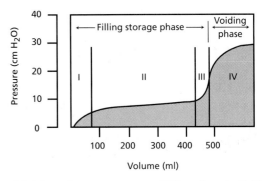

Fig. 4-8 Normal cystometrogram. Filling phase is divided into an initial slight rise in bladder pressure (phase I), followed by a tonus limb reflecting bladder accommodation (phase II). At maximum capacity, the detrusor muscle and elastic bladder wall tissue are stretched to their limits causing a rise in bladder pressure (phase III). A detrusor contraction is voluntarily initiated and the patient voids (phase IV). *(Modified from Wein AJ:* Voiding function and dysfunction. *In Walters MD:* Clinical urogynecology, *St. Louis, 1993, Mosby.)*

obtained by subtracting the abdominal pressure measurement from the intravesical pressure reading.

This examination is useful in determining bladder capacity, bladder wall compliance, detrusor muscle stability, filling sensations, and the ability of the bladder to contract during voiding. The procedure is also adaptable to evaluate the characteristics of continent diversions and the competence of continence mechanisms postoperatively, the presence of extravasation of contrast material or reflux of urine into the kidneys, in addition to the evaluation of the bladder contour. The presence or absence of bladder or urethral diverticuli during voiding may be discovered as well.

A **voiding pressure study** is a pressure flow study that measures intravesical pressure and flow by combining uroflowmetry and CMG data to assess micturition in detail and is obtained immediately following the filling CMG. Intravesical pressure, detrusor pressure, and uroflowmetry are measured simultaneously with or without fluoroscopy as the patient urinates into the urinary flowmeter (Fig. 4-10). A graphic comparison is then available to evaluate detrusor contractility, urinary flow rate, and pelvic floor muscle response to voiding.

Sphincter electromyogram (EMG) measures the activity of the pelvic floor muscles (Fig. 4-11). Data about the gross pelvic muscle or bulbocavernosus response to bladder filling and micturition is provided. It is necessary to attach one of three types of electrodes to the patient. Patch electrodes (ECG), percutaneous wire electrodes, or bipolar needle electrodes are placed over the perineal area. This procedure is performed during the filling CMG and voiding flow study when employed in combination with any of the other studies.

A **urethral pressure study** produces a depiction of sphincter closure pressure, functional length, continuous response to bladder filling and voiding, or response to a specific mechanism such as coughing. A urethral pressure profile (UPP) is achieved by slowly withdrawing a catheter through the urethra as the side ports perfuse the urethral wall and measure urethral closure pressure (Fig. 4-12). Maximum urethral closure pressure

(MUCP) offers a static measure of the dynamic sphincter mechanism while functional length provides an estimate of the length of urethra affected by the sphincter mechanism.

The **Whitaker test** (upper tract urodynamics) gives graphic tracings of the pressure gradient between the renal pelvis and UVJ (see Fig. 3-32). A percutaneous cannula attached to a constant-rate infusion pump and pressure transducer is inserted into the kidney. A second catheter is placed urethrally into the bladder and attached to another pressure transducer. Fluid is instilled until the renal pelvis, ureter, and bladder are full, or until flank pain and obvious obstruction are displayed. The recorded cannula (perfusion) pressure and bladder pressure are subtracted to establish the existence of any upper urinary tract obstruction.

Urethrocystograms (UCGs) are voiding x-ray studies of the process of micturition (Fig. 4-13). The bladder is filled with contrast material from a retrograde aspect and a series of films are taken as the patient voids. Bladder compliance to the voiding process as well as postvoiding residual urine can be determined with this examination.

Nephrograms or nephrotomograms require that a tract be created through which a catheter is fed into the kidney (Fig. 4-14). The renal pelvis and calyces may be visualized in this manner. Contrast material is injected and films rapidly taken before the dye reaches the urinary collecting system. This is frequently done when obstruction of the collecting system is suspected. A nephrotomogram employs computed tomography and may be indicated when the anatomic properties of the renal system are obscured by extra renal shadows (bone, feces) on standard radiographic images.

Duplex Doppler ultrasonographic evaluation of penile erections is performed using a high-frequency transducer that localizes the deep cavernosal artery by ultrasonographic scanning. The velocity of blood flow through these arteries is then measured by utilizing Doppler principles (Fig. 4-15). This is generally performed before and after injecting a vasoactive substance such as papaverine hydrochloride or prostaglandin E_1. The

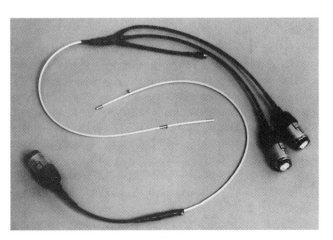
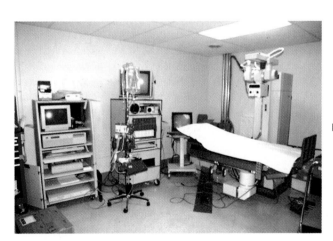

Fig. 4-9 **A,** Microtransducer catheters. One has a single microtransducer for estimating abdominal pressure. The other has two microtransducers, and a fluid filling port, for measuring intravesical and intraurethral pressure. *(From Walters MD:* Clinical urogynecology, *St. Louis, 1993, Mosby.)* **B,** VUD equipment.

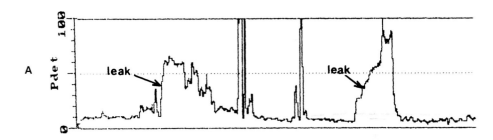

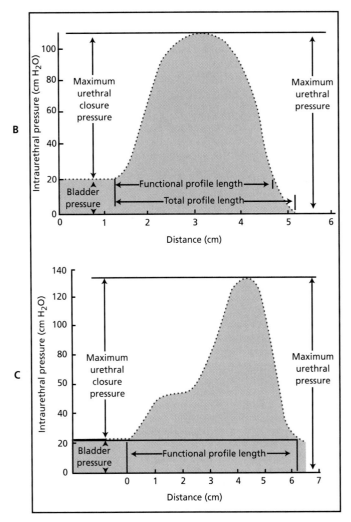

Fig. 4-10 **A,** Pressure flow showing involuntary detrusor contractions, which occur as a result of overt neurologic disease representing an upper-motor neuron lesion or as an idiopathic phenomenon. These contractions cause frequency, urgency, or frank incontinence. Alternatively, lower-motor neuron lesions result in low pressure autonomic detrusor contractions and ineffective bladder emptying. **B,** Normal male urethral pressure profile. **C,** External sphincter spasm on urethral pressure profile. *(From Gillenwater et al: Adult and pediatric urology, ed 3, St. Louis, 1996, Mosby.)*

velocity of blood flow through the deep cavernosal artery should be at least 30 cm per second unless the patient has not responded to the injection (high anxiety will prevent this), or there is significant arterial insufficiency. In some cases patients may not respond to vasoactive substances though the mechanism for this

is still unclear. If priapism (persistent erection) has developed as a result of the injected drug, one will not see normal arterial pulsations because of the inability of the cardiac system to pump additional blood into the already filled erectile bodies.

The patient may also be assessed at this time for the likelihood of an abnormality of the venous trapping mechanism. The presence of blood flow between the cardiac cycles is observed in the face of a normal arterial inflow, or the deep dorsal vein of the penis is assessed for significant outflow with normal arterial flow. At the same time, the urologist can evaluate the patient's response to an injection of a test dose of a vasoactive substance. This study may aid the genitourinary surgeon in determining whether or not the patient has erectile dysfunction that is likely to be psychologically mediated, secondary to neurologic deficits such as those found in diabetics, because of arterial or venous insufficiency, or a combination of these causes. Therefore the study can be used to streamline the patient's investigation and treatment. It is also useful in evaluating the penile shaft for scarring (Peyronie's disease) or masses as occasionally seen with metastasis.

Dynamic infusion cavernosometry and cavernosography (DICC) studies the venous trapping mechanism of penile erection (Fig. 4-16). There are four phases to the examination. Initially, after injection of a local anesthetic, a vasodilator (papaverine hydrochloride or prostaglandin E_1) is injected into the corpus cavernosum through butterfly needles placed dorsally on each side just above the penile head. Cavernosal responses are measured after 10 minutes with a pressure transducer recording through one of the needles in the erectile body.

Penile venous competence is measured in the second phase. Heparinized saline is rapidly infused into the penis until a preestablished suprasystolic pressure is obtained. The infusion is stopped and the rate of venous runoff is assessed. In phase three, arterial compliance is measured, again with heparinized saline. Several infusions are performed in both corporal bodies, and right and left cavernosal artery occlusion pressure is determined with a Doppler transducer. In the final phase, contrast material is infused slowly into the corpora cavernosa and serial x-ray images are obtained.

Erectile dysfunction can be evaluated for venous leakage or incompetence, arterial insufficiency, neuropathic dysfunction, and psychogenic dysfunction. It is particularly useful for those who are not successful with the standard pharmacologic injection program.

Transrectal ultrasonographies and biopsies (TRUS Bxs) are commonly performed in the urologist's office using a high frequency transrectal ultrasonographic transducer to assess the prostate gland. The size, volume, and shape of the prostate may be assessed in addition to the likelihood of the presence of a

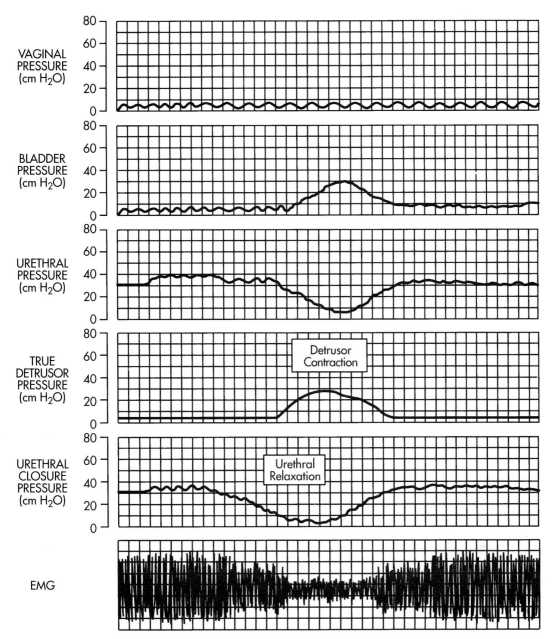

Fig. 4-11 Urethrocystometry, multi-channel showing detrusor instability. Observe urethral relaxation and quieting of EMG activity. *(From Walters MD:* Clinical urogynecology, *St. Louis, 1993, Mosby.)*

malignancy (Fig. 4-17). Suspicious areas or lesions may be biopsied with a needle passed under ultrasonographic guidance across the rectal wall. Color flow imaging may also be utilized to help in the identification of areas that are likely invaded with prostatic carcinoma or acute and chronic inflammation. A full bladder helps delineate the base of the prostate.

The prostate is visualized in three dimensions allowing more accurate localization of abnormalities and extent of disease. For the axial view, the transducer (probe) is placed deeply in the rectum, just proximal to the seminal vesicles. Here the vas deferens may be distinguished. The transducer is slowly withdrawn to the level of the base of the gland, enabling visualization of the inner gland. To obtain the longitudinal per-

spective, a side-viewing transducer is placed to the level of the prostate, where the midline image (inner gland) is obtained. Seminal vesicles are seen in cross section. To evaluate the lateral lobes the transducer may be rotated clockwise or counterclockwise. A series of "sextant" (six) biopsies is generally taken with a disposable "core biopsy" needle. These are taken from the right and left apex, the right and left midline, and the right and left base.

Although digital rectal examination is the first step following PSA in detecting prostate abnormalities, all lesions are not palpable. An elevated PSA, the patient's history, and what is visualized during the ultrasonogram may indicate the need for a biopsy.

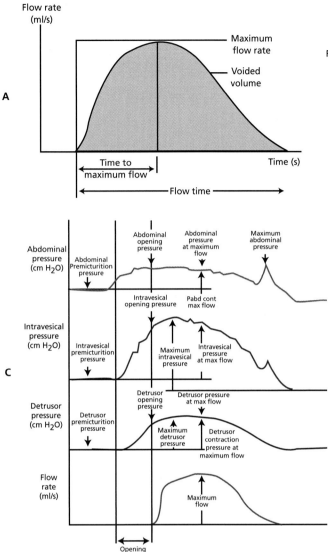

Flow rate
(ml/s)

Maximum
flow rate

Voided
volume

A

Time to
maximum flow

Time (s)

Flow time

Flow rate
(ml/s)

B

Voiding time

Time (s)

Abdominal
pressure
(cm H₂O)

Abdominal
opening
pressure

Abdominal
pressure at
maximum
flow

Maximum
abdominal
pressure

Abdominal
Premicturition
pressure

Intravesical
opening pressure

Pabd cont
max flow

Intravesical
pressure
(cm H₂O)

Intravesical
premicturition
pressure

Maximum
intravesical
pressure

Intravesical
pressure
at max flow

C

Detrusor
pressure
(cm H₂O)

Detrusor
opening
pressure

Detrusor pressure
at max flow

Detrusor
premicturition
pressure

Maximum
detrusor
pressure

Detrusor
contraction
pressure at
maximum flow

Flow
rate
(ml/s)

Maximum
flow

Opening
time

Fig. 4-12 **A,** Continuous urine flow recording with ICS (International Continence Society) recommended nomenclature. **B,** Interrupted urine flow recording with ICS recommended nomenclature. **C,** Pressure flow recording of micturition with ICS recommended nomenclature. *(From Walters MD:* Clinical urogynecology, *St. Louis, 1993, Mosby.)*

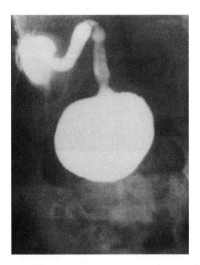

Fig. 4-13 Normal micturating cystogram in a male with contrast inside prepuce. *(From Lloyd-Davies W:* Color atlas of urology, *ed 2, London, 1994, Mosby-Wolfe.)*

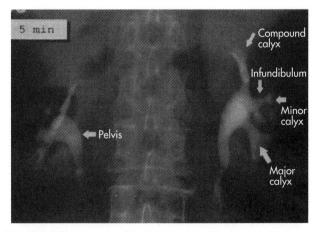

5 min

Compound
calyx

Infundibulum

Minor
calyx

Pelvis

Major
calyx

Fig. 4-14 Tomogram of both kidneys at 5 minutes. *(From Gillenwater et al:* Adult and pediatric urology, *ed 3, St. Louis, 1996, Mosby.)*

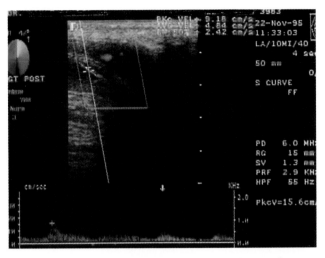

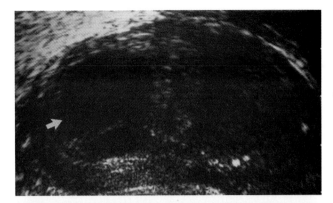

A

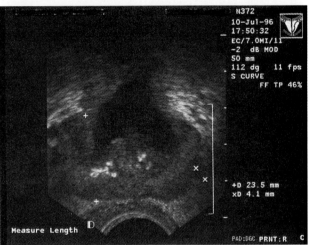

B

Fig. 4-15 Normal papaverine-stimulated penile Doppler ultrasonogram. The deep cavernosal arteries are identified by color Doppler *(red line)* and the spectral wave form measured. In this study, maximum arterial flow in systole is 15.6 centimeters/sec.

Fig. 4-17 A, Sagittal transrectal ultrasonogram using the end-firing transducer. Dark area right of center is a portion of the prostate anterior to the urethra. Prostate is seen as a clam shell shape partially surrounding the bladder (dark area left of center). Hyperechoic foci may be visualized in lower right of prostate near the apex. **B,** Transverse axial transrectal ultrasonogram using end-firing transducer. Prostate is seen as a horseshoe shape surrounding bladder (darkened area in center). Hyperechoic foci are again seen in the lower middle of the gland.

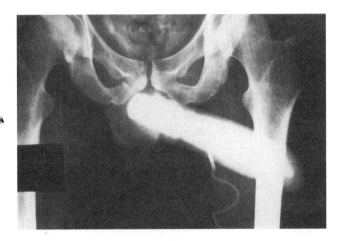

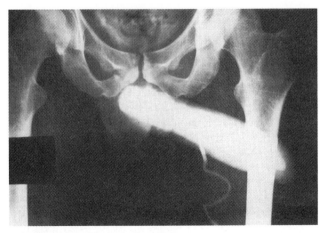

Fig. 4-16 A, Normal corpora cavernosum. *(From Whitehead ED:* Impotence and infertility, *Philadelphia, 1994, Lippincott.)* **B,** Pump for DICC. *(From Gray M:* Genitourinary disorders, *St. Louis, 1992, Mosby.)*

The most important potential complication of a biopsy is systemic infection. This can be eliminated by providing antibiotic coverage pre- and postprocedure and by the use of an enema before the examination. The patient is placed on antibiotic therapy 24 hours before the procedure and requested to use a Fleets enema 2 to 3 hours before the test is performed. Before the examination, antiseptic solution mixed with a viscous local anesthetic is often instilled in the rectum and allowed to coat the tissues for 5 to 15 minutes.

NONINVASIVE DIAGNOSTIC PROCEDURES

The patient's chart may also contain the results of several noninvasive diagnostic examinations. The following are those most often found.

Ultrasonography (ultrasound) uses high-frequency sound waves, rather than radionuclide counts (radiation), to visualize the urinary system (Fig. 4-18). A number of images can be

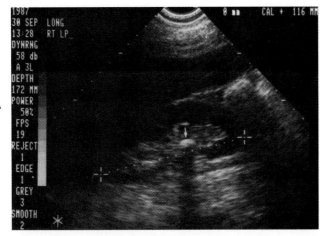

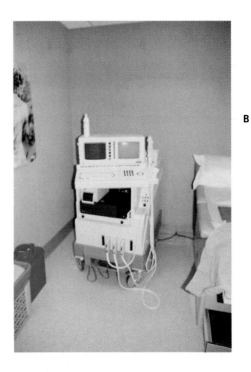

Fig. 4-18 **A,** Transrectal ultrasound of prostatic abscess with large echopenic region in the right prostate *(arrow).* *(From Drach GW:* Common problems in infections and stones, *St. Louis, 1992, Mosby.)* **B,** Ultrasound unit.

obtained and the tests can be repeated without threat of radiation exposure. Often, these examinations may be carried out in the urologist's office, lowering the cost to the patient.

Common indications for ultrasonographic examination are urinary calculi, recurrent urinary tract infections with or without fever, asymmetric prostate enlargement, testicular irregularities, and abdominal masses. The procedure holds no risk to the patient. This study may also be performed to assess for the presence of areas that appear to be involved with chronic prostatitis or occupied by prostatic calculi and, in cases of male infertility, for congenital absence of seminal vesicles, and ejaculatory duct obstruction.

Ultrasonography may be utilized intraoperatively to locate renal and prostatic calculi, to evaluate the extent of intrarenal tumor, or to insert percutaneous nephrostomy tubes.

Renal ultrasonography (scan) allows images of the kidneys, renal pelvis, and ureters in the prone and supine positions. Conducting jelly is placed on the patient's abdomen or back and images are obtained with the transducer. Transverse (axial) and sagittal (longitudinal) views and measurements can be obtained.

Hydronephrosis can be detected as well as dilatation of the upper ureters. In addition, calculi (Fig. 4-19), solid tumors, and renal cysts may be seen or suspected by virtue of the ultrasonographic presentation. Hydronephrosis and renal cysts produce a dark area on ultrasonographic examination as a result of the absence of an acoustic interface in the fluid contained inside the kidney or cyst. Calculi, on the other hand, produce a bright echo with shadowing behind them because they block the transmission of the ultrasonic waves. Solid tumors cause distortion of the normal renal architecture on ultrasonogram and are therefore unmasked, and can be appreciated, by ultrasonographic examination when they are present. Renal cysts are very common and if all of the criteria for a renal cyst are fulfilled then no further investigation is required. Renal masses that do

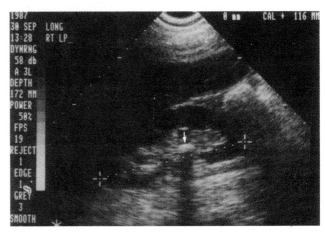

Fig. 4-19 Renal ultrasonogram, calculus right kidney *(arrow)* with characteristic acoustic shadowing. *(From Drach GW:* Common problems in infections and stones, *St. Louis, 1992, Mosby.)*

not fulfill all of the requirements for a cyst necessitate at least a follow-up ultrasonographic examination or computed tomography (CT) scan to rule out malignancy.

Bladder scan produces sonolucent bladder images when there is urine present in the lower urinary tract (Fig. 4-20). The suprapubic area is scanned with the conducting jelly and transducer with the patient in the supine position.

Although a normal ureter cannot be distinguished, dilated ureters become visible. A comparison of full and post voiding bladder volumes allows evaluation of the efficiency of micturition. An estimate of bladder volume can also be measured.

Prostate scan is achieved by the gentle insertion of a transrectal transducer into the rectum. A fluid-filled condom is

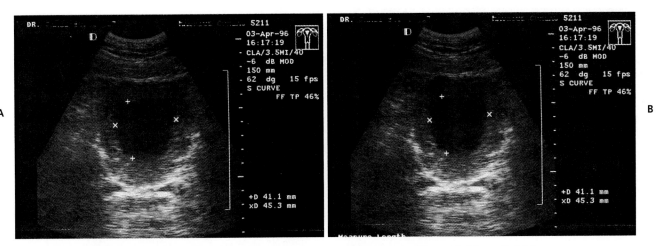

Fig. 4-20 A, Full bladder in male patient on ultrasonogram, displaying bladder wall thickening as a result of long-term bladder outlet obstruction. **B,** Full bladder in female patient on ultrasonogram. *(From Lloyd-Davies W: Color atlas of urology, ed 2, London, 1994, Mosby-Wolfe.)*

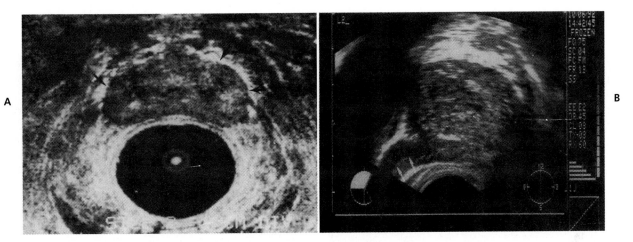

Fig. 4-21 A, Transverse axial transrectal ultrasonogram of a well-defined and predominantly homogenous prostate gland. **B,** Sagittal transrectal ultrasound of the prostate. *(From Gillenwater et al: Adult and pediatric urology, ed 3, St. Louis, 1996, Mosby.)*

placed over the probe to enhance the images. Both axial and longitudinal views may be obtained (Figs. 4-21). It is considered noninvasive because body membranes are not violated. If a biopsy becomes necessary, the procedure falls into the realm of invasive diagnostics. Refer to the previous discussion of TRUS Bx for further information.

Testicular scan allows detection of masses by producing images over the testicular parenchyma with a Doppler transducer (Fig. 4-22).

CT scan affords computer-generated axial images of the abdominal contents as well as the male genitalia (Figs. 4-23 and 4-24). The kidneys, ureters, bladder, major renal vessels, and pelvic lymph nodes may all be viewed through this technique. Tumors of the urinary system, pelvic abscess, primary pelvic masses, and enlarged lymph nodes caused by metastatic invasion may be detected with this procedure.

The patient is placed supine on a conveyor-belt mechanism. The entire body is moved at precise distances to obtain the images needed. A measurement of tissue density is computed allowing for further diagnosis.

Magnetic resonance imaging (MRI) creates computer-generated films that rely on radio waves and alteration of the magnetic field produced by human tissue (Fig. 4-25). Living tissue emits a small electron field that may be altered by exposure to a stronger energy field. When the exposure is discontinued, the human protons return to a lower energy state and produce a signal that is detected and subsequently generated on an image. Coronal, transaxial, and sagittal views of the kidney, pelvic structures, prostate gland, scrotal contents, and penis may be obtained. Generally, MRI is employed when an abdominal, pelvic or renal mass is suspected or when a genitourinary system tumor may be present.

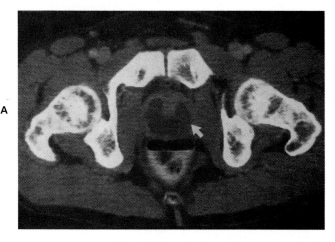

Fig. 4-22 A, Longitudinal scan of testis. *(From Gillenwater et al:* Adult and pediatric urology, *ed 3, St. Louis, 1996, Mosby.)*

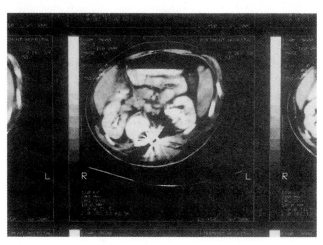

Fig. 4-23 Precontrast axial CT scan, normal anatomy of kidneys and surrounding tissues and organs. *(From Gray M:* Genitourinary Disorders, *St. Louis, 1992, Mosby.)*

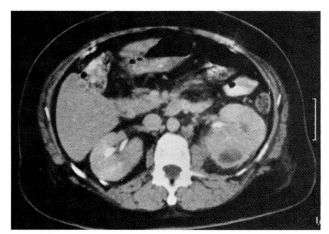

Fig. 4-24 A, CT scan of large prostatic abscess *(arrow).* **B,** CT scan with contrast, left intrarenal abscess, displayed by intrarenal mass in posterior portion of left kidney with blurring of the overlying cortical outline. *(From Drach GW:* Common problems in infections and stones, *St. Louis, 1992, Mosby.)*

Patients with a pacemaker in place are at risk for interference with the pacemaker's function. Surgical clips of stainless steel or other metallic implants may also alter the imaging.

KUB is an anteroposterior x-ray film of the kidneys, ureters, bony pelvis, and urinary bladder achieved without the use of contrast material (Fig. 4-26). It is common before genitourinary intervention and is used to detect the presence of radiopaque urinary calculi or abnormal bowel gas patterns. The latter may be present when there is a large abdominal, pelvic, or renal mass. Because the spine is also seen in the view provided, defects in the bony spinal column that could indicate neuropathic bladder dysfunction may also be apparent.

GLOSSARY

Amyloidosis Condition characterized by the deposit of a waxy, translucent substance of protein and polysaccharides (amyloid).

Analog Similar to in function but different in structure and origin.

Antegrade Performed in the usual direction of conduction or flow.

Artifact An artificial character caused by extraneous interference; an ECG or EEG wave arising from a source other than the heart or brain.

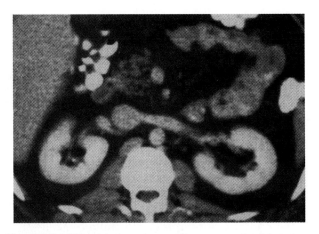

Fig. 4-25 MRI axial view. *(From Gillenwater et al: Adult and pediatric urology, ed 3, St. Louis, 1996, Mosby.)*

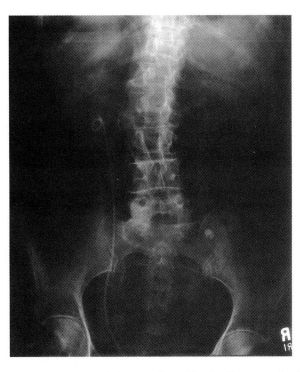

Fig. 4-26 KUB with left ureteral, double pigtail stent and calcification on the right.

Atrioventricular Situated between an atrium and a ventricle.

Bulbocavernosus Muscle surrounding and compressing the bulb of the penis and the bulbar urethra in the male; muscle that divides into lateral halves and extends from behind the clitoris along each side of the vagina to the central tendon of the perineum compressing the vagina in the female.

Calyces Cuplike divisions in the kidney pelvis surrounding one or more renal papillae.

Contractility Capability of shrinking or contracting; the power of muscle fibers to shorten into a more compact form.

Contralateral Acting in conjunction with similar parts on the opposite side.

Coronal Relating to the frontal plane that passes through the long axis of the body; relating to the upper section of a body part.

Corpus cavernosum A mass of erectile tissue with large interspaces capable of being distended with blood; forms the bulk of the penis or clitoris.

Diverticulum Abnormal pouch or sac opening from a hollow organ; a blind tube or sac branching off from a canal or cavity of the body.

Doppler Utilizing a shift in frequency according to the Doppler effect; used in anatomic measurements and in radar and navigation.

Doppler effect A change in the frequency in which waves from a given source reach the observer when in rapid motion with respect to each other; the frequency increases or decreases according to the speed at which the distance is decreasing or increasing.

Duplex Two waves of sound where one is used to measure the velocity of blood flow through a vessel and the other measures the rate of reflection of that sound; double ultrasound, one focusing on the vessel and the other on the area of interest.

Dysuria Painful or difficult discharge of urine.

Electromyogram A tracing made with an instrument that converts the electrical activity associated with functioning skeletal muscle into a visual record or audible sound; used to diagnose neuromuscular disorders and in biofeedback training.

Fibrillation Muscular twitching involving individual muscle fibers acting without coordination; very rapid irregular contractions of the muscle fibers of the heart resulting in a lack of synchronism between heartbeat and pulse.

Fistula An abnormal passage leading from an abscess or hollow organ to the body surface, or from one hollow organ to another, permitting passage of fluids or secretions.

Fluoroscopy Observation of internal structures by means of the shadow cast on a fluorescent screen when placed between the screen and a source of x-ray.

Fossa navicularis A depression between the posterior margin of the vaginal opening and the small fold of membrane covering the labia minora in the posterior vulva.

Gradient Change in the value of a quantity with change in a given variable per unit on a linear scale; a graded difference in physiologic activity along an axis.

Hypertonic Exhibiting excessive tone or tension; having a higher osmotic pressure than the surrounding medium or fluid.

Hyperuricuria Excretion of excessive amounts of uric acid in the urine.

Intravesical Occurring within the bladder.

Ionic Functioning by means of ions, free electrons or charged subatomic particles; radiopaque contrast material (Hypaque, Renografin, Conray) with a high concentration of iodine.

Ipsilateral Appearing on or affecting the same side of the body.

Ischemia Localized tissue anemia caused by obstruction of the inflow of arterial blood.

Longitudinal Occurring in the lengthwise dimension; extending along the anteroposterior axis of a body or part.

Morphology The form and structure of an organism or any of its parts.

Myeloma A primary tumor of the bone marrow formed of bone marrow cells usually involving several different bones at one time.

Nephric phase In renal arteriogram, when the injection of contrast material creates an image of the functioning kidney tissue before the contrast reaches the collecting system.

Neuropathic Abnormal or degenerated state of the nervous system or nerves.

Nonionic Water-soluble, iodine-bearing compound with low osmolality, characterized by the ratio of the number of atoms of iodine to the number of particles in solution for each molecule; radiopaque contrast material (Amnipaque, Omnipaque, Isovue 30) considered safer for patients with potential allergy to contrast material.

Opacification Process of becoming opaque or radiopaque, impervious to the rays of light.

Peyronie's disease Formation of fibrous plaques in one or both corpus cavernosa of the penis resulting in distortion or deflection of the erect organ.

Priapism Abnormal, persistent, painful penile erection caused by disease or injection therapy.

Radionuclide Radioactive nuclide, a species of atom.

Radiopaque Obstructing the transmission of radiation by absorption or reflection.

Reflex Automatic nerve response; vasovagal reaction.

Reflux Flowing backward, regurgitation.

Residual Remaining in a body cavity after maximum normal expulsion has occurred.

Retrograde Performed in the opposite direction of conduction or flow; catheterization.

Rhonchi Whistling or snoring sound heard on auscultation of the chest when air channels are partly obstructed.

Sagittal Being of the median plane of the body or any plane parallel to it.

Sequential In a sequence.

Sinogram X-ray study of a sinus following injection of contrast medium.

Sonolucent Giving passage to ultrasonic waves without producing echoes as a result of reflection of some of the waves.

Sonogram An image produced by ultrasonographic scanning.

Stricture An abnormal narrowing of a body passage as from inflammation, cancer, or formation of scar tissue.

Suprasystolic At a pressure above systolic blood pressure.

Tachycardia Relatively rapid heart action, physiologic (after exercise) or pathologic.

Thrombosis Formation or presence of a blood clot within a blood vessel.

Thrombus A clot of blood within a vessel that remains attached to its place of origin.

Tomography A diagnostic technique using x-rays where the shadows of structures before and behind the area under investigation do not show.

Transaxial Across an axis.

Transducer A device actuated by power from one system and supplying power in another form to a second system.

Transrectal Passing through the rectum.

Transverse Lying across, at right angles to the anteroposterior axis of the body.

Ultrasonography Diagnostic or therapeutic involving a two-dimensional image used for examination and measurement of internal body structures and the detection of abnormalities.

Ultrasound Rations of the same physical nature as sound but with frequencies above the range of human hearing.

Ureteropelvic Involving the ureter and adjoining renal pelvis.

Ureterovesical Relating to the ureteral juncture with the urinary bladder.

Urodynamic Measurement of the dynamic parameters of lower urinary tract function as in the intravesical pressure of urinary flow during the voiding cycle.

Urticaria An allergic disorder marked by raised edematous patches of skin or mucous membrane; intense itching caused by contact with a precipitating factor externally or internally; hives.

Vasoactive Affecting the blood vessels in respect to the degree of their relaxation or contraction.

Venous phase Stage during renal arteriogram (renogram) when veins fill with contrast material.

Bibliography

1. Bennett AH: *Impotence: diagnosis and management of erectile dysfunction*, Philadelphia, 1994, WB Saunders.
2. Brundage DJ: *Renal disorders*, St. Louis, 1992, Mosby.
3. Coussons TR, McKee PA, Williams GR: *Manual of medical care of the surgical patient*, Boston, 1990, Little, Brown.
4. Davidson AJ, Hartman DS: *Radiology of the kidney and urinary tract*, Philadelphia, 1994, WB Saunders.
5. Drach GW: *Common problems in infections and stones*, St. Louis, 1992, Mosby.

6. Droller MJ: *Surgical management of urologic disease,* St. Louis, 1992, Mosby.

7. Gray M: *Genitourinary disorders,* St. Louis, 1992, Mosby.

8. Kirby R, Christmas T: *Benign prostatic hyperplasia,* London, 1993, Gower.

9. Lloyd-Davies W et al: *Color atlas of urology,* London, 1994, Mosby-Wolfe.

10. Meeker MH, Rothrock JC: *Alexander's care of the patient in surgery,* ed 10, St. Louis, 1995, Mosby.

11. O'Reilly PH, George NJR, Weiss RM: *Diagnostic techniques in urology,* Philadelphia, 1990, WB Saunders.

12. Resnick MI, Kursh E: *Current therapy in genitourinary surgery,* St. Louis, 1992, Mosby.

13. Resnick MI: *Prostatic ultrasonography,* Philadelphia, 1990, WB Saunders.

14. Resnick MI, Novick AC: *Urology secrets,* St. Louis, 1995, Mosby.

15. Rifkin MD: *Ultrasound of the prostate,* New York, 1988, Raven.

16. Smith JA: *The urologic clinics of North America,* Philadelphia, 1990, WB Saunders.

17. Tanagho EA, McAninch JW: *Smith's general urology,* Norwalk, 1995, Appleton & Lange.

18. Walters MD, Karram MM: *Clinical urogynecology,* St. Louis, 1993, Mosby.

5

Perioperative Nursing Care

The Physician, the Drugs, the Nurse, and the Patient constitute an aggregate of four. Of what virtues each of these should be possessed, so as to become causes for the cure of the disease, should be known.
Physician. Thorough mastery of the scriptures, large experience, cleverness, and purity ...are the principal qualities of the physician.
Drugs. Abundance of virtue, adaptability to the disease under treatment, the capacity of being used in diverse ways, and undeterioration are attributes of drugs.
Nurse. Knowledge of the manner in which drugs should be prepared or compounded for administration, cleverness, devotedness to the patient waited on, and purity ... are the four qualifications of the attending nurse.
Patient. Memory, obedience to direction, fearlessness, and communicativeness ... are the qualities of the patient....
Like clay, stick, wheel, threads, in the absence of the potter, failing to produce anything by their combination, the three others, viz., drugs, nurse, and patient cannot work out a cure in the absence of the physician. [Team concept of medical care]

Kaviratna, n.d.

THE GENITOURINARY SURGICAL TEAM

The success of any surgical intervention is in direct relation to the efficiency of the perioperative team. The influence of advanced diagnostic measures and high-tech equipment has resulted in an expansion of that team beyond the intraoperative setting. It is imperative that communication extend beyond the patient. Collaboration is necessary to ensure continuity of care to the genitourinary patient population.

Direct communication between the perioperative nurse, surgeon, and office personnel allows for accurate preoperative preparation, so that both procedural and specific patient needs are addressed. Other disciplines are often involved in some aspect of genitourinary surgery. Collaboration with other departments within the hospital or ambulatory surgery setting affords the perioperative nurse a concise patient profile. Precise transfer of information will decrease potential delays, improve patient care, and favorably affect the surgical outcome. An understanding of the roles that these services play allows a "person-oriented" approach to care.

Scheduling requires providing staff members with the appropriate skills and knowledge to afford patient safety, decrease intraoperative and anesthesia time, and limit tissue exposure. The genitourinary staff includes personnel to assist with patient transport, transfer, preparation, and positioning in addition to those fulfilling the circulating, scrub, assistant, and anesthesia roles.

Genitourinary Surgeon

Finally let me say that a great surgeon cannot be recognized by the public. They have no way of judging between a good doctor and a quack or between a real surgeon and a mere pretender. The cardinal way of judging of a surgeon's work is to see it done and to be allowed to see the final results of the operations. A great surgeon will therefore always be willing to invite colleagues, young ones as well as prominent ones, to witness his operations, to watch his after-treatment, and to study his results. An infallible sign of a great surgeon is his willingness not only to show his results, but to teach and demonstrate his methods to students and colleagues from any or all quarters of the globe .... Great surgeons owe it to mankind to make the art of surgery as accessible and free as the science.

August Charles Bernays

The role of the urologist is ever changing as a result of new innovations and advanced technology. Surgical procedures are being refined to provide optimum outcome with minimal invasion and surgical stay. Continual perfection of equipment, instrumentation, supplies, and surgical procedures presents the genitourinary surgeon with a constant challenge. Public media has caused an increase in patient demand for new procedures. This has led to increased specialization and individualized patient care. Urologists now find the field opening new vistas that include management of erectile dysfunction, infertility treatment, cancer therapies, incontinence management, stone management, and correction of congenital and degenerative conditions.

The genitourinary surgeon has become increasingly dependent on the knowledge and expertise of the genitourinary perioperative team. This dependence results in a multidisciplinary environment providing nurses with opportunities for extended practice through their expanded role. It is therefore ever more important for perioperative nurses to refine their practice to facilitate the surgical course.

A relatively new subspecialty, that of the urogynecologist, has appeared on the surgical scene. Board-certified gynecologists have now expanded their practice to include minor urologic interventions in female patients, such as cystoscopy and suprapubic catheter insertion.

Perioperative Genitourinary Nurse

Woman is an instinctive nurse, taught by Mother Nature. The nurse has always been a necessity, and thus lacked social status. In primitive times she was a slave, and in the civilized era a domestic. Overlooked in the plans of legislators, and forgotten in the curricula of pedagogues, she was left without protection and remained without education. She was not an artisan who could obtain the help of an hereditary guild; there was no Hanseatic League for nurses. Drawn from the nameless and numberless army of the poverty, the nurse worked as a menial and obeyed as a servant. Denied the dignity of a trade, and devoid of professional ethics, she could not rise above the degradation of her environement. It never occurred to the Aristotles of the past that it would be safer for the public welfare if nurses were educated instead of lawyers. The untrained nurse is as old as the human race; the trained nurse is a recent discovery. The distinction between the two is a sharp commentary on the follies and prejudices of mankind.

Victor Robinson

Perioperative nursing encompasses the preoperative, intraoperative, and postoperative stages of direct patient surgical care. Registered nurses specializing in perioperative genitourinary nursing perform nursing activities in these phases in various health care settings. Some of these are acute and long-term care facilities, ambulatory care and inpatient hospital settings, research or teaching centers, home or hospice care, and urology clinics or offices. Because treatment options have expanded dramatically as a result of innovative technologies for diagnostic and surgical purposes, genitourinary surgery has become more complex.

The perioperative genitourinary nurse is challenged to keep abreast of these advancements through the certification processes and educational opportunities available. Competency is defined as "the knowledge, skills, and abilities necessary to fulfill the professional role functions of a registered nurse in the operating room."[4] The nurse specializing in urology serves as educator and resource to other members of the health care team with commitment to excellence a priority.

Perioperative nurses need to validate their practice by certification through the NCB:PNI (National Certification Board of Perioperative Nursing, Inc., Denver, Colo.) and by attaining a CNOR (certified nurse operating room). The genitourinary nurse may also keep abreast of current trends in urology through SUNA (Society of Urologic Nurses and Associates, Pitman, New Jersey), formerly known as the American Urological Association Allied, Inc. A CURN (certified urology registered nurse) may be attained through the CBUNA (Certification Board for Urologic Nurses and Associates, Pitman, N.J.).

Because of advancements in genitourinary surgery, more procedures are being done on an outpatient basis. The holistic approach to patient care becomes increasingly important, involving the family in the teaching process. Individuals of all ages suffer from congenital, traumatic, infectious, endocrinologic, metabolic, degenerative, inflammatory, and oncologic conditions. The registered nurse specializing in genitourinary surgery has the opportunity to influence this ever-increasing population by promoting self-care, wellness, and prevention of injury.

Corrective genitourinary procedures often allow the patient to return to a lifestyle and activity level that would have otherwise resulted in aggravation of their condition. Through implementation of the nursing process, patient care can be individualized and surgical outcomes enhanced.

In many settings, the perioperative genitourinary nurse functions in the capacity of the circulating nurse. The primary role of the circulating nurse is to implement the nursing process. Perioperative planning, assessment, implementation, and evaluation are integral to the role. He or she functions as the patient's advocate as nursing activities are planned and implemented. The genitourinary nurse also has the ability to function in the role of scrub nurse, preceptor for new employees, and RN first assistant if the appropriate training has been accomplished.

Registered Nurse First Assistant

We claim, and I think justly, the status of a profession; we have schools and teachers, tuition fees and scholarships, systems of instruction from preparatory to postgraduate; we are allied with technical schools on one hand and here and there a university on the other; we have libraries, a literature, and fast-growing numbers of periodicals owned, edited, and published by nurses; we have societies and laws. If therefore we claim to receive the appurtenances, privileges, and standing of a profession, we must recognize professional responsibilities and obligations which we are in honor bound to respect and uphold.

M. Adelaide Nutting

The RN first assistant (RNFA) role involves a unique set of competencies based on a didactic and supervised clinical learning regimen. In 1980 the American College of Surgeons issued statements supporting the appropriateness of qualified RNs to first assist. Intraoperative responsibilities of the RNFA are a refinement of perioperative nursing practice and include but are not limited to the following:

- Handling tissue
- Providing exposure
- Using instruments
- Suturing
- Providing hemostasis

The RNFA demonstrates behaviors that progress on a continuum from basic competency to excellence.[2] Functioning in a collaborative relationship with the operating surgeon, the RNFA performs a single role, under the direct supervision of the surgeon, to assist in the safe performance of procedures and achieve optimum patient outcome. Certification is available to RNFAs through the NCB:PNI.

Many genitourinary procedures require assistance beyond the scrub technician or nurse, and the RNFA will generally be called on. When there is an RNFA assigned, the patient communication process can be enhanced. This process can be handled by the RNFA, allowing more time for exchange of information to take place, while the balance of the team prepares the room. The RNFA assisting in genitourinary surgery should have a thorough knowledge of genitourinary anatomy and the procedure to be performed as well as of the potential risks and expected outcome for the patient. This expanded understanding will augment the communication and teaching process. Attention to the details of instrumentation, equipment, positioning requirements, and the principles of the procedure are essential to practice. Genitourinary surgery frequently requires assistance to maintain exposure of the surgical site. The RNFA must be able to anticipate and meet needs as they occur. When managed appropriately, the activities of the RNFA benefit the patient and the urologist for a timely and uneventful procedure with minimal tissue trauma.

Surgical Technologist

In dwelling upon the vital importance of sound observation, it must never be lost sight of what observation is for. It is not for the sake of piling up miscellaneous information or curious facts, but for the sake of saving life and increasing health and comfort.

Florence Nightingale

The surgical technologist functions in the sterile scrub role for most genitourinary procedures. Responsibilities include maintaining an aseptic field and a comprehensive understanding of surgical procedures as well as the required supplies and instrumentation. A knowledge of the anatomy involved in the procedure is important for the surgical technologist to remain attuned to the needs of the surgeon.

The surgical technologist complements the activities of the perioperative and anesthesia teams. Technical skills should encompass safe handling and preparation of equipment, maintaining a safe environment, and assisting in patient care as deemed appropriate by the perioperative nurse. Surgical technologists may attain certification through the Association of Operating Room Technicians (Littleton, Colo.).

Anesthesia Team

The vocation of nursing goes hand in hand with that of the physician and surgeon, and they are absolutely indispensable one to the other. Incompetency on the part of the nurse renders negatory the best efforts of the doctor in the most critical moments, and has frequently resulted in the loss of life. All the most brilliant achievements of modern surgery are dependent, to a great extent, upon careful and intelligent nursing. . . . The skilled nurse, by minutely watching the temperature, conditions of the skin, pulse, respiration, and the functions of all the organs, and reporting faithfully to the attending physician, must increase the chances of recovery two-fold.

Gibbon and Mathewson 1947, p. 145

The anesthetic of choice in genitourinary surgery is determined according to the surgical procedure being performed, the pre-

operative interview with the anesthesiologist, and both patient and surgeon preference. Many genitourinary procedures are done with a spinal or regional anesthetic accompanied by intravenous sedation.

The patient may be monitored by the anesthesiologist or by a certified registered nurse anesthetist (CRNA). It is the role of the anesthesia department to maintain the patient in a safe and pain-free state for the duration of the surgical procedure. Therefore the anesthesia personnel need to have a working knowledge of the procedure being performed and the average time needed to complete the procedure. Often the position required for the procedure places an undesirable stress on the patient's cardiac status. The anesthetist is responsible for closely monitoring the patient and controlling the speed at which positions are changed to avoid any undesirable reactions.

The genitourinary patient is frequently at risk for alterations in his or her hemodynamic status. The perioperative nurse specializing in urology should be aware of common anesthetic side effects and be alert to any changes in the patients status. Communication and teamwork will afford a smooth surgical course for the patient.

Other Care Providers

Genitourinary surgery requires support personnel from various services within the hospital or ambulatory surgery setting as well as providers of care or services from outside the facility. All are necessary collaborators in providing satisfactory patient care. The support personnel may include the pathologist, laboratory technician, radiologist, radiology technologist, oncologist, product representative, laser technician, enterostomal therapist, home health care provider, and other assistive personnel.

Laboratory personnel

The majority of genitourinary procedures require some or all of the following preoperative laboratory studies: complete blood count (CBC); prothrombin and partial thromboplastin time (PT, PTT); bleeding time; blood chemistry profiles that include blood urea nitrogen (BUN), serum glucose, and creatinine; cardiac enzymes; serum and urine electrolytes; urinalysis and urine cultures; special studies for fertility; and prostate specific antigen (PSA). Intraoperatively, arterial blood gases, hemoglobin, and hematocrit may be required. Laboratory personnel play a key support role by responding to the needs of the surgical team in a timely and accurate manner. It is important that preoperative laboratory results are made available before the start of any genitourinary procedure.

It is not uncommon to rely on frozen-section biopsy evaluations during genitourinary interventions. The pathologist plays a key role in establishing a rapid and accurate diagnosis. Procedures for the eradication of carcinoma are often predicated upon the pathologist's consultative and diagnostic abilities. Diagnosis is officially confirmed with histologic examinations.

Radiology personnel

Radiographic studies of the genitourinary system are required for almost every procedure. Some of these are intravenous urography (IVU), computed tomography (CT scan), magnetic resonance imaging (MRI), KUB (genitourinary flat plate of kidneys, ureters, and bladder), and radiographic examinations utilizing fluoroscopy such as angiography and cavernosography. Additionally, many genitourinary procedures require use of the portable x-ray unit or C-arm fluoroscopy intraoperatively.

The role of the radiologist is specialized, and his or her expertise in evaluating the studies done by means of written reports is important to a satisfactory surgical encounter. This expanded specialization may include the uroradiologist and the interventional radiologist, though intraoperatively the surgeon often assumes this role.

An experienced urologist with access to ultrasonographic and radiographic equipment often performs procedures himself. Frequently, however, the interventional radiologist or uroradiologist is responsible for the placement of percutaneous nephrostomy tubes, renal cyst aspirations, dilation of stenotic ureters, renal angiography, and renal or ureteral stenting procedures.

The certified radiology technologist plays a key support role during those procedures requiring C-arm fluoroscopy or radiography. A knowledge of aseptic technique, patient size and position, and the desired surgical outcome allows the technologist to function in synchronization with the operative team. A technologist who can anticipate the surgical needs enhances the final outcome.

Oncologist

Many genitourinary procedures are performed on patients with carcinoma. The oncologist plays a key role in the preoperative, intraoperative, and postoperative care of these patients. Communication with the surgeon and perioperative nurse will establish a framework for developing a patient-specific plan of care.

Product representative

The role of the product representative has become increasingly important as genitourinary surgery expands in new directions, requiring costly and specialized equipment and implants that many facilities cannot afford to purchase. The representative who is attuned to the needs of hospitals and ambulatory facilities, in addition to the needs of the surgeon, performs a valuable service to the patient.

Communication between the product representative and the perioperative genitourinary nurse must clearly establish the needs of the team. The availability of implants and other devices needs to be assured through the product representative. Ensuring that stock supplies are maintained and at appropriate levels for the volume of procedures performed must be a priority for the genitourinary team. As new products are developed, the registered nurse has a responsibility to become involved in the evaluation process. An objective attitude toward the available products will ultimately benefit the patient, surgeon, and facility.

Laser technician

Many facilities cannot afford the purchase of the laser units required for genitourinary surgery. These procedures are then scheduled with advance notice, and a laser unit from an outside source is rented. A certified laser technician always accompanies these units and functions within the operative setting. Knowledge of the specialty and the procedures being performed and an understanding of aseptic technique and laser safety are crucial to the expected surgical outcome.

Enterostomal therapist

When major genitourinary surgery involves the removal of the urinary bladder, a urostomy, or stoma, will be fashioned on the patient's abdomen. When this surgery is planned the certified wound, ostomy, and continence nurse (WOCN) assesses the patient for proper placement of the stomal site. These nurses are extended-practice nurses and are certified in wound and ostomy care through the International Association for Enterostomal Therapy (IAET; Irvine, Calif.). Collaboration with the surgeon and perioperative genitourinary nurse allows for a patient-specific placement and results in a smooth postoperative course. An improperly placed stoma will cause unnecessary restrictions on the patient and may lead to breakdown of the site.

Home health care providers

Genitourinary procedures are increasingly being done on an outpatient basis. Some of these procedures require postoperative pain or antibiotic management. Various home health care agencies offer this service, commonly known as PCA (patient-controlled analgesia or antibiotics). Outpatient PCA programs offer subcutaneous injection of the required medication.

Before the procedure the health care worker meets with and interviews the patient to set up an appropriate program of care based on the surgeon's choice of medication. Immediately after the procedure the health care provider attends to the patient while in the recovery unit, placing the PCA unit and reviewing its operation. This service allows the patient to return home earlier and be involved in managing his or her own care. Overall cost to the patient is potentially decreased by removing the necessity for inpatient management.

Assistive personnel

Caring for the genitourinary patient can be physically and mentally demanding. The variety of positions employed obviates the need for personnel trained in proper body mechanics, for both the patient and themselves, to accomplish proper patient transfer and positioning. Knowledgable support personnel within the department can play a key role in meeting desired surgical outcomes.

The opportunity for collaborative nursing care extends to all individuals providing care to the genitourinary patient. Recognition of the unique skills each individual can provide, concise and accurate communication of the patient's needs, and a sense of common purpose among the caregivers enhances the role each person plays and benefits everyone. Genitourinary patients have special and frequently unique needs that will benefit from this approach. Commitment to quality and excellence, patient advocacy, and dedication to the same common goal will achieve the very best result for each patient.

STANDARDS OF PERIOPERATIVE NURSING

"Standards are authoritative statements that describe the responsibilities for which nursing practitioners are accountable".[4] These standards reflect the values and priorities of the nursing profession and serve as a method for directing and evaluating nursing practice. The "Standards of Perioperative Nursing"[4] are generic and applicable to all nurses in perioperative nursing practice, no matter what the educational preparation, clinical specialty, or employment setting. The standards are intended to be implemented within the framework of the American Nurses Association (ANA) "Code for Nurses with Interpretive Statements" and its "Explications for Perioperative Nursing." The Agency for Health Care Policy and Research (AHCPR, Rockville, Md.) has also established clinical practice guidelines for perioperative nursing practice.[4]

AORN's perioperative nursing standards are categorized into structure, process, and outcome standards. The process and outcome standards and their correlating competency statements are the guide for those in clinical practice. Process standards include "Standards of Perioperative Clinical Practice," "Standards of Perioperative Professional Performance," and "Quality Improvement Standards for Perioperative Nursing." The outcome standards are encompassed in the "Standards of Perioperative Care."

SUNA's basic tenets include high standards of patient care that are continually updated, competence and excellence in varied practice settings through education, research for growth and expertise in practice, a team approach to patient care through interdisciplinary communication, and responsibility to respond to the public and private sectors concerning issues that affect urologic nursing practice. "The purpose of the American Urological Association Allied, Inc., is to unite urologic allied health professionals to promote the highest quality of urologic education and professional standards for the better and safer care of the urologic patient/client."[1] The "Standards of Urologic Nursing Practice" define the optimal levels of care, assessment, and intervention by means of eight nursing diagnoses that represent those most commonly occurring among the urologic patient population. Embracing a holistic approach to patient care, the standards are meant to be implemented within the framework of the "Standards of Nursing Practice," published by the American Nurses Association.

Incorporating the nursing process with the technical skills necessary for perioperative care changes the focus to center on the patient as a unique individual. Perioperative nurses are expected to assess, diagnose, plan, intervene, and evaluate within a limited time frame. The role of a specialist in genitourinary surgery requires independent judgment and action initiated by the nurse for the benefit of the patient.

The genitourinary population is unique in its diversity as it spans age, race, gender, socioeconomic status, and cultural and ethnic background. Individuality of the genitourinary patient is also apparent in his or her anatomic structure, psychosocial condition, and physiologic integrity. When those caring for the genitourinary patient have a comprehensive understanding of the genitourinary system, physiologic limitations and needs, and the procedures designed to correct dysfunctions, care can be individualized.

Care of Special Populations

It is a very common error among the well to think that "with a little more self-control" the sick might, if they choose, "dismiss painful thoughts" which "aggravate their disease," etc. . . . Almost any sick person who behaves decently well exercises more self-control every moment of his day than you will ever know till you are sick yourself."

Florence Nightingale

The genitourinary population varies from infants with congenital anomalies to the elderly with physiologic limitations. Staff must be attuned to the specific demands each patient poses and be prepared to tailor the plan of care accordingly.

When dealing with the pediatric patient, it is critical to include the parents or caregivers in the process. To allay the stress and fear that parents unknowingly transfer to the child, preoperative teaching must be specific, concise, and diplomatically honest. During the assessment phase, questions should be directed to the parents as well as to the child, if at all possible, and expressed in a nonjudgmental manner. Perceptions about the surgical experience and the recovery period need to be determined, clarified, and confirmed or corrected as necessary. Pediatric patients tend to recover rapidly, and it is valuable that the parents be aware of this. Intraoperative care must also be structured to address pediatric concerns such as fluid volume and the increased need for warmth and comfort.

Care of the elderly genitourinary patient must incorporate an understanding of the normal aging process. As people age, bones develop a tendency toward osteoporosis, joints may be inflamed with arthritis, and cardiopulmonary status may be compromised with accompanying peripheral or cardiovascular disease. Intraoperative care should be planned to avoid further damage to these systems through the use of protective measures and a coordinated team approach. Genitourinary procedures often involve the flank or lithotomy position, raising the risk for brachial plexus injury, pressure on the vena cava, and vascular or pulmonary compromise.

Thorough assessment of the adult patient will determine what coping mechanisms are firmly in place and what unaddressed fears or anxieties should be dealt with. Fear of cancer or altered lifestyle is common among this population, and the perioperative nurse is afforded a unique opportunity to assist these people toward wellness. The elderly patient should be assessed for the ability to ambulate early and perform self-care to avoid postoperative embolus or thrombosis. Dependency on others often leads to lowered self-esteem and depression. Efforts toward independence need to be encouraged to avoid this psychologic complication. Alterations in sight or hearing may also be present and require special attention.

Communication

In all diseases it is important, but in diseases which do not run a distinct and fixed course, it is not only important, it is essential that the facts the nurse alone can observe, should be accurately observed, and accurately reported.

Florence Nightingale

Communication is an art form and a basic necessity for the nursing process to function properly. The perioperative environment does not afford a lot of time, and concise, accurate communication skills must be honed. To plan patient care with a person-oriented approach, both verbal and nonverbal techniques need to be employed. Tension, anxiety, and embarrassment are often increased when there is a noticeable absence of privacy or space. The perioperative genitourinary nurse has the responsibility to eliminate as many environmental distractions as possible to enhance the communication process.

Data collected by the preoperative nurse should be reviewed and clarified when necessary. The plan of care should be discussed with the anesthesiologist and anesthetist who will be attending the patient. Any physiologic limitations need to be incorporated into the intraoperative plan.

Assessment

The most important lession that can be given to nurses is to teach them what to observe—how to observe—what symptoms indicate improvement—what the reverse—which are of importance—which are of none—which are the evidence of neglect—and of what kind of neglect.

Florence Nightingale

Patient assessment usually begins in the urologist's office. Because of the potential for compromise to other organ systems, this preoperative evaluation is generally quite thorough from both a physiologic and a psychologic standpoint.

The goal of perioperative assessment is collection of data to identify the nursing diagnosis, to communicate pertinent information, and to provide continuity of the nursing process. Beginning the planning phase of the perioperative experience requires a thorough nursing assessment. Perioperative genitourinary nurses should always perform their own physical and psychologic evaluation of the patient. This will provide accurate measures of health and function at the time of surgery that can be compared with the preoperative work-up completed in the office setting. Often patients forget significant details such as medication allergies in one setting but mention them in another. To maintain continuity of care it is beneficial for the intraoperative nurse to establish contact with those performing the initial patient assessments.

Synthesis of information and individualized patient care plans are necessary because of the wide range of urologic procedures. Accurate information will decrease confusion and increase the success of intraoperative interventions. General guidelines to be met for every genitourinary procedure include the following:

- Verification of the patient and operative procedure
- Understanding of the surgical procedure to be performed
- Complete and accurate consent form for the procedure
- Complete consent for the administration of blood products if applicable
- Presence of living will if applicable
- Understanding of the anesthetic to be administered

Information pertinent to the care of the genitourinary patient includes but is not limited to the following:

- Presence of allergies
- Physical limitations or presence of prosthetics
- Previous surgery and anesthetics
- Medical status (including lab studies)
- Radiologic and other diagnostic findings
- Psychosocial status
- Presence of learning disabilities or impairments
- Anticipated surgical outcome

Each of these are discussed in the sections to follow.

Presence of allergies

As a rule, establishing the presence of allergies is a part of the medical work-up. However, the importance of discovering any patient allergies and the clinical reaction cannot be stressed enough. Allergies are frequently forgotten and therefore omitted by the patient when communicating his or her history during the preoperative work-up. Of importance to the perioperative team are any allergies to medications, soaps, tapes, material (linens, metals), sutures, contrast material, foods (shellfish usually indicates an iodine allergy), latex, and other chemicals. Equally important, from an anesthesia standpoint, are allergies to suntanning products, environmental allergies such as hay fever, asthmatic responses, and a family history of an anesthetic reaction. Adverse responses to contrast material are discussed in further detail under invasive diagnostic procedures in Chapter 4.

Every effort should be made to determine the presence of allergic mechanisms so that perioperative care can be coordinated and adjusted before the patient enters the operating room suite.

Physical limitations and presence of prosthetics

To plan and prepare a safe perioperative experience for the genitourinary patient it is important to consider the physical limitations that may be present. Since many of the patients seen in this specialty are elderly, limited range of motion is often a factor. Additionally there may be patients with other physical impairments. Some of the conditions not infrequently encountered include impaired sight, hearing, or speech; language barriers; loss of a limb; chronic back conditions; altered mental state as with Alzheimer's disease, retardation, or senile dementia; peripheral vascular disease; chronic obstructive pulmonary disease (COPD); renal disease; and heart disease. Each of these physical states requires a unique plan of care. Special paddings, Allen stirrups, and thromboembolism-deterrent sequential compression stockings should be utilized as necessary. Proper placement of the electrosurgical dispersive pad is also crucial, avoiding excessively hairy areas or sites with altered skin or vascular integrity. The pad should be positioned so that the wide expanse opposite the cord faces the operative site.

Prosthetics may also be in place and need to be assessed for location and type. Patients with valvular heart disease or cardiac prosthetics (e.g., a history of endocarditis, mitral valve prolapse (MVP), valvular replacements, pacemakers, and so forth) and those with prosthetic orthopedic joints or other implants will require a course of antibiotic therapy. Those with metal implants, such as a knee, hip, or fixation plates, will require extra caution during positioning and the placement of electrocardiogram (ECG) electrodes or the electrosurgical dispersive pad. If silicone implants are present, the area needs additional protection from violation of the implant integrity. These devices may include breast implants or testicular, penile, or urinary sphincter prostheses. If a patient presents with a pacemaker in place, care must be taken to place the electrosurgical dispersive pad as far from the site as possible. Ideally, electrocautery should not be employed at all, but this is often not a feasible alternative. A good choice might be a bipolar cautery unit. A magnet should be available in the event of disruption in the pacemaker's function.

Previous surgery and anesthetics

Patients about to undergo genitourinary intervention have either had no prior surgical experiences to draw on or are influenced by past encounters, favorable or adverse. It is important to understand their perceptions and memories so that the genitourinary perioperative nurse may include supportive measures in the plan of care. Information about any prior operative procedures should be elicited from the patient and from family and significant others. Data that will prove valuable to the assessment includes the types of previous surgeries, the patient's response both physically and emotionally, complications of any anesthetics used and type (if known), the postoperative recovery experience, and any other significant recollections.

Medical status

Genitourinary procedures frequently require positions that create both anatomic and physiologic stress. Renal, cardiac, pulmonary, and neurovascular histories are usually obtained in addition to routine admission information. A current cardiac and serum electrolyte profile should be evaluated to determine the patient's ability to tolerate the potential stress. Common preoperative genitourinary laboratory studies include CBC, PT, PTT, blood chemistry profiles (including BUN, serum glucose, and creatinine), cardiac enzymes, serum and urine electrolytes, urinalysis and urine cultures (Table 5-1) as well as ECG, and an x-ray study of the chest.

Routine admission information should include vital signs, height and weight, allergies, the presenting problem according to the patient, history of the current condition, nature of symptoms, limitations resulting from the presenting disease process, history of any infectious process, medication history, nutritional state, skin conditions, past or present medical

Table 5-1 **Common Preoperative Laboratory Analyses for Patients with Genitourinary Disorders**

LABORATORY STUDIES	NORMAL RANGE (ADULT VALUES)	LABORATORY STUDIES	NORMAL RANGE (ADULT VALUES)
COAGULATION PROFILES		**SERUM PROFILES (LOW: FEMALE; HIGH: MALE)—CONT'D**	
Bleeding time	1-9 min	Creatinine	0.5-1.2 mg/dl
Partial thromboplastin time (PTT)	60-70 sec	Glucose (blood sugar)	70-105 mg/dl
Platelet count	150,000-400,000/mm^3	Osmolality	285-295 mOsm/kg H$_2$0
Prothrombin time (PT)	11-12.5 sec	Potassium (K)	3.5-5 mEq/L
		Phosphorus (P)	3-4.5 mg/dl
FERTILITY PROFILES (MALE)		Prostate specific antigen (PSA)	<4 ng/ml
Follicle-stimulating hormone (FSH)	1-15 mIU/ml	Prostatic acid phosphatase (PAP)	0.11-0.6 U/L
Luteinizing hormone (LH)	7-24 mIU/ml	Protein	6-8 g/dl
Testosterone (total)	300-1000 ng/dl	Sodium (Na)	136-145 mEq/L
Sperm count	50-200 million/ml, 60%-80% motile	Uric acid	2-8.5 mg/dl
		URINE PROFILES (VALUES NOT LISTED SHOULD BE NEGATIVE)	
HEMATOLOGIES (LOW: FEMALE; HIGH: MALE)		Calcium (Ca)	100-300 mg/day
Hematocrit (Hct)	37%-52%	Chloride (Cl)	110-250 mEq/L
Hemoglobin (Hgb)	12-18 g/dl	Creatinine clearance	88-137 ml/min
Red blood cells (RBCs)	4.2-6.1 million/mm^3	Glucose (24 hr)	0.5 g/day
White blood cells (WBCs)	5000-10,000 million/mm^3	Hyaline casts	Occasional
		Osmolality (random)	50-1400 mOsm/kg H$_2$O
		Phosphorus	4.5-8
SERUM PROFILES (LOW: FEMALE; HIGH: MALE)		Potassium (K)	25-120 mEq/L/day
Bicarbonate	21-28 mEq/L	Protein	30-150 mg/day
Blood urea nitrogen (BUN)	10-20 mg/dl	Red blood cells (RBCs)	0-2
Calcium (Ca)	9-10.5 mg/dl	Sodium (Na)	40-220 mEq/L/day
Chloride (Cl)	90-110 mEq/L	Uric acid	250-750 ml/day
Cholesterol	150-200 mg/dl	White blood cells (WBCs)	0-4
HDL (high-density lipids)	>45-55 mg/dl	pH	4.6-8 (ave. 6)
LDL (low-density lipids)	60-180 mg/dl	Specific gravity	1.005-1.30
VLDL (triglycerides)	25%-50%		

From Pagana K: *Diagnostic and laboratory test reference,* St. Louis, 1990, Mosby; Tanagho E, McAninch JW: *Smith's general urology,* Norwalk, Conn., 1995, Appleton & Lange; and Gray M: *Genitourinary disorders,* St. Louis, 1992, Mosby.

needs, social habits (alcohol, smoking, drugs), family history of disease, and sensory or physical impairments. Past or chronic medical conditions can increase the perioperative risk for the patient undergoing genitourinary intervention. Some of the entities that raise the surgical and anesthetic risk are blood dyscrasias, diabetes mellitus, chronic respiratory disease (COPD, asthma), heart disease, fever, and infection. Nutritional status can directly affect the integrity of the skin and should be evaluated to determine specific requirements for positioning and protective measures. Medications often have a direct effect on the patient's physiologic response to anesthesia and surgery. Common over-the-counter medications that can affect perioperative bleeding are aspirin products and non-steroidal antiinflammatory agents (Naprosyn, ibuprofen). Allergies influence the use of certain skin preparation agents, anesthetics, contrast material, and tapes. Abrasions or rashes, especially near the surgical site, may increase the potential for postoperative infection. The presence of implantable devices requires adjustment in the position employed or the placement of ECG leads and dispersive pads.

The results of specific genitourinary diagnostic studies will also be found in the chart. These bear review and may include some or all of the following: CT scans, MRIs, IVPs, KUBs, urinary flow studies, fluoroscopic examinations (angiography, cavernosography), PSA, videourodynamics, and ultrasonograms. Other pertinent laboratory or radiologic tests relevant to the planned intervention may also be present.

Radiologic and other diagnostic findings

Preoperative studies can provide valuable information to the perioperative nurse. Results of laboratory tests can often indicate the presence of an insidious infection, an undetected cardiac condition, or the need for potassium or blood supplements. Many urologic procedures are elective and may be rescheduled to allow correction of a previously undiscovered medical problem. It is important for the perioperative genitourinary nurse to recognize subtle alterations in laboratory values that could indicate a medical state requiring attention.

Diagnostic examinations for genitourinary disease help determine the extent of the surgery to be performed. These results need to be available before the patient's arrival in the operating room. IVUs that have been done for the presence of renal calculi may be repeated in the surgical suite as a retrograde pyelogram (RGP) to ascertain any movement of the calculi along the urinary tract. An RGP may be performed intraoperatively in lieu of an IVU in those patients with iodine allergies or a complicating renal condition.

Psychosocial status

It is a matter of painful wonder to the sick themselves how much painful ideas predominate over pleasurable ones in their impressions; they reason with themselves; they think themselves ungrateful, it is all of no use. The fact is that those painful impressions are far better dismissed by a real laugh, if you can excite one by books or conversation, than by any direct reasoning; or if the patient is too weak to laugh, some impression from nature is what he wants. I have mentioned the cruelty of letting him stare at a dead wall. In many diseases, especially in

convalescence from fever, that wall will appear to make all sorts of faces at him; now flowers never do this. Form, colour, will free your patient from his painful ideas better than any argument.

Florence Nightingale

Patients undergoing genitourinary procedures must be assessed for their response to the anticipated surgical event. Their understanding of the recovery process and their willingness to cooperate in their own care directly influence the final outcome. Preparation should include a frank discussion of the pain that may be experienced. They should learn about mechanisms for pain control and their role in the ultimate return to health. Patient-controlled analgesia (PCA) is being employed more frequently as more procedures are taking place on an outpatient basis. This is an excellent way for the patient to be in control of his or her comfort level, promoting a sense of autonomy that can lead to good self-esteem and allowing for a more realistic yet optimistic outlook postoperatively. It is important to assess the other support systems available to the urologic patient by determining the family's response to the surgery and postoperative needs. During the teaching process the perioperative genitourinary nurse needs to meet the comprehension levels of all those involved in the learning phase and thereby influence any anxiety or fear and resultant postoperative response.

Preoperative preparation is part and parcel of the teaching element in perioperative nursing care. The genitourinary patient may require antibiotic therapy several days before surgery. The importance of remaining faithful to the prescribed regimen should be stressed. Oral intake, especially fluids, should be encouraged to ensure a well-hydrated and nutritionally sound patient at the time of the surgical intervention. However, it is equally important to emphasize the need for stopping food and fluid intake at the time recommended by the anesthesiologist and surgeon. Often the patient will be encouraged to eat a normal breakfast and lunch and a high caloric liquid or small dinner on the day before surgery. He or she will also be encouraged to drink 8 ounces of non–caffeinated liquid every 2 hours until midnight (one half as fruit juice).

If a patient is following a routine regimen of medication for a separate medical condition, such as heart disease, diabetes, or ulcers, it is necessary to clarify which medications should be discontinued before surgery. Aspirin products and other over-the-counter medications that can alter the effects of anesthesia and surgery should be discontinued approximately 7 to 10 days before the surgery.

Presence of learning disabilities or impairments

All these things require common sense and care. Yet perhaps in no one single thing is so little common sense shown, in all ranks, as in nursing.

Florence Nightingale

When learning disabilities or mental impairments are present, the perioperative genitourinary nurse is faced with a unique challenge. At these times, the family or primary caregivers must be the focus of the teaching. The comprehension level of the patient should be established and teaching geared accordingly. Often when dealing with a patient that is at the learning level of a child it is best to make it a game or small challenge for the patient. The anticipation of a reward for cooperation is frequently an appropriate incentive to elicit a positive response. Approaching a patient stricken with Alzheimer's disease is more difficult because the cognitive level can change from moment to moment and requires constant adjustment of the presentation.

Expected surgical outcome

What the genitourinary patient expects to gain from the anticipated surgical intervention must be determined. Patients may have unrealistic or unfounded beliefs and preconceptions as to what will take place intraoperatively and how they will feel postoperatively. One of the best approaches to determine understanding of the intended surgery and postoperative period is to have the patient explain to you what he or she thinks is going to take place. As discrepancies or misconceptions are exposed, clarification can immediately take place through a question-and-answer style of exchange of information.

Honesty tempered with tact is usually the best approach. Pain should not be emphasized but neither should it be downplayed. Discussion regarding the options available for postoperative pain management is often beneficial. Frequently a brief, concise discussion of the anatomy involved in the planned procedure will aid understanding. Explanations that are worded in layman's terms must be employed. Assurances that positioning will be done in a manner to ensure the most optimal comfort level possible are appropriate.

Diagnosis

If you find it helps you to note down such things on a bit of paper, in pencil, by all means do so. I think it more often lames than strengthens the memory and observation. But if you cannot get the habit of observation one way or the other, you had better give up being a nurse, for it is not your calling, however kind and anxious you may be.

Florence Nightingale

To determine the nursing diagnosis, assessment data must be analyzed. Individualized nursing diagnoses based on the information gathered during the interview process can be established. Through documentation of the diagnoses chosen as the primary foci, a nursing plan of care can be developed. The chosen diagnoses should be validated with the patient and other health care providers as well as significant others. Examples of nursing diagnoses from the accepted list developed by the North American Nursing Diagnosis Association (NANDA) that may be utilized for the genitourinary patient include the following:

- Altered body temperature
- Altered nutrition
- Altered patterns of urinary elimination
- Altered sexuality patterns
- Altered thought processes
- Altered tissue perfusion (specify type)
- Anticipatory grieving
- Anxiety
- Body image disturbance
- Diarrhea/constipation
- Fluid volume excess/deficit
- Functional incontinence
- High risk for infection
- High risk for injury
- Hyperthermia/hypothermia
- Impaired gas exchange
- Impaired physical mobility
- Impaired skin integrity
- Ineffective individual coping
- Knowledge deficit (specify)
- Pain
- Potential autonomic dysreflexia
- Potential for altered acid-base balance
- Potential for sensory alterations
- Potential for trauma
- Potential noncompliance (specify)
- Reflex/extraurethral incontinence
- Sexual dysfunction
- Situational low self-esteem
- Social isolation
- Stress/urge incontinence
- Urinary retention

Outcome Identification

In surgical wards, one duty of every nurse certainly is prevention.

Florence Nightingale

Expected outcomes, unique to each genitourinary patient, are based on the nursing diagnoses chosen and the anticipated results of the plan of care. These are formulated by the perioperative nurse, with deference given to the patient's goals and preferences to promote involvement and independence. These may include the following:

- Absence of adverse response to positioning
- Absence of infection
- Anxiety/fear expressed and controlled
- Appropriate body temperature maintained
- Maintenance of adequate pulmonary exchange
- Maintenance of fluid/electrolyte balance
- Management of pain
- Participation in the recovery process
- Skin integrity maintained
- Understanding of the surgical experience
- Return of normal alimentary processes

Outcomes should be realistic and achievable, with consideration given to the resources that are available to the patient and those resources provided for if necessary. They should be couched in measurable terms that communicate clearly to other caregivers what the desired results should be. This will afford ongoing intraoperative and postoperative evaluation.

Planning

Excellence in perioperative nursing care requires critical thinking. Each situation and each patient cared for will differ. Therefore nothing should be taken as rote but rather refined and adapted to meet the needs at the moment. When this is the focus, the optimal level of nursing care will be achieved for each patient through a truly holistic, person-oriented approach.

The plan of care should stipulate prescribed interventions designed to meet expected outcomes. The perioperative nurse develops this plan using the data collected during the assessment stage of the patient interview, establishing diagnoses and identifying patient goals and needs. The plan should incorporate the following:

- A teaching plan that includes providing information specific to the planned surgical intervention is ensured.
- The surgical site and the patient's understanding of the surgical procedure is verified.
- Competent personnel, properly functioning equipment, and appropriate supplies are available and utilized.
- Transportation needs are clarified.
- The type of anesthetic to be employed is confirmed.
- Positioning and special protective needs are provided.
- Policies and procedures based on the AORN Recommended Practices for Perioperative Nursing Care are adhered to.[4]

Planning patient care begins when the case is scheduled and must be a coordinated effort between the surgeon, office staff, nurses, and the anesthesia team to meet the unique requirements of each patient. The organization and efficiency of the implementation of care by the genitourinary perioperative nurse will be enhanced with planned patient care. The resurgence of old, revised surgical techniques along with the advent of new, highly technical procedures has put greater responsibility on the perioperative genitourinary nurse. It is now necessary to be a computer and video wizard as well as a competent caregiver. A typical care plan for the genitourinary patient follows (Table 5-2).

Patient teaching

Teaching begins in the urologist's office when the patient makes the conscious decision to have the surgical procedure. The perioperative nurse's involvement in the entire process will vary according to the practice setting. After preoperative assessment, teaching plans for the genitourinary patient are individualized. Thought must be given to the specific psychosocial, physical, and spiritual demands of each individual being cared for. If these are incorporated into the teaching process, needs will be met, and the final surgical outcome will be improved. The following information, covering all phases of the surgical experience, will prepare the patient for the procedure and expected postoperative results.

Preoperative stage
- Cause of condition, disease process, or injury
- Diagnostic examinations
- Surgical procedure and expected outcome
- Anticipated preoperative requirements
- Operating room environment

Intraoperative stage
- Preoperative area, operating room, postanesthesia care unit (PACU)
- Waiting area for family and friends
- Anticipated length of surgery
- Anticipated length of PACU stay

Postoperative stage
- Expected body response
- Symptoms of complications
- Recovery process and limitations
- Care of drains and catheters
- Care of dressings and packs
- Anticipated discharge

Many patients with genitourinary problems have dealt with their condition for long periods. This may be particularly true for women with incontinence and men with erectile dysfunction. Only in recent years has the stigma associated with these complaints been lifted. These patients must be prepared for short-term and long-term postoperative management even though they are aware of the limits that their condition has imposed on them.

Postoperative pain requiring effective pain management may be encountered. Often, large doses of a local anesthetic will be administered intraoperatively and at the time of wound closure. These attempts at affording pain control during the early postoperative hours have proved to be extremely beneficial in many instances, significantly decreasing the need for postoperative pain medication. PCA by subcutaneous or epidural infusion are viable options for most genitourinary patients postoperatively and should be discussed in detail during the preoperative teaching phase. The patient should be instructed to initially use their pain medication regularly and before the onset of severe discomfort and before treatments or bladder-training exercises. As the need for pain management decreases, the medication may be spread out over longer periods of time. Complementary strategies for pain management should also be discussed. These may include guided imagery, subliminal tapes, mediation and stress-reduction techniques, therapeutic touch, reflexology and massage, yoga, herbal remedies, hypnosis, *reiki*, and aromatherapy.

Postoperative infection may also occur because of the violation of fluid-filled organs and accompanying bacteria that may be present. Antibiotic therapy is usually prescribed and, depending on the patient history and specific procedure, may range from 8 days preoperatively to 5 to 14 days postoperatively. The importance of remaining faithful to the regimen prescribed cannot be stressed enough.

Procedure verification

Verification of the intended surgical assault should be one of the initial steps for every genitourinary procedure. The patient should be able to verbalize an understanding of what intervention is planned. Many times, through miscommunication, a procedure will be scheduled incorrectly or the patient will be misinformed. It is important to ascertain well ahead of time what instrumentation and equipment will be required to avoid intraoperative delays. The planned surgical approach should be

Table 5-2 **Care Plan for Transurethral Resection of the Prostate**

Key Assessment Points:

1. Serum sodium/potassium values
2. Pedal pulses: qualify
3. Urinalysis/urine culture
4. Preoperative urinary flow pattern

Nursing Diagnosis:

All generic nursing diagnoses apply, with the addition of altered patterns of urinary elimination.

Patient Outcome:

All generic outcomes apply, with the addition of:

Urine flow through the indwelling catheter will be unobstructed.

The urinary drainage system will remain patent.

1. Catheter will remain patent and drain tension free.
2. Collecting system will be below level of patient's bladder.
3. The catheter will be secured in place; connections will be secure.
4. There will be no complaints of dysuria.
5. Urinary output will be at least 0.5 to 1 ml/Kg/hr without obstruction

Nursing Actions:	Yes	No	N/A
1. Equipment properly aerated or rinsed?			
2. ESU checked/functioning?			
3. Fiberoptic light system checked/functioning?			
4. Irrigation solution/warming system prepared?			
5. Special equipment/supplies available?			
6. Patient assessment performed?			
7. Perioperative care explained?			
8. Privacy maintained?			
9. Positioned correctly?			
10. Alternating compression stockings applied?			
11. Prep per institutional protocol with warmed solution?			
12. Dispersive pad site checked?			
13. Return flow monitored?			
14. Patient observed for signs of TUR syndrome?			
15. Catheters secured and documented?			
16. Specimen to lab in formalin?			
17. CBI connected?			

Nursing Actions (continued)	Yes	No	N/A
Document additional nursing actions/generic care plans initiated:			

Evaluation of patient outcomes:

1. Urinary flow through the catheter/drainage system was maintained.
2. The patient met outcomes for additional generic care plans as indicated under Nursing Actions.

Outcome met:	Outcome met with additional outcome criteria:	Outcome met with revised nursing care plan:	Outcome not met:	Outcome not applicable to this patient:
—	—	—	—	—
—	—	—	—	—

Signature: _____   Date: _____

CBI, Continuous bladder irrigation; ESU, electrosurgical unit; TUR, transurethral resection.

confirmed with the patient and with the genitourinary surgeon. Any special precautions also need to be reconfirmed at this time to ensure that planning is complete. Willingness of the patient to discuss the intended operation will aid the teaching and support mechanisms chosen.

Equipment and supplies

The advanced technology and innovative procedures available to the genitourinary surgeon require nursing staff knowledgable about the anatomy and physiology of the genitourinary system as well as the surgical intervention and required equipment.

Equipment and supplies vary according to the intended procedure. Video units, ultrasound machines, electrohydraulic (EHL) or ultrasonic lithotriptors, electrosurgical units, laser equipment, smoke evacuators, operating microscopes, flexible and rigid endoscopy instrumentation, and open surgical instrumentation may be employed. C-arm fluoroscopy and a compatible operating room bed are often needed. Chest or axillary bolsters, gel pads, stirrups, beanbag devices, alternating sequential compression stockings, x-ray aprons and patient shields, and laser eyewear may also need to be available and utilized.

Anesthetics

The administration of anesthesia for the genitourinary patient is a specialized activity. The perioperative nurse is required to have a functional awareness of the medication, mode of delivery, possible side effects, and duration of action. The patient should also be aware of the anesthetic planned, the procedure required for its delivery, and the expected effects. Physiologic effects differ with the type of anesthetic employed. The choice of anesthetic is based on several factors, which include surgeon preference, patient preference, site of intended surgical approach, anatomic features, coexisting disease or physiologic limiting factors, absence or presence of contraindications to a given type of anesthesia, length of procedure, surgical position, and length of hospital stay.

General anesthesia is usually necessary for patients undergoing laparoscopic intervention and perineal prostatectomy and for procedures requiring a thoracoabdominal, flank, or lumbar approach. Airway management and maintenance of adequate pulmonary and cardiovascular exchange are key priorities during general anesthesia. The more involved interventions (i.e., cystectomy, laparoscopic nephrectomy) may require insertion of an atrial line, a central venous pressure line, or both. Since extreme positioning is often involved, proper padding needs to be available to avoid compromise of critical pressure areas (vena cava, bony prominences, nerve pathways).

Regional anesthesia includes spinal, epidural, and regional block. Continuous epidural anesthesia affords the ability to control postoperative pain and is often chosen for involved surgical interventions, such as radical retropubic prostatectomy and radical cystectomy with urinary diversion. An epidural catheter is inserted preoperatively in the operating room, and a local anesthetic or narcotic is injected into the epidural space. With continuous infusion, supplemental anesthetic may be added periodically as needed. The site of insertion needs to be protected from being dislodged or kinked during positioning

and transfer of the patient. These patients will require postoperative monitoring beyond the PACU stay.

"Single-shot" spinal anesthesia may be the method of choice for implantation of a penile prosthesis or artificial urinary sphincter and certain pelvic procedures. The anesthetic is injected into the subarachnoid space and provides a more profound block than does epidural anesthesia. The anesthetic, however, has a finite duration, and dosages must be calculated accurately according to the length of the procedure. Spinal anesthesia may reduce blood loss, decrease thromboembolic complications, and preserve mental acuity and respiratory exchange. The major complications from spinal anesthesia are epidural hematoma and postoperative headache. Ambulation after spinal anesthesia should not be discouraged, and the patient should be advised to maintain adequate fluid intake.[7] When spinal anesthesia is contemplated, it is especially important that the patient has refrained from using aspirin and anti-inflammatory agents for 7 to 10 days before surgery.

Regional block, with continuous intravenous sedation (monitored anesthesia care [MAC]), may be selected for procedures expected to cause less postoperative discomfort. Regional block may also be employed by the surgeon, in conjunction with general, spinal, or epidural anesthesia, to decrease bleeding and to augment postoperative comfort levels.

Before induction of any anesthetic it is imperative for the perioperative team to rule out medication allergies and investigate family history for indications of risk for malignant hyperthermia or other adverse anesthesia-related complications. Anesthetic drugs may alter renal blood flow, glomerular filtration, or tubular function. These effects may be direct or secondary to changes in cardiovascular function or neuroendocrine activity. Mechanical ventilation and positive end-expiratory pressure (PEEP) has been associated with decreased urinary output and may be reversed through volume expansion.

Patients with renal disease may exhibit hypocapnia and potential hypoxemia because of compensatory hyperventilation brought on by systemic acidosis. Long-term diuretic therapy has been known to result in hypokalemia (serum potassium depletion) with resulting arrhythmias. Severe hypertension intraoperatively, though generally controlled, can be the result of undiagnosed pheochromocytoma or intraoperative distention of the urinary bladder. Pheochromocytoma may also precipitate mild to severe hyperthermia because of the profound catecholamine release common with the condition. The patient presenting with known uremia and acute, severe hyponatremia will exhibit an increased incidence of postoperative nausea and vomiting. The exact mechanism accounting for this is still under debate.

When the anesthetic for the procedure is local injection only, knowledge of drug interactions and contraindications becomes critical, rather than merely important, for the perioperative genitourinary nurse. Most complications are attributed to high levels of local anesthetic secondary to inadvertent intravascular injection rather than a true allergic reaction. Symptoms common with an untoward intravenous reaction are tinnitus, restlessness, diaphoresis, blurred vision, numbness around the mouth, and drowsiness. As blood levels rise, symptoms become more severe, and the patient may experience central nervous system depression, seizure activity, apnea, cardiac dysrhythmias, and cardiovascular collapse. When there is an allergic response, it is most likely caused by the preservative in the anesthetic. With the esters, PABA (*para*-aminobenzoic acid) has been found to be the causative agent. Local anesthetics may potentiate the effects of neuromuscular agents and exacerbate an infectious process. An awareness of the patient's medical history can ward off inherent danger.

Progressive hypothermia results in diuresis and a subsequent decrease in renal blood flow and glomerular filtration rate. This can cause a cessation in tubular reabsorption thereby impairing the urinary concentrating and diluting ability of the kidney. A consequence of this will be noted by a slowing of urinary output. Use of warming devices intraoperatively will aid the anesthetic management of the genitourinary patient. These devices may include water-filled warming blankets, forced warm air blanket units, special metal-coated coverings, plastic coverings, and warming units for intravenous, blood, and irrigation solutions.

Acute hemolysis occurring after blood transfusion is a life-threatening complication that is often preventable. Renal vascular ischemia and activation of the coagulation mechanism that leads to disseminated intravascular coagulopathy (DIC) are characteristic of the physiologic process of a hemolytic reaction. Renal vascular ischemia is the most important mechanism of renal failure, and symptoms may be masked by general anesthesia. If fever, hemoglobinuria, tachycardia, and hypotension occur after a transfusion, a hemolytic reaction must be investigated.

A final, little-discussed complication is malignant hyperthermia (MH). Although it is not a common occurrence, the genitourinary nurse should be cognizant of the warning signs and be prepared to assist anesthesia with management of any crisis. Symptoms include but are not limited to hypercapnia, tachypnea, tachycardia, hypoxia with dark blood in the operative field, metabolic and respiratory acidosis, cardiac dysrhythmia, and a body temperature that continues to rise 1 to 2° C every 5 minutes.

Intraoperative planning

Inappropriate planning can turn the simplest procedure into a major undertaking. To decrease surgical time, provide safe patient care, and ascertain ways to improve on current routines, an effective intraoperative plan should be developed.

Policies and procedures are written guidelines for implementation of care and must be utilized when planning for any genitourinary procedure. These guidelines should be developed according to the standards of care recommended by AORN and SUNA. Coordination of the key sources for perioperative nursing care and genitourinary patient care will allow for an individualized treatment plan that focuses on the human factor. Both may be adapted to meet the needs specific to each patient undergoing genitourinary intervention. Activities to be implemented necessitate organization of knowledgable personnel, control of traffic patterns, and provisions for patient safety. Infection control practices such as aseptic technique and implant handling, manufacturer's criteria for safe equipment usage and care, and documentation of pertinent intraoperative data, should be established and adhered to.

Aseptic practices and traffic patterns are intended to decrease the opportunity for infections. Room setup and activities should be planned to minimize movement of personnel around the sterile field. Air currents through the room are accelerated as a result of movement, increasing bacteria counts and the shedding of contaminated particles from the patient, personnel, and draping materials. Proper placement of ancillary equipment before the patient's entry into the operating room and prioritizing patient care activities will ease traffic flow and the progression of the procedure. Equipment should be checked for proper functioning and arranged to minimize traffic near the field while maximizing visualization by the surgical team before the sterile field is prepared.

Physician preference plays a vital role in the planning and implementation of patient care. To plan activities geared toward improving the surgical outcome, the perioperative genitourinary team should be aware of the surgeon's rationale, understand the procedure that is planned, and be cognizant of specific patient needs. If the physician has confidence in the operating room personnel, the entire intraoperative phase will function like a well-oiled machine. Preoperative planning must involve all team members and the physician for the benefit of the patient.

Implementation

The interventions outlined in the plan of care are proactively implemented by the perioperative genitourinary nurse. The individualized plan of care and the actual interventions undertaken should be in harmony. Each step is implemented, documented, evaluated, and adjusted during patient care according to changing needs. The procedures mentioned in this text are intended to be used as a guide for implementation by those caring for the genitourinary patient. The individual practice setting, physician preference, and the role played by the caregivers will necessitate variations in the implementation of care. Activities to be incorporated include patient teaching, safety assurances, proper positioning techniques, documentation of interactions and interventions, and infection control measures.

Patient teaching

Patient teaching is a continuous process from the initial visit to the physician through the recovery process. Collaboration of effort must span across the range of caregivers who will be providing for the patient. This will provide continuity of care and strengthen the total perioperative experience. A teaching program may be developed to offer both emotional and informational support to the patient and family. The perioperative nurse should always be attuned to special needs as they present themselves and be prepared to seek additional resource personnel when necessary. These may include the surgeon, primary medical physician, anesthesiologist, oncologist, cardiologist, social services department, mental health department, financial aid, rehabilitation or ostomy clinicians, and home health care agencies.

Immediately before surgical intervention, a review of previous instructions regarding postoperative sequelae, expected outcome, potential complications, and the recovery process should take place. Nursing personnel may review deep-breathing and coughing techniques, drain and dressing care, postoperative oral intake, and medication therapy. Those undergoing procedures in an ambulatory care setting or those with learning deficits will benefit from the repetition provided and from preoperative and postoperative return demonstration.

Safety

All personnel functioning in a genitourinary service need to be trained in equipment safety measures, Universal Precautions, Occupational Safety and Health Administration (OSHA) guidelines, and environmental hazards during the orientation process. Education should include the proper use of skin preparation solutions, glutaraldehydes, and irrigation solutions and any accompanying precautions in their application. MSDSs (material safety data sheets) should be available to all personnel and updated as products are added or removed.

Safety measures during patient transport, transfer, and positioning require personnel with the proper training in sound body mechanics and correct patient body alignment. Adequate personnel should be available to perform these tasks to avoid injury to the patient or to themselves. Safe practice must also incorporate the appropriate precautions during laser treatments, x-ray procedures, and C-arm fluoroscopy.

Laser precautions

Laser stands for "light amplification by the stimulated emission of radiation." Lasers used clinically produce nonionizing radiation and are not considered hazardous from that perspective. Laser light energy is delivered within a small portion of the electromagnetic spectrum. Some waves are visible; some are not. Energy may extend from the near-ultraviolet to the far-infrared region. Laser light differs from ordinary light in three ways. Laser light is collimated, monochromatic, and coherent. The collimated property of a laser beam minimizes loss of power as it passes through a lens. This enables the beam to be focused into a small spot that concentrates the energy and allows for precision. The focal length of the lens determines the size of the beam spot: the shorter the beam, the smaller the spot, and the greater the intensity of that beam. Laser energy is composed of photons all the same color, hence monochromatic, or highly purified color. All waves travel in phase and in the same direction, making the light coherent, adding to the amplitude, or power, effect.

The distribution of laser light energy is altered when the beam is scattered through the tissue. If the energy is absorbed, it will be converted to heat. The potential hazard lies in the ability of the laser to backscatter. The beam could backscatter up the endoscope and cause damage to the optics and distal end of the scope. When calculating power density, backscatter must be taken into consideration because of the loss of energy it may cause.

Some wavelengths are transmitted through certain tissues, or solutions, with little thermal effect, as with the Nd:YAG laser in a cavity distended by solution. Thermal damage is directly related to the wavelength, beam fluence, tissue color and consistency, and water content. As the laser cuts through tissue, it continues to heat and destroy deeper layers, causing concern for adjacent structures. With the newer contact fibers this risk is decreased but not avoided. Approximately 85% of the lasers in use produce an effect by a photon (noncontact), thermal (contact), or acoustical (sonic) interaction at the tissue level. They coagulate, vaporize, and ablate from the site where the tissue interaction begins. The beam also generates sonic energy creating a mechanical effect, as when calculi are imploded.

The **Nd:YAG (neodymium:yttrium-aluminum-garnet)** laser is the most commonly used laser to treat bladder tumors and prostatic hyperplasia because of the greater depth of penetration. It consists of a solid crystal of yttrium-aluminum-garnet laced with neodymium to produce laser light energy. At tissue impact with a contact fiber there is a considerable scatter effect and a homogeneous coagulative response. During noncontact tissue interaction large tissue volumes are heated slowly followed by deep progressive coagulation. The Nd:YAG laser light is transmitted through clear structures or fluids easily, whereas its path is stopped by dark colors (Fig. 5-1). It has a color selectivity for darker tissues and an absorption depth of 2 to 6 mm. It is in the near-infrared spectrum with a wavelength of 1060 nm. Historically the required goggles have been tinted green or blue. Clear eyewear for the Nd:YAG laser are now being manufactured, making color coding of the lenses insufficient by itself for determining the appropriate goggles. The wavelength and optical density for the specific laser must be clearly marked on the eyewear.

The medium in the **CO_2 laser** is a combination of CO_2, nitrogen, and helium gases designed to increase output efficiency. It is strongly absorbed by water in the tissue and produces a very superficial effect. Independent of tissue color, it is absorbed to a depth of 0.1 to 0.2 mm with little scattering. The CO_2 laser finds the highest success with treatment of external conditions such as condylomas and penile carcinoma. It is not practical for treating intraluminal or intravesical conditions

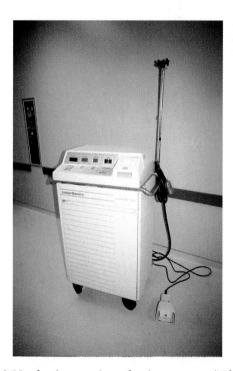

Fig. 5-1 Neodymium: yttrium-aluminum-garnet (Nd:YAG) laser.

because of absorption by fluid and short beam length. The CO_2 laser is readily adapted for use with the microscope or free handpiece. A smoke evacuator should always be used with the laser (Figs. 5-2 and 5-3). It is in the far-infrared spectrum with a wavelength of 10,600 nm. The goggles are generally clear or pink and again must be marked according to the wavelength and optical density of the particular laser.

The **tunable dye** *laser* has as its primary function the treatment of ureteral and renal calculi. The flashlamp-excited pulsed dye, or tunable dye, laser produces a dye of coumarin green that is well absorbed by the pigment of most calculi (Fig. 5-4). It will not cause damage to soft tissue but causes more concrete matter to implode without causing bulk heating. The light absorption created results in a small cloud (plasma) of ions and electrons. The fluid environment confines the acoustic waves of this plasma affording a more direct impact on the stone. Its spectrum is visible with a wavelength of 400 to 1000 nm. Orange to orange-red goggles are generally used but must be marked with the wavelength and optical density specific to the laser to be employed.

The **argon** and **KTP lasers** are generally employed for more superficial lesions within the bladder, prostate, or urethra. The KTP-532 (frequency-doubled YAG) utilizes a potassium-titanyl-phosphate crystal. Energy is delivered through a fiber made of a quartz core that is surrounded by silicone and nylon to prevent damage or breakage. It may be easily connected to a microscope or endoscope. It is in the "green" range of the infrared spectrum with a wavelength of 532 nm. The glasses are usually tinted green or blue but must be wavelength and optical-density specific for the laser in question. The argon laser produces blue and green lights to allow for more complex tissue absorption. High energy passes down a plasma tube through the argon gas and is readily absorbed by melanin, hemoglobin, or other pigmentation to a depth of 0.5 to 2 mm. Upon absorption the laser energy converts to heat, producing coagulation or vaporization. It is in the blue range of the visible spectrum with a wavelength of 488 nm. Goggles have generally been tinted orange to orange-red but need to be wavelength and optical-density specific.

The **holmium:YAG (Ho:YAG) laser** produces a vapor bubble in a fluid medium that allows beam transmission to the tissue. This laser fiber must be held in close contact to the target site and results in a thermal response similar to that of the CO_2 laser. It has been used successfully to fracture ureteral calculi. It is in the infrared spectrum with a wavelength of 2100 nm. Goggles tend to be clear but must be clearly identified with wavelength and optical density for the laser to be used.

Ophthalmic safety is critical when laser energy is employed because the eye is extremely sensitive to laser radiation. Low levels of laser emission can result in significant and permanent eye damage. The wavelength of the laser and the energy absorption of the tissue determine the potential hazards and the required eyewear. The optical density and wavelength filtering ability should be inscribed on the goggles and must correspond with specifications for the laser to be used. The patient, as well as all perioperative personnel, must be protected.

Argon, tunable dye, KTP, and Nd:YAG laser light beams pass easily through the cornea to focus on the retina. This increases the beam's power density and results in severe retinal destruction. The lights from the CO_2 and Ho:YAG lasers are readily absorbed by the surface of the eye and cause corneal or scleral damage. Eye protection with side shields that filters the specific wavelength is necessary. Prescription glasses and contact lenses are not adequate to ensure protection.

Laser goggles are extremely expensive and must be properly cared for and stored. The eyewear should be routinely cleaned in

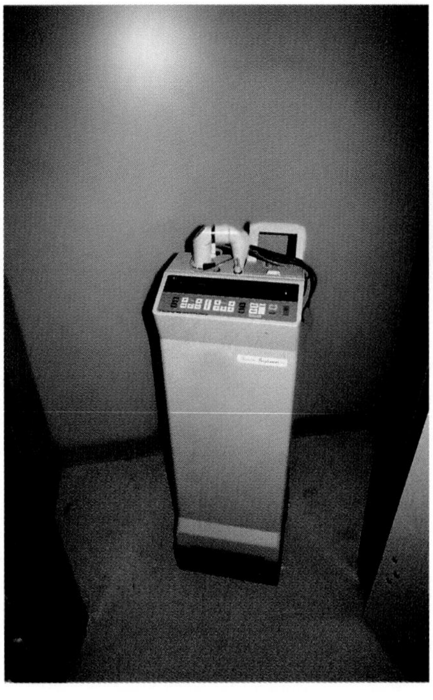

Fig. 5-2 CO_2 laser.

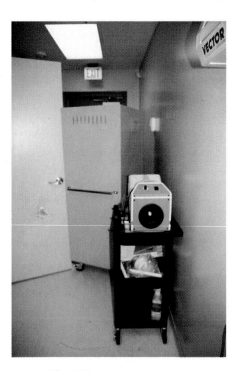

Fig. 5-3 Smoke evacuator.

mild detergent and stored in soft cloth containers or eyeglass or goggle cases. Even a small scratch on the lenses of these goggles can render them ineffective and unsafe for use. Enough goggles should be available for all personnel in the room, plus one or two additional pairs for any others who may need to enter during the procedure. The extra goggles should be outside the entrance to the operating room suite.

Every operating room should have a laser-safety committee, an established training program, and appropriate standards of care in place for each type of laser utilized. Laser protocols need to be adhered to and procedures need to be logged according to the guidelines established. Doors are to remain closed during laser treatments with signs displayed that indicate the type of laser in use. A low- or no-residue fire extinguisher and sterile water should be readily available in the event of a laser fire. Flammable prep solutions, those containing alcohol or acetone, should not be utilized during laser interventions. Prep solutions should be dried by patting with a sterile towel, ensuring that any pooled solutions are removed. Pooled solutions retain laser heat and can result in a tissue burn. If the laser energy is absorbed by pigmentation, iodophor solutions should be rinsed off. All laser procedures should have a designated laser nurse in attendance. Whenever a laser is used externally, a smoke evacuator and special high-filtration masks should be used.

Radiology precautions

Fluoroscopy with image intensification (**C**-arm) converts an x-ray beam onto a television screen to produce an image. The radiology technologist operates the equipment and needs to be consulted regarding timing of the procedure, special positioning requirements, and sterility requirements. As a rule, most **C**-arm beams penetrate the proposed site of application from below, so that the beam is directed upward. This necessitates that any protective shields should be placed under the patient.

If a portable x-ray unit is to be used, a grid containing the x-ray film must be placed under the patient. Most operating room beds have elevated x-ray cassette compartments that allow for easy placement of the grid.

When radiologic activities occur it is important to protect the patient and personnel from undue exposure to radiation. Lead shields and thyroid collars should be placed under or on top of the patient whenever possible. Unfortunately, genitourinary procedures do not allow that the reproductive system be protected in this manner. The thyroid and chest areas usually can be, however. Perioperative, anesthesia, and radiology personnel should be attired in lead aprons and thyroid collars for these procedures. The surgeon should be afforded the opportunity to wear sterile lead-impregnated surgical gloves in addition to the lead apron and thyroid collar. Doors should remain closed during all operative procedures and especially so during radiography or laser interventions.

Other safety requirements include but are not limited to surgical counts (instruments, sponges, needles, and so forth), proper containment of sharps (blades, needles, sharp instruments), maintaining Universal Precautions such as the use of protective apparel as indicated by the wound classification/task categories established by OSHA (goggles, gloves, and so forth), and electrical cords placed away from traffic flow.

Positioning

A careful nurse will keep a constant watch over her sick, especially the weak, protracted, and collapsed cases, to guard against the effects of the loss of vital heat by the patient himself. In certain diseased states much less heat is produced than in health; and there is a constant tendency to the decline and ultimate extinction of the vital powers by the call made upon them to sustain the heat of the body. . . . The feet and legs should be examined by the hand from time to time. . . . Patients are frequently lost in the latter stages of disease from want of attention to such simple precautions.

Florence Nightingale

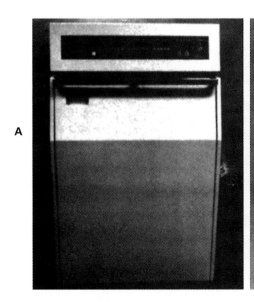
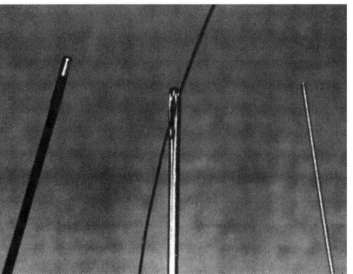

Fig. 5-4 Candela laser, **A,** and fibers **B.** *(From Gillenwater JY et al: Adult and pediatric urology, ed 3, St. Louis, 1995, Mosby.)*

A working understanding of the urologic operating room bed and its uses is imperative to provide optimum patient positioning for each operative procedure. The position chosen is dependent upon the procedure to be performed. The patient may require lithotomy, supine, prone, or lateral position. Lithotomy position may be exaggerated to provide maximum exposure of the organ involved, as in radical prostate and bladder surgery. Precautions must be taken to avoid compromise to the patient's pulmonary and cardiovascular circulation. It is essential to avoid displacement of joints and undue tension on ligaments or neurovascular structures. Elderly patients are at increased risk for injury and extra care should be taken when maneuvering them on the operative bed. If an epidural catheter is in place, it must be protected from dislodging or kinking.

Because of the threat of compromise to anatomic structures, the genitourinary surgeon is closely involved with the positioning of the patient for surgery. Thorough assessment of nutritional status, other medical conditions, any physical limitations, and the skin and peripheral vascular integrity will dictate what ancillary equipment will be needed.

The RNFA involved with the procedure, because of the advanced level of expertise in nursing practice, should be a guiding force for the surgical team. In collaboration with the surgeon, optimum care can be afforded through safe, patient-oriented positioning maneuvers, utilizing all available resources and protective devices deemed appropriate.

Lithotomy position is often the position of choice for bladder and prostate procedures (Fig. 5-5). The safest stirrups to use are the boot style (Allen stirrup), where the foot fits neatly into a padded, carved-out form and allows for plantar and calf support without compression on the peroneal nerve and vessels, or the popliteal vessels. The stirrups should be adjusted to avoid undue calf pressure and attached so that they promote normal alignment of the legs. The boot stirrup is extremely versatile and allows for extreme positioning without vascular compromise. They are especially beneficial with the patient who has limited hip mobility and altered peripheral vascular status. Other stirrups include the standard "knee-crutch" style and the "candy-cane" style, which allows high lithotomy by means of a narrow canvas loop that fits over the Achilles area and the arch of the foot. When the knee-crutch stirrups are employed, the curve of the yoke suspension should flow outward, as do the patient's legs (Fig. 5-6, A). Padding the stirrups will be beneficial in relieving pressure on the popliteal space, lateral femoral nerve, and peroneal nerve and vessels. With the candy-cane (sling) style, padding attached to the post and under the sling to prevent pressure on the peroneal nerve and constriction across the Achilles area (Fig. 5-6, B). Anterior and dorsal pedal pulses and inguinal and radial pulses must be assessed before and after placement, as well as postoperatively. Alterations in status may require repositioning of the involved extremity.

Two people should slowly raise the feet simultaneously while supporting the back of the knee. The patient should be protected from hyperextension of the knee and hip joints and thereby avoid damage to the sciatic or femoral nerve complexes. The feet are removed from the stirrups in the same manner. It is often in the patient's best interest to place a small foam or gel pad under the sacrum to alleviate potential lumboscral plexus and sciatic injury. This relieves sacral pressure and avoids potential stress on the lower back. The buttocks should extend at least 2 inches beyond the break in the bed, sometimes more for extreme positioning. The arms are extended on bilateral

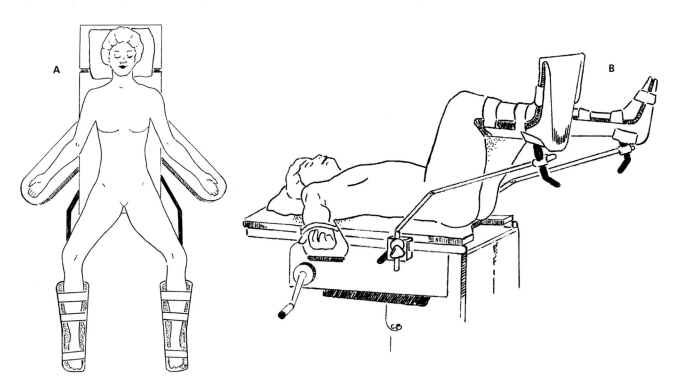

Fig. 5-5 **A,** Lithotomy position viewed from above, with Allen stirrups. **B,** Lithotomy position, viewed from the side, with Allen stirrups. *(Artwork by Cindy J. Bollinger.)*

armboards at less than a 90 degree angle with the palmar surface up and are padded to maintain a level support surface, thereby avoiding brachial plexus and supraclavicular nerve damage. If it is necessary to elevate the arms at a greater angle, the elbow may be bent cephalad, palmar surface up, with the hands placed near the head, after being appropriately padded. Care must be taken not to abduct the shoulders posteriorly. If the arms must be tucked at the side, the palmar surface should face inward with the arm supinated and the elbows well padded to avoid ulnar or radial nerve injury. The arms may be tucked inside a draw sheet, which is then tucked smoothly under the patient or placed inside protective "toboggan" arm guards. When cracking the foot of the bed, close attention must be paid to confirm that the fingers are free of constriction. The head and neck are protected from extension and pressure with a neck roll and formed head support. If the patient will be in this position for longer than 1 hour, it is appropriate to utilize sequential compression stockings. One contraindication for these stockings is the presence of a synthetic vascular graft in the lower extremities. A warming blanket under the patient and additional warming devices across the upper torso and surrounding the head should be utilized to help maintain body temperature.

Supine (dorsal recumbent) position will be utilized for many abdominal and suprapubic procedures (Fig. 5-7). It is a misconception that this position requires no particular precautions. All bony prominences need to be protected from undue pressure. The patient should always be lifted because dragging will cause skin shearing. The heels of the feet need to be within the confines of the mattress and not resting on the edge. If the patient is above 6 feet tall, a well-padded foot extension should

be attached to the end of the bed. It may be necessary to place a bolster under the knees to avoid hyperflexion and alleviate low back strain. Padding for the torso, head, and upper extremities is like that for lithotomy position. If the arms are placed at the side, the palmar surface should be inward with the elbow padded to avoid hyperflexion and assault to the bony aspect. Often, toboggan style arm slides are placed to keep the arms securely at the side. On a thin patient, the arms may be wrapped inside the draw sheet, with the sheet tucked smoothly under the patient. Sequential compression stockings should be employed for longer procedures and for patients with peripheral vascular compromise. Radial and pedal pulses should be assessed for integrity before and after positioning and postoperatively. Alterations in status after positioning may require realignment. The patient is at risk to damage of the same nerve complexes as discussed under lithotomy position. A warming blanket under the patient and warming devices across the torso and around the head should be employed.

Prone position is not often utilized and may be modified so that the patient is semilateral, or prone-oblique, on the operating room bed (Fig. 5-8). This is seen when the operative procedure requires a lumbar approach. At least four people are needed to properly transfer and position the patient. The patient should be log-rolled by one person facing the posterior side of the torso into the arms of a second person on the opposite side and then lifted onto supportive chest pads, with the dependent arm straight at the side, palmar surface inward. A third person guides the legs while the anesthesiologist or anesthetist guards the head and neck from injury. Close attention is paid to maintaining the airway and keeping the head and neck in proper body alignment. The head is gently turned to

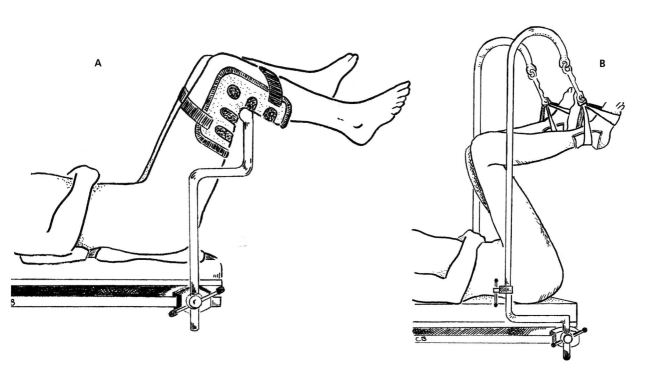

Fig. 5-6 **A,** Proper positioning in knee-crutch stirrups. **B,** Proper positioning in candy-cane stirrups. *(Artwork by Cindy J. Bollinger.)*

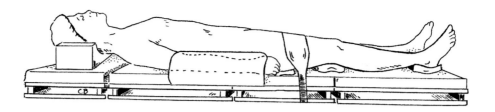

Fig. 5-7 Supine position, side view. *(Artwork by Cindy J. Bollinger.)*

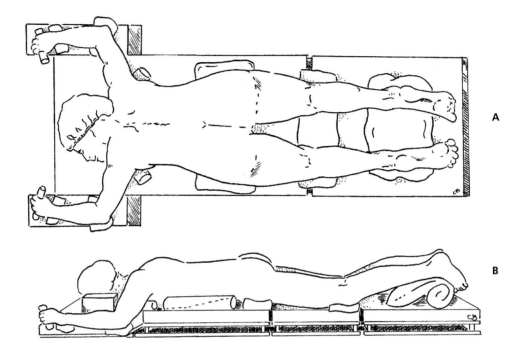

A

B

Fig. 5-8 A, Prone position viewed from above. **B,** Prone position, side view. *(Artwork by Cindy J. Bollinger.)*

one side and placed on a formed support assuring that the eyes and ears are free from undue compression. Once the patient has been turned, the dependent arm is carefully freed by bringing the arm down and outward in a smooth motion while the elbow and wrist are supported. When the arm is at a 45-degree angle, the elbow is bent and the forearm is raised cephalad. The hands are pronated, and padding is placed under the shoulders, axillae, elbows, wrists, and hands. Specially designed padded prone armboards are ideal for this position. Additional rolls are placed under the iliac crests (upper thighs) and foam or gel pads are placed under the knees. Attention must be paid to protecting the female breasts and the male genitalia properly. The feet and ankles are elevated over several folded blankets or a large padded bolster, making sure that the toes hang freely. Assessment of radial and pedal pulses before and after positioning will determine if repositioning is neces-

sary to maintain vascular integrity. Pulses are again checked postoperatively. Sequential compression stockings are of benefit to the patient. A warming device across the upper torso is appropriate.

Lateral (flank or **lateral decubitus) position** is the most common position for renal surgery (Fig. 5-9). The spine is extended for greater access to the retroperitoneal space. Padding and gel pad supports, as well as pillows, sandbags, beanbags, safety straps, and tape, should be available to offer precise anatomic positioning, safety, and stabilized support. A warming blanket under the patient will assist in controlling intraoperative body temperature. The patient is positioned so that the area of the tenth to the twelfth ribs are over the kidney rest. The bottom leg should be flexed at the knee with the heel of the foot drawn toward the patient's buttocks without hyperflexion of the knee. Pads are important below the dependent

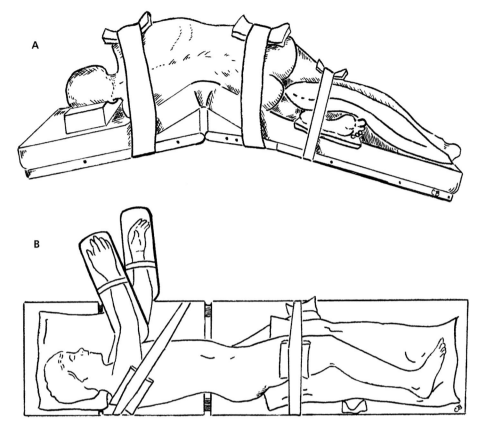

Fig. 5-9 **A,** Lateral position, side view. **B,** Lateral position from above. *(Artwork by Cindy J. Bollinger.)*

ankle and knee to prevent pressure, nerve damage and footdrop. Pillows or similar padding should be placed under the length of the upper part of the leg to prevent peroneal or tibial nerve damage. The top leg is extended over the padding with the knee just slightly bent to avoid stress on the joint. The patient's back, buttocks, and hips are aligned and approach the edge of the bed to allow optimum access to the surgical site. After blankets are applied over the legs, the safety strap should be placed across the thighs. The patient's dependent shoulder is brought slightly forward with an axillary roll under the dependent axilla and padded from below if necessary. Padding must be provided for the neck and head to maintain proper alignment of the cervical spine and avoid pressure damage. The lower ear and eye are subject to compression and should also be carefully protected. The lower arm is extended, palmar surface up, with the elbow slightly bent cephalad and protective padding provided for the elbow, wrist, and hand. The upper arm is extended outward and pronated on a pillow, padded Mayo stand, or gel-padded lateral armboard with the elbow slightly bent and the joints padded to avoid wristdrop and pressure injury. To prevent the torso from rolling out of position, tape is placed across the shoulder area and upper rib cage. Protective gauze or thin cloth should be against the skin to prevent shearing and tape burns. Radial and pedal pulses need to be assessed before and after positioning as well as intraoperatively and immediately postoperatively. It is prudent to apply sequential compression stockings before the induction of general anesthesia and resulting

vasodilation to promote peripheral vascular circulation and help prevent phlebitis, or thrombus formation. It may be necessary to attach a padded foot extension to the end of the bed. A blanket or warming device covers the patient's shoulders, neck, and often the head. The exact position of the upper extremities will vary by the intended incisional site. The kidney rest should be elevated slowly and the patient observed for any fluctuations in blood pressure or changes in respiratory status. This also holds true when the operating room bed is "cracked" or jack-knifed as the patient's head is lowered and the lower extremities are extended downward.

Trendelenburg position is frequently required during genitourinary surgery. Well-padded shoulder braces, when used, must be placed over the bony aspect of the shoulders (Fig. 5-10). Improper positioning will cause supraclavicular and brachial plexus nerve damage. **Reverse Trendelenburg,** though less often employed, may also be utilized (Fig. 5-11). When the patient is placed in this position, there is a tendency for the body to slide on the operating room bed. To avoid this and protect the posterior aspect from shearing and potential damage, a well-padded foot extension should be placed perpendicular to the flat bed surface.

A potential cause of nerve damage and skin shearing that is often overlooked is crumpled linen. As the patient is positioned, the sheets on the bed tend to slide and bunch up. It is important to smooth them out as much as possible to avoid the damage that uneven surfaces and ridges can cause.

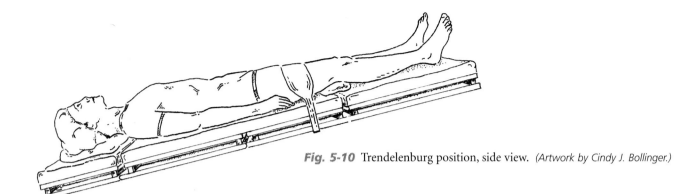

Fig. 5-10 Trendelenburg position, side view. *(Artwork by Cindy J. Bollinger.)*

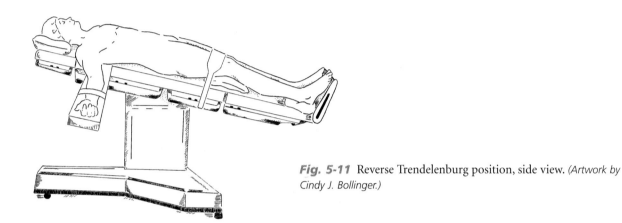

Fig. 5-11 Reverse Trendelenburg position, side view. *(Artwork by Cindy J. Bollinger.)*

To avoid burns when an electrosurgical unit is employed, the patient must not be in contact with metal. It is equally important to prevent pooling of skin preparation solutions because chemical burns may result. This holds true for any position employed.

Documentation

To demonstrate accountability, it is necessary to document all nursing care and actions and patient responses throughout the perioperative nursing process. Proper documentation should indicate the level and quality of care provided and the provisions made to protect the patient's rights. Documentation specific for the genitourinary patient includes the following:

- Operative procedure, preoperative and postoperative diagnoses
- Additional procedures performed
- Names with titles of persons in attendance during the procedure (include visitors: radiology technician, product representative, and so forth)
- Room (in and out), operation, and anesthesia times
- Counts performed: sharps (needles, blades), sponges, instruments, vessel loops, umbilical tapes, rubber shods, signatures of those involved
- Anesthetic: type, caregiver; with local anesthetic the AORN recommendations for monitoring the patient under local anesthesia should be followed
- Surgical wound classification
- Radial and pedal pulses: character, site

- Prepping agents: type, site, skin status before and after application
- Specimens: description, studies requested
- Medications administered in the sterile field: time, drug, dosage, site, route, provider of care
- Irrigations: site, type, amount
- Urinary output and estimated blood loss, replacement therapy: type, amount
- Drain or catheter placement: time and date, type, size, site, character of return flow, one collection device, method of securing, provider of care; when more than collection devices are labeled
- Equipment and tracking codes
- Appliances (electrosurgical dispersive pad, sequential stockings): skin status before and after, site, provider of care
- Implants: type, size, lot number, site
- Positioning devices: type, site
- Radiologic exposure: type, patient protected, site
- Dressings: site, type, tape type or securing method, provider of care

Genitourinary procedures often necessitate the use of C-arm fluoroscopy or a portable x-ray machine. When these are employed, it is usually not feasible to protect the patient from exposure to the reproductive organs. The thyroid gland, however, is extremely x-ray sensitive and should always be protected, as well as the chest when possible, with a small leaded shield. Documentation of equipment includes the Biomed number for the electrosurgical unit, laser unit, smoke evacuator, electrohydraulic machine, ultrasound machine, ultrasonic lithotriptor, x-ray unit, solution-warming units, and video equipment.

Implants used are documented on the operative record, the implant log, and the implant-tracking form. Typical products that are in this category are penile implants, artificial urinary sphincters, collagen implants, stents, and graft material (synthetic material, fascia lata).

Genitourinary surgery is known for its high utilization of irrigating solutions. Because of the large volume often instilled, the use of warming units is advisable. The type and amount of irrigation should be noted on the operative record. The patient is at risk for dilutional hyponatremia and needs to be observed. Symptoms need to be noted in the operative record and reported to the operating surgeon. Irrigations are discussed in greater detail in another section.

When the procedure takes place under local anesthesia only, it is important that one nurse be assigned to monitor the patient. Blood pressure, respiratory, and radial pulse readings are recommended every 10 to 15 minutes. The patient should be attached to the oxygen-saturation monitor and ECG machine and closely observed for untoward effects. If necessary, nasally administered O_2 at 4 L may be used. The time, type, amount, and site of the anesthetic and the patient's response should be recorded.

Asepsis

Do not for instance explain away deaths after . . . nephritis or other pathological processes. The pneumonia or nephritis would probably not kill the patient if there were no septic infection.

Augustus Charles Bernays

Infection control measures to maintain aseptic technique and minimize wound and instrument contamination must be emphasized. Much of the genitourinary population is at risk for infection because of the high incidence of elderly patients, the violation of fluid-filled organs, and the compromised state the disease process has caused. Procedures should be established and carried out according to the recommended standards and practices of perioperative nursing care as stated by AORN.

Activities that affect wound and instrument integrity include traffic-flow patterns, air currents, skin shaving and cleansing techniques, instrumentation methods, and draping products and procedures. In general, airborne contamination is responsible for the majority of postoperative wound infections. In the case of urologic surgery, instrumentation of the genitourinary system poses an almost equal risk.

When a shave prep is mandated for a surgical procedure, the preparation of the patient should take place preoperatively. Current thought proposes that the shave be done as close to the time of surgical intervention as possible. However, the presence of loose hairs within the confines of what will become the sterile field should be avoided. This can be achieved in the patient's room or the preoperative examination and assessment area, with privacy assured. When shaving the patient in the operating room is unavoidable, a wet shave should be done. The area is dried well, and all loose hairs are retrieved with tape. A preop-

erative scrub should then be performed before the application of the prepping solution.

One must assure that during meticulous cleansing of the female perineal area the sponges are not reused once they have contacted the rectum. Prepping solutions should be warmed and applied with downward strokes from the outer perineal edge inward. Agents selected for use should have broad-spectrum, antimicrobial action, be nontoxic, and provide long-acting protection. When urinary catheters are inserted, care must be taken to maintain their sterility in a confined space. If the catheter is inadvertently compromised, it must be discarded in favor of a new one. When catheterizing women it is not uncommon to mistakenly insert the catheter into the vagina. When this occurs, it should not be reused. It is frequently helpful to place one of the iodophor-soaked prep sponges at the vaginal opening before attempting to insert the catheter.

Proper cleansing of the male genitalia begins at the penile prepuce. Sponges should used in a circular motion, beginning with the meatus and working outward. The solution is applied to the penile shaft last. Men are also at risk because of enlarged prostate glands. If this is the case, difficulty inserting the catheter may result, causing kinking and rolling of the catheter. The tendency to force the catheter past the obstructing sphincter should be avoided. Slow manipulation of the catheter and the angle of the penile shaft will usually allow smooth passage.

Endoscopy is the most common genitourinary procedure. Instrumentation of the urethral and ureteral orifices must be gentle to avoid trauma to the linings, which will raise the opportunity for organisms to proliferate. When possible, it is wise to drape off the rectal area before instrumentation. Irrigations employed must be sterile with closed administration systems that prevent the risk of cross-contamination.

Other activities that have high priority in reducing the incidence of contamination include the following:

- Conscientiously following Universal Precautions
- Reducing traffic and limiting the number of visitors
- Wearing appropriate operating room apparel properly
- Ensuring minimal talking and laughing
- Keeping doors and cabinets closed
- Planning room setup to achieve optimal traffic flow away from sterile field
- Avoiding procedures on patients with altered skin integrity caused by infection or abrasion
- Maintaining sterile technique with gentle, minimal tissue handling and effective hemostasis
- Double gloving or donning puncture-proof sterile gloves for implant procedures
- Encouraging preoperative bathing for the patient
- Performing wet shave preps outside the confines of the operating room suite
- Keeping environment and equipment clean and free of dust and particulate matter
- Following recommended guidelines for disinfection of endoscopy instrumentation
- Providing appropriate antibiotic coverage
- Utilizing water-repellent draping materials
- Observing for breaks in technique and rectifying situation (hole in glove)

When prepping other anatomic sites, the solution should be warmed and applied in a circular fashion from the interior aspect to the outside without returning to the incisional site with the same sponge. The prepped area should extend beyond the fenestration in the drape to be employed. Protective, absorbent pads or towels tucked around and under the patient will help prevent pooling of prep solutions. The towels should be removed after prepping and before draping.

Drapes that are water repellent and disposable afford more protection against bacterial migration than provided by cloth draping materials. Adherence to aseptic technique during draping is the most cost-efficient method of controlling contamination and decreasing the possibility of wound infection. After the drape is applied it should not be readjusted to lie closer to the wound. Fanning of draping products and gowns increases the air currents and should be avoided. Clips that do not puncture the draping material should be utilized for securing suctions and electrosurgical pencils.

If prophylactic antibiotics are planned, they should be administered 1 hour before the scheduled surgery time to be at peak effect at the time of the actual incision or instrumentation.

Irrigations

Commercially prepared sterile irrigation products with closed administration sets are recommended for genitourinary interventions. These are available in collapsible bags or rigid plastic containers in volumes of 3000, 4000, or 5000 ml. Both function independently of air, may be hung in series providing continuous flow, and eliminate the distorted visibility caused by air bubbles prevalent with other systems. During the more extensive endoscopic procedures, large volumes of irrigation are used. When instilled at room temperature, they may cause a shock to the patient's internal thermostat and create hypothermia. Solution-warming units are available and provide a controlled temperature that may decrease this risk. The drawback is that clotting is delayed, therefore potentially increasing blood loss.

During cystoscopy the bladder is distended with sterile water for irrigation to increase visualization. Water is also appropriate for a simple retrograde pyelogram and bladder tumor fulguration without undue risk of complication from extravasation and fluid overload. During transurethral resection of the prostate (TURP), however, venous sinuses may be opened allowing varying amounts of solution to be absorbed into the circulation. The use of distilled water for TURP may cause hemolysis of erythrocytes and possible renal failure. Other complicating effects are dilutional hyponatremia and cardiac decompensation.

For TURP and transurethral resection of the bladder neck (TURBN), a clear, nonelectrolytic, and isosmotic solution is ideal. The most widely accepted are 3% sorbitol (an isomer of mannitol), and 1.5% glycine (an aminoacetic acid). At slightly hypotonic concentrations, sorbitol and glycine do not produce hemolysis. Their nonelectrolytic properties prevent the dispersion of high-frequency current and the resultant loss of electrosurgical cutting ability as caused by saline solutions. Other acceptable solutions include 5% mannitol, 1.8% urea, and 4% glucose.

It is important to have a comprehensive knowledge of the risks encountered during transurethral surgery. Although complications more commonly appear in the postoperative stage, close observation intraoperatively is essential. Sudden restlessness, irritability, apprehension, and slow pulse with rising blood pressure may be indicative of transurethral resection (TUR) syndrome. In this condition a decrease in the volume of extracellular sodium causes a shift of body fluids and electrolytes, causing cerebral edema. Serum electrolyte studies should be drawn if the onset of symptoms occurs. Minimal amounts of intravenous fluids and irrigations should be administered at low pressure and the bladder emptied before full capacity is reached, to prevent intravesical pressure. Hypertonic sodium or a diuretic (furosemide/Lasix) may be added to the intravenous line if a low serum sodium value is reported.

During ureteroscopy and nephroscopy, 0.9% saline is the irrigant of choice. When it is necessary to visualize the collecting system fluoroscopically, a radiographic contrast material is used. Saline approximates a physiologic solution, and absorption will not alter osmolality or electrolyte composition. Fluid overload can still occur, however, and the patient should be observed for early symptoms. Systemic absorption may occur if there is a perforation with extravasation and pyelolymphatic, pyelorenal, or pyelovenous backflow from the ureter or renal collecting system.

If bipolar electrosurgery is employed, it is prudent to remain with saline by means of simple gravity flow. When monopolar electrosurgery is chosen, the irrigation should be changed to sorbitol, glycine, or water.

Evaluation

The patient's attainment of established outcomes is evaluated on a continuing basis throughout the perioperative experience. The process is systematic, resulting in altering the plan of care as determined through assessment. Collected data is compared against the outcome criteria to discover the level of goal achievement reached. For continuity of care it is necessary to not only document the care provided but also to verbalize it to other pertinent caregivers. Evaluation is accomplished immediately postoperatively, in the PACU unit, on the inpatient surgical unit, and through follow-up communication with the patient after discharge from the ambulatory care facility or hospital. Each patient care situation is unique, and the evaluation process must be adjusted accordingly. The information gleaned allows for the implementation of improved methods of patient care. A Critical Pathway appropriate for TURP is found in Table 5-3.

Postoperative complications

Under the best of circumstances, complications will occur. The genitourinary patient is frequently at increased risk for intraoperative and postoperative complications. The ones posing the greatest effect over the long term are briefly discussed. They include pulmonary embolus, myocardial infarction, congestive heart failure, hemorrhage, brachial plexus injury, and infection (including cardiac implications). Additionally, mention should be made of paralytic ileus and cerebral vascular accident (CVA).

Pulmonary embolus (PE) occurs as a result of deep vein thrombosis and has a significant occurrence in the postopera-

Table 5-3 **Critical Pathway for TURP without Complications**

DRG 336; expected LOS 4 days	Day of surgery Day of admission			Day of discharge
	DAY 1	**DAY 2**	**DAY 3**	**DAY 4**
Diagnostic tests	*Preoperative:* Chest x-ray film, CBC, ECG, PT/PTT, PSA, electrolytes, chemistries *Postoperative:* CBC, electrolytes	CBC, electrolyes		
Medications	*Preoperative:* IV antibiotic *Postoperative:* IVs; IV antibiotic; PRN: IV or IM analgesic, B& O suppository, stool softener	IV to saline lock; IV/PO antibiotic; PRN: PO analgesic, B&O suppository, stool softener	D/C saline lock; PO antibiotics; PRN: PO analgesics, B&O suppository, stool softener	PO antibiotic; PRN: PO analgesic, stool softener; no ASA or non-steroidals until cleared
Treatments	I&O q8h including Foley catheter and CBI, tension on Foley catheter as indicated; VS q4h; alternating compression stockings until ambulatory; assess peripheral vascular circulation q2h.	I&O q8h including Foley catheter; D/C CBI, Foley catheter to DD; VS q6h; D/C compression stockings if fully ambulatory; assess peripheral vascular circulation q4h	I&O q8h; D/C Foley catheter; VS q8h, assess peripheral vascular circulation q8h	D/C I&O; VS q8h
Diet	*Preoperative:* NPO *Postoperative:* clear liquids, advance to regular as tolerated; force fluids: 8 oz q2h (1/2 juice, 1/2 water).	Regular diet; force fluids; 8 oz q2h (1/2 juice, 1/2 water).	Regular diet; force fluids: 8 oz q3h if urine clear (1/2 juice, 1/2 water).	Regular diet, force fluids: 8 oz q3h (1/2 juice, 1/2 water), no alcohol until cleared
Activity	Bedrest; assess neuromotor return after spinal anesthesia; assist with ambulation when functional	Up ad lib to chair; assist with ambulation	BR privileges; ambulate ad lib; no lifting >10 lb	Ambulate ad lib, stairs 1-2 day max, no strenuous exercise or lifting >10 lb, 10 min ride as tolerated, no sexual activity until cleared
Consultations		Social service, home health		

ASA, Acetylsalicylic acid; *B&O,* belladonna and opium; *BR,* bathroom; *CBC,* complete blood cell count; *CBI,* continuous bladder irrigation; *D/C,* discontinue; *DD,* differential diagnosis; *DRG,* diagnosis-related group; *ECG,* electrocardiogram; *IM,* intramuscular; *I&O,* intake and output; *IV,* intravenous; *LOS,* length of stay; *NPO,* nothing by mouth; *PO,* by mouth; *PRN,* as required; *PSA,* prostate specific antigen; *PT/PTT,* prothrombin and partial thromboplastin time; *VS,* vital signs.

tive urologic patient. Many of the predisposing factors are found in the genitourinary patient and include the presence of malignancy, advanced age, obesity, long-term estrogen therapy, and immobility both intraoperatively and postoperatively. Symptoms of onset are sudden apprehension, tachycardia, dyspnea, and rales. Dilation of the hemorrhoidal veins also occurs and is displayed by a sense of urinary urgency. Unfortunately, many procedures are performed under general anesthesia, removing the patient's ability to verbalize these sensations.

Prostatectomy and pelvic lymph node dissection pose the greatest threat for the development of PE. There is a 40% occurrence with open prostatectomies compared with 10% for TURP. The best treatment is prevention, and efforts should focus on therapies to reduce the risk. The use of alternating compression stockings has been shown to offer the greatest

benefit to the urologic patient. Placing the patient in Trendelenburg position intraoperatively aids venous return and prevents venous pooling in the lower extremities. These two modalities probably afford the best chance of decreasing this potential complication. Postoperatively, early ambulation, passive exercises of the feet and ankles (dorsiflexion, plantar flexion), and anticoagulants such as heparin will assist the patient toward an uneventful recovery. Thrombolytic agents, often employed for pulmonary embolus, are contraindicated in the postoperative genitourinary patient because of the already high incidence of bleeding complications.

Myocardial infarction (MI) has a low incidence in patients with no prior history (0.15%) but rises to a range of 5% to 6% in those with a remote history of MI and to as much as 30% for those who have suffered an attack 3 months or less preoperatively. The prevalence of heart disease and disturbances in the patient's physiologic state is high in the genitourinary population. Additionally, many of the patients are elderly with cardiac impairments that present more subtly. Often the hemodynamic and metabolic stress of anesthesia and surgery exceed the reserve of homeostatic responses in patients with cardiac disease and increase the burden on a circulatory system that is already impaired. The best preventive measure is to postpone elective surgery for 6 months after onset of the last MI. When surgery is undertaken, it is wise to interrupt aspirin therapy (common in these patients) for 7 to 10 days preoperatively. The risks of bleeding and the potential imbalance between myocardial oxygen demand and supply takes precedence over the chance of a major change in any cardiac atherosclerotic lesion.

Congestive heart failure (CHF) generally will develop very early in the postoperative period and may be related to the patient's functional state preoperatively. Symptoms include systolic dysfunction, pulmonary congestion, hypoxia, vasoconstriction, hypotension, and decreased peripheral perfusion. Major organ dysfunction can result if left unrecognized and not properly treated.

The most common surgical causes are blood transfusions and absorption of irrigation solutions through the venous circulation during transurethral resections. The use of a continuous low-pressure flow of irrigants will decrease the incidence of major extravasation, even if perforation occurs. Other intraoperative preventive measures include avoiding fluid overload, cautious administration of anesthetic agents, controlling hypertension, and correcting myocardial ischemia. Intraoperative hemodynamic monitoring of patients with circulatory instability and potential left ventricular dysfunction, when shifts in intravascular fluid volume are anticipated, as during prostate or bladder tumor resection, is advisable. This can be accomplished easily with a peripheral arterial line. Treatment with diuretic therapy and intravenous hypertonic sodium chloride may be required.

Hemorrhage is always a risk during genitourinary interventions and may entail significant cardiac consequences, particularly with transurethral bladder tumor resection, radical prostate surgery, and radical cystectomy. The bladder is highly vascular, and most tumors contained within it are well vascularized. To prevent overt and extensive bleeding, all vessels should be cauterized, as they appear, during tumor resection. The prostate gland also has a copious vascular supply and typical blood loss could reach 1 L. Additionally, hemodilution often occurs because of intravascular fluid shifts as a result of the large amounts of irrigating solutions employed. Radical cystectomy is associated with extensive blood loss that is poorly tolerated by frail or elderly patients. When hemorrhage occurs during the recovery period, the best treatment is often a return to the operating room to establish control of bleeding sites. The use of a traction catheter in the fossa of the bladder neck may also provide adequate control until coagulation occurs. Intraabdominal hemorrhage leaves little option but to reoperate.

Brachial plexus injury is one of the most painful and potentially long-term complications that can occur during genitourinary surgery. The extreme positioning frequently employed puts the patient at high risk for injury. Many surgeons refuse the use of shoulder braces because of the potential untoward results. Improperly placed shoulder braces stretch the brachial plexus by forcing the shoulders downward or damage the nerves through direct compression. If the braces are applied correctly over the bony acromial process, the risk is dramatically reduced.

Hyperabduction of the arm and severe extension and flexion of the neck are the most common causes intraoperatively. If the arm is hyperabducted with the shoulder posteriorly displaced and forced downward during positioning, the costoclavicular space is narrowed. As a result, the subclavian artery is occluded by the costoclavicular compression. The absence of a radial pulse warns of potential nerve compression. Palsy postoperatively can be attributed to stretch or compression for extended periods of time. When the neck is extended and flexed to the opposite side or if the arm is in any extreme position, especially if abducted and externally rotated, the plexus is stretched.

Infection prevention remains a primary goal no matter what the surgical undertaking. In genitourinary interventions, the risk is ever present because many patients are presenting to the operating room for that very reason. Any obstruction of the genitourinary canal poses the possibility of the presence of infection.

Infectious endocarditis carries an incidence of 10% in genitourinary patients with valvular heart disease. Conditions include aortic stenosis, aortic regurgitation, mitral stenosis, rheumatic heart disease, mitral regurgitation, and the presence of prosthetic heart valves. The need for prophylactic antibiotics begins preoperatively to reduce the chance of infective endocarditis whenever procedure-associated bacteremia may be present.

Protocol for techniques to reduce the risk begin with the patient assessment. A well-hydrated patient will better be able to withstand surgical violation. A review of the medical record along with the patient interview should ascertain if any inflammatory process is occurring. Urinary tract infections or genital lesions that are infected may necessitate cancelation, especially if implantation of a prosthetic device is planned. Other steps to include are maintenance of meticulous aseptic technique, provision of intravenous antibiotic therapy, utilization of antibiotic wound-irrigating solutions, prevention of surface contaminants from contacting the prosthesis, verifying the integrity and sterility of all prosthetics before actual implantation, and following of the manufacturer's recommendations for the implant.

Paralytic ileus is not an uncommon event after major abdominal or pelvic intervention. It is usually associated with manipulation of the intestines. Ileus is characterized by a reflex loss of bowel function caused by diminished peristaltic activity, believed to be attributable to transient diminished autonomic function. It often does not manifest itself until after the patient has been discharged.

Cerebrovascular accident (CVA) is an additional but little discussed untoward event. Many genitourinary patients have labile blood pressures along with undiagnosed carotid insufficiency. Because of the known relation of atherosclerotic disease to cardiovascular disease, it is important to investigate the cardiovascular status during the preoperative workup. Recent history of an acute MI may be associated with carotid artery disease. Total operative deaths from CVA average about 5% overall. Intraoperatively the best course is the prevention of hypertension, hypotension, and hypocapnia.

Quality improvement

The overall success of direct and indirect nursing care is assessed through quality review and improvement. The Joint Commission on Accreditation of Healthcare Organizations (JCAHO)[21] encourages the provision of high-quality health services through a generic 10-step model that assesses patient care outcomes and guides the process leading to improved patient care activities. The Association of Operating Room Nurses has published standards consistent with JCAHO guidelines.[4]

Each key aspect of patient care has identified quality indicators that focus on structure, process, and outcome. These indicators should be objective, measurable, and based on current knowledge and clinical experience. The criteria are drawn from the Standards of Perioperative Administrative Practice; the Standards of Perioperative Clinical Practice; the Standards of Perioperative Professional Performance; Quality Improvement Standards for Perioperative Nursing; Patient Outcomes: Standards of Perioperative Care; and the Recommended Practices for Perioperative Nursing.[3,4] Additionally, within the specialty of genitourinary surgery, criteria based on the Standards of Urologic Nursing Practice[1] should be incorporated.

Each indicator is independent of any others and should measure appropriate protocols. Data to be collected for each indicator is defined according to determined criteria. Once the data has been gathered, it is evaluated to identify ongoing needs for improved patient care or other areas for improvement. The methods of data collection are specific for each listed indicator. The goal of this ongoing monitoring is improved patient care.

Patient care activities are broad in their scope and include the patient population, customers served, clinical care activities, services provided, and physical site. Important aspects of care in the genitourinary field include high risk, high volume, and increased anxiety.

Emphasizing quality improvement (QI) links the continuum of caregivers who interact with the genitourinary population. As a result, a standard of excellence may be achieved in an objective and comprehensive manner for the patient's benefit. There are numerous opportunities for the perioperative genitourinary nurse to directly affect patient care through the QI process and monitor the results for unaddressed issues and needed improvements.

GLOSSARY

Abduct To draw away from a position parallel to the median axis of the body.

Apnea Transient cessation of respiration, either normal or abnormal; asphyxia.

Autonomic dysreflexia (hyperreflexia) Manifested by cardiovascular symptoms occurring involuntarily in patients with transverse lesions of cervical and thoracic spinal cord, above the sixth thoracic vertebra; syndrome of exaggerated sympathetic activity in response to stimuli below the level of the lesion (usually bladder or rectum); symptoms: pounding headache, hypertension (may be severe enough to cause seizure or cerebral hemorrhage), flushing of face and body above the level of the lesion, diaphoresis, bradycardia or tachycardia.

Bacteremia Transient presence of bacteria in the blood.

Brachial plexus Complex network of nerves formed chiefly by the lower four cervical nerves and the first thoracic nerve, partly in the axilla, supplying nerves to the chest, shoulder, and arm.

Bradycardia Relatively slow heart action, physiologic or pathologic.

Cephalad Toward the head.

Dementia Condition of deteriorated mentality characterized by a sharp decline from a former intellectual level and by emotional apathy.

Diaphoresis Profuse perspiration artificially induced.

Disseminated intravascular coagulopathy (DIC) All clotting factors, including fibrin, are used up, or coagulated, resulting in uncontrollable bleeding widely dispersed throughout the body; treatment is difficult, requiring anticoagulants, such as heparin, to stop the clotting propensity.

Dyscrasia An imbalance of components of the blood.

Dyspnea Difficult or labored respirations.

Echopenic Decreased reflections on ultrasonography; fewer echoes.

Embolus Abnormal particle, such as an air bubble, circulating in the blood.

Endocarditis Inflammation of the lining of the heart and its valves.

Epidural Administered outside the dura mater.

Erythrocyte Red blood cell.

Extraurethral Occurring outside the urethra.

Femoral nerve Largest branch of the lumbar plexus, from the second to the fourth lumbar nerves, supplying the extensor muscles of the thigh, skin on the front of the thigh, medial surface of the leg and foot with articular branches to the hip and knee joints.

Hemodynamics Functioning mechanics of circulating blood.

Hemoglobinuria Free hemoglobin in the urine.

Hemolysis Lysis of red blood cells with release of hemoglobin.

Homogeneous Same echo pattern throughout structure.

Hypercapnia Presence of an excess of carbon dioxide in the blood.

Hyperextension Angle between bones of a joint is greater than normal.

Hyperflexion Angle between bones of a joint is smaller than normal.

Hypocapnia Deficiency of carbon dioxide in the blood.

Hypokalemia Deficiency of potassium in the blood.

Hyponatremia Deficiency of sodium in the blood.

Hypotonic Deficient tone or tension; a lower osmotic pressure than the surrounding medium or fluid.

Hypoxia Deficiency of oxygen to the tissues of the body.

Ileus Obstruction of the bowel, commonly characterized by painful distension of the abdomen, vomiting of dark or fecal matter, toxemia, and dehydration; occurs when intestinal contents back up due to peristaltic failure although the lumen is open; not uncommon after manipulation of the bowel.

Isosmotic Having the same osmotic pressure, as a solution to a protoplasm.

Labile Frequently changing; continually undergoing physical, biologic, or chemical breakdown, characterized by wide fluctuations.

Lateral decubitus Position in which patient lies on his or her side.

Lumbosacral plexus Network of nerves comprising the lumbar plexus and the sacral plexus.

Mitral valve prolapse (MVP) Bicuspid valve displaced down from its anatomic position.

Palsy Uncontrollable tremor or quivering of the body or one of its parts.

Peroneal nerve Between the fibula and peroneus longus muscle innervating the muscles of the anterior part of the leg and skin on the lower anterior leg, dorsum of the foot, lateral and medial aspects of the foot, and between the toes.

Phlebitis Inflammation of a vein.

Popliteal nerve Common peroneal nerve, behind the knee joint.

Pyelolymphatic Urine flow from the kidney pelvis into the lymphatic system; abnormal.

Pyelorenal Urine flow from the kidney pelvis into the kidney; abnormal.

Pyelovenous Urine flow from kidney pelvis to renal venous system; backflow abnormal amounts of pressure in a direction opposite to normal.

Rales Abnormal rattle heard on auscultation of chest.

Retroperitoneal Behind the peritoneum.

Sciatic nerve Either of the pair of the largest nerves in the body arising from each side of the sacral plexus, passing out of the pelvis down the back of the thigh where it divides into the tibial and common peroneal nerves.

Sequelae Aftereffect of disease, injury, procedure, or treatment.

Shearing Shaving action.

Subarachnoid Under the arachnoid membrane where cerebrospinal fluid circulates.

Supraclavicular Above the clavicle.

Tachycardia Relatively rapid heartbeat action physiologic or pathologic.

Tinnitus Sensation of noise, ringing or roaring, caused by a bodily condition, heard only by the one affected.

Uremia Accumulation in the blood of constituents eliminated in the urine producing severe toxicity.

Bibliography

1. American Urological Association Allied: *Standards of urologic nursing practice,* Richmond, Va., 1990, AUAA.
2. Association of Operating Room Nurses: *Core curriculum for the RN first assistant,* Denver, 1990, AORN.
3. Association of Operating Room Nurses: *Quality improvement in perioperative nursing,* Denver, 1992, AORN.
4. Association of Operating Room Nurses: *Standards and recommended practices,* Denver, 1996, AORN.
5. Bagley DH: *Techniques with the flexible ureteroscope,* Stamford, Conn., 1991, Circon-ACMI.
6. Bennett AH: *Impotence: diagnosis and management of erectile dysfunction,* Philadelphia, 1994, WB Saunders.
7. Benumuf JL, Saidman LJ: *Anesthesia and perioperative complications,* St. Louis, 1992, Mosby.
8. Bernays AC: *Golden rules of surgery,* St. Louis, 1906, Mosby.
9. Brundage DJ: *Renal disorders,* St. Louis, 1992, Mosby.
10. Coussons TR, McKee PA, Williams GR: *Manual of medical care of the surgical patient,* Boston, 1990, Little, Brown.
11. Davidson AJ, Hartman DS: *Radiology of the kidney and urinary tract,* Philadelphia, 1994, WB Saunders.
12. Donahue MP: *Nursing—the finest art,* St. Louis, 1985, Mosby.
13. Doughty DB: *Urinary and fecal incontinence: nursing management,* St. Louis, 1991, Mosby.
14. Drach GW: *Common problems in infections and stones,* St. Louis, 1992, Mosby.
15. Droller MJ: *Surgical management of urologic disease,* St. Louis, 1992, Mosby.
16. Gillenwater JY et al: *Adult and pediatric urology,* ed 3, St. Louis, 1996, Mosby.
17. Gray M: *Genitourinary disorders,* St. Louis, 1992, Mosby.
18. Hampton BG, Bryant RA: *Ostomies and continent diversions,* St. Louis, 1992, Mosby.
19. Horne MM, Swearingen PL: *Pocket guide to fluid, electrolyte, and acid-base balance,* St. Louis, 1993, Mosby.
20. Huffman JL, Bagley DH, Lyon ES: *Ureteroscopy,* Philadelphia, 1988, WB Saunders.
21. Joint Commission on Accreditation of Healthcare Organizations: *Quality improvement in ambulatory care,* Oakbrook Terrace, Ill., 1994, JCAHO.
22. Kirby R, Christmas T: *Benign prostatic hyperplasia,* London, 1993, Gower.
23. Litwack K: *Core curriculum for post-anesthesia nursing practice,* Philadelphia, 1995, WB Saunders.
24. Lloyd-Davies W et al: *Color atlas of urology,* London, 1994, Mosby-Wolfe.
25. McCarthy JR: *Registered nurse first assistant what's that? The Nursing Spectrum* 4-8, 1995.
26. Meeker MH, Rothrock JC: *Alexander's care of the patient in surgery,* ed 10, St. Louis, 1995, Mosby.
27. Nightingale F: *Notes on nursing,* London, 1859, Harrison & Sons.
28. O'Reilly PH, George NJR, Weiss RM: *Diagnostic techniques in urology,* Philadelphia, 1990, WB Saunders.
29. Pagana KD, Pagana TJ: *Diagnostic and laboratory test reference,* St. Louis, 1992, Mosby.
30. Pfister J et al: *The nursing spectrum of lasers,* ed 2, Denver, 1996, Education Design.
31. Phipps WJ, Long BC, Woods NF: *Medical-surgical nursing,* St. Louis, 1991, Mosby.
32. Resnick MI, Kursh E: *Current therapy in genitourinary surgery,* St. Louis, 1992, Mosby.
33. Resnick MI, Novick AC: *Urology secrets,* St. Louis, 1995, Mosby.
34. Resnick MI: *Prostatic ultrasonography,* Philadelphia, 1990, WB Saunders.
35. Rifkin MD: *Ultrasound of the prostate,* New York, 1988, Raven.
36. Rothrock JC: *Perioperative nursing care planning,* St. Louis, 1995, Mosby.
37. Salerno E, Willens JS: *Pain management handbook,* St. Louis, 1996, Mosby.
38. Smith JA: *The urologic clinics of North America,* Philadelphia, Nov., 1990, WB Saunders.
39. Tanagho EA, McAninch JW: *Smith's general urology,* Norwalk, Conn., 1995, Appleton & Lange.
40. Vaiden RE, Fox VJ, Rothrock JC: *Core curriculum for the RN first assistant,* Denver, 1990, Association of Operating Room Nurses.
41. Walters MD, Karram MM: *Clinical urogynecology,* St. Louis, 1993, Mosby.

6

Genitourinary Supplies

ASSESSMENT OF NEEDS

Collaboration between patient care disciplines to provide the necessary equipment and supplies for a surgical procedure begins when the case is scheduled for the operating room. Preoperative assessment information received from the surgeon's or primary physician's office evaluation and the anticipated procedure should concur with the perioperative assessment performed on the patient's arrival in the preparation area or operating room (OR). Assessment should include consideration of the activities that will take place for each given operative intervention. Some of the needs common to genitourinary surgery are required positioning devices and their relation to the patient's physical and physiologic status, the use and placement of specific table attachments, warming units mandated by the intended event, and employing ancillary machinery.

If x-ray or C-arm fluoroscopy is indicated, the radiology department must be informed so the timing of the procedure may be coordinated with them. When implantable devices are to be employed the appropriate product representative needs to be contacted to provide for any special needs. Suppliers of any unusual or special equipment should be apprised of the scheduled surgery and requested to be available.

Room preparation should focus on optimal traffic patterns in relation to the size and types of equipment to be used. Video units should be placed to provide the operative team with the best possible viewing angle without compromising the sterile field or interfering with nursing functions. Equipment should be tested before the patient's arrival to ensure patient and team safety and effective function. Electrical cables should lie flush with the floor and preferably not in traffic pathways.

To prevent injury to the patient and the staff, proper body mechanics must always be employed. Patient transfer and positioning should be performed with care and consideration should be given to potential neurovascular and peripheral pressure areas. Positioning devices should be clean, in good condition, and placed appropriately.

Routine inspection of electrical components, video units, endoscopy attachments, and laser machines should be done daily. A maintenance program for periodic inspection and calibration adjustments that may be necessary should be in place and utilized.

EQUIPMENT

Genitourinary surgery requires varied types of equipment. To properly function within this specialty, the perioperative nurse must understand the operation and maintenance of these specific electrical devices and the supplies that complement them.

To improve the management and performance of perioperative care, procedural needs must be assessed and organized.

Radiographic equipment may be used at any point before or during a genitourinary procedure. Most commonly radiography will be employed during endoscopic interventions that require visualization of the urinary tract as well as documentation of the condition encountered, and treatments performed. C-arm fluoroscopy is utilized most frequently and can provide hard data to place in the patient record as well as live images. The portable x-ray unit may also be mandated if kidneys-ureters-bladder (KUB) or other large radiographs are necessary for documentation. The OR bed must be compatible with the use of C-arm fluoroscopy and portable x-ray .

Laser units employed in genitourinary surgery include the Nd:YAG, CO_2, tunable dye, argon, KTP-532 (frequency doubled Yag), and Ho:YAG. When the laser treatment is performed outside of a fluid environment, the smoke evacuator must be utilized. No matter what type of laser energy is utilized, precautions appropriate to its action must be in place and adhered to. Refer to Chapter 5 for a detailed discussion of lasers and related safety precautions.

Electrical equipment often employed during genitourinary interventions include electrosurgical units, argon enhanced electrosurgical units, bipolar cautery units, fiberoptic light systems, headlights, electrohydraulic and ultrasonic lithotriptors (Fig. 6-1, *A* and *B*), Doppler units, CO_2 insufflators, tissue morselizers, and ultrasound machines. The perioperative nursing staff must be knowledgeable in the use and care of this equipment and be able to troubleshoot when difficulties arise. Manufacturer's guidelines for appropriate settings and safety precautions should be available and followed.

Photography (and videography) has become extremely popular in genitourinary surgery. Endoscopic, ureteroscopic, nephroscopic, laparoscopic, and microscopic interventions now employ camera units for optimal visualization, elimination of eyepiece contamination, and interventional documentation. If still photographs or videotaping is to occur, the patient must be informed. Most operative permits include this possibility but it is often best to make the patient aware that this will indeed take place. Most systems consist of a small camera that mounts on the scope, a monitor, VCR, and printer (Figs. 6-2 and 6-3).

Warming units have become popular during transurethral resection (TUR) procedures (Fig. 6-4). Their use has helped to eliminate the hypothermic effect of the copious amounts of irrigation instilled. The warmed solution may, however, decrease tissue coagulation thereby increasing blood loss. Intravenous solutions and blood products may also be delivered through these units or special warming coils, thereby assisting in the maintenance of internal body temperature.

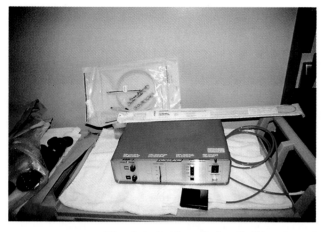
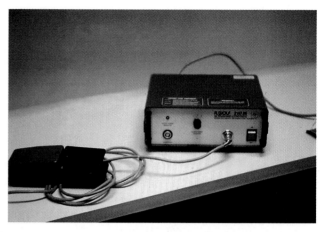

A

Fig. 6-1 **A,** Electrohydraulic lithotriptor (EHL) unit. **B,** Ultrasonic lithotriptor (USL) unit.

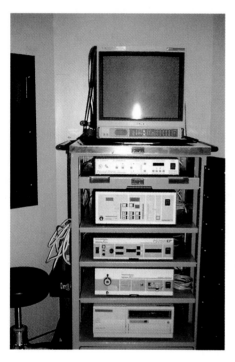

Fig. 6-2 Video system.

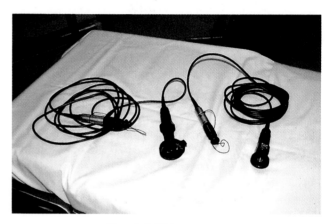

Fig. 6-3 Video camera.

Suction units and **pulse irrigation systems** are generally involved with open or laparoscopic urologic procedures, more recently with transurethral resection of the prostate (TURP), utilizing the continuous flow resection system, and with cryotherapy. Care must be taken to ensure that the vacuum control is adjusted appropriately for the tissue involved.

Power equipment has entered the realm of urology. With some of the newer bladder neck suspension techniques, and more specifically the pubofascial sling, power drills are being employed. The perioperative nurse must be aware of the proper pounds per square inch (psi) setting for the drill being used. These drills run on compressed air or nitrogen through tanks or wall outlets. At the completion of the procedure the power supply should be turned off and the system bled of remaining pressure.

Microscopes are utilized during laser CO_2 ablation and microscopic intervention. Laser vaporization of penile lesions often requires that the microscope or colposcope be attached to the laser arm for optimal visualization of small condylomatous lesions. The microscope need not be draped for laser interventions. It must, however, be thoroughly wiped down following all procedures with a germicidal or 9 to 1 concentration of bleach solution. Alcohol should be used on the lens and binoculars (Fig. 6-5).

Vasovasostomy and vasoepididymostomy mandate use of a microscope designed for plastic or reconstructive surgery. This microscope is equipped with two inclinable binocular heads located across from each other (Fig. 6-6). During reconstructive procedures it should be covered with a sterile microscope drape. Sterile operating handles may be attached to the adjustable knobs if draping is not possible.

Microscopes tend to be top heavy and cumbersome and must be handled with care. During storage they should be covered for protection from particulate matter and guarded from jarring.

Positioning devices used in genitourinary surgery include vacuum packs (Vacpac), gel pads, stirrups, prone frames, standard arm boards, lateral arm boards, prone arm boards, shoul-

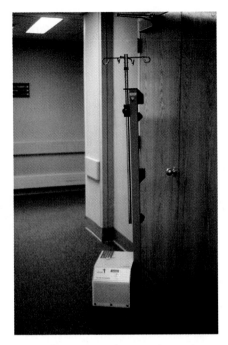

Fig. 6-4 Level 1 warming unit

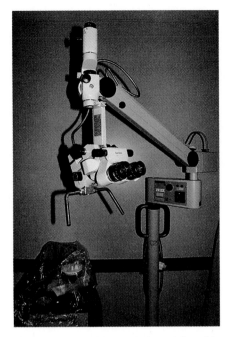

Fig. 6-5 ENT microscope, laser adaptable.

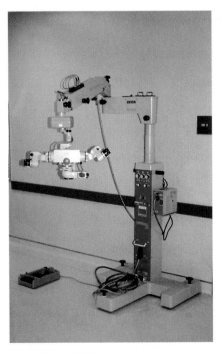

Fig. 6-6 Plastic microscope.

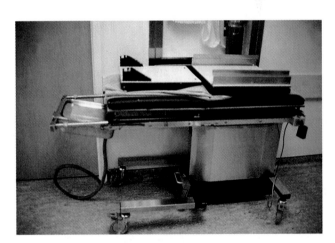

Fig. 6-7 Cystoscopy bed.

der braces, three-point hip positioner, pillows, blankets, foam bolsters, sandbags, head supports, and foot extensions. The patient may be positioned in lithotomy, supine, prone, lateral, semi-lateral (prone-oblique), Trendelenburg, or reverse Trendelenburg positions depending on the intended procedure. Three types of stirrups are depicted in Figs. 5-5 and 5-6.

Endoscopic procedures require an OR bed designed for urologic procedures. This bed has a drainage pan with a removable screen that may be pulled out to catch resected tissue (Fig. 6-7). The pan should be thoroughly cleaned after each use. When the procedure requires lateral or exaggerated lithotomy positioning, an electric OR bed with an adjustable kidney rest is preferable (Fig. 6-8). Electric beds afford a smoother action when extreme positioning is necessary, as is common in perineal prostatectomy and laparoscopic nephrectomy. It is important to charge the electric bed at the end of each operative day to ensure proper function.

INSTRUMENTATION

Instrumentation for the specialty of genitourinary surgery has become extremely sophisticated and costly. As a result of the advanced technology available, the operating room that handles genitourinary surgery must have a healthy budget. The

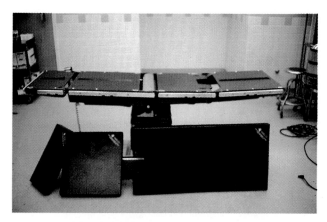

Fig. 6-8 Electric operating room bed.

fiberoptics and video equipment currently employed are constantly improving in quality and capabilities, requiring periodic updating. Perioperative genitourinary nurses cannot function efficiently within the specialty without current knowledge of the instrumentation and equipment, as well as a good understanding of proper care and operation. Inherent in this understanding should be the ability to troubleshoot, maintain, sterilize, and operate the various components. Repairs are costly and proper handling of the delicate instrumentation is essential.

CARE AND HANDLING

Open urology procedures do not require instrumentation that differs greatly from general surgery. Instruments will be employed on varied anatomic structures and must accommodate diverse needs as they present themselves. A knowledge of anatomy and the intended interventions will allow the perioperative nurse to plan properly when selecting instruments for the procedure. Needs will range from large retractors to delicate microsurgical scissors. It is important that instruments be used for the purpose for which they were designed in order to avoid unsafe patient care, unnecessary damage, and costly replacement. Some common misuses include the following:

- Failure to check instruments routinely for damage and flaws
- Using Metzenbaum scissors to cut sutures
- Using hemostats that are too small to accommodate the tissue mass
- Failure to clear the lumens of suction tips and other channeled instruments
- Improper storage of instruments and endoscopes

The genitourinary surgeon has the right to expect instruments that are in good working order and the appropriate size and type for the task. Instruments of good quality that have been properly maintained will afford many years of useful service. The instrument quality is as important as the care given to them. When purchasing instruments it behooves the perioperative nurse to choose instruments that are cost effective by evaluating quality versus price and company guarantee. The goal should be the highest quality for the best value.

Proper instrument care necessitates cleaning during the operative procedure by rinsing blood and other debris in sterile distilled water. Foreign matter that has been allowed to dry will adversely affect the box locks and jaws, leading to compromise in sterility and instrument corrosion and malfunction. Channeled instruments should be periodically cleared with a syringe and obturator. Instruments should never be cleaned or soaked in saline solution because of its corrosive properties. Damage can also be avoided by ensuring that lighter weight or delicate instruments are not stacked below heavier items. It is wise to separate sharps, retractors, and general instruments into different containers during the clean-up process.

All instruments that have been in the surgical field, whether used or not, are considered case-contaminated and require routine decontamination. Soiled instruments should be opened and immersed in water, preferably with a mild detergent added, until appropriate precautions can be taken. It is standard practice to place the instruments in an ultrasonic washer or washer-sterilizer for initial cleaning. Scissors, hemostats, forceps, and channeled instruments generally require additional attention to remove gross blood and debris before placing them in the washing unit. After the initial washer-sterilizer cycle, instruments should be placed in an ultrasonic rinsing unit, which will remove any remaining particles. This may be followed by an ultrasonic dryer in some institutions. Any instruments that appear stiff or tight in their ratchet or jaw action should be placed in an instrument lubricating solution to eliminate freezing of the jaws and box locks. Following decontamination, all instruments should be evaluated for proper function and alignment. Stained, pitted, or rusting instruments should be removed from service; these are the preliminary signs of instrument damage and require correction.

BASIC INSTRUMENTS

Instruments are generally arranged in sets designed to accommodate intraabdominal, retroperitoneal, inguinal, perineal, suprapubic, retropubic, flank, endoscopic, laparoscopic, and microscopic approaches. Figure 6-9 displays microscopic instrumentation specific to urology. The instrument sets may serve more than one approach, are composed of basic general surgery instrumentation, and are interchangeable with the addition of more specific specialized instrumentation (Figs. 6-10 to 6-19). Large self-retaining retractors are frequently employed for major intraabdominal, perineal, and flank surgery (Figs. 6-20 to 6-26) These are packaged separately because of their size and weight.

Basic soft tissue instruments are required for all open genitourinary surgery. The exact procedure will determine the need for case-specific (larger, deep, microscopic, vascular) instrumentation (Figs. 6-27 and 6-28). The trays should contain enough instrumentation to accommodate anatomic requirements and the surgeon's specific preferences.

ENDOSCOPY

Endourology instrumentation is in the domain of fiberoptics. This instrumentation differs greatly from that employed in open surgery. A minimal amount of soft tissue instrumentation needs to be included. The basic cystoscopy tray contains all items used routinely for endoscopy (Fig. 6-29). When ureteral catheterization is planned, specialized catheterizing instrumen-

Text continues p. 125.

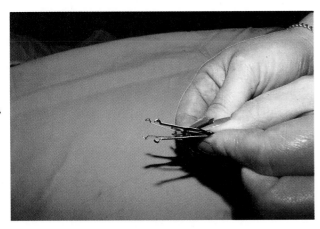
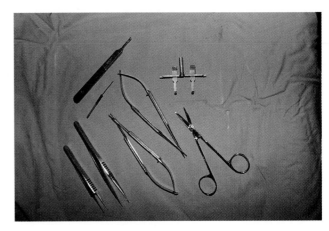

Fig. 6-9 **A,** Microspike for vasovasostomy. **B,** Microsurgery instruments.

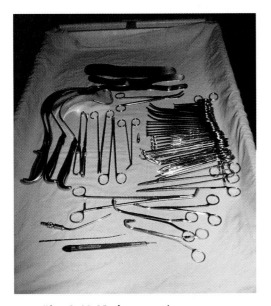

Fig. 6-10 Nephrectomy instruments.

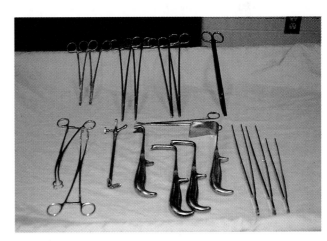

Fig. 6-11 Perineal instruments.

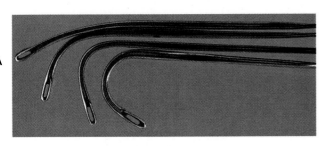
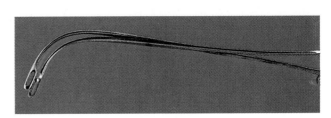

Fig. 6-12 Randall forceps *(From Brooks Tighe SM:* Instrumentation for the operating room, *St. Louis, 1994, Mosby.)*

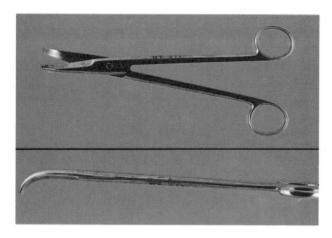

Fig. 6-13 Jorgenson (long, curved-tip) scissors. *(From Brooks Tighe SM:* Instrumentation for the operating room, *St. Louis, 1994, Mosby.)*

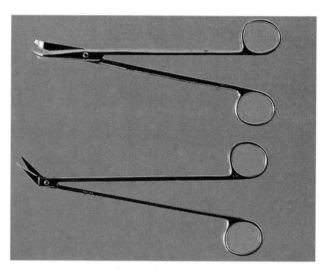

Fig. 6-14 Thorek-Feldman scissors, Potts scissors. *(From Brooks Tighe SM:* Instrumentation for the operating room, *St. Louis, 1994, Mosby.)*

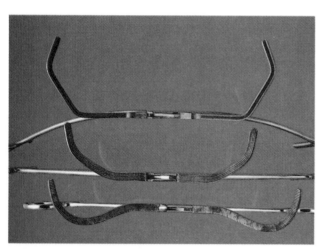

Fig. 6-15 Nephrectomy clamps. *(From Brooks Tighe SM:* Instrumentation for the operating room, *St. Louis, 1994, Mosby.)*

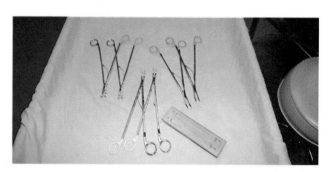

Fig. 6-16 Clip appliers, standard and right angle, and clip base.

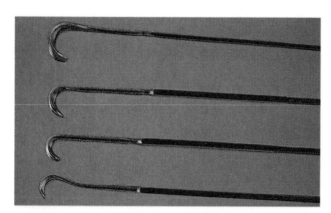

Fig. 6-17 Vein retractors. *(From Brooks Tighe SM:* Instrumentation for the operating room, *St. Louis, 1994, Mosby.)*

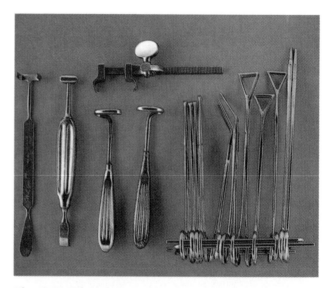

Fig. 6-18 Rib instruments. *(From Brooks Tighe SM:* Instrumentation for the operating room, *St. Louis, 1994, Mosby.)*

tation and supplies may easily be added. Instruments for transurethral resection should be packaged or stored separately (Fig. 6-30).

The ideal is gas-sterilized endoscopy instrumentation that is separately packaged. However, many institutions cannot afford the cost of, or space for, an ETO (ethylene-oxide, "gas") sterilizer. Other options available are soaking in glutaraldehyde (Cidex), employing a hydrogen peroxide or plasma sterilizing unit; and high-vac or gravity steam autoclaving for those components that may be sterilized in this manner. The manufacturer's recommendations should always be followed. If soaking is chosen, it is imperative that the instrumentation be thoroughly rinsed in sterile distilled water. Residue of Cidex remaining in the channels or on the lens can result in chemical burns for the patient and the surgeon. Endoscopy of the genitourinary tract is considered a Class II (clean-contaminated) procedure and, according to Centers for Disease Control and Prevention (CDC) and Association for Practitioners in Infection Control (APIC) guidelines, presently requires disinfection rather than sterilization. Many institutions are treating endoscopic interventions as a sterile procedure, however. Whatever method chosen should be adhered to for every patient treated to provide consistency of care.

Endourology frequently requires the addition of varied instrumentation. In the armamentarium of urology products there are baskets, biopsy forceps, graspers, scissors, stone crushers, visual obturators, laser adapters, urethral sounds, filiforms and followers, evacuators, ureteral pumping systems, fulgerating electrodes, ureteral and urethral catheters, and ureteral stents. Figures 6-31 through 6-34 display some of the ancillary items utilized in endourology.

LAPAROSCOPY

Genitourinary surgery has been modified and improved in the last years with laparoscopic techniques. Procedures now being successfully performed with the laparoscope include nephrectomy, nephroureterectomy, pelvic lymph node dissection, varicocelectomy, orchiectomy, bladder neck suspension, orchiopexy, adrenalectomy, and lymphocelectomy. Other procedures are being attempted but have not progressed beyond the clinical trial stage at this writing.

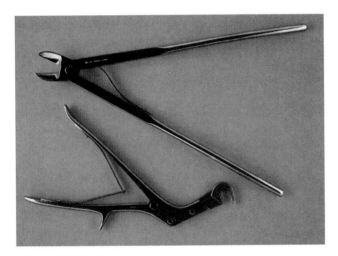

Fig. 6-19 Rib shears. *(From Brooks Tighe SM:* Instrumentation for the operating room, *St. Louis, 1994, Mosby.)*

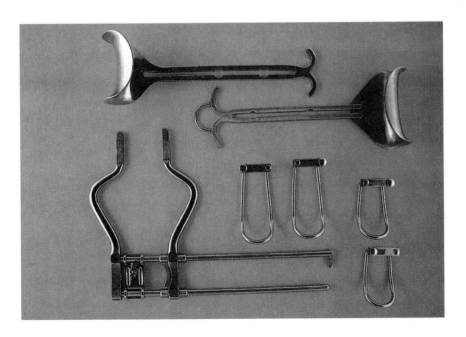

Fig. 6-20 Balfour retractor. *(From Brooks Tighe SM:* Instrumentation for the operating room, *St. Louis, 1994, Mosby.)*

Laparoscopic instrumentation is identical to that employed in general surgery with the addition of a few select instruments not needed in other specialty areas. Care of the laparoscope must be conscientious to avoid damage to the delicate lenses and fiberoptic cables. Laparoscopic instruments frequently utilized include a 10 mm laparoscope, 5 mm laparoscope, 30-degree laparoscope, Metzenbaum scissors with coagulating ability, locking and nonlocking nontoothed graspers, dissectors, Allis forceps, Babcock forceps, suction-irrigators, fulgurating electrodes, suture ligatures, hemoclips, morcelizers, and entrapment sacs. The routine gamut of disposable trocars are also utilized; usually they include insufflation needles, 10- to 12-mm trocars, and 5-mm trocars. Figures 6-35 through 6-39 demonstrate some of the laparoscopic devices employed. During laparoscopic nephrectomy endo-gastrointestinal anastomosis (GIA) staplers and endovascular

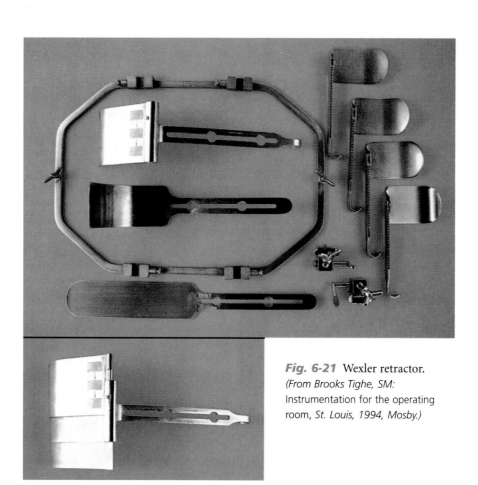

Fig. 6-21 Wexler retractor.
(From Brooks Tighe, SM: Instrumentation for the operating room, St. Louis, 1994, Mosby.)

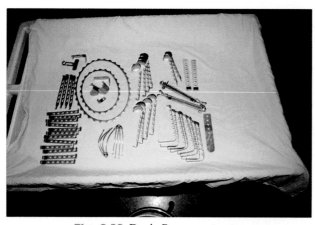

Fig. 6-22 Denis-Browne retractor.

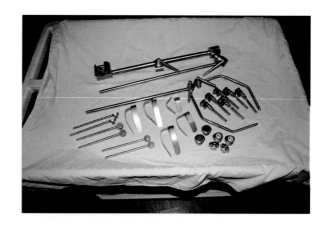

Fig. 6-23 Omni-Tract retractor.

stapling devices will also be employed. Preperitoneal lymphadenectomy and Burch bladder neck suspension utilize the preperitoneal balloon system along with a blunt 10-mm trocar and sharp 5-mm trocar. (Fig. 6-40).

ANCILLARY SUPPLIES

Ureteral catheters are generally provided as presterilized, disposable products. Most are packaged double-wrapped in peel open packages to allow aseptic handling during insertion. Some common indications for ureteral catheters include retrograde pyelography, identification of structures during open gastrointestinal or gynecologic surgery, to provide patency to a strictured or obstructed ureter, and to maintain patency after stone extraction or fracturing. These catheters may be inserted through flexible or rigid cystourethroscopes or ureteropyeloscopes (Figs. 6-41 and 6-42).

The most commonly used ureteral catheter is the simple 5 Fr open-ended catheter. Other frequently needed catheters include the whistle tip, Braasch bulb, spiral-tip, cone-tip, and olive-tip. The spiral-tip Blasucci is often useful when difficulty at the ureterovesical junction (UVJ) occurs. The Braasch bulb or cone tip catheter allows occlusion of the UVJ when retrograde pyelography is inadequate with the open-ended catheter (Fig. 6-43). If a ureteral catheter is left indwelling during open abdominal surgery, it may be connected to a special adapter and attached to a collection bag. A small slit may also be created in the Foley catheter and the distal end of the ureteral catheter slipped in and secured with tape.

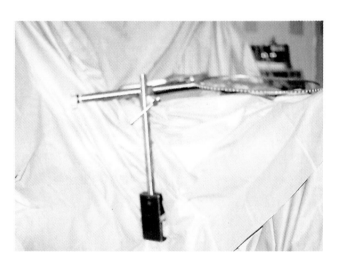

Fig. 6-24 Bookwalter retractor.

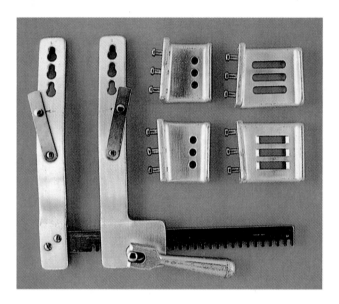

Fig. 6-25 Burford rib spreader. *(From Brooks Tighe SM: Instrumentation for the operating room, St. Louis, 1994, Mosby.)*

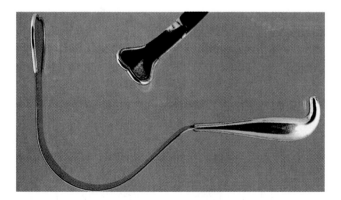

Fig. 6-26 Harrington retractor. *(From Brooks Tighe, SM: Instrumentation for the operating room, St. Louis, 1994, Mosby.)*

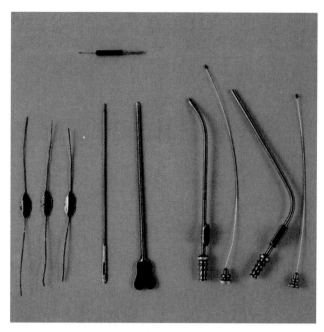

Fig. 6-27 Tear duct probes, suction tips. *(From Brooks Tighe SM: Instrumentation for the operating room, St. Louis, 1994, Mosby.)*

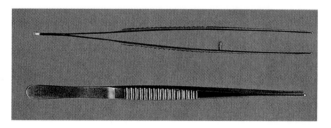

Fig. 6-28 DeBakey forcep. *(From Brooks Tighe SM: Instrumentation for the operating room, St. Louis, 1994, Mosby.)*

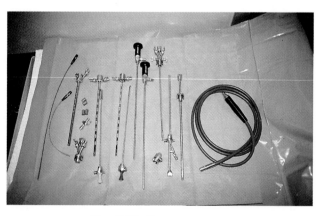

Fig. 6-29 Cystoscopy setup.

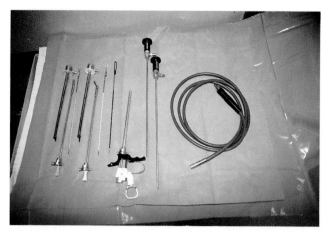

Fig. 6-30 Transurethral resection (TUR) setup.

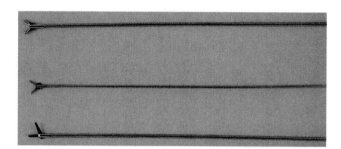

A

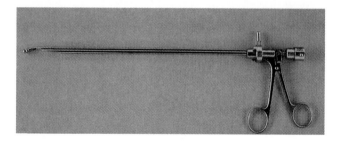

B

Fig. 6-31 A, Flexible endoscopic biopsy forceps and scissors. *From Brooks Tighe SM: Instrumentation for the operating room, St. Louis, 1994, Mosby.)* **B,** Rigid endoscopic biopsy forceps. *(From Brooks Tighe SM: Instrumentation for the operating room, St. Louis, 1994, Mosby.)*

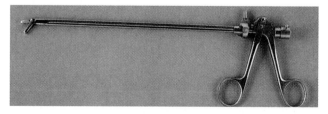

Fig. 6-32 Endoscopic stone crusher. *(From Brooks Tighe SM: Instrumentation for the operating room, St. Louis, 1994, Mosby.)*

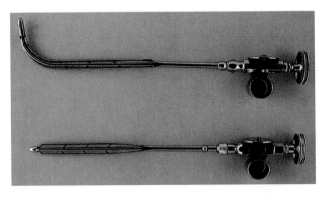

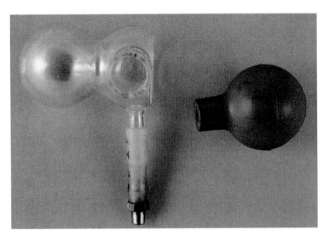

Fig. 6-34 Ellik evacuator. *(From Brooks Tighe SM: Instrumentation for the operating room, St. Louis, 1994, Mosby.)*

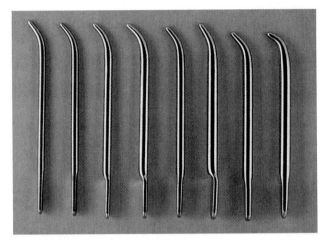

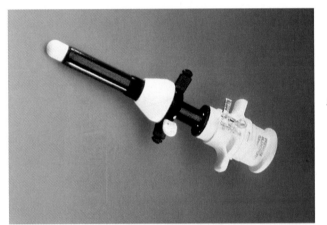

A

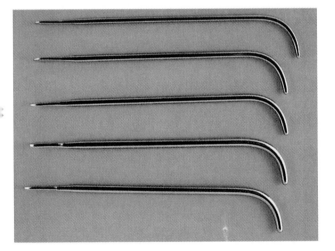

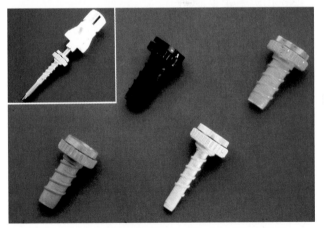

B

Fig. 6-33 Urethral dilators (sounds). **A,** Kollman expandable dilators, curved and straight. **B,** McCrea curved female dilators. **C,** Van Buren curved male dilators. *(From Brooks Tighe SM: Instrumentation for the operating room, St. Louis, 1994, Mosby.*

Fig. 6-35 A, Laparoscopic trocars. **B,** Trocar stabilizers. *(Courtesy United States Surgical Corp., Norwalk, Conn.)*

Ureteral stents generally employed are indwelling pigtail or double-J stents to maintain patency when there is stricture or obstruction of the ureteral canal, or for postoperative extracorporeal shock-wave lithotripsy (ESWL) management. These are generally passed retrograde through the cystoscope or uretero-

scope but may be placed through a percutaneous antegrade (nephroscopic) approach. After ileal diversion stents of this variety are often placed. When the guidewire is removed, a proximal and distal curl (pigtail or J) forms, allowing retention of the stent within the ureter. A nonabsorbable suture may be attached

A

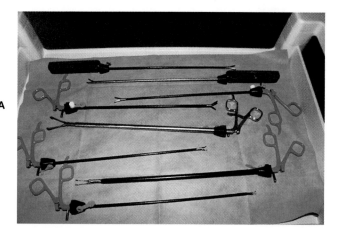

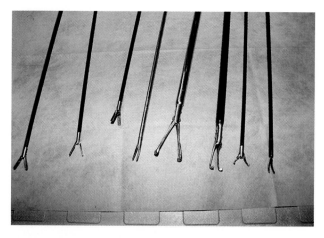

Fig. 6-36 A, Laparoscopic graspers and scissors. **B,** Tip view, laparoscopic graspers, and scissors.

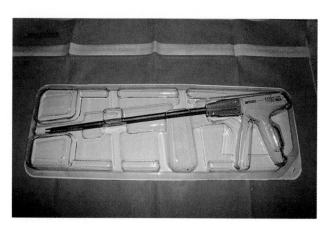

Fig. 6-37 Laparoscopic clip applier.

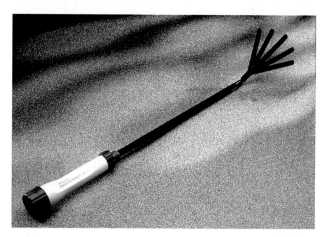

Fig. 6-38 Laparoscopic fan retractor. *(Courtesy United States Surgical Corp.,* Norwalk, Conn.)

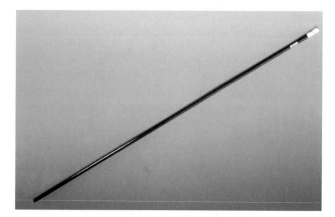

Fig. 6-39 Laparoscopic suction-coagulator. *(Courtesy United States Surgical Corp., Norwalk, Conn.)*

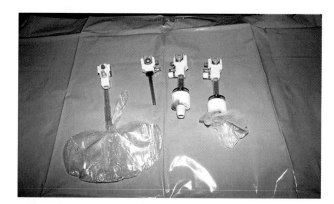

Fig. 6-40 Preperitoneal balloon trocar system, open.

to the distal end before placement (some stents have them already attached) (Fig. 6-44). This suture extends through the urethral meatus, allowing ease of removal in the office setting.

Urethral catheters are utilized for a multitude of purposes. Some of the common indications are stents, drainage tubes,

hemostatic traction, and intraoperative diagnostic studies. They are divided into two categories: indwelling (retention) and plain or straight, ranging in size from 8 to 30 Fr. The most common indwelling catheter is the Foley catheter, available in a variety of tip styles, balloon sizes, lengths, diameters, and eye configura-

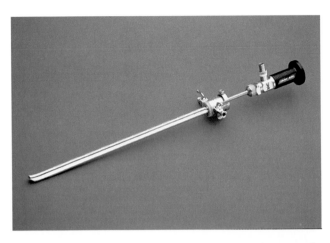

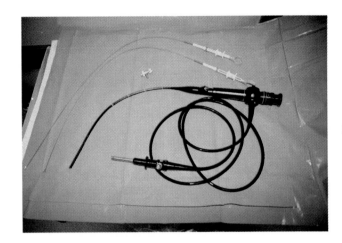

B

Fig. 6-41 **A,** Rigid cystourethroscope. **B,** Flexible cystourethroscope.

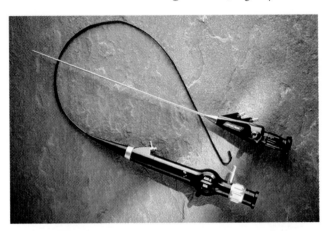

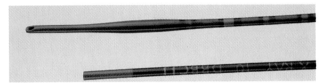

Fig. 6-43 Braasch bulb ureteral catheter. *(Courtesy CR Bard, Urological Division, Covington, Ga.)*

Fig. 6-42 Flexible ureteropyeloscope and rigid ureteropyeloscope. *(Courtesy Circon Corp., Santa Barbara, Calif.)*

be employed. This catheter contains a reinforcing stretch spiral wire within the lining, allowing for more vigorous clot aspiration without lumen collapse.

Diagnostic studies may necessitate the use of a Davis double-balloon urethrography catheter. This catheter is employed for diagnosing lesions of the female urinary tract such as urethral diverticula, stricture, and fistula. The catheter balloons are inflated, one at the external urethral orifice and one within the bladder, isolating the urethra. The entire urethra may be visualized under fluoroscopy by the injection of a contrast medium (Fig. 6-45).

The Pezzar's (mushroom) catheter is a self-retaining catheter primarily used for suprapubic bladder drainage for poor-risk patients suffering from uremia, neurogenic bladder syndrome, or long-standing urinary retention. The Pezzar catheter has a flexible, preformed mushroom-shaped tip, and is a large single-channel catheter (Fig. 6-46).

The Malecot four-winged catheter is often used as a nephrostomy tube to provide temporary or permanent urinary diversion following renal surgery and to restore damaged renal tissue. It may also be used for suprapubic drainage, like the Pezzar catheter (Fig. 6-47). A Foley catheter will also serve either purpose.

Wound drainage may be used after major genitourinary procedures to minimize dead space and provide a method for monitoring postoperative blood loss or wound drainage. These are generally closed suction-drainage systems with a drain whose lumen is large enough to prevent inactivation by coagulated material. Suprapubic drains are also commonly utilized to provide urinary drainage thereby avoiding the need for, or assisting the drainage of a urethral catheter (Fig. 6-48). For simpler surgeries such as testicular approaches a penrose drain

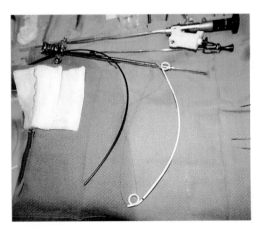

Fig. 6-44 Ureteral stent with tether.

tions. It is common after transurethral resection of the prostate to leave a 3-way Foley with a 30-ml balloon in situ, possibly under traction, to provide hemostasis of the prostatic fossa by placing pressure against the bladder neck. The 3-way catheter also allows for continuous bladder irrigation (CBI) postoperatively. When a patient tends to develop excessive clots postoperatively, a special 3-way Foley, called the hematuria catheter, may is often utilized. The drain should be sutured to the skin to prevent migration. Drains are easily removed in the office setting postoperatively.

Dressings placed over the incision following genitourinary interventions will vary to some degree. After procedures involving the perineum, large, soft, bulky, compressive dressings are usually placed and secured with a supportive device. Laparoscopic procedures may require as little as Steri-Strips or a gauze pressure dressing. Major abdominal interventions generally necessitate gauze dressings and compressive abdominal pads. Many surgeons prefer to place Montgomery straps instead of tape after major surgeries that will require frequent postoperative dressing changes.

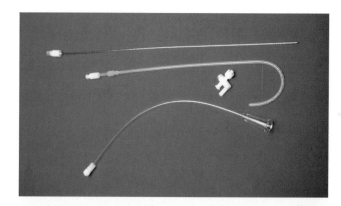

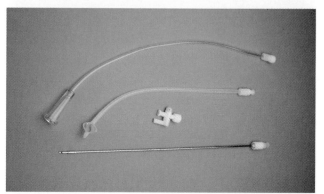

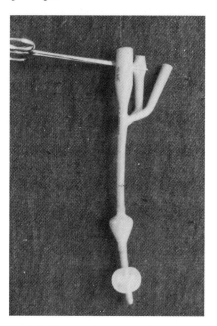

Fig. 6-45 Davis balloon catheter. *(From Meeker MH: Alexander's care of the patient in surgery, ed 10, St. Louis, 1995, Mosby.)*

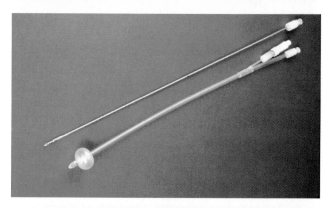

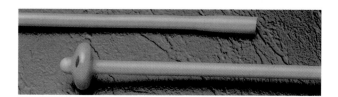

Fig. 6-46 Mushroom Pezzar catheter. *(Courtesy CR Bard, Urological Division, Covington, Ga.)*

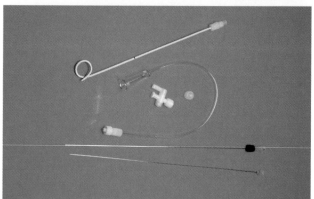

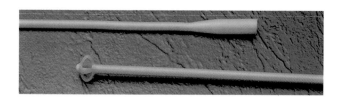

Fig. 6-47 Malecot catheter. *(Courtesy CR Bard, Urological Division, Covington, Ga.)*

Fig. 6-48 **A,** Stamey percutaneous loop suprapubic catheter set. **B,** Stamey malecot percutaneous suprapubic catheter set. **C,** Rutner percutaneous suprapubic balloon catheter set. **D,** Percutaneous pigtail suprapubic catheter set.

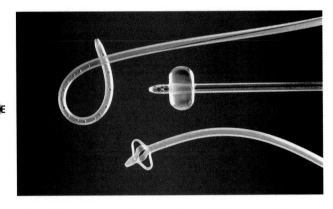

E

Fig. 6-48—cont'd Closeup of pigtail, Ratner and Stamey malecot. **E,** suprapubic drainage tubes. *(Courtesy Cook Urological, Spencer, Ind.)*

IMPLANTS

Prosthetic implantation is a common procedure in genitourinary surgery. Implants that may be placed include the artificial urinary sphincter, malleable and inflatable penile prostheses, fascia lata allografts, "mycro-mesh" grafts (Gore-Tex), and autografts obtained from the dorsal penile shaft or thigh. Synthetic grafts are prepackaged sterile products and the manufacturer's guidelines must be followed when caring for and handling them. Fascial lata graft is available as fresh frozen or freeze-dried cadaver allograft. Proper procedure for tracking all implantable devices must be carried out as mandated by the Food and Drug Administration (FDA) and the manufacturer or bone bank.

GLOSSARY

Electrohydraulic Device that employs electric shock waves generated by a spark plug that may be transmitted through a coupling agent (water).

Homogenous Uniform, from same species.

Insufflator Device used to blow a gas, powder, or vapor into a body cavity.

Intraluminal Within a lumen.

Lithotriptor Noninvasive device that pulverizes calculi by focusing shock waves at a patient.

Morcelizer Instrument that surgically cuts or divides tissue into small pieces for removal.

Veress (Verres) Small needle used for insufflation of carbon dioxide into peritoneal cavity before laparoscopic intervention.

Bibliography

1. Association of Operating Room Nurses: *Standards and recommended practices,* Denver, 1996, AORN.
2. Bagley DH: *Techniques with the flexible ureteroscope,* Stamford, 1991, Circon-ACMI.
3. Ball KA: *Lasers: the perioperative challenge,* ed 2, St. Louis, 1995, Mosby.
4. Brooks Tighe SM: *Instrumentation for the operating room,* St. Louis, 1994, Mosby.
5. Didusch WP: *Anatomy, pathology, and instrumentation of the urogenital tract,* New York, 1973, ACMI.
6. Gershenson DM, DeCherney AH, Curry SL: *Operative gynecology,* Philadelphia, 1993, WB Saunders.
7. Gregory B: *Orthopedic surgery,* St. Louis, 1994, Mosby.
8. Huffman JL, Bagley DH, Lyon ES: *Ureteroscopy,* Philadelphia, 1988, WB Saunders.
9. Kirby RS, Christmas TJ: *Benign prostatic hyperplasia,* London, 1993, Gower.
10. Lytton B, et al: *Advances in urology,* vol 4, St. Louis, 1994, Mosby.
11. Meeker MH, Rothrock JC: *Alexander's care of the patient in surgery,* St. Louis, 1995, Mosby.
12. Smith JA, Stein BS, Benson RC: *Lasers in urologic surgery,* ed 2, Chicago, 1989, Mosby.

SURGICAL INTERVENTIONS

7   Endoscopic Interventions

Endoscopy was originally intended for the diagnostic evaluation of urinary tract dysfunction. The discovery of new technology has allowed for improved methods and subsequently increased knowledge of how the system functions. Education has steadily advanced, resulting in a steady progression of new or revised surgical interventions. Endoscopy now enables the genitourinary surgeon to perform corrective procedures for urinary incontinence; ureteral calculi; bladder, prostate, and ureteral lesions; urethral irregularities; and renal alterations.

Surgical interventions can correct existing problems but will not necessarily alter the progression of certain disease processes. Thorough patient evaluation and teaching is necessary before any proposed surgical treatment.

Laser interventions have become common in endourology. The possibility is mentioned during later discussion of those procedures amenable to its use. Specific laser interventions are addressed separately. A detailed review of laser theory and safety precautions can be found in Chapter 5. A brief overview and information specific to each intervention accompany the procedures discussed in this chapter.

NURSING CARE

Nursing diagnoses will vary according to the procedure intended and the patient history. Patient-specific nursing diagnoses, preoperative planning, and perioperative interventions for a patient requiring endoscopy might include the following:

NURSING DIAGNOSIS	PREOPERATIVE PLANNING AND INTERVENTION

Risk of altered pattern of urinary elimination related to:
Instrumentation
or
Type of procedure, i.e.,
  Cystoscopy
  Ureteroscopy
  Transurethral resection of the prostate (TURP) or transurethral resection of the bladder (TURB)
  Urethral dilation
  Collagen (Contigen) injection
  Litholapaxy
  Lithotripsy
  Bladder biopsies
	Maintain patent, tension-free urinary catheter by securing to leg.
	Secure all connections.
	Keep collection device below bladder level.
	Assess and document return flow of urine, include character and color.
	Observe for and document signs of dysuria.
	Observe and document any abdominal distention.
	Irrigate catheter if output <30 ml/hr, excessive clots/tissue/mucus, or color darker than pink.
	Maintain adequate hydration (IVs, 8 oz oral fluid q2h, half in form of fruit juices until urine remains clear for 24 hours).
	Teach intermittent catheterization.
	Discuss indications of retention, infection, or hemorrhage (<30 ml of urine/hr; fever, pyuria, dysuria; clots; urine darker than pink).
	Suggest use of stool softeners to avoid constipation.
	Discuss use of medication to control initial dysuria (e.g., phenazopyridine HCl, Pyridium).
	Teach Kegel exercises.

Risk of fluid volume excess related to fluid absorption	Document amount of irrigation employed. Observe and document cardiovascular status, noting alterations.

Nursing Diagnosis	Perioperative Planning and Intervention
Risk of fluid volume excess related to fluid absorption—cont'd	Observe and record respiratory status, noting any changes. Observe for abdominal distention and discomfort; assess for rigidity. Note alterations in mental status. Discontinue procedure as indicated and insert Foley catheter. Administer diuretics as ordered. Postoperatively notify surgeon.
High risk for infection related to instrumentation	Maintain aseptic environment and properly disinfect instrumentation. Use appropriate technique during surgical prep. Drape patient according to aseptic standards. Insert catheter aseptically and maintain closed urinary drainage system. Observe for indications of fever, pyuria, dysuria, or bacteriuria. Provide adequate hydration through IVs or oral fluids (8 oz q2h, half as fruit juices). Administer antibiotic therapies as ordered.
Altered tissue perfusion related to: Medical status/ vascular integrity *or* Position	Assess bilateral pedal and radial pulses perioperatively. Adjust position as necessary to maintain peripheral circulation. Utilize alternating compression stockings for procedures lasting beyond 1 hour or if preoperative status indicates need. Observe and document status of capillary refill and extremity temperature.
Risk of urinary retention related to surgical intervention	Assess abdomen for distention. If no catheter is in place, straight catheterize as necessary (anesthetize urethral meatus with topical anesthetic if necessary). Maintain patent, tension-free urinary catheter. Evaluate catheter position by determining length of catheter protruding from urethra, reposition catheter as necessary (in male one half or less of catheter length should be visible, in female approximately two thirds). Determine status of gross sensory motor function, particularly after spinal anesthesia. Irrigate catheter as necessary, observe for clot formation, note amount and character of urinary output.
High risk for injury related to: Position Prep Electrosurgery	Correctly position patient in proper body alignment after adequate relaxation of leg and perineal muscles; avoid severe hip and arm flexion. Reduce pressure on sensitive neurovascular areas such as popliteal space, peroneal nerve, calf area, and acromioclavicular region by padding as necessary. Assess character and presence of bilateral pedal pulses perioperatively. Utilize alternating compression stockings for procedures lasting beyond 1 hour or for patients with already altered peripheral circulation. Avoid pooling of prep solutions under buttocks, sacrum, or back. Avoid hairy areas or areas where prosthetic joint implants are in place when placing electrosurgical grounding pad (if necessary shave small area).
Anxiety related to: Knowledge deficit regarding procedure and outcome (may include fear of altered sexuality or urinary pattern) *or* Immediate discharge home	Encourage patient to express concerns. Document expressions of anxiety by the patient or family. Provide explanations and reassurance to the patient and family. Reinforce and review patient teaching; answer questions as necessary. Encourage participation in discharge planning; review discharge instructions. Keep family informed during intraoperative and postoperative stages. Verify understanding of signs and symptoms to be reported. If patient-controlled analgesic or antibiotic (PCA) is to be utilized, confirm that contact has been established with home care provider.
Pain related to: Medical status *or* Extent of procedure	Place follow-up call, or visit if inpatient, the day after surgery. Provide adequate assistance when moving patient. Assess and maintain comfort during positioning. Provide procedural and positional explanations. Discuss postoperative expectations. Offer comfort measures to alleviate pain as appropriate.

Nursing Diagnosis	Perioperative Planning and Intervention
Pain related to—cont'd Medical status or Extent of procedure	Collaborate with health care team to plan pain control management. Administer medication as ordered; explain side effects. Assist patient to implement strategies to control pain through emotional and informational support.
Fluid volume deficit related to blood loss	Assess nutritional status, skin turgor, and medications affecting fluid balance. Observe for and report significant blood loss intraoperatively. Record all solutions administered from the surgical field. Maintain adequate hydration through IVs, blood products, or oral fluids. Observe for and report significant drainage and excessive or diminished urinary output. Evaluate electrolytes postoperatively compared with perioperative studies.
Hypothermia related to: Irrigation temperature or Room temperature	Provide warmed irrigations and intravenous solutions. Keep patient covered as much as possible; provide warm blankets (pillowcases over legs; plastic or metallic head covers are helpful). Adjust room temperature to afford comfort to patient as well as surgical team. Utilize warming blanket units as indicated (i.e., water-coil units under patient, "bear hugger" type over patient).
Risk of laser injury	Adhere to laser precautions for specific laser employed. Provide undamaged goggles, or glasses with side shields, appropriate for laser wavelength. Hang laser signs and extra goggles on doors to room. Have fire extinguisher available. Have acetic acid and smoke evacuator available for CO_2 laser. (Any external procedures with other lasers require smoke evacuator also.) Perform laser check, and fiber check if indicated, before patient enters room. (Disposable prepackaged fibers do not require calibration.) Provide one trained employee to run laser unit. Keep doors to room closed. Cover windows if Nd:YAG, KTP, or argon lasers are used. Keep other foot pedals free of surgeon's foot. Keep laser in standby mode when not being fired or when being repositioned. Keep liquids away from laser unit. Enclose foot pedal in waterproof bag. Complete laser log correctly. Properly clean or dispose of laser supplies. Return laser keys to designated area.

As perioperative patient care is implemented, the plan of care will be subject to adjustment on a continual basis based on data collected through the preoperative assessment and changing intraoperative circumstances. This ongoing evaluation and revision of care allows for an individualized approach. Once care has been implemented the postoperative assessment is completed, but it is not always possible to properly determine long-term outcomes. Immediate postoperative assessment allows for a baseline determination of the effect of the nursing interventions provided. Priority postoperative assessment data appropriate for the continual evaluation of nursing care may include the following:

- Review of catheter and drain care
- Understanding of the medication regimen
- Discussion of reportable signs and symptoms
- Awareness of postoperative appointments with physician
- Knowledge of the need for high fluid intake
- Readiness for discharge

An overview of the care provided and the subsequent evaluation is recorded to provide for the continuity of care throughout the recovery period. This documentation should be individualized according to the procedure and the needs of the patient. Surgical settings differ and perioperative documentation will have guidelines appropriate for the specific institution. A summary of the intraoperative activities designed to achieve certain outcome criteria should be reported to the perianesthesia care nurse. Information to be recorded and reported will vary according to the procedure performed. Reports may differ between an outpatient and inpatient setting depending on the amount of preoperative instruction afforded the patient and services available to meet each patient's requirements.

Priority information for the genitourinary endoscopy patient may include the following:

- Catheters inserted (include location, type, size, method of securing, collection device)

- Patency of catheters at discharge from the operating room
- Precautions pertinent to the patient's physical condition (i.e., allergies, disabilities)
- Fluid loss and replacement
- Level of comprehension and apprehension during preoperative instruction
- Information taught to the patient preoperatively
- Nursing care provided

The text and photographs to follow in this chapter are intended to be generic for the specific endoscopic interventions. Each is subject to alteration depending on the practice setting and the involvement of the procedure. Common surgical techniques and instrumentation are depicted and intended as an overview to enable the perioperative nurse to anticipate patient care needs. Instrumentation and actual equipment in practice will vary according to physician preference and the procedural setting. It is important to focus on the principles involved in each procedure and consider the instrumentation listed as suggestions for the specialty of genitourinary endoscopy.

CYSTOSCOPY

The term *cystoscope* refers to the Brown-Buerger endoscopic instrument designed in 1909 for passage into the urinary bladder.[8] The lens of this instrument provides only a 90-degree view of the bladder with respect to the shaft of the scope, and the incandescent lens system provides limited optical visualization (see Fig. 1-4). Adequate visualization of the bladder neck may be achieved with this cystoscope, however. The cystoscope is configured with an angled bend at the tip to allow careful passage through the membranous urethra, with an opening for a lens on the convex side. It is passed into the urethra much as one would pass a urethral sound in a male patient. The instrument is used with a deflecting mechanism when ureteral catheterization is necessary but will not allow for biopsy with a rigid forceps.

Presently, the panendoscope (cystourethroscope) is the rigid instrument most commonly used. This is a straight endoscope that may be passed with direct visualization of the urethra or with an obturator. The panendoscope may be used with a 0-, 30-, 70-, or 120-degree lens allowing for examination of the entire lining of the urinary bladder and urethra. It will accommodate a rigid biopsy forceps, an insulated electrical fiber (Bugbee electrode) for coagulation or fulguration, a laser fiber, and an electrohydraulic lithotriptor fiber. Additionally, endoscopic scissors, graspers, and biopsy forceps may be employed. Access to the upper urinary tract may be accomplished when dilators are passed through the panendoscope. Panendoscopes are available in sizes ranging from 8 to 25 Fr as well as smaller diameters and lengths specifically designed for pediatric applications.

Flexible cystoscopes have been available since the mid-1980s. The primary advantage of these instruments is that they allow for endoscopic examination of the bladder in the supine or, in some cases, prone position. It is generally accepted that flexible cystoscopy is less traumatic to the patient. It is an excellent choice for patients with a rigid prostatic urethra, for those with obstructive symptoms resulting from severe prostatic hyperplasia, and for those who cannot assume lithotomy position (because of spinal cord injury or severe arthritis, for example). With the use of a topical anesthetic alone, cystoscopic examination may be done in an office setting, or any hospital setting, provided that the patient is properly prepared.

Other advantages include the ability to use any flexible fiber through the instrument including laser, electrohydraulic lithotriptor, or fulgurating electrode (Bugbee). In addition, the instrument can be turned down to view the bladder neck area completely and can be used for ureteral catheterization for retrograde pyelography and access to the upper tracts.

Disadvantages include the inability to easily evacuate blood clots and to use rigid instruments such as biopsy forceps. In the past it was believed that the fiberoptic endoscopes did not provide visualization equivalent to rigid lens systems. Because of advancements that have been made, they are now believed to be of the same quality as the rigid endoscopes (Fig. 7-1).

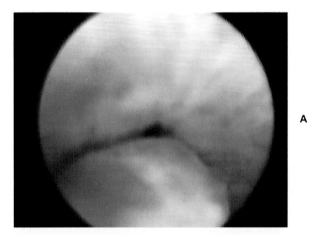

A

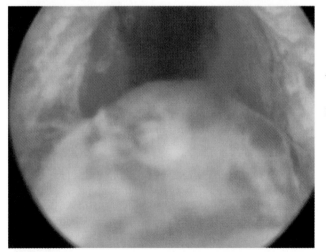

B

Fig. 7-1 **A,** Verumontanum viewed through flexible cystourethroscope. **B,** Verumontanum viewed through rigid cystourethroscope.

Description. To perform cystoscopy or panendoscopy with rigid instrumentation the patient is placed in dorsal lithotomy position. The patients hips must be flexed at least 45 degrees and abducted approximately 30 degrees. If flexible instrumentation is employed, the patient may be supine or in frog-leg position. Flexible cystoscopy is also amenable to unusual circumstances, such as when the patient is prone or in lateral decubitus position. Contraindications to endoscopic examination include the presence of severe urinary tract infection, urethritis, and symptoms of bladder outlet obstruction. In these cases cystoscopy may exacerbate symptoms, making intravenous antibiotics or Foley catheterization necessary.

Any irrigation solution may be used for investigative cystoscopy. Water is typically used for biopsy or fulguration of bladder tumors because it has the ability to lyse tumor cells. Nonelectrolyte solutions are also used in cases where electrical energy will be used so that the current is concentrated and not dispersed by the bladder irrigant. If the procedure is expected to be lengthy, the irrigant may be warmed by the use of specially designed intravenous and irrigant warming units. This will assist in preventing hypothermia, which, particularly in the case of patients with known cardiac disease, can increase the incidence of intraoperative cardiac arrhythmia.

Indications. **Diagnostic cystoscopic investigative examination** may be done to evaluate the lower urinary tract for causes of gross or microscopic hematuria, urinary retention or incontinence, and the presence of bladder calculi and to rule out interstitial cystitis or symptoms that cannot be explained by noninvasive techniques. The male and female bladder, bladder neck, and urethra may be examined for stricture, inflammation, posterior urethral valves, and abnormal growths such as condylomas, diverticula, or carcinoma. Additionally the verumontanum and the median and lateral lobes of the prostate may be examined in the male patient. Frequently, what was intended as a diagnostic procedure will become a therapeutic maneuver. The perioperative genitourinary nurse should be prepared for this adjustment in the planned surgical intervention.

Operative, (therapeutic) cystoscopy requires the implementation of electrocautery or the use of varied instrumentation. Procedures that may be carried out through the cystoscope include bladder biopsies, fulguration of bleeding sites, distal ureteral stone retrievals, insertion of ureteral stents, biopsies or fulguration of urethral and meatal lesions, collagen injections, hydraulic bladder distention, litholapaxy (crushing and evacuation of bladder calculi), and lithotripsy (fracturing and evacuation of bladder calculi).

Perioperative risks. Possible complications surrounding cystoscopy include trauma to the urethra resulting in stricture formation, introduction of bacteria leading to infection, trauma to the sphincter with possible transient incontinence, and perforation of the bladder or urethra. Anesthetic risks may include adverse reaction to local anesthetics, cardiopulmonary compromise caused by the patient's position or large amounts of irrigation, and hypothermia. The majority of these procedures may be performed with monitored sedation and the instillation of a local anesthetic.

Equipment and instrumentation
(Refer to Chapter 6 for basic cystoscopy table setup.)
Equipment
C-Arm–compatible cystoscopy bed
Allen stirrups
Fiberoptic light source
Positioning pads and pillows
Head and neck support
Armboards, padded
Instruments
Panendoscope—17 and 23 Fr with obturators and light cable, *or*
Flexible cystourethroscope
Stopcock with Luer-Lok connection
Suture scissors
Adson forceps with teeth
Hemostat, 2
Needle holder
Knife handle
Miscellaneous supplies
Cytoscopy pack with gown, or apron, and gloves
Sterile water irrigant—3000 ml bag or rigid container
Sterile water, 500 ml bottle
Sterile saline, 500 ml bottle
Cystoscopy irrigation tubing
Lubricating jelly, water soluble
Prep solution and sponges with forceps
Sterile screwtop containers for urine specimens
Open-ended catheter, 4 to 6 Fr
Cone-tip ureteral catheter, 8 Fr
Absorbent drape for prep
Additional for local anesthesia
Penile clamp or applicators
Cystoscopic injection needle
Uro-Jet of 2% lidocaine or other topical, viscous anesthetic
Lidocaine 1% or 2% solution without epinephrine
Urethral syringe (in place of Uro-Jet)
Syringe, 10 or 20 ml
Contingent on intended procedure
Solution warmer
Electrosurgical unit (ESU)
Electrosurgical dispersive pad
Bugbee electrode and high-frequency cable (3 to 6 Fr)
Electrohydraulic lithotriptor
EHL probes, 1 to 9 Fr
Sterile 0.9% saline irrigant, 1000 ml or 3000 ml bag or rigid container
Video camera, monitor, printer, and VCR
Unit for alternating compression stockings
Alternating compression stockings, thigh length
C-arm fluoroscope
X-ray aprons, collars, gloves
Laser unit of choice (KTP, Nd:YAG, Ho:YAG, argon), goggles, signs
Albarren deflecting mechanism or detachable bridge
Rubber nipples for ureteral catheterization or Bugbee insertion

Endoscopic forceps and scissors
Hendrickson-Bigelow lithotrite
Lowsely forceps
Laser adapter and fiber
Urethral dilators
Urethrotomes
Balloon dilator
Pressure syringe
Phillips filiforms and followers
Guidewires, 0.038 inches
Ellik evacuator
Toomey syringe
Luer-Lok syringes, 3 or 5, 10, 20 ml
Sterile container and 20 ml syringe for contrast material
Contrast solution (e.g., Hypaque 50% , Renografin 30%, or Conray)

Pressure bag for 1000 ml or 3000 ml of saline
Urethral catheter: Foley, #16-5 ml and #18-5 ml; Council or coudé, #18-5 ml
Urinary drainage bag
Specimen containers with and without formalin
Collagen or fat injection supplies
Collagen and transurethral (TU) or periurethral (PU) needle
Stabilizer for TU needle
Cystoscopic (Williams) injection needle (may be used in place of TU needle)
Lukens trap or Ellik evacuator
Suction lipectomy probes and tubing
Suction lipectomy machine
Knife blade, #15

PREOPERATIVE

Nursing Care and Teaching Considerations

Generic for All Cystoscopic Interventions

1. Incorporate generic nursing diagnoses and interventions that apply to the specific patient as well as procedure.
2. Gather needed equipment and positioning devices.
3. Check endoscopy instrumentation and equipment (e.g., electrosurgical unit, video unit and camera, warming unit, electrohydraulic lithotriptor [EHL]) for proper function preoperatively.
4. Check sterile supplies for package integrity.
5. Check medications for dose and outdate.
6. If video system is to be used, place it for appropriate visualization.
7. If C-arm fluoroscopy is scheduled, ensure that x-ray protection is available for the patient and all personnel (lead aprons, thyroid collars, small chest and neck shield for patient, sterile lead gloves if indicated).
8. If laser is to be used, hang appropriate signs, provide sufficient eyewear, perform routine laser check, collect appropriate fibers, and follow other established guidelines for the specific laser.
9. Thoroughly rinse endoscopic equipment that has been disinfected in glutaraldehyde solution.
10. Review patient record for reports of preoperative studies (complete blood count [CBC], urinalysis and/or urine culture, chest x-ray, electrocardiogram [ECG], others pertinent to patient history and planned procedure).
11. Assess patient for comprehension of planned procedure and anxiety level. Address concerns expressed by patient and clarify misconceptions. Assure patient that alterations in sexuality are not generally an issue with cystoscopic procedures.
12. Evaluate patient for skin integrity, range of motion, physical limitations (e.g., hearing, vision, low back syndrome).
13. Assess cardiopulmonary status (chronic obstructive pulmonary disease [COPD], obesity, asthma, heart disease, etc.) and peripheral vascular circulation (radial and pedal pulses).
14. Determine presence of any allergies and implants.
15. Review expected postoperative course (e.g., Foley catheter, stent/tether, flank discomfort, mild hematuria, burning, urgency, frequency) and signs and symptoms to be reported (i.e., fever, pyuria, excess hematuria, distention, output <30 ml/hr or >200 ml/hr that persists more than 24 hours). Include family when able.
16. Position patient appropriately for the planned intervention. If the patient has low back or hip disabilities, position legs in stirrups before the administration of anesthesia to determine comfort range. Place padding as appropriate (sacral pad, elbow and wrist pads, stirrup pads, head support). The legs may be returned to supine position for the induction of general anesthesia or the injection of spinal anesthesia.
17. Employ alternating compression stockings if patient's condition or length of procedure warrant use. Apply before vasodilation caused by induction of anesthesia occurs. Explain purpose to patient.
18. Apply electrosurgical dispersive pad, if indicated, as close to perineal region as possible, avoiding excessively hairy areas or prosthetic implants. Anterior thigh area is the common site. Attach high-frequency cable to electrosurgical unit.
19. Aseptically prep and drape patient according to Association of Operating Room Nurses (AORN) guidelines.
20. Connect light cable and adjust intensity, attach irrigation tubing to appropriate solution, and allow surgeon to clear system of air.
21. Connect irrigant warming unit if indicated.
22. Connect laser fiber if indicated.
23. Document assessment findings and nursing interventions.

DIAGNOSTIC CYSTOSCOPY
Procedural Steps

1. After ascertaining that the patient understands the procedure and indications for examination are appropriate, properly position the patient in dorsal lithotomy position for rigid cystoscopy. For flexible cystoscopy, men may be in supine position and women may be in a supine, frog-legged position.

STEP **1-1**

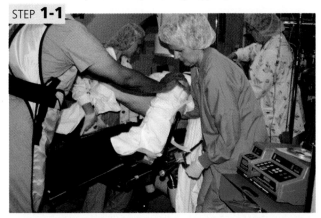

STEP **1-2**

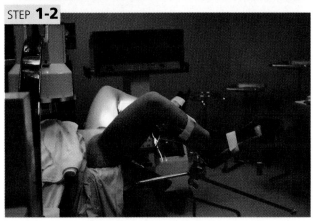

2. After application of an antiseptic skin preparation and sterile draping, inject 20 to 30 ml of water-soluble topical anesthetic into the urethra.

STEP **2-1**

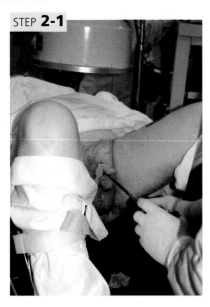

STEP **2-2**

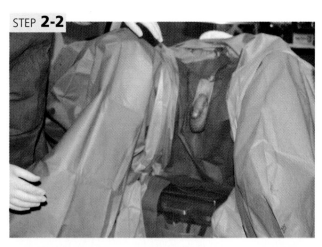

STEP **2-3**

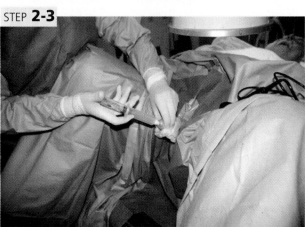

A penile clamp is employed to ensure retention of the anesthetic solution in the male patient.

STEP **2-4**

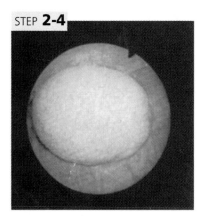

In the female patient, local anesthesia may be instilled by inserting applicators soaked in the anesthetic, or by inserting the tip of the Uro-Jet into the urethral meatus.

STEP **2-5**

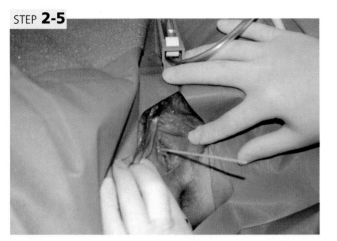

STEP **2-6**

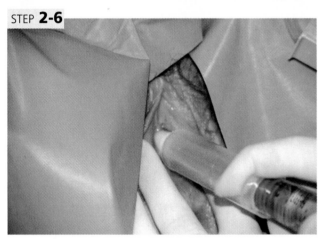

CONSIDERATIONS If the patient is anxious, intravenous sedation will probably be necessary. The use of a video system with projection on a monitor may make complete visualization easier and allows the patient to observe the procedure (Fig. 7-2).

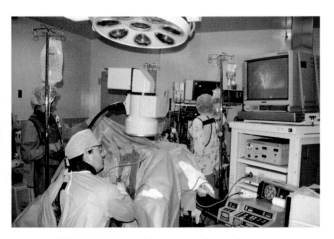

FIG. 7-2 Using video system for endoscopy.

Rigid Cystoscopy

3. The smallest rigid panendoscope, well lubricated, which will be adequate to achieve the desired result (investigative versus therapeutic), is passed into the bladder. Use an obturator unless passing the scope under direct vision.

STEP **3-1**

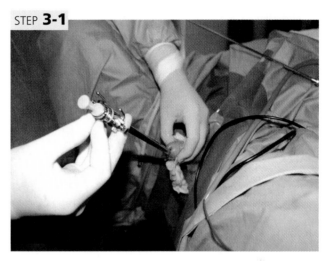

CONSIDERATIONS If a urethral disorder is likely or possible, passage under direct vision with a visual obturator or the endoscope is desirable to avoid altering urethral abnormalities. Use a 0- or 30-degree lens to visualize the urethra and evacuate bloody or cloudy urine if present.

4. The urethra is visualized with a 0- and 30-degree panendoscope; the bladder is then examined with 30-, 70- , 90, or 120-degree lenses to systematically examine all surfaces. The ureteral orifices are viewed for efflux of urine, and its color is noted (localizes site of hematuria).

STEP **4-1**

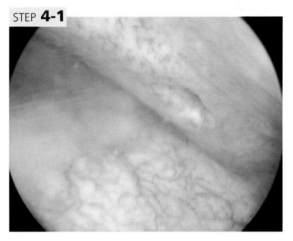

Efflux of clear urine from ureteral orifice.

STEP **4-2**

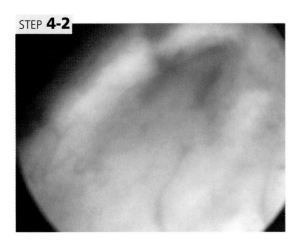

Efflux of bloody urine from ureteral orifice.

5. The topography of the urinary bladder is observed (trabeculation may indicate alteration of the normal smooth appearance because of obstruction or neurogenic bladder dysfunction).

STEP **5-1**

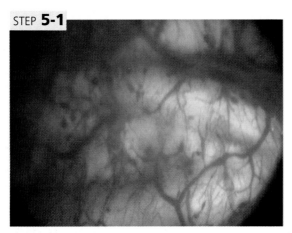

Trabeculation of bladder wall, cystitis.

6. The color of the bladder mucosa is noted (erythematous mucosa is present in inflammatory conditions or carcinoma in situ). Bladder capacity and residual volume is calculated, and urine specimens for culture and cytologic testing are collected if appropriate.

STEP **6-1**

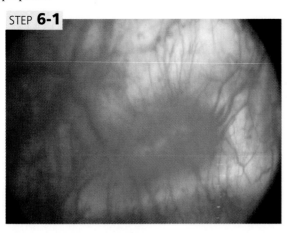

Inflammatory bladder wall, cystitis.

Flexible Cystoscopy

3. The penis is stretched slightly to straighten the urethra. The flexible scope is guided under direct vision while the urethra is inspected for possible abnormalities.

STEP **3-1**

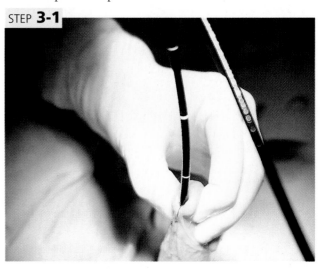

4. The entire bladder interior is inspected, including the bladder neck area, by rotating the flexible scope into the sagittal plain.

STEP **4-1**

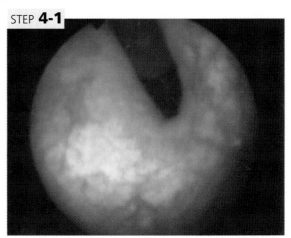

CONSIDERATIONS Cloudy or bloody urine and clots will obscure findings and are not so easily removed with the flexible cystoscope as with the rigid instrument. For further evaluation of hematuria, obstruction, or hydronephrosis, a retrograde pyelogram may be performed. The procedure is discussed under operative cystoscopies.

OPERATIVE CYSTOSCOPIES

Cystoscopy with Urethral Dilatation and Internal Urethrotomy

Description. Periodic dilatation is performed utilizing Phillips filiforms and followers or graduated urethral dilators (sounds). Balloon dilation catheters (Fig. 7-3) and expandable dilators are also available for intermittent dilation of the bulbomembranous urethra (see Fig. 6-33). Generally, urethral sounds are used; curved van Buren sounds are employed for the

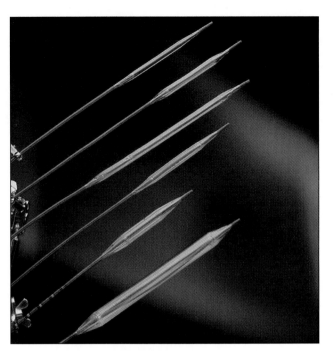

FIG. 7-3 Balloon dilation catheters. *(Courtesy CR Bard, Urological Division, Covington, Ga.)*

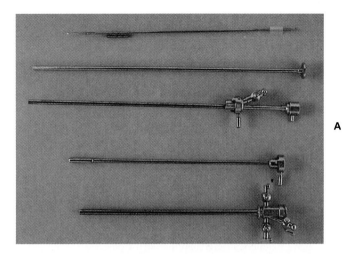

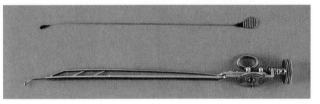

A

B

FIG. 7-4 **A,** Optical internal urethrotome. *(From Brooks Tighe SM: Instrumentation for the operating room, St. Louis, 1994, Mosby.)* **B,** Otis urethrotome. *(From Brooks Tighe SM: Instrumentation for the operating room, St. Louis, 1994, Mosby.)*

male patient, and angled McCrea or straight McCarthy sounds for the female patient (see Fig. 6-33). Internal urethrotomy is an incision of scar tissue, at the point of stricture, with the optical internal or Otis urethrotome (Fig. 7-4).

Indications. Urethral strictures or narrowing of the urethra caused by congenital malformation (generally located at the external urinary meatus), and stricture of the membranous or pendulous urethra resulting from infection or trauma with the formation of scar tissue.

Perioperative risks. Problems encountered may include difficult dilation, hematuria, creation of a false passage, hemorrhage, recurrence of stricture, and infection. Anesthetic risks are generally patient specific and include those previously mentioned.

Procedural Steps

1. The male patient may be supine; the female patient is placed in lithotomy position. After application of antiseptic solution and draping, a local anesthetic is instilled into the urethra.

2. Phillips filiforms of gradually increasing size are introduced to attempt passage beyond the urethral stricture. Followers of increasing diameter are then attached to the distal end of the largest filiform that successfully passes and are pushed gently through the stricture to stretch the scarred area.

CONSIDERATIONS When urethral sounds are used, the same approach is followed, increasing the size and allowing the largest desirable instrument diameter to remain in place for a short time.

CONSIDERATIONS

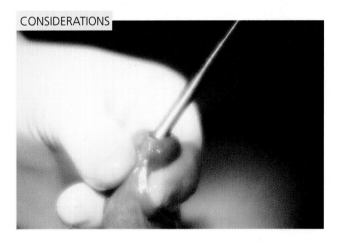

In a male patient, after instillation of a local anesthetic, a rigid guidewire can be passed into the bladder from the point of stricture through the flexible cystoscope. Dilatation may be accomplished with coaxial dilators or with a 12 mm balloon catheter inflated in coaxial fashion to 12 atm for 1 to 2 minutes. Both techniques allow extensive dilation. After balloon dilatation, a #18 Council catheter may be inserted over the guidewire and left in place for several days to promote healing and maintain a patent urethral channel.

3. For an optical internal urethrotomy, the urethrotome is passed through the urethroscope and advanced to the strictured area. A blade in the instrument incises the scar tissue. The urethra is incised to a point 1 cm proximal and distal to the stricture.

CONSIDERATIONS Because of the availability of the optical internal urethrotome, the Otis urethrotome is rarely used. It is designed for treatment of a long, strictured segment, whereas the optical urethrotome may be used on virtually any stricture. The Otis urethrotome is inserted past the stricture and opened by turning the ring until the urethrotome is snug; the knife is then pulled back to make a longitudinal incision in the strictured segment.

4. A Foley catheter may be left in place for several days after treatment to serve as a tamponade to minimize bleeding from the incision and keep the urethra open during the initial healing.

Cystoscopy with Bladder Biopsies

Description. The procedure is approached in the same manner as diagnostic cystoscopy. Endoscopic biopsy forceps are generally employed.

Indications. Bladder biopsies are indicated for hematuria that cannot be explained by other findings; the presence of abnormal urine cytologic findings ruling out associated bladder carcinoma in situ in the presence of other known transitional cell, squamous cell, or adenocarcinomas; accounting for symptoms unexplained by other studies; or determining the histologic features of a suspicious lesion found on cystoscopy.

Perioperative risks. Concerns surrounding bladder biopsy may include perforation of the bladder wall, uncontrolled bleeding, inadequate biopsy size for histologic verification, postoperative hematuria, bladder spasm, and infection. Anesthetic concerns include but are not limited to reaction to the local anesthetic, cardiac dysrhythmia, compromised respiratory exchange, and blood loss.

Procedural Steps

The procedure begins as described for cystoscopy.

1. A cold biopsy forceps should be used if the lesion is small and likely to be altered by electrosurgery.

2. After excision of the suspicious tissue, cauterize or laser fulgurate the biopsy site to prevent postoperative bleeding.

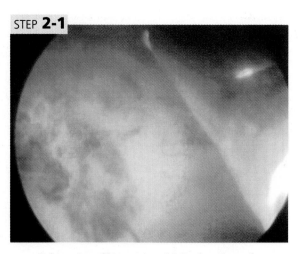

STEP **2-1**

Fulguration of biopsy site with Bugbee electrode.

CONSIDERATIONS. If laser fulguration is chosen, the Nd:YAG, KTP-532, or Ho:YAG, with a right-angled or end-firing fiber, may be used. Precautions applicable to the specific laser must be employed. Refer to Chapter 5 for more detailed safety considerations.

3. Specimens should be sent in separate containers of formalin to the laboratory to "map" areas of abnormality. (Some institutions have a bladder map; the surgeon marks the sites biopsied, referenced by the specimen number on the diagram, and places it in the patient record.)

CONSIDERATIONS If frozen sections are to be performed, the tissue is sent immediately to the histology lab on a small piece of nonadherent material in a container free of formalin (saline in small amounts may be used to keep the tissue moist).

Cystoscopy with Litholapaxy and Lithotripsy

Description. Litholapaxy is the manual destruction of intravesical calculi. Calculi are most readily destroyed in this manner with the the Hendrickson-Bigelow lithotrite (Fig. 7-5). Bladder calculi tend to be very hard (Fig. 7-6), and multiple modalities may be necessary to fragment the calculus. The EHL is one modality that may be used. When this is chosen the procedure is called a lithotripsy.

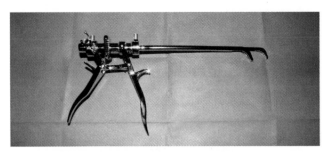

FIG. 7-5 Hendrickson-Bigelow lithotrite.

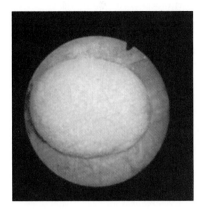

FIG. 7-6 Large bladder calculus. *(From Lloyd-Davies W: Color atlas of urology, London, 1994, Mosby-Wolfe.)*

Indications. Litholapaxy is employed when intravesical calculi are too large to pass spontaneously, generally identified with ultrasonography, cystography, or cystoscopy. Associated contributory findings such as urethral stricture, a large obstructing prostate adenoma (benign prostatic hypertrophy [BPH]), and bladder diverticulum, which may require open surgical correction, should be ruled out. Alternative therapy such as cystolithotomy must be considered.

Perioperative risks. Concerns applicable to litholapaxy include hematuria, retained fragments leading to dysuria or retention, infection, bladder perforation, urethral trauma, bladder spasm, and electrical shock (or burn if the EHL is used). Anesthetic risks are the same as previously mentioned.

Procedural Steps

1. The procedure begins as described for a routine cystoscopy.

2. The 23 Fr panendoscope will be employed, frequently after insertion of the 17 Fr panendoscope and possibly urethral dilation.

3. If the lithotrite is the instrument of choice, sterile water irrigant may be used. The surgeon should test the instrument for ease of operation before inserting it into the bladder. The jaws must be appropriately positioned around the calculus before crushing and should be angled away from the bladder wall.

The Bugbee electrode should be available to control any bleeding sites in the bladder wall.

STEP **3-1**

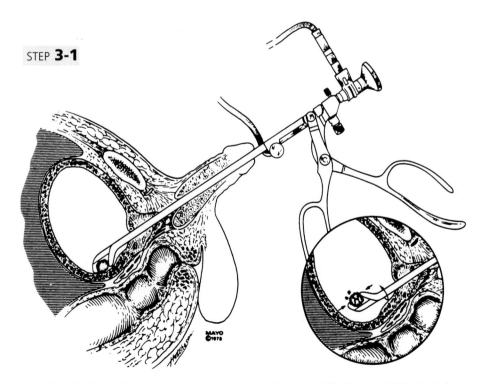

(From Droller M: Surgical management of urologic disease, ed 10, St. Louis, 1995, Mosby.)

4. All stone fragments are evacuated from the bladder with a Toomey syringe or Ellik evacuator or by gravity drainage. The bladder is reexamined to be certain that its integrity has been maintained.

5. Any bleeding sites may be coagulated with the Bugbee electrode.

CONSIDERATIONS Laser fulguration is also an option, but the cost to the patient should be considered because laser fibers are expensive. Its use may not be applicable to minor bleeding sites.

6. The largest EHL probe available (9 Fr) is passed through the panendoscope.

CONSIDERATIONS Normal saline irrigation must be used with the EHL. This may be in place from the beginning of the procedure provided that treatment is anticipated beforehand. At least three extra probes should be available.

7. The EHL probe is placed squarely against the calculus before the power generator is activated.

CONSIDERATIONS It is important that the patient, surgeon, anesthetist, and nursing personnel are separated from the metal of the table to avoid an inadvertent shock or burn when the probe is activated. All other foot pedals should be distanced from the surgeon's foot.

8. Any bleeding sites may be coagulated with the Bugbee electrode after the irrigation system has been flushed and converted to sterile water.

9. Insertion of a Foley catheter is dependent on the patient's status and the surgeon's preference after either procedure.

All fragments are again flushed from the bladder in the same manner as after use of the EHL.

Cystoscopy with Retrograde Pyelogram and Ureteral Stent Insertion

Description. Either rigid or flexible instrumentation may be used to perform retrograde pyelograms (RGP) and insert ureteral stents. Flexible cystoscopy may be used if the procedure is likely to be straightforward and uncomplicated, as in temporary relief of obstruction caused by a ureteral calculus.

Before stent insertion it should be determined if the ureteral stent will be temporary or remain in place for more than 1 to 2 weeks. Stents are available with or without a tether suture (see Fig. 6-44, showing a tethered stent). The former is generally used when the stent is considered temporary or short term and allows for ease of removal in the office setting. The suture is usually taped to the penis, or to the mons pubis or inner thigh of the female patient, to prevent dislodgment. If containing inventory is an institutional issue, it is not necessary to maintain a stock of both types. The tether is easily removed from a stent if the surgeon prefers there not be one.

It is preferable to avoid placement of a Foley catheter. Ureteral stents by their very nature are a common cause of urinary tract infection. The presence of a Foley catheter adds to the risk by the potential introduction of bacteria, which may ascend and precipitate infection.

Indications. To relieve obstruction, demonstrated on intravenous pyelography (IVP), computed tomography (CT) scan, or ultrasonography resulting from a progressive or permanent cause such as periureteral fibrosis or tumor; to relieve transient obstruction caused by calculus where sepsis or colic is present; to stabilize the patient before definitive therapy such as extracorporeal shock-wave lithotripsy (ESWL), ureteroscopic, or percutaneous stone removal.

Perioperative risks. Concerns surrounding RGP and stent insertion may include difficulty of stent insertion, ureteral perforation with extravasation, hemorrhage, flank discomfort after insertion, ureteral colic, stent migration or accidental dislodgment, occlusion of stent, fever, nausea, postobstructive diuresis, and infection. The patient is generally placed on antibiotic therapy while the stent is in place. Anesthetic risks have included cardiac dysrhythmia, respiratory insufficiency, reaction to anesthetic agents, and fluid volume imbalance. Nonionic contrast material may be employed for patients who are highly allergic to iodine, shellfish, or ionic contrast material. Nonionic contrast material is more expensive than an ionic product, making the use individualized by patient history and relative risk.

Procedural Steps

A routine cystoscopy initiates the procedure. Sterile water irrigant may be employed.

1. An RGP is performed to determine the course, caliber, and contour of the ureter. To avoid retrograde displacement of a ureteral calculus or distortion of the ureter, it may be advisable to use an 8 Fr cone catheter to occlude the ureteral orifice before contrast is injected.

STEP **1-1**

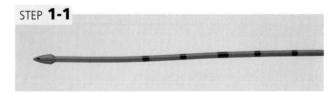

Cone ureteral catheter. *(Courtesy CR Bard Urological Division, Covington, Ga.)*

STEP **1-2**

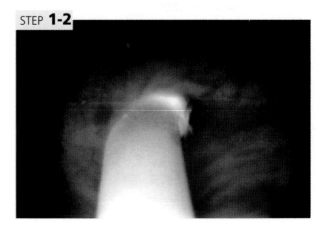

Cone ureteral catheter entering ureter.

2. A 5 Fr open-ended ureteral catheter is often sufficient for a simple RGP to evaluate conditions other than calculi.

STEP **2-1**

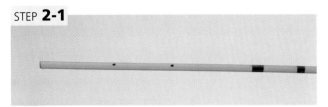

Open-ended ureteral catheter. *(Courtesy CR Bard Urological Division, Covington, Ga.)*

STEP **2-2**

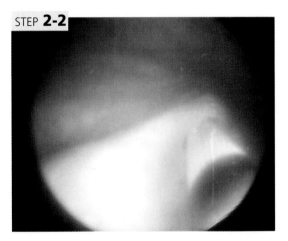

Open-ended ureteral catheter entering ureter.

CONSIDERATIONS The Albarren deflecting mechanism, or detachable bridge, is employed if the procedure is performed with rigid instrumentation.

3. A guidewire is passed into the ureter under fluoroscopic control. Once an RGP has been performed and the collecting system has been demonstrated, a stent of the appropriate length and diameter is passed and positioned with fluoroscopic and cystoscopic control.

STEP **3-1**

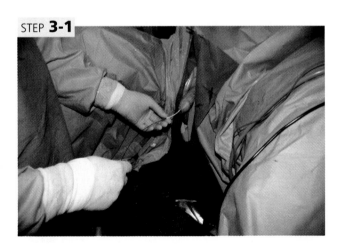

Indications for possible alternative regimens. Some patients may not be appropriate candidates for ureteral stent insertion because of certain underlying medical conditions. These patients will require alternative approaches to alleviate obstruction. Included in this category are terminally ill patients who may require concentrated postoperative pain management because they are likely to experience increased pain after stent placement, patients with renal insufficiency where close monitoring of renal function is necessary, and patients with lower urinary tract disease and high resting bladder pressures because they may not be able to achieve adequate drainage with ureteral stenting alone, mandating insertion of a Foley catheter.

Periurethral-Transurethral Injection of Collagen (Contigen)

Description. Collagen injection was developed as an outpatient procedure achievable under local anesthesia with or without sedation. Contigen is cross-linked dermal collagen. Collagen is packaged in sterile syringes containing 2.5 ml of the material. The injection needles are packaged separately. It is advisable to have extra injection needles or a cystoscopic injection needle available. Collagen must be kept under refrigeration, and the Food and Drug Administration (FDA) guidelines for its use and documentation followed (Fig. 7-7). If the patient has an allergy to eggs he or she may be an inappropriate candidate for the procedure.[28]

An alternative, somewhat less effective, but less costly approach is the injection of subcutaneous fat. Both procedures generally need to be repeated at periodic intervals over time. It is optimal to utilize a video system for the procedure.

Indications. Female patients with intrinsic sphincter deficiency (ISD) demonstrated by urodynamic evaluation and male patients (usually after prostatectomy) with incontinence lasting more than 1 year are candidates. Other indications may include stress urinary incontinence secondary to previous stricture treatment, trauma, or myelodysplasia. Patients selected for collagen injection must be evaluated with a skin test dose of the material 1 month before treatment to rule out allergic reaction. A urine culture and sensitivity will be done approximately 10 days preoperatively.

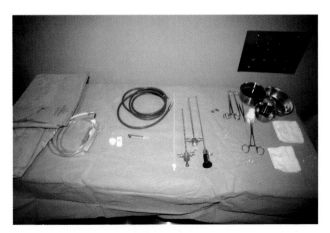

FIG. 7-7 Collagen setup with transurethral needle.

Perioperative risks. The possible side effects the patient may experience include the inability to urinate, requiring intermittent catheterization, bleeding, suprapubic and urethral soreness, and postanesthesia nausea. Patients are placed on antibiotic therapy preoperatively and postoperatively but should remain alert to signs of infection.

Procedural Steps

1. Urethral anesthetic is instilled and a perineal block of 1% or 2% lidocaine may be injected. Cystoscopic examination is performed before collagen injection to rule out any associated findings.

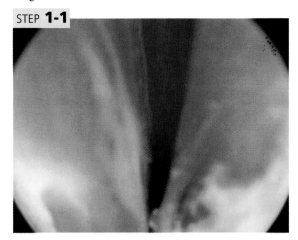

STEP **1-1**

Bladder neck before injection.

CONSIDERATIONS The manufacturer suggests that the irrigation be instilled utilizing a pressure bag to increase the intraurethral pressure and minimize extravasation of the material.

2. In men, the transurethral injection needle provided by the manufacturer is introduced through the cystoscope and the tip is placed below the urethral mucosa, just distal to the bladder neck. In women the periurethral needle provided is shorter and is introduced perneally, outside the scope and along the urethra at 3 and 9 o'clock positions. Positioning of the needle tip is accomplished by endoscopically observing a protrusion of the urethra, where the tip contacts the outer wall, as the needle is manipulated by the surgeon.

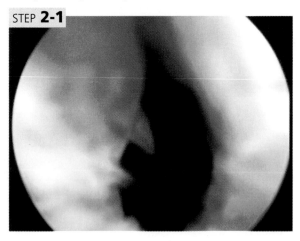

STEP **2-1**

Inserting transurethral needle.

3. Collagen is injected until the urothelium coapts in the midline, approximating the appearance of lateral lobe enlargement of the prostate.

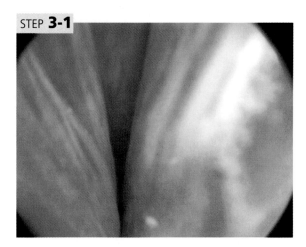

STEP **3-1**

Bladder neck after partial injection on the left.

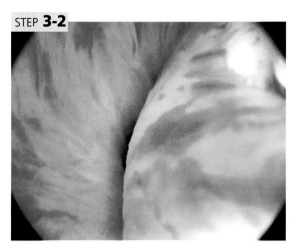

STEP **3-2**

Bladder neck after full injection on the left.

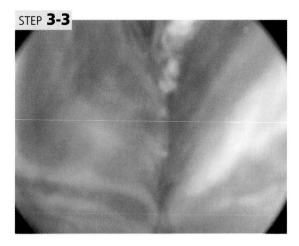

STEP **3-3**

Bladder neck after full bilateral coaptation.

4. Generally, no more than 4 to 6 syringes are injected at one time. It may not be possible to achieve coaptation of the urothelium during the first application. It may be possible to do so on subsequent injections, however, once the pockets of collagen established originally have congealed and become compact.

5. The alternative technique is the injection of subcutaneous fat. Subcutaneous fat is aspirated under sterile technique much as in suction lipectomy. A suction lipectomy cannula on a Lukens trap or Ellik evacuator is inserted into the lower abdomen subcutaneously after the application of an antiseptic prepping solution. The Lukens trap or Ellik evacuator is then attached to the suction lipectomy machine with the wide-bore tubing designed for it. The aspirated material is transferred to a 3 or 5 ml syringe and attached to a cystoscopic, or collagen, injection needle. The same procedure is then carried out.[18]

CONSIDERATIONS Insertion of a Foley catheter is common but not routine. It is usually removed in 1 or 2 days.

POSTOPERATIVE

Nursing Care and Discharge Planning

Generic for All Cystoscopic Interventions
1. Cleanse patient of prep solutions.
2. Secure any catheters or stents.
3. Evaluate peripheral vascular circulation and skin integrity.
4. Assess Foley output if applicable.
5. Provide instruction to patient and family:
   - Patient must void before discharge if no catheter is in place.
   - Patient may resume normal diet as tolerated.
   - Patient should increase fluid intake (8 oz q2h until urine clear, half as fruit juice to prevent potassium depletion) to assist voiding process, ward off infection, and promote recovery from spinal anesthesia, if used.
   - Patient may resume nonstrenuous activity in 2 or 3 days and strenuous activity in 2 weeks. Time frame will vary by extent of procedure.
   - Aspirin and other nonsteroidal antiinflammatory agents should be avoided for 48 hours unless advised by surgeon as medically necessary.
   - Medications ordered should be taken as directed. Stool softeners should be used to prevent constipation if the patient is receiving narcotic analgesia. Antibiotics should be taken as directed.
   - Reinforce and review catheter and stent care if indicated. Foley catheters are usually removed within 2 days; stents vary by purpose of insertion. Collaboration with surgeon is important to properly inform patient.
   - Reinforce intermittent self-catheterization if indicated (after collagen injection).
6. Review symptoms of infection or retention (fever, pyuria, dysuria, clots, urine darker than pink, output <30 ml/hr, unrelieved flank pain).
7. Document nursing assessment and interventions.

URETEROPYELOSCOPY (URETEROSCOPY)

Transurethral ureteropyeloscopy began as an endoscopic exam of the ureters and renal pelvis. The use of rigid and flexible instrumentation now allows access to the entire collecting system and provides for the inspection, diagnosis, and immediate treatment of conditions involving the ureter and renal pelvis.

A critical factor in successful implementation is careful dilation of the ureter with video monitoring and C-arm fluoroscopy. Techniques for ureteral dilation first implemented ureteral catheters. As expertise improved, the metal bougie dilator was introduced, followed by the use of long fascial dilators. Currently the instrumentation of choice is a balloon dilator or coaxial dilators.[30]

Hopkins is credited with the greatest achievements in the development of instrumentation for the upper urinary tract. Fiberoptic technology of the 1950s led to the creation of the flexible fiberscope and enhanced the illumination of the rigid endoscope. Further invention of rigid-rod lens systems dramatically changed light transmission and visualization. Transurethral ureteropyeloscopy may employ the use of rigid or flexible instrumentation and is amenable to the outpatient setting (see Fig. 6-42).[13]

The flexible ureteropyeloscope has an inherent 160-degree active-tip mobility and passive infundibular deflection allowing for a more panoramic view of the entire ureteral circumference and renal parenchyma. In 1964 Marshall was the first to successfully use a 9 Fr flexible ureteropyeloscope developed by American Cystoscope Makers, Inc. through a transurethral approach. Since that time smaller ureteropyeloscopes, 2.3 to 3.6 Fr, have been developed. This has allowed a progression of minimally invasive operative interventions, resulting in an increase in the number of procedures performed that allow the patient to be treated on an outpatient basis.[27]

The first rigid ureteropyeloscope, modeled after a juvenile cystoscope, was designed in 1977 by Lyon and Goodman in collaboration with Richard Wolf Instruments.[13] The modern endoscope now has a total light transmission of about 80 times that of the traditional endoscope. Commonly, 0- and 70-degree interchangeable telescopes with a 65-degree field of view, available in 33 and 41 cm lengths, are used. One of the newer rigid ureteropyeloscopes is constructed with an inherent dilatory effect. The 33 cm scope allows for visualization of the distal ureter to the level of the external iliac vessel in men and the lumbar ureteral region in women. The longer scope reaches into the upper urinary tract and allows diagnosis and treatment of the renal pelvis and calyces.

A variety of operative instrumentation may be utilized depending on the working diameter of the ureteropyeloscope being employed. The smaller flexible scopes are currently more limited in their applications. Fibers for EHL or laser treatment are available for use through any of the present-day instrumentation, but only the rigid ureteropyeloscope currently accepts the probe for ultrasonic lithotripsy. The operative bed must be

C-arm compatible and allow for ease of adjustment to the lateral position, as well as to alterations in the height level.

Description. Transurethral ureteropyeloscopy has been performed using all anesthetic modalities. Access to the ureter is gained through the bladder utilizing a flexible or rigid ureteropyeloscope. The approach will be consistent regardless of the intended intervention, be it diagnostic or therapeutic. The pattern of examination is dependent on the purpose of the intervention. When evaluating the cause of unilateral hematuria discovered on cystoscopic examination, a systematic approach through the ureter to the lower pole and into each individual infundibulum is indicated. Any defects or calculi found are treated first.

Transurethral ureteropyeloscopy is a far more sensitive diagnostic tool than radiography. Documented case histories demonstrate that tumors of the papillae and calyces have been discovered through surgical intervention in patients with essentially normal radiographic data. Ureteropyeloscopy also has advantages over open therapies, resulting in shorter hospitalization and recovery time, decreased postoperative pain, and overall cost savings to the patient as well as the institution. Many of the following interventions are being successfully performed on an outpatient basis.

When working in the ureter and renal pelvis, normal saline is the irrigant of choice for all but procedures employing electrosurgery. This solution approximates a physiologic solution, important should perforation occur with extravasation and absorption of fluid into the circulatory system. If electrosurgery is used, the irrigant should be converted to sorbitol, glycine, or, as a last resort, sterile water. Dispersion of electric current will occur should saline remain in place. The irrigant will best serve the surgeon if it is administered under pressure. This may be accomplished with a pressure bag, such as that used when instilling blood transfusions (Fig. 7-8), with a three-way stopcock and two 50 ml syringes, or with a refilling syringe that attaches to the scope and irrigant by a specially constructed split tubing. C-arm fluoroscopy routinely accompanies ureteropyeloscopy.

Since the approach to ureteropyeloscopy is consistent, the description to follow concentrates on involved therapeutic intervention. The perioperative genitourinary nurse may use this as a guide and adjust intraoperative needs according to the exact procedure scheduled. It is important for the perioperative nurse to know the size of the instrumentation that the ureteropyeloscope to be employed will accommodate.

Indications. **Diagnostic:** Ureteropyeloscopy is performed to evaluate and locate filling defects of the ureter and renal pelvis, congenital anomalies, ureteral obstruction, hematuria, ureteral calculi, a ureteral fistula, trauma-related defects, and ureteral stricture as well to perform tumor surveillance (Fig. 7-9). The entire ureter, renal pelvis, calyces, and papillae may be visualized with the patient in supine or lithotomy position.

Operative: Achievable interventions include manipulating, fragmenting, and basketing of ureteral and renal calculi; retrieval of foreign bodies; lithotripsy with EHL, laser, or ultrasonic probes; management of residual calculus sludge *(steinstrasse)*; biopsy of tumors of the ureter and renal pelvis; treatment of low-grade tumors; fulguration of bleeding sites; inser-

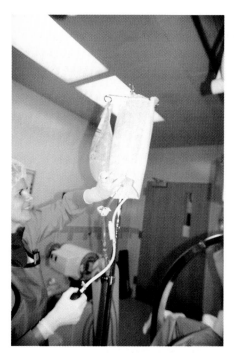

Fig. 7-8 Setting up the pressure bag for irrigation during endourologic procedure.

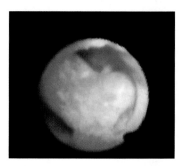

Fig. 7-9 Compound calyx.

tion of ureteral and nephrostomy stents; and dilation or lysis of ureteral strictures (endopyelotomy). The most common purpose for operative ureteropyeloscopy is stone management.

Perioperative risks. Procedural concerns include damage to ureteral mucosa, ureteral perforation with extravasation, hemorrhage, infection, ureteral stricture formation, creation of a false passage, ureteral avulsion, periureteral fluid collection, thermal injury, vesicoureteral reflux, ureteral colic, ureteral reflux, fever, urinary retention, nausea and vomiting, lower quadrant pain, abdominal pain or distention, intraureteral instrument breakage, stent migration or obstruction, and stent dislodgment. Anesthetic issues include the possibility of tachycardia or bradycardia, hypotension or hypertension, hypervolemia, and respiratory compromise.

Equipment and instrumentation

All items listed under cystoscopy may be employed in addition to the following:

Ureteroscope, rigid or flexible, with light cables
Ureteral forceps and scissors, 2 to 3 Fr

Endopyelotomy system of choice

Ureteral coaxial dilators

Ureteral stone baskets, 2.4 to 3 Fr

Ureteral Bugbee electrode, 2 to 3 Fr, and high-frequency cable

Ureteral stents

Ureteral guidewires, 0.025 to 0.038 inches, Bentson and J tipped

Ureteral balloon dilators

Dual-lumen injection catheter

Pressure gauge

Sealing port adapter (i.e., Urolok)

Pressure bag, refilling syringe with tubing, *or* syringe, 50 ml (2), with three-way stopcock

TUR irrigation tubing (instead of cystoscopy tubing)

Sorbitol or glycine, 1000 ml, or 3000 ml bag or rigid container

URETEROPYELOSCOPY WITH DILATION, CALCULUS EXTRACTION, AND BIOPSY

Description. **Ureteropyeloscopy with dilation** involves four important steps: access to the upper part of the ureter, placement of a dilating balloon catheter or coaxial dilators, activation of the dilating balloon or sequential dilation, and removal of the device at completion. Fluoroscopy is essential to the procedure to ensure proper positioning and activation of the balloon catheter. The patient is given general or regional anesthesia and placed in lithotomy position. **Ureteropyeloscopy with calculus extraction** involves obtaining access to the calculus by passing a guidewire beyond the stone, advancing the ureteroscope to the level of the calculus, and mechanically removing the calculus with a basketing device. **Ureteropyeloscopy with biopsy** allows the surgeon to obtain preoperative tissue diagnosis. The combined results of cytologic, histologic, and radiologic studies are used to determine treatment options. Flexible instrumentation affords access to

PREOPERATIVE

Nursing Care and Teaching Considerations

Generic for All Ureteroscopic or Ureteropyeloscopic Interventions

1. Incorporate applicable generic nursing diagnoses and interventions.
2. Gather needed equipment and positioning devices.
3. Check equipment and instrumentation for proper function preoperatively.
4. Check sterile supplies for package integrity.
5. Check medications for dose and expiration dates.
6. Place video system to be used in position for appropriate visualization.
7. Ensure that C-arm protection is available for the patient and personnel.
8. If laser will be used, perform laser check and gather goggles and signs.
9. Thoroughly rinse endoscopic equipment that has been disinfected in glutaraldehyde solution.
10. Review patient record for reports of preoperative studies (e.g., [CBC] prothrombin time [PT], partial thromboplastin time [PTT], bleeding profile, urinalysis and urine culture, serum chemistry values and electrolytes, cardiac enzymes by patient history, IVP, CT scan, renogram, chest x-ray, and ECG). Patient should be free of or under treatment for urinary tract infection.
11. Review patient record for preoperative orders and confirm that they have been accomplished: administration of antibiotics or enemas if indicated, cessation of oral intake of fluid or food (NPO). Patient may have stent in situ.
12. Interview patient to determine understanding of procedure and postoperative course. Review expectations and clarify misconceptions. Explain that sexuality is rarely affected by the procedure.
13. Assess patient anxiety level and provide support measures.
14. Include family in teaching process whenever able.
15. Examine and assess patient for disabilities, peripheral vascular circulation, skin integrity, obesity, range of motion, cardiopulmonary status. Review medical and surgical history: COPD, asthma, allergies, prosthetics, heart disease, etc.
16. Review common postoperative course (stent, antibiotics, pain management, reportable signs and symptoms).
17. Position patient appropriately for the planned intervention. If the patient has low back or hip disabilities, position legs in stirrups before the administration of anesthesia to determine comfort range. The legs may be returned to the supine position for the induction of general anesthesia or the injection of spinal anesthesia.
18. Apply alternating compression stockings before anesthetic induction, before vasodilation occurs. Explain purpose to patient.
19. Apply electrosurgical dispersive pad, if indicated, as close to perineal region as possible, avoiding excessively hairy areas or prosthetic implants. Anterior thigh is the common site. Attach high-frequency cable to electrosurgical unit.
20. Aseptically prep and drape patient according to AORN guidelines.
21. Connect light cable and adjust intensity, attach irrigation tubing to normal saline solution, and allow surgeon to clear system of air. Have solution appropriate for electrosurgery available.
22. Place irrigation in pressure bag if indicated.
23. Connect irrigant to warming unit if indicated.
24. Connect EHL unit, or laser fiber, if indicated, and ensure that no metal contacts the patient, surgeon, or staff members.
25. Monitor fluid volume instilled intraoperatively.
26. Document assessment findings and nursing interventions.

the entire intrarenal collecting system. The latter two interventions have been successfully accomplished with monitored anesthesia care (MAC), sedation, and instillation of a local anesthetic.

Indications. **Ureteral dilation** is commonly performed before operative ureteropyeloscopy to increase the size of the ureter and reduce the chance of intimal damage, to enhance the flow of irrigant, and to improve visualization. Additionally, dilation may be performed to alleviate stricture disease, afford spontaneous passage of stone fragments, and allow placement of a ureteral stent during healing. **Ureteroscopic calculus extraction** is no longer limited to the distal or middle third of the ureter. It allows definitive treatment versus the high chance of retained fragments after ESWL, particularly if a large calculus is involved. Success rates average 90% to 100% compared with 80% to 85% for ESWL. Patients are generally given options. It is often performed after ESWL to remove retained fragments that will not pass spontaneously. It is also indicated where ESWL is contraindicated: pregnant women, small poorly visualized calculi, and cystine calculi greater than 1 cm. **Ureteroscopic biopsy** is primarily indicated for the diagnosis and staging of intrarenal tumors and for posttreatment surveillance. Possible detrimental effects on the patient's disease and survival must be weighed against the other options available.

Perioperative risks. In addition to the risks previously discussed, other concerns include balloon breakage, postoperative ureteral edema, difficulty with retrograde passage of the ureteroscope, ureteroiliac stricture, ureteral fibrosis, inaccurate staging of tumor, potential for seeding of cancerous cells, and recurrence of tumor if ureteroscopic excision and fulguration are chosen. The same anesthetic risks apply as previously discussed.

Procedural Steps

The procedure begins as described for routine cystoscopy; the ureteropyeloscope may be employed immediately, however.

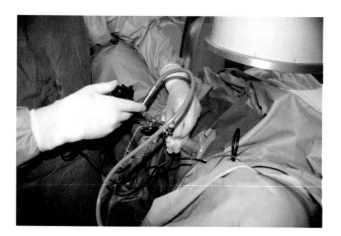

1. Once the ureteropyeloscope has been inserted, access to the ureter is gained by passing a guidewire under fluoroscopic control.

STEP **1-1**

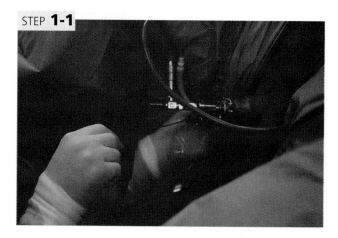

The ureter should be irrigated as the guidewire is advanced. The assistance of a scrub nurse to hold the wire on slight tension will allow for a smoother course of operation.

2. The ureter is dilated to 10 to 12 Fr with a balloon dilator or coaxial dilators.

STEP **2-1**

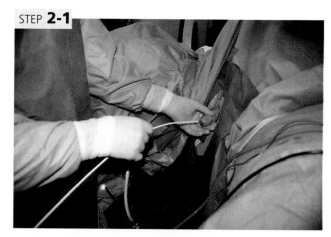

Placing balloon dilation catheter.

STEP **2-2**

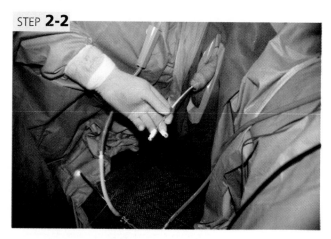

Balloon catheter in position.

If a balloon dilator is chosen, the balloon should be inflated with contrast material and a pressure syringe to ensure not exceeding the maximum allowable atm (burst pressure).

3. A working guidewire to be used as a safety wire is placed in addition to the initial guidewire.

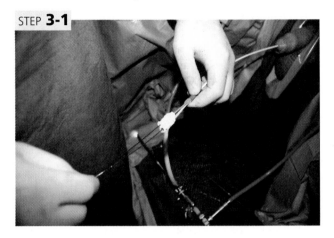

4. The ureteroscope is passed over the working guidewire to the location of interest.

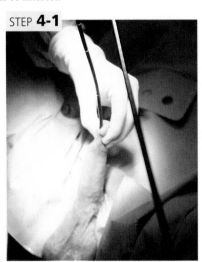

5. Biopsy of suspicious lesions and diagnostic pyeloscopy and ureteroscopy are performed. The characteristics of calculi are observed to determine the best treatment approach. Urine may be obtained for cytologic and microbiologic examination.

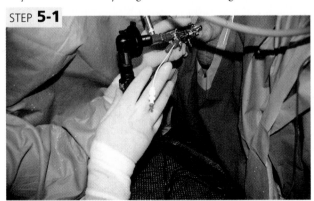

Efflux of renal urine.

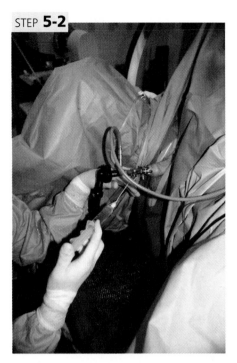

Collecting urine sample for laboratory analysis.

6. If a calculus is small enough to be delivered through the ureter, it is engaged in a retrieval basket and removed under both visual and fluoroscopic control.

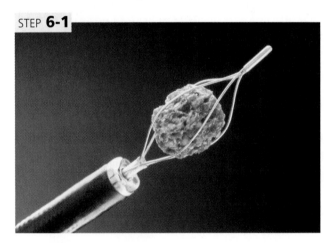

(Courtesy Circon Corporation, Santa Barbara, Calif.)

If after ureteral dilation the calculus does not appear to be small enough for delivery, lithotripsy (fragmentation) must be performed through the ureteroscope, or ESWL may be performed later.

Lithotripsy may be performed with the ultrasonic (through a rigid ureteroscope) or electrohydraulic lithotriptors, or with the pulse-dyed or Ho:YAG lasers. Appropriate laser precautions must be enforced. Chapter 5 discusses laser safety issues in more depth.

7. After the completion of the procedure, the ureter is assessed for integrity (perforation or laceration) with RGP. A ureteral stent is placed over the remaining safety guidewire, and the guidewire is removed.

URETEROPYELOSCOPY WITH LITHOTRIPSY

Description. The procedure previously described precedes lithotripsy. If the safety wire is Teflon coated, it may remain in place. The calculus is fragmented using a probe that is passed through the working channel of the ureteropyeloscope.

Ultrasonic waves do not damage the ureteral wall and are not diffused by the metal wires of a stone basket. The ultrasound probe will only pass through the larger, rigid ureteropyeloscope. The procedure can tend to be tedious and lengthy.

The EHL is capable of fragmenting calculi of a harder consistency than the ultrasound unit can manage. A rapid expansion of vapor is generated by a high-voltage spark that crosses two copper wires. A shock wave that disintegrates the stone is created. The probe is amenable to the flexible ureteropyeloscope but carries more inherent danger for ureteral injury. The use of a stone basket is not recommended, and fragments tend to disperse in the ureter because the probe does not allow for suction to be attached. It is necessary to place an occlusion catheter proximal to the stone before use of the device. The operative time is generally shorter, however.

Indications. Uretural stones too large to remove intact require disintegration. Ultrasonic and electrohydraulic lithotripsy are two techniques that may be employed.

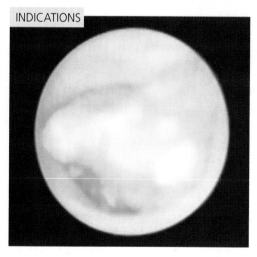

INDICATIONS

Calculus to be fragmented.

Perioperative risks. Problems encountered with ultrasonic lithotripsy include occlusion of the aspirating device by stone fragments, ureteral perforation, and migration of the calculus cephalad. Concerns indigenous to EHL include a high incidence

of ureteral perforation; less effectiveness on hard stones, often requiring more than one probe and grasping instrument; and the precautions that must be taken to prevent shock to the patient. EHL is not recommended for impacted calculi. Bleeding with either procedure is generally minimal, though postoperative hematuria is not uncommon as a result of trauma from the calculus. The general risks previously discussed may apply as well.

Procedural Steps
Ultrasonic lithotripsy

1. Ureteropyeloscopy is performed as previously described.
2. The calculus is immobilized with a stone basket, and the ultrasonic probe is brought into direct contact.

The probe is hollow and provides for the application of suction and irrigation.

3. Short bursts of ultrasonic energy disintegrate the stone while it is under direct visual control. Irrigation followed by suction is applied to the probe to dissipate the heat produced by the ultrasonic waves and to aspirate stone fragments.

Aspiration also prevents proximal migration of the calculus by maintaining stone-to-probe contact.

4. Should fragments escape, it may be necessary to insert a balloon catheter proximal to the stone, occlude the upper part of the ureter, and prevent further migration.
5. Attempts are made to render the ureter stone and fragment free using irrigation and stone baskets, or forceps style retrievers.
6. A ureteral stent is placed at the conclusion of the procedure

Electrohydraulic Lithotripsy (EHL)

1. Ureteropyeloscopy is carried out as previously described.
2. An occlusion balloon catheter is placed and inflated proximal to the calculus to be treated.
3. The probe is passed through the ureteropyeloscope and brought within 1 mm of the stone.

Before firing, one must assure that no persons are in contact with metal. The unit may be set on pulse or continuous fire, with hard or soft power, and at a pulse duration determined by the surgeon.

4. Attempts are made to render the ureter stone and fragment free with irrigation, stone baskets, or forceps-style retrievers.
5. A ureteral stent is placed at the conclusion of the procedure.

URETEROSCOPY WITH RESECTION OR ENDOPYELOTOMY-ENDOURETEROTOMY

Description. **Segmental endoscopic resection** is performed, as an alternative to nephroureterectomy, to completely remove low-grade tumors without penetration of the ureteral wall. **Endopyelotomy** is the reconstruction of the ureteropelvic junction endoscopically using a cold endopyelotomy knife or endopyelotomy electrosurgery instrumentation (Fig. 7-10).

Endoureterotomy is the controlled recanalization of the ureteric segments. In this procedure the ureteroscope is passed proximally, as the narrowed, scarred ureter is incised and dilated, until the normal area of the ureter is encountered.

For procedures involving electrosurgery it is important to use sorbitol or glycine irrigant. This may be diluted with contrast material to allow continuous fluoroscopic visualization.

Indications. **Resection:** Tumor accessible by ureteroscopic intervention, tumor less than 1.5 cm that does not extend circumferentially on the ureteral wall. **Endopyelotomy-endoureterotomy:** Upper ureteral obstruction caused by stricture or vessel compression.

Perioperative risks. Complications documented with these procedures include ureteral avulsion, hemorrhage, blood transfusion, ureteral obstruction, stent obstruction and malposition, and ureterovesical junction (UVJ) stenosis. Other potential risks include ureteral perforation with extravasation, infection, stent dislodgment, tumor recurrence, and intraluminal or intrarenal instrument breakage. Anesthetic risks are as previously discussed.

Procedural Steps

The procedure begins as previously described.

Tumor resection

1. The operating ureteroscope is passed into the ureter after dilation under fluoroscopic guidance.

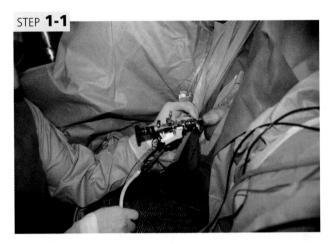

STEP **1-1**

2. The tumor is visualized through the ureteroscope and resected systematically with the cutting electrode of the instrument.

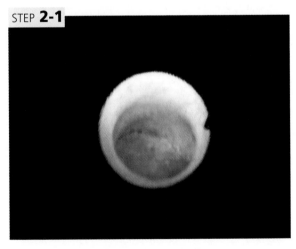

STEP **2-1**

Hemorrhagic papillae.

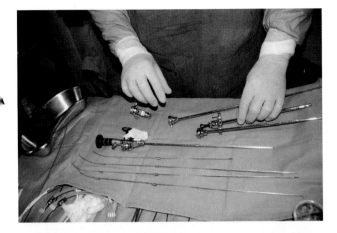

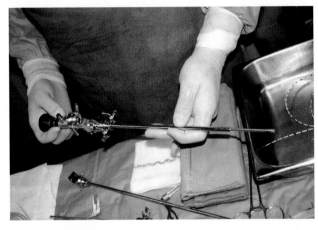

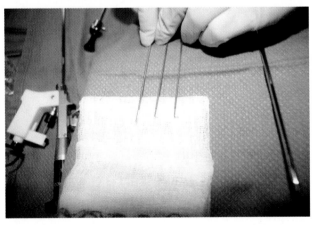

Fig. 7-10 **A,** Operating ureteropyeloscope components **B,** Operating ureteropyeloscope. **C,** Cutting elements for operating ureteropyeloscope.

STEP **2-2**

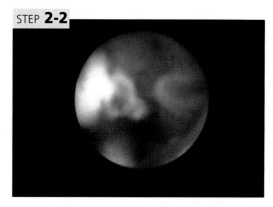

Location of ureteral tumor for resection.

STEP **2-3**

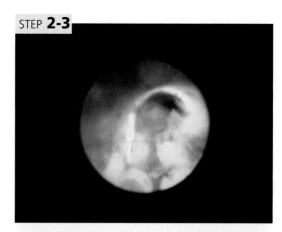

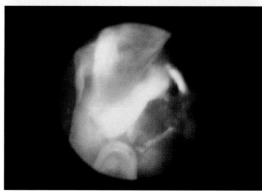

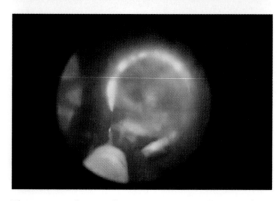

Three stages of ureteral tumor resection with cutting loop.

CONSIDERATIONS As an alternative, Nd:YAG fulguration of ureteral tumors may pose less risk of stricture and perforation. Theories differ regarding this.

3. The integrity of the ureter must be documented after resection.

4. The ureter is stented.

Endopyelotomy-endoureterotomy

1. Access may be achieved ureteroscopically or percutaneously.

2. Access to the upper ureter is gained by coaxial or balloon dilation of the ureter.

CONSIDERATIONS Percutaneous access should be established through a calyx in the midportion of the kidney, allowing introduction of a rigid instrument into the upper ureter.

3. The obstructing portion is identified endoscopically after the location has been demonstrated by RGP. Visualization of the obstructing segment includes observation for pulsations caused by an arterial branch passing behind the ureter and supplying the lower pole of the kidney.

4. A longitudinal incision, posterolaterally at the level of the ureteropelvic junction (UPJ), is made in the ureter extending beyond the area of obstruction. The incision must extend through the ureter but avoid vessels lying just outside the ureteral wall.

STEP **4-1**

Safety Guidewire Through UPJ   Posterior Incision

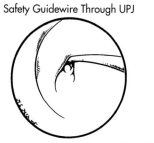
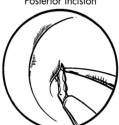

Posterior Incision View of Periureteral Tissue

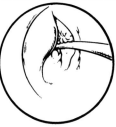

(From Resnik MI: Current therapy in genitourinary surgery, *ed 2, St. Louis, 1992, Mosby.)*

5. The ureter is stented with an endopyelotomy stent that is left in place for 6 weeks. A Foley catheter may be placed and removed in 1 to 2 days.

CONSIDERATIONS An alternative to the endopyelotomy knife is the "Acucise" endopyelotomy balloon-electrocautery wire.

POSTOPERATIVE

Nursing Care and Discharge Planning

Generic for All Ureteropyeloscopic Interventions
1. Cleanse patient of prep solutions.
2. Secure any catheters or stents.
3. Evaluate peripheral vascular circulation and skin integrity.
4. Assess Foley catheter output if applicable.
5. Provide instruction to patient and family:
   - Patient must void before discharge if no catheter is in place.
   - Patient may resume normal diet as tolerated.
   - Patient should increase fluid intake (8 oz q2h until urine clear, half as fruit juice to prevent potassium depletion) to assist voiding process, ward off infection, and promote recovery from spinal anesthesia, if used.
   - Patient may resume nonstrenuous activity in 2 to 3 days and strenuous activity in 2 to 6 weeks. Time frame will vary by extent of procedure.
   - Aspirin and other nonsteriodal antiinflammatory agents should be avoided for 48 hours unless advised by surgeon as medically necessary.
   - Medications ordered should be taken as directed. Stool softeners should be used to prevent constipation if patient is receiving narcotic analgesia. Antibiotics should be taken as directed, often until stent is removed.
   - Reinforce and review catheter and stent care if indicated. After endopyelotomy or endoureterotomy, Foley catheter will be placed and remain for approximately 2 days; stents will remain 4 to 10 weeks. After lithotripsy, stents often remain until ureter is fragment free. After tumor resection, stents remain about 4 to 7 days.
   - Patient will have follow-up IVPs as decided by physician: approximately 1 to 2 weeks after lithotripsy, in 3 months after endopyelotomy-ureterotomy.
   - Postoperative diuretic scans and ultrasonograms will be performed about 4 to 6 weeks after endopyelotomy-ureterotomy.
   - Commonly, patient will experience some ureteral colic, flank pain, hematuria, and dysuria.
6. Review symptoms of infection or retention (fever, pyuria, unremitting dysuria, clots, urine darker than pink, abdominal distention, output <30 ml/hr, unrelieved flank pain).
7. Review technique for straining urine for stone fragments.
8. Document nursing assessment and interventions.

NEPHROSCOPY

Description. Nephroscopy is the endoscopic, systematic investigation and treatment for abnormalities located in the collecting system and pelvis of the kidney. Access to the upper part of the ureter and kidney has been most commonly achieved by an antegrade, percutaneous route through a previously established nephrostomy tract. More recently the kidney and the renal collecting system have become accessible through retrograde passage of a flexible or rigid ureteropyeloscope. This approach is less invasive, but its application may be somewhat limited, but advancements are continuously being made. The retrograde approach is virtually identical to ureteropyeloscopy. The procedure described is the classic antegrade nephroscopy. The procedure requires C-arm fluoroscopy and general anesthesia.

Indications. Operative nephroscopy may be indicated to investigate and treat the source of hematuria localized to the side in question; to locate filling defects associated with hematuria; to rule out and treat papillary lesions, flat carcinoma, nonopaque calculi, blood clots, and inflammatory debris. The only definite contraindication to nephroscopy is an uncorrected bleeding diathesis.

Perioperative risks. Concerns specific to nephroscopy may include hemorrhage, renal laceration, pleural invasion, laceration of the ureter, possible need for blood transfusion, perforation of the ureter or collecting system, urinoma formation, UPJ stricture, large or small bowel perforation, duodenal perforation, splenic injury possibly leading to splenectomy, fistula formation, abscess formation, peritonitis, retroperitoneal or intraperitoneal extravasation of fluid, residual stone fragments, infection, fever, sepsis, UVJ stenosis, and obstruction necessitating stent repositioning.

Anesthetic concerns are most commonly a result of intraoperative problems and may include hypotension, shock, renal failure, hydrothorax, pneumothorax, hemothorax, cyanosis, respiratory compromise, urinothorax, atelectasis, intravascular extravasation, bradycardia, hypertension, and myocardial infarction.

Equipment and instrumentation

All items listed under ureteroscopy in addition to the following:

Equipment
Suction unit
Prone positioning pads *or*
Beanbag *or*
Kidney braces
Lateral armboard

Instruments
Nephroscope, rigid and flexible
Minor instrument set

Miscellaneous supplies
Sterile pack with draping system of choice (laparotomy pack)
Amplatz dilators
Cobra catheter
Cope mandril guidewire
Kaye tamponade balloon catheter
Suction tubing
Nephrostomy tube
Endopyelotomy stent
Cannulated injection needle, 18 gauge, 6 to 8 inches long

Nursing Care and Teaching Considerations for Nephroscopy

1. Incorporate all generic nursing diagnoses that apply.
2. Gather equipment and positioning devices.
3. Check instrumentation and equipment for proper function preoperatively.
4. Check sterile supplies for package integrity.
5. Check medications for dose and expiration dates.
6. Place video system to be used in position for appropriate visualization.
7. Ensure that C-arm protection is available for the patient and personnel.
8. Check laser and provide goggles and signs if indicated.
9. Thoroughly rinse endoscopic equipment that has been disinfected in glutaraldehyde solution.
10. Review patient record for reports of preoperative studies (e.g., CBC, PT, PTT, coagulation profile, serum electrolytes and chemistries, urinalysis and urine culture, cardiac enzymes, blood gases, pulmonary function studies, chest x-ray, ECG, IVP, CT scan, magnetic resonance imaging [MRI], and renogram.
11. Confirm that preoperative orders are accomplished: NPO, enema, antibiotics.
12. Assess patient for peripheral vascular circulation, skin integrity, range of motion, presence of disabilities, pulmonary status, heart disease, allergies, obesity, diabetes, etc.
13. Discuss intended procedure with patient and family. Address concerns and anxieties, clarify misconceptions.

14. Review common postoperative course: coughing and deep breathing, ambulation, antibiotic and pain therapies, catheter and stent care.
15. Positon patient appropriately for the planned intervention. Patient will be in modified lateral or prone position on a C-arm–compatible operating room bed.
16. Apply electrosurgical dispersive pad, if indicated, as close to flank region as possible, avoiding excessively hairy areas or prosthetic implants. Posterior area of thigh is the common site.
17. Prep and drap patient aseptically according to AORN guidelines.
18. Attach high-frequency cable to electrosurgical unit.
19. Connect light cable and adjust intensity, attach irrigation tubing to normal saline solution, and allow surgeon to clear system of air. Have solution appropriate for electrosurgery available.
20. Place irrigation in pressure bag if indicated.
21. Connect irrigant to warming unit if indicated.
22. Connect EHL unit, if indicated, and ensure that no metal contacts the patient, surgeon, or staff members.
23. Connect laser fiber if indicated.
24. Monitor amount of irrigant instilled.
25. Document assessment findings and nursing interventions.

Procedural Steps

1. With the patient prone, a 5 to 6 Fr open-ended ureteral catheter is placed using a retrograde approach under fluoroscopic guidance either in radiology or the operating room.

2. The patient is turned onto the operating room bed into a 30-degree prone-oblique position.

3. Contrast material is infused through the catheter to visualize the collecting system.

4. The 18-gauge cannula needle is introduced into the affected calyx, with efforts made to create a nephrostomy tract below the twelfth rib to avoid the pleural cavity.

5. Once access is accomplished a Bentson or small J-tipped guidewire is introduced into the dilated calyx.

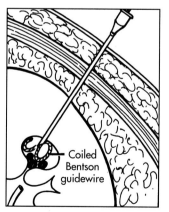

STEP **5-1**

(From Drach GW: Infections and stones, St. Louis, 1992, Mosby.)

6. An additional safety guidewire is introduced during dilatation.

CONSIDERATIONS If the only objective is to place a nephrostomy tube for drainage, dilation does not need to go beyond 8 to 10 Fr.

7. Sequential dilatation of the tract is performed to a 34 Fr size with Amplatz dilators or a fascial balloon dilator.

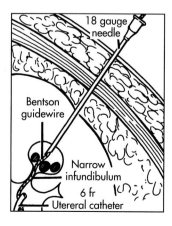

STEP **4-1**

(From Drach GW: Infections and stones, St. Louis, 1992, Mosby.)

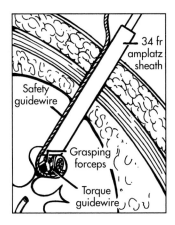

STEP **7-1**

(From Drach GW: Infections and stones, *St. Louis, 1992, Mosby.)*

8. The rigid nephroscope is introduced through the 34 Fr Amplatz sheath to visualize the collecting system.

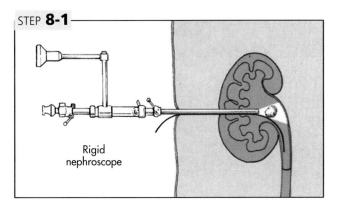

STEP **8-1**

CONSIDERATIONS If portions of the collecting system cannot be visualized through the rigid nephroscope, the flexible scope may be used through the Amplatz sheath.

CONSIDERATIONS

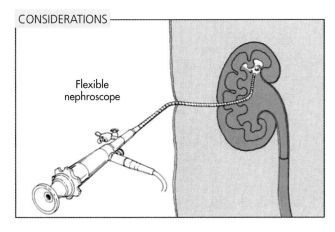

(From Brundage D: Renal disorders, *St. Louis, 1992, Mosby.)*

If a lesion is found, it should be biopsied, if not done already, and treated by resection or laser fulguration.

9. If a calculus is seen and is small enough to be withdrawn, it is removed with a grasping forceps. If larger, it must be fragmented with ultrasound, EHL, or laser.

CONSIDERATIONS Every effort must be extended to render the kidney completely stone free.

Endopyelotomy may be performed by passing an endoscopic knife across the UPJ and incising it longitudinally in the posterolateral position. This is followed by insertion of an endopyelotomy stent and nephrostomy tube.

CONSIDERATIONS After the procedure has been completed, the integrity of the collecting system and ureter should be documented with a nephrostogram before insertion of the nephrostomy tube.

POSTOPERATIVE

Nursing Care and Discharge Planning for Nephroscopy

1. Cleanse patient of prep solution.
2. Assess peripheral circulation and skin integrity.
3. Secure catheters and stents.
4. Apply nephrostomy disc or dressing.
5. Provide instruction to patient and family.
6. Patient should void before discharge if no catheter is in place.
7. Patient may resume normal diet as tolerated.
8. Patient should increase fluid intake postoperatively to assist voiding process and ward off infection (8 oz q2h until urine clear, half as fruit juice to prevent potassium depletion).
9. Aspirin and other nonsteriodal antiinflammatory agents should be avoided until advised by surgeon.
10. Medications ordered should be taken as directed: antibiotics, analgesics, stool softeners.
11. Reinforce and review catheter and stent care. Stent is removed or exchanged in 4 to 6 weeks. If a Cope catheter is used, it is clamped in 12 to 24 hours to test drainage and removed if systems are functioning.
12. A nephrostogram is performed in 2 days to document stent placement and urinary drainage. Stent may be clamped overnight to assess leakage and tolerance.
13. Review urine straining techniques for the collection of stone fragments.
14. Review postoperative course to expect bloody urine, ureteral colic, and dull flank pain.
15. Review symptoms of infection, diuresis, or retention (fever, pyuria, redness at site, output >200 ml/hr, orthostatic hypotension, output <30 ml/hr, abdominal distention, unrelieved flank pain).
16. Document nursing assessment and interventions.

TRANSURETHRAL RESECTION (TUR)

McCarthy, in collaboration with Wappler, is credited with development of the Foroblique resectoscope in 1932. It was sold by American Cystoscope Makers, Inc., as the complex oscillator. The resectoscope is an endoscope that allows for removal of tissue from the prostate, as in cases of bladder outlet obstruction

PREOPERATIVE

Nursing Care and Teaching Considerations for Transurethral Resections

1. Incorporate generic nursing diagnoses appropriate for intervention planned.
2. Gather equipment and positioning devices.
3. Check equipment and instrumentation for proper function preoperatively.
4. If video system is to be used, place it for appropriate visualization.
5. Thoroughly rinse endoscopic equipment that has been disinfected in glutaraldehyde solution.
6. If laser is to be used, gather goggles, signs, and appropriate fiber and perform laser check.
7. Check sterile supplies for package integrity.
8. Check medications for dose and expiration dates.
9. Review patient record for reports of preoperative studies (e.g., CBC, PT, PTT, coagulation profiles, cardiac enzymes, serum electrolytes and chemistry values, urinalysis and urine culture, chest x-ray, prostate specific antigen [PSA], ECG).
10. Confirm that preoperative orders were accomplished (enema, NPO, antibiotics, etc.)
11. Review patient's medical and surgical history (COPD, diabetes, asthma. heart disease, etc.)
12. Assess patient for physical limitations, range of motion, peripheral vascular circulation, skin integrity, allergies, presence of implants, presence of infection.
13. Discuss intervention with patient and family. Address concerns and clarify misconceptions.
14. Discuss common postoperative course, possibility of alteration in sexual function, presence of Foley catheter.
15. Review signs and symptoms to be reported (fever, abdominal distention, output <30 ml/hr or >200 ml/hr, pyuria).
16. Position patient appropriately for the planned intervention. If the patient has low back or hip disabilities, position legs in stirrups before the administration of anesthesia to determine comfort range. The legs may be returned to the supine position for the induction of general anesthesia or the injection of spinal anesthesia.
17. Apply alternating compression stockings before induction of anesthesia and subsequent vasodilation.
18. Apply electrosurgical dispersive pad as close to perineal region as possible, avoiding excessively hairy areas or prosthetic implants. Anterior area of thigh is the common site. Attach high-frequency cable to electrosurgical unit.
19. Perform aseptic prep and drape patient according to AORN guidelines.
20. Connect light cable and adjust intensity; attach irrigation tubing to sorbitol or glycine and allow surgeon to clear system of air.
21. Connect irrigant to warming unit.
22. Monitor amount of irrigation used.
23. Document assessment findings and nursing interventions.

caused by prostatic hyperplasia, or the bladder, as with bladder tumors. Because of the combination of two types of current, coagulating and cutting, it is possible to cut away tissue from the bladder or prostate and to coagulate the resulting bleeders.

Equipment and instrumentation

Equipment
Irrigation warming unit
Electrosurgical unit
Allen stirrups
Cystoscopy bed
Fiberoptic light source
Alternating compression machine
Armboards
Head and neck support
Positioning pads (e.g., gel pad for sacrum)

Instruments
Deflecting (Timberlake) resectoscope sheaths and obturators, standard or continuous flow, 24, 26, and 28 Fr
Iglesias or Stern-McCarthy working element
Panendoscopes, 30 and 70 degrees
Urethral dilators (van Buren sounds)
Cystoresectoscope spacer
Stopcock with Luer-Lok connection

Miscellaneous supplies
Cystoscopy pack with gown or apron and gloves
TUR rectal drape (optional but preferable)

Resectoscope loops, knives, roller balls, Vaportrode, or Sled
High-frequency electrosurgical cable
Patient dispersive pad
TUR irrigation tubing, or irrigation tubing compatible with warming unit
Sterile sorbitol or glycine irrigant, 3000 ml bag or rigid container (2 to 4)
Lubricating jelly, water soluble
Prep solution and sponges with forceps
Absorbent drape for prep
Specimen containers with formalin
Screwtop containers for urine specimens
Luer-Lok syringes, 10 and 20 ml
Toomey syringe or Ellik evacuator with adapter
Urethral catheter: Foley, #22-30 cc balloon or #24-30 cc balloon three-way
Urinary drainage bag
Alternating compression stockings, thigh length

Additional for local anesthesia
Penile clamp
Uro-Jet of 2% lidocaine or other topical anesthetic

Contingent on intended procedure
Video camera, monitor, printer, and VCR
Albarren deflecting mechanism or detachable bridge
Rubber nipples for ureteral catheterization or Bugbee insertion

Bugbee electrode
Panendoscope, 17 and 23 Fr with obturators and light cable
Flexible cystourethroscope
Endoscopic forceps and scissors
Cold knives
Urethrotomes
Pressure bag
Telescope adapter
Laser bridge
Laser fiber, lateral firing or end firing
Nd:YAG laser machine
KTP laser unit if indicated
Cystoscopic injection needle
10 ml injection syringe

TRANSURETHRAL RESECTION OF BLADDER TUMOR (TURBT)

Description. Diagnosis is made by flexible or rigid cystoscopy. The size and position of the lesion is established. The urethral caliber, amount of tumor tissue requiring resection, and the anesthetic time necessary to complete the procedure should be considered when selecting the resectoscope sheath and elements (Fig. 7-11). The sheath chosen should be adequate for tumor removal but also the smallest diameter feasible. This will decrease the amount of urethral dilation needed for scope passage and the incidence of altered patterns of urinary elimination postoperatively.

Replacement components such as electrodes and electrosurgical cords must be available before the procedure is begun. Position the patient appropriately in the stirrups, keeping in mind the potential for sudden medial flexion of the thighs caused by inadvertent obturator reflex during the procedure.

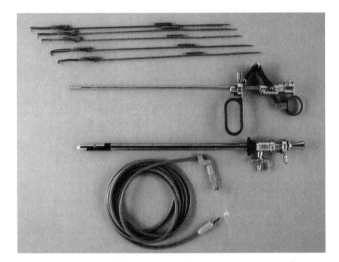

Fig. 7-11 Resectoscope and cutting elements. *Top to bottom,* Cutting loops with round wire tip; cutting knife with pointed tip (Collings knife); coagulating ball end electrode. *(From Brooks Tighe SM: Instrumentation for the operating room, St. Louis, 1994, Mosby,)*

Indications. Eradication, staging, and follow-up management of transitional cell carcinoma (TCC) and carcinoma in situ (CIS) of the bladder (Fig. 7-12). Existing tumor may be eradicated, but the development of recurrent tumors cannot be prevented.

Perioperative risks. The most common problem associated with TURBT is hemorrhage. Additionally, bladder perforation may occur because of elevation of intravesical pressure, resection into the bladder wall, necrotic tumors, or stimulation of the obturator nerve. In the female patient, resection of a vesical neck tumor carries the risk of postoperative vesicovaginal fistula formation. Other concerns, from both a surgical and an anesthetic standpoint, include intraperitoneal extravasation of fluid (abdominal pain with distention and rigidity, cold sweats, hypotension, tachycardia, pallor), hyponatremia, hypervolemia, ureteral orifice injury, ureteral stenosis or obstruction, and bladder neck stricture.

Procedural Steps

The procedure may begin as a routine cystoscopy.

1. The patient's urethra and the resectoscope sheath are generously lubricated with water-soluble jelly. The resectoscope

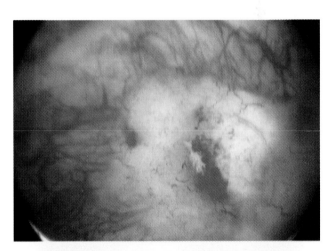

A

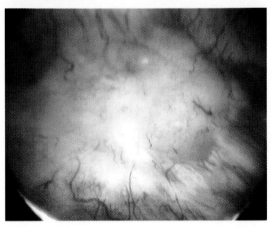

B

Fig. 7-12 **A,** Flat transitional cell carconima of bladder. **B,** Carcinoma in situ of bladder.

sheath is inserted either with a deflecting obturator, or under direct vision with a visual obturator.

STEP **1-1**

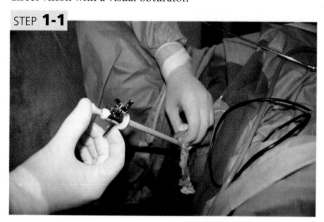

If urethral dilation is necessary at this time, it should not be more than is adequate for scope passage.

CONSIDERATIONS Areas suspicious for carcinoma in situ are biopsied and sent to the histology lab in separate containers of formalin labeled according to their location in the bladder.

2. The size and position of the lesion is observed and assessed through the resectoscope.

STEP **2-1**

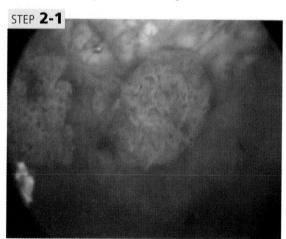

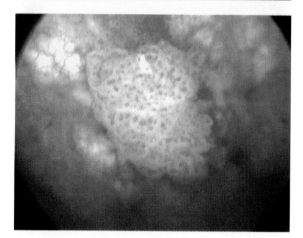

Two views of tumor assessment before resection.

3. The lesion is resected from its furthermost extension into the lumen of the bladder, toward its base to avoid releasing large pieces of tumor into the bladder which will be difficult to remove. Bleeding vessels are coagulated as they occur.

STEP **3-1**

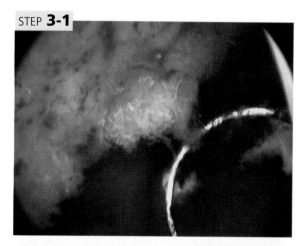

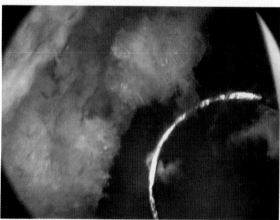

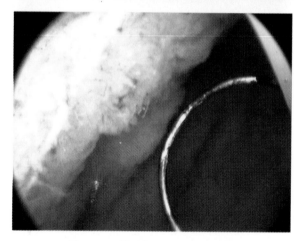

Three-step bladder tumor resection.

4. The need for a biopsy from the base of the tumor after resection should be considered to assess for muscle invasion. Laser fulguration either before or after resection may be performed.

5. A bimanual examination is accomplished to assess for any pelvic masses caused by tumor invasion outside the bladder and for possible fixation of the bladder to the pelvic side wall. This may be performed before or after resection.

6. Once hemostasis has been achieved a catheter large enough to accommodate blood clots is inserted if significant bleeding is a potential complication during the postoperative period (24 to 48 hours).

TRANSURETHRAL INCISION OF THE BLADDER NECK (TUIBN)

Description. Flexible or rigid cystoscopy precedes TUIBN to rule out residual prostatic nodules and urethral stricture. Incision is made into the scarred bladder neck with a cold knife, resectoscope, or internal urethrotome. Transurethral incision is preferable to resection of a scarred bladder neck to prevent recurrent bladder neck contracture. Injection of a steroid preparation (methylprednisolone acetate, Depo-Medrol) through a cystoscopic injection needle may help prevent recurrence.

Indications. Bladder neck contracture after TURP with symptoms of severe obstructive voiding, usually appearing around 6 weeks postoperatively. It may be applicable to patients with bladder outlet obstruction (BOO) localized to the bladder neck, without prostatic enlargement or with a small prostate, and to patients concerned about retrograde ejaculation.

Perioperative risks. Problems encountered have included perforation, recurrent stricture, and minimal bleeding. Anesthetic concerns are related to the patient's presenting medical status.

Procedural Steps

1. The procedure is initiated in the same manner as cystoscopy and TUR.

   CONSIDERATIONS Any appropriate anesthetic may be employed.

2. The bladder neck is incised with a cold knife or electrocautery knife at the 5 and 7 o'clock positions through a 24 Fr resectoscope (or with a Bugbee electrode through the cystourethroscope).

3. An indwelling catheter is not routinely required.

TRANSURETHRAL RESECTION OF THE PROSTATE (TURP)

Description. Diagnosis is again confirmed by flexible or rigid cystoscopy. Transurethral resection of obstructing prostatic tissue (adenoma) within the surgical capsule is removed utilizing electrosurgery. The median and lateral lobes of the prostate are resected with specialized endourologic cutting instrumentation.

If a continuous-flow resectoscope is used intravesical pressure is reduced, a "still" bladder is created, and a clearer field of vision provided. Operative time may be decreased because of the constant inflow and outflow of irrigant (Fig. 7-13).

Indications. Bladder outlet obstruction (infravesical obstruction) secondary to BPH and symptoms of prostatism. These may include weak stream, abdominal straining, hesi-

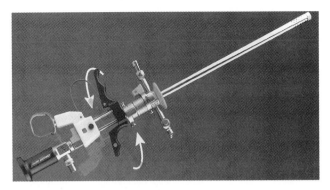

Fig. 7-13 Continuous flow resectoscope. *(Courtesy Circon Corp., Santa Barbara, Calif.)*

tancy, intermittency, incomplete bladder evacuation, and dribbling at termination of voiding. Irritative urinary outflow symptoms include hematuria, chronic or acute urinary tract infection, chronic or acute urinary retention often with outflow incontinence, and acute or chronic renal failure as a result of backflow of urine into the kidneys.

Perioperative risks. The most frequently encountered complications with TURP continue to be fluid-load shifts and hemorrhage. Sexual dysfunction after TURP includes retrograde ejaculation and possible impotence. Other concerns include intraperitoneal extravasation of fluid (abdominal pain with distention and rigidity, cold sweats, hypotension, tachycardia, pallor), hyponatremia, hypervolemia, and bladder neck stricture.

Procedural Steps

1. The urethra is lubricated generously with water-soluble jelly and dilated with van Buren sounds.

2. The smallest resectoscope sheath, consistent with removal of the amount of hyperplastic prostate tissue present in a reasonable period of time (1 to 1 1/2 hours or less), is chosen.

3. Resection of prostatic tissue begins with the middle lobe to the crossing fibers of the bladder neck. This opens the prostatic urethra proximally to facilitate the balance of the resection.

STEP **3-1**

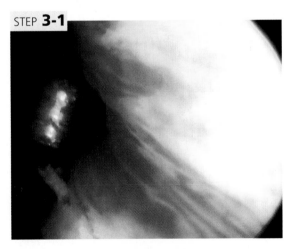

Vaportrode resection.

4. Resection of the lateral lobe component is begun at the anterior aspect of the prostatic urethra to allow the lobes to "fall" into the prostatic urethra. This allows for an easier resection. The lateral lobes are resected to their attachment in the surgical capsule.

STEP **4-1**

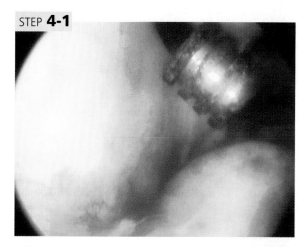

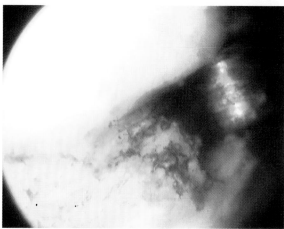

Vaportrode resection.

5. The distal resection is limited to the level of the verumontanum to prevent injury of the intraprostatic continence mechanism (sphincter).

STEP **5-1**

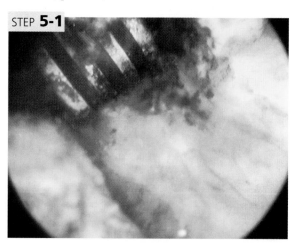

Vaportrode resection.

6. All prostatic chips are evacuated from the bladder with a Toomey syringe or Ellik evacuator to prevent catheter obstruction in the early postoperative period. If a continuous-flow resectoscope is used, suction is attached to the outflow. This removes the need to periodically clear the bladder of tissue and fluid.

7. Residual arterial bleeders and significant venous bleeders in the prostatic urethra are located and cauterized.

8. A three-way Foley catheter with a 30 cc balloon, large enough to accommodate blood clots that may form during the postoperative period, is inserted and generally attached to continuous irrigation. If the resection is small and only a small volume of tissue is removed, a two-way catheter may be sufficient, or no catheter may be needed at all.

9. The Vaportrode (Fig. 7-14) and Sled are also being used with increasing frequency to promote hemostasis and ablate tissue in place of the standard attachments or Nd:YAG laser ablation. An adequate prostatic urethral channel must be created to allow for voiding.

CONSIDERATIONS The Vaportrode requires an electrosurgical unit that is able to deliver energy at high levels of resistance (1500 to 2500 ohms). Conventional electrosurgical units may not be capable of handling the Vaportrode, resulting in "burnout" of the unit. The manufacturer should be consulted to determine the unit's capability.

10. Blood for serum electrolytes, hemoglobin, and hematocrit is drawn in the immediate postoperative period if blood loss is significant or the operative time is more than 1 hour.

TRANSURETHRAL INCISION OF THE PROSTATE (TUIP)

Description. Transurethral incision of the prostate is a procedure in which the prostate is incised at the 5 and 7 o'clock positions. This provides relief of obstruction with results similar to those provided by a complete transurethral resection, with a lower incidence of bladder neck contracture and retrograde ejaculation. The shorter operative time inherent with the procedure minimizes fluid absorption and may decrease postoperative pulmonary and cardiovascular complications. The procedure may be performed with cold or hot knives as well as the standard resectoscope or laser fiber.

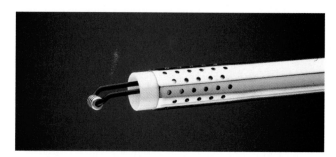

Fig. 7-14 Vaportrode electrode. *(Courtesy Circon Corp., Santa Barbara, Calif.)*

Indications. This procedure is appropriate for sexually active patients with moderate to small obstructive prostates without a significant middle lobe component. One major disadvantage is the potential of missing occult prostatic cancer that may be present. Despite this, some clinicians view this as an underused, valuable form of treatment.

Perioperative risks. Risks with this procedure appear to be minimal. Issues encountered include possibility for recurrence of obstructive symptoms, a 2% to 6% incidence of urethral stricture, a less-than 45% occurrence of retrograde ejaculation, inability to treat a large gland or median lobe hyperplasia, and lack of tissue for histologic examination. There have been no documented cases of bladder neck obstruction, and bleeding and extravasation of fluid have been minimal.

Procedural Steps

1. After the patient is appropriately anesthetized, a 24 Fr resectoscope sheath is passed transurethrally.

2. The cutting instrument of choice is inserted into the working element. Incisions are made at the 5 and 7 o'clock positions.

3. Incisions are carried from above the bladder neck to the verumontanum.

POSTOPERATIVE

Nursing Care and Discharge Planning for TUR

1. Cleanse patient of prep solution.
2. Assess peripheral circulation and skin integrity.
3. Connect and secure Foley catheter.
4. Assess urinary output.
5. Provide instruction to patient and family.
6. Patient may resume normal diet as tolerated.
7. Review activity level allowed postoperatively.
8. Patient should increase fluid intake postoperatively to assist voiding process, ward off infection, and promote recovery from spinal anesthesia if used (8 oz fluid q2h until urine clear, half as fruit juice to prevent potassium depletion).
9. Aspirin and other nonsteriodal antiinflammatory agents should be avoided until approved by surgeon.
10. Medications ordered should be taken as directed. Antibiotics for full regimen, analgesics as needed before onset of pain, stool softeners if narcotics are used.
11. Reinforce and review catheter care, including irrigation techniques.
12. Review symtpoms of infection, retention, and diuresis (fever, pyuria, abdominal distention, output <30 ml/hr, urine darker than pink, presence of clots, output >200 ml/hr, hypotension, weakness, pallor and chills.)
13. Review possibility of retrograde ejaculation or impotence. Provide support; seek additional resources if indicated.
14. Discuss possibility of transient incontinence after Foley catheter removal. Foley will be removed in 2 to 7 days after 24 hours of clear urine and a successful voiding trial.
15. Document nursing assessment and interventions.

4. The prostatic urethra is inspected to ensure that obstructing prostatic tissue is not present and bleeding has been controlled.

5. A two-way Foley catheter is generally necessary.

LASER APPLICATIONS

When laser therapy is performed, additional safety issues must be addressed. The laser has the ability to incur ophthalmic damage. Despite the fact that the fiber is inside a body cavity, fiber breakage may occur to the section extending from the endoscope.

Lasers that have had successful genitourinary applications are the Nd:YAG, holmium:YAG (Ho:YAG), KTP-532 (frequency-doubled YAG), argon, tunable dye, and CO_2. The CO_2 laser is the only one not applicable internally. Precautions will differ slightly between these lasers based on their wavelength and tissue absorption of the respective beam. Wattages mentioned are not intended to be recommendations. The wattage chosen is determined by the operating surgeon, the specific laser, and the fiber to be employed.

The Nd:YAG and argon are absorbed by clear fluids or structures and can cause damage to the retina. The CO_2 and Ho:YAG are easily absorbed by the surface tissue of the eye, resulting in corneal or scleral damage. Standard glasses are not considered adequate protection. The KTP and tunable dye lasers are absorbed by hemoglobin and melanin but can also be transmitted through clear fluids or structures. Windows must be covered with nonflammable shutters or shades for all lasers except the CO_2 and Ho:YAG.

A smoke evacuator that filters 0.1 to 0.5 μm should be utilized for any external, or open, laser procedures to purify the laser plume. The plume carries bacteria or viruses from the site and may also cause eye irritation and nausea. A no-residue fire extinguisher should be readily available because an inadvertent impact from a stray beam may ignite flammable materials. Additionally, sterile water should be handy to douse small fires. Sponges used during treatment should always be moistened, and an alcohol-based prep solution should be avoided.

Benefits have been reported as a result of laser techniques to ablate, vaporize, coagulate, and cut tissue. They include the following:

- Dry field of surgery because of sealing of small vessels
- Decreased postoperative edema and seeding of malignancy because of sealing of lymphatics
- Decreased postoperative pain because of sealing of nerve endings
- Sterilization of tissue resulting from heat buildup at the site of interest
- Decreased scarring and subsequently decreased postoperative stenosis
- Shorter recovery period and earlier return to daily routine
- Decreased surgery time
- Ability to perform more procedures on an outpatient basis with local or minimal anesthesia

Benefits of contact Nd:YAG therapy have also been reported:

- Less power than previously needed to deliver laser energy
- Direct coagulation yielding less blood loss
- Less smoke production in fluid-filled cavities
- Less backscatter and beam reflection
- Less adjacent tissue damage
- Uniform performance in all soft tissue
- Tactile sense enhanced

The cost of laser therapy remains a controversial issue. Do the benefits override the expense? Does laser therapy really decrease surgical time? These issues continue to be debated, making the use of a laser a selective treatment that must be carefully weighed for each patient.

ENDOSCOPIC LASER FRAGMENTATION OF CALCULUS

Ureteropyeloscopic-Nephroscopic

Description. A tunable dye (pulse-dyed or Candela) or Ho:YAG laser is utilized to disintegrate calculi without risk of damage to the soft tissue. A continuous flow of normal saline irrigant is employed. The procedure may be used with ureteropyeloscopy or nephroscopy. The fibers for both are reusable. The pulse-dyed laser probe is discharged in direct contact with the stone, releasing a nonionized plasma gas that coats the surface of the calculus. As the plasma expands and collapses through repeated firings, mechanical shock waves fracture the stone. It may not be necessary to immobilize the calculus. The Ho:YAG emits a pulsed beam producing a vapor bubble. It drills holes into the calculi, causing it to fracture. The fiber must be touching the target. Further discussion of laser safety may be found in Chapter 5.

Indications. To manage ureteral calculi, particularly fragile and impacted stones, instead of using ureterolithotomy or nephrolithotomy, and to disimpact *steinstrasse* after ESWL treatment. It has the ability to reach any stone in the collecting system.

Perioperative risks. Concern generally centers around laser safety issues. Although the fiber is activated inside the lumen of the ureter, laser goggles should be worn by everyone in the room in the event of fiber damage external to the ureteroscope. The laser pedal should be the only foot pedal within the surgeon's reach to prevent inadvertent firing of any ancillary electrical equipment (e.g., electrosurgery). The pulse-dyed laser wavelength is about 1000 nm and requires yellow- to orange-tinted eyewear rated for its use. The Ho:YAG has a wavelength of 2100 nm and requires clear eyewear rated for it. Since it is absorbed by water, the Ho:YAG may hold more risk to ureteral tissue if the fiber is directed at the ureteral wall or the guidewire. Other risks would the same as those discussed for ureteroscopy or nephroscopy and for lithotripsy.

PREOPERATIVE

Nursing Care and Teaching Considerations for All Laser Interventions

1. Incorporate laser risk diagnosis and any others applicable to the procedure and patient.
2. Gather all equipment and instrumentation; examine for proper function.
3. Set up laser and do mandatory laser check; hang signs, goggles; cover windows. Collect ancillary needs.
4. Assess sterile packaging for integrity.
5. Check medications for dose and expiration dates.
6. Place video system in position for appropriate visualization.
7. If C-arm fluoroscopy is scheduled, ensure that x-ray protection is available for the patient and personnel.
8. Thoroughly rinse endoscopic equipment that has been disinfected in glutaraldehyde solution.
9. Review patient record for medical history (COPD, diabetes, heart disease, etc.)
10. Review patient record for reports of preoperative studies (e.g., CBC, urinalysis and urine culture, PT, PTT, cardiac enzymes, serum electrolytes and chemistry values, PSA, IVP, ECG, chest x-ray, urodynamics).
11. Assess patient for peripheral vascular circulation, physical limitations, range of motion, skin integrity, presence of allergies or implants.
12. Discuss procedure with patient. Clarify misconceptions; explain laser precautions.
13. Review postoperative course (Foley catheter, less chance of sexual alteration, possibility of recurrence). Involve family; allay anxieties.
14. Discuss risks detailed under specific intervention.
15. Position patient appropriately for the planned intervention. If the patient has low back or hip disabilities, position legs in stirrups before the administration of anesthesia to determine comfort range. The legs may be returned to the supine position for the induction of general anesthesia or the injection of spinal anesthesia.
16. Apply alternating compression stockings before induction of anesthesia and subsequent vasodilation.
17. Provide laser goggles to patient and personnel. Make sure one person is available to run laser.
18. Apply electrosurgical dispersive pad as close to perineal region as possible, avoiding excessively hairy areas or prosthetic implants. Anterior area of the thigh is the common site. Attach high-frequency cable to electrosurgical unit.
19. Perform aseptic prep and drape patient according to AORN guidelines.
20. Connect light cable and adjust intensity, attach irrigation tubing to irrigant of choice (water or saline), and allow surgeon to clear system of air.
21. Connect irrigant to warming unit.
22. Monitor amount of irrigation used.
23. Document assessment findings and nursing interventions.

Procedural Steps

1. The patient is placed in dorsal lithotomy position for a transurethral approach and in lateral position for the nephroscopic approach. Any appropriate anesthetic modality may be employed.

2. A routine cystoscopy and retrograde pyelogram is performed with a cone-style ureteral catheter to assess the extent of impaction and the patency of the distal ureter.

3. The stone may be entrapped in a basket or allowed to sit free in the ureter.

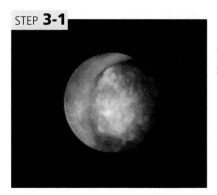

Ureteral calculus free in ureter.

4. Two 0.025 to 0.038 inch guidewires are passed into the ureter. Ideally the wires are passed into the renal pelvis. If they cannot be inserted beyond the calculus, they are placed at that level and advanced as fragmentation occurs.

5. The 7 Fr rigid ureteropyeloscope is introduced into the ureteral orifice over one guidewire and alongside the other, generally without the need for ureteral dilation.

CONSIDERATIONS Several approaches are possible. The ureteroscope may be placed directly on the wire and slowly advanced, or the guidewire may be passed through the working channel of the scope and a second wire used to open the ureter enough to allow passage. If the ureter is still too narrow, a balloon dilation catheter is placed and inflated to stretch the canal.

6. Once the ureteroscope is in place, irrigation is propelled through one channel as the laser fiber is passed through the other.

7. The fiber is placed directly on and perpendicular to the stone's surface and aimed at the junction of any nodules or cracks.

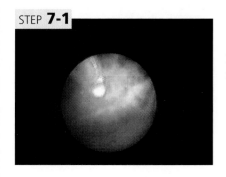

Ho: YAG laser fiber impacting calculus.

8. The stones are fractured to a size that may be easily passed spontaneously. If this is not achievable, fragments may be trapped in baskets and removed manually.

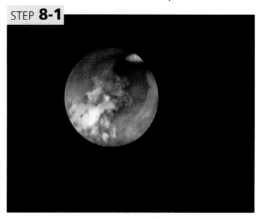

9. The ureter is stented over the safety wire after the treatment.

INTRAURETHRAL LASER ABLATION
Condyloma/Papillary Tumor/Caruncle

Description. Tangential application of the laser beam is applied until a white discoloration occurs. The laser chosen depends on surgeon preference and the specific site of application.

Indications. Unsuccessful results with electrosurgery and other conventional treatment modalities.

Urethral Condyloma/Papillary Tumor

Description. Circumferential intraurethral Nd:YAG or KTP-532 laser treatment (accompanied by intraurethral instillation of 5-fluorouracil cream 3 to 4 weeks postoperatively for condylomas) is most commonly employed. The Ho:YAG and argon lasers have also shown some success for these conditions. Local anesthetic with monitored sedation is generally adequate to afford a pain-free procedure for the patient.

Indications. Lesions of the fossa navicularis; and differentiation between condylomata acuminata and papillary tumor must be determined through histologic diagnosis to afford appropriate follow-up care (Fig. 7-15).

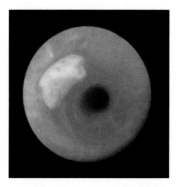

Fig. 7-15 Urethral tumor with condylomatous appearance. (*(From Lloyd-Davies W:* Color atlas of urology, *London, 1994, Mosby-Wolfe.)*

Perioperative risks. Risks include injury to the corpora or damage to the penile neurovascular bundles resulting from urethral perforation and recurrence. Risk for urethral stricture exists but has been found to be lower than that after treatment with electrosurgery. Anesthetic risks are few and may include hypertension, reaction to the local anesthetic, and positional nerve injury. The Nd:YAG, KTP, and argon lasers require wavelength-rated tinted goggles; the wavelengths are 1064, 532, and 488 nm respectively. The same laser precautions apply as previously discussed.

Procedural Steps

1. Meatotomy or visualization with a pediatric cystoscope or nasal speculum is necessary.

2. The entire lesion, including the base, is treated. Excessive penetration into the urethra is avoided.

3. The lesions are removed with biopsy forceps after treatment or allowed to slough.

Urethral Caruncle

Description. Laser is applied at low to medium wattage determined by the surgeon until the lesion undergoes a characteristic white discoloration. The CO_2 laser may be used as well as the KTP, argon, and Ho:YAG or Nd:YAG lasers. A contact tip is usually employed. Acetic acid, 4%, and cotton balls are used to define the tissue to be treated. The microscope may also be utilized if the laser used is adaptable to it. This procedure is commonly done under local anesthetic instillation with monitored sedation.

Indications. Painful inflammatory masses of the female urethra treated unsuccessfully by other methods (Fig. 7-16).

Perioperative risks. The same risks as previously discussed apply. Bleeding is the most common difficulty because of the vascularity of the tissue. If the CO_2 laser is used, the risk of laser fire is increased.

Procedural Steps

1. Local anesthetic is instilled into the urethra by infiltration.
2. Laser is applied without penetration into the urethra.
3. Antibiotic ointment may be applied.

TRANSURETHRAL LASER ABLATION
Transurethral Laser Ablation of Bladder Tumor

Description. Commonly the Nd:YAG and a contact fiber at low wattage is used. A side-firing fiber is safer with respect to avoiding damage to adjacent small bowel, but an end-firing fiber may also be used. The power setting and power density most appropriate for the application and fiber are chosen. Delivery of energy depends on the power setting, distance of the laser beam from the target, and the length of time the laser energy is delivered. Concentrated power delivery to the bladder dome, which is adjacent to the small bowel, should be avoided. The effect of energy delivery is determined by the appearance of the tissue lased. Tissue should turn a characteristic white discoloration (Fig. 7-17). This procedure is easily performed in an outpatient setting with local anesthetic and monitored anesthesia care, or sedation only.

A noncontact Nd:YAG fiber at medium power (average 35 to 45 W) on continuous mode has been successful with superficial tumors. Argon, KTP, and Ho:YAG lasers have also shown some promising results.

Indications. Bladder tumor known to be superficial or tumor in a difficult-to-reach location such as inside a bladder diverticulum and on the anterior bladder neck, anterior to the urethral opening. Laser ablation may be employed as the primary treatment of superficial tumors less than 2 cm in diameter. In instances of superficially invasive tumor greater than 2 cm, it is performed to deliver destructive energy to the tumor cells at deeper levels before transurethral resection and to prevent the spread of tumor by sealing lymphatic and vascular channels. Laser ablation may be used to minimize blood loss in patients with coagulopathy.

Perioperative risks. Complications revolving around laser ablation of bladder tumors have been few but may include recurrence, penetration of the bladder wall with perforation, inadequate depth of ablation, postoperative reflex paralytic ileus, fever and infection, seeding of tumor cells during therapy, bowel perforation, and pelvic pain.

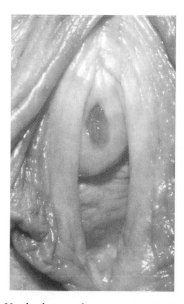

Fig. 7-16 Urethral caruncle. *(From Lloyd-Davies W: Color atlas of urology, London, 1994, Mosby-Wolfe.)*

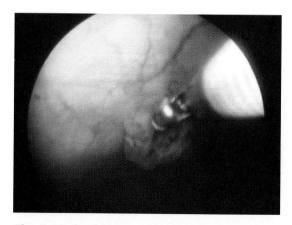

Fig. 7-17 Graphic tissue ablation with Nd:YAG laser.

Procedural Steps

1. Cystoscopy with a rigid or flexible instrument is accomplished to determine the size, extent, location, and appearance of the lesions and to form an impression of its level of invasiveness and biologic potential. The bladder is thoroughly inspected for evidence of carcinoma in situ and other malignant conditions.

2. Before treatment, biopsy specimens are taken from the tumor base and tissue within 1 cm of the tumor at 3, 6, 9, and 12 o'clock positions.

3. The exophytic (protruding) portion of the tumor is resected deeply into the bladder wall after laser coagulation of the tumor margins. The fiber chosen should have a beam that fires laterally to lower the risk of injury to organs adjacent to the bladder, in particular, the small bowel, which lies directly above the dome of the bladder.

CONSIDERATIONS The patient may be placed in Trendelenburg position to allow the bowel to ride upward and avoid potential perforation. The lateral, or right-angle, laser fiber works tangentially. The beam is directed through the tumor with more energy concentrated into the bladder wall rather than across the bladder. A forward-firing fiber aims directly at the small bowel if dome tumors are being addressed. Additionally a flexible cystoscope or lateral-firing fiber may reach the lateral walls of the bladder or the bladder neck with greater ease.

4. The edges and base are ablated with the laser.

5. Smaller lesions are totally ablated linearly with the laser fiber after a sealing pass at 0.5 cm surrounding each tumor. The sealing pass coagulates efferent vessels and lymphatics.

6. The tumor is removed with biopsy forceps after coagulation to be sent for tumor classification.

7. A catheter is usually unnecessary because bleeding is minimal after laser treatment.

Transurethral Laser Incision of the Bladder Neck

Description. Laser incision down to the muscle or the capsule of the prostate-bladder neck. Either the Nd:YAG or KTP-532 laser may be used for treatment. An end-firing or right-angle fiber may be chosen.

Indications. Post-TURP bladder neck contracture.

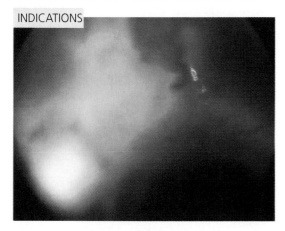

INDICATIONS

Bladder neck contracture.

Perioperative risks. Complications have been minimal and may include stricture recurrence and fiber breakage. Potential problems include perforation, extravasation, and bleeding.

Procedural Steps

1. The laser fiber is passed through the cystourethroscope.

2. The scarred bladder neck is touched with the fiber at the 5 and 7 o'clock positions. A 3-second pulse at medium power (usually 30 to 40 W) is generally sufficient for adequate incision with the Nd:YAG laser. With the KTP laser, low power (approximately 5 to 10 W) in continuous mode will commonly achieve the desired result.

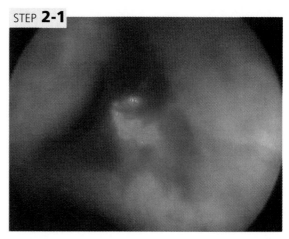

STEP **2-1**

Nd:YAG laser fiber incising bladder neck at 7 o'clock.

3. Additional incisions at 11 and 2 o'clock positions will minimize the risk of rectal injury resulting from the forward scatter of energy.

4. Any anesthetic modality may be used. Postoperative catheterization is not routine.

Visual Laser Ablation of the Prostate (VLAP)

Description. Visual laser ablation of the prostate is an endoscopic procedure in which laser energy is delivered to the prostate gland. This is done by delivering laser energy through a contact side-firing (right-angle) laser fiber passed through a panendoscope to a mirror at the end of the fiber (Fig. 7-18). Here the laser light is reflected onto the prostate tissue. A noncontact end-firing fiber may also be used, as well as a right angle noncontact fiber. A combination technique may also be employed. The advantage of VLAP is that coagulation of potential bleeding sites and ablation of tissue can be achieved as an outpatient or one night stay in the hospital. Additionally the risk of retrograde ejaculation, impotence, incontinence, and postoperative TUR syndrome is significantly reduced.

The procedure can be performed in about 30 minutes. Anesthesia may be provided by any modality. Patients have returned to normal activity and employment on the first postoperative day.

Indications. Tissue lasing for coagulation to achieve blanching of the prostatic tissue at the lase site facilitates resection with less blood loss as long as the depth of resection is not

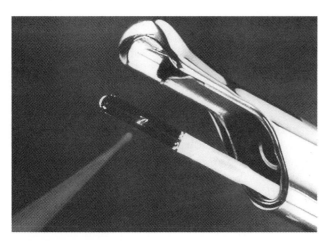

Fig. 7-18 Side-firing laser fiber. *(Courtesy Circon Corp., Santa Barbara, Calif.)*

carried below the level of laser penetration. Lasing for destruction of prostatic tissue at a more superficial level to create vaporization of tissue as demonstrated by the release of bubbles at the lased site and a disappearance of obstructing tissue as the procedure is carried out. Generally the more laser energy expended during the procedure and the closer the depth of laser penetration to the surgical capsule, the greater the irritative symptoms of the patient will be in the postoperative period. Patients require treatment with antiinflammatory agents postoperatively.

Earlier catheter removal may make this a more attractive option for patients with cardiac implants, lessening the chance of secondary infection caused by the presence of a catheter.

Perioperative risks. Problems encountered have included postoperative edema, lack of tissue for histologic confirmation without performing a biopsy, urinary tract infection, bladder neck stenosis, sloughing of tissue for 6 to 12 weeks with possible obstruction, epididymo-orchitis, and urinary retention. Because few vessels are affected, the risk of bleeding, fluid absorption, and electrolyte shifts is low. Anesthetic concerns tend to be patient specific and related to the patient's preoperative medical status.

Procedural Steps

1. The patient is positioned in the dorsal lithotomy position, under intravenous sedation, spinal injection, or general anesthesia. A topical anesthetic is administered if intravenous sedation is being used.
2. A panendoscope large enough to accommodate the laser fiber, generally 23 Fr, is introduced under direct vision or with a visual obturator. A deflecting mechanism is used to aid in proper fiber placement.
3. The size of the obstructing adenoma is determined so that the number of lased zones can be decided, generally four, at 2, 4, 8, and 10 o'clock positions.

STEP **3-1**

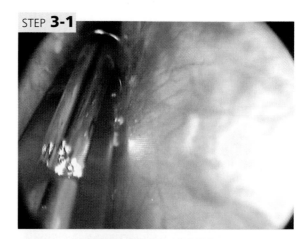

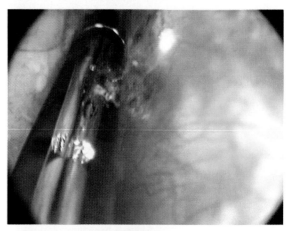

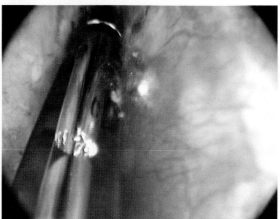

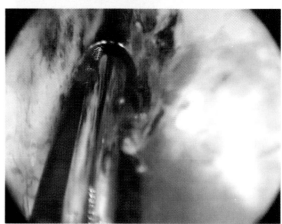

Four-step VLAP procedure.

If the prostatic urethra is longer than 4 cm, an additional four zones may be necessary at a more distal site above the verumontanum. The fiber tip is distanced slightly from the obstructing adenoma, in the prostatic urethra, proximal to the verumontanum

4. The laser energy level is chosen depending on the philosophy of the operating surgeon and may range from 30 to 80 W.

CONSIDERATIONS If it is desirable to coagulate the prostatic tissue deeply, a medium setting of around 30 W, for a lasing period of 1 to 2 minutes, in continuous mode in each zone, has historically been preferable. If it is desirable to ablate the tissue as a primary objective, a higher setting ranging from 60 to 100 W, in continuous mode for 30 to 90 seconds, has been found to be appropriate.

5. Patients who are treated with laser ablation primarily, without resection of a channel for voiding, may not be able to void for several weeks and may require a Foley catheter or intermittent catheterization. A Foley catheter is placed for the immediate postoperative period.

POSTOPERATIVE

Nursing Care and Discharge Planning for Laser Interventions

1. Cleanse patient of prep solution.
2. Assess skin integrity and peripheral circulation.,
3. Patient must void before discharge if no catheter is in place.
4. Patient may resume normal diet as tolerated.
5. Normal activity may resume as tolerated. Strenuous activity in 2 to 4 weeks.
6. Patient should increase fluid intake postoperatively to assist voiding process, ward off infection, and promote recovery from spinal anesthesia, if used. Fruit juice should be included to prevent potassium depletion.
7. Aspirin and other nonsteriodal antiinflammatory agents should be avoided for 48 hours unless advised by surgeon as medically necessary.
8. Medications ordered should be taken as directed.
9. Teach intermittent catheterization.
10. Sexual activity may resume in 1 to 2 weeks as tolerated.
11. Review symptoms of infection or retention. Discuss risks detailed under specific intervention.
12. Document nursing assessment and interventions.

Bibliography

1. Bagley DH: *Techniques with the flexible ureteroscope*, Stamford, 1991, Circon-ACMI.
2. Ball KA: *Lasers—the perioperative challenge*, ed 2, St. Louis, 1995, Mosby.
3. Crowe H, Costello A: Laser ablation of the prostate: nursing management, *Urol Nursing*, 14:2, 38-40, June 1994.
4. Davidson AJ, Hartman DS: *Radiology of the kidney and urinary tract*, ed 2, Philadelphia, 1994, WB Saunders.
5. Drach GW: *Common problems in infections and stones*, St Louis, 1992, Mosby.
6. Dretler SP: An evaluation of ureteral laser lithotripsy: 225 consecutive patients, *J Urol* 143, 267-272, 1990.
7. Droller MJ: *Surgical management of urologic disease*, St. Louis, 1992, Mosby.
8. Eaton Laboratories: *A bicentennial history of the practice of urology in the United States.* Northfield, 1976, Medical Communications.
9. Emmett JL, Witten DM: *Clinical urography*, vol 2, Philadelphia, 1971, WB Saunders.
10. Getz, BJ: Interstitial cystitis, *Nursing Spectrum*, 12-13, April 3, 1994.
11. Gillenwater JY et al: *Adult and pediatric urology*, ed 3, St. Louis, 1996, Mosby.
12. Gray M: *Genitourinary disorders*, St. Louis, 1992, Mosby.
13. Huffman JL, Bagley DH, Lyon ES: *Ureteroscopy*, Philadelphia, 1988, WB Saunders.
14. Kirby RS, Christmas TJ: *Benign prostatic hyperplasia*, London, 1993, Gower.
15. Lepor H, Lawson RK: *Prostate diseases*, Philadelphia, 1993, WB Saunders.
16. Meeker MR, Rothrock JC: *Alexander's care of the patient in surgery*, ed 10, St. Louis, 1995, Mosby.
17. Pfister J et al: *The nursing spectrum of lasers*, ed 2, Denver, 1996, Education Design.
18. Raz S: *Atlas of transvaginal surgery*, Philadelphia, 1992, WB Saunders.
19. Resnick MI, Kursh ED: *Current therapy in genitourinary surgery*, ed 2, St. Louis, 1992, Mosby.
20. Resnick MI, Novick AC: *Urology secrets*, St. Louis, 1995, Mosby.
21. Seidman EJ, Hanno PM: *Current urologic therapy 3*, Philadelphia, 1994, WB Saunders.
22. Smith AD: *Controversies in endourology*, Philadelphia, 1995, WB Saunders.
23. Smith JA, Stein BS, Benson RC: *Lasers in urologic surgery*, ed 2, Chicago, 1989, Mosby.
24. Soloway MS, Wajsman Z: *Superficial bladder cancer*, Miami, 1993, University of Miami School of Medicine.
25. Walsh PC ET AL: *Campbell's urology*, ed 6, Philadelphia, 1992, WB Saunders.
26. Watson G, Wickham J: Initial experience with a pulse dye laser for ureteric calculi, *Lancet* 1: 1357, 1986.

Videos

27. Bagley DH: *Flexible ureteroscopy: use and application*, Stamford, Conn., 1991, Circon-ACMI.
28. Bard Urological Division: *Contigen-Collagen implant nursing care*, Covington, Geo., 1993, CR Bard Inc.
29. Circon-ACMI: *USA series endourology systems*, "less is more," Stamford, Conn., 1991, Circon-ACMI.
30. Daughtry J: *Urethral dilatation*, Oakland, Calif., undated, Meadoxurgimed Inc.
31. Heraeus Surgical, Inc: *The new gold standard—Uroline Nd:YAG laser system.* Milpitas, 1993, Heraeus Surgical, Inc.
32. Huffman J: *Balloon dilatation of the ureter for ureteroscopy procedures*, Oakland, Calif., undated, Meadox-Surgimed, Inc.

8

Laparoscopic Interventions

Genitourinary laparoscopy has afforded the urologic patient new treatment options. Through laparoscopy, procedures that once required large incisions, lengthy recovery time, and hospital confinement are now achievable with minimal invasion. Although the cost of supplies is increased, the patient's postoperative recovery has been shortened dramatically and the need for hospitalization has been decreased. In most instances, these procedures may successfully be performed in the outpatient setting. Additionally, when indicated, laser intervention may be utilized.

Use of a video monitor frees the surgeon from the need to utilize direct visualization through the laparoscope. Fatigue is also avoided with correct placement of the monitor or monitors to afford comfortable viewing. When only one monitor is needed, it is best placed at the patient's feet to allow adequate viewing without requiring the surgeon or assistant to contort their stance (Fig. 8-1). If two monitors are employed, as with nephrectomy, they are best placed along the sides, one opposite the surgeon and one opposite the assistant (Fig. 8-2).

Since postoperative recovery will differ from open interventions, patient education must be revised to meet the anticipated surgical outcome after laparoscopy. Rather than the deep incisional and muscular pain that occurs after open surgery, the patient is likely to experience the discomfort of diaphragmatic pressure and distention caused by gas instillation and, in the male patient, symptoms of pneumoscrotum.

When general anesthesia is employed, the patient should have an endotracheal tube, Foley catheter, and nasogastric tube in place to maintain airway control and to avoid trocar perforation of the bladder, stomach, and intestinal tract (Fig. 8-3).

These should be placed before establishing the pneumoperitoneum. Depending on the intended intervention, the patient may be placed in the supine, lateral, modified lithotomy, Trendelenburg, or reverse Trendelenburg positions. A bolster may be placed under the patient in the sacral or subumbilical region to afford maximum access to the pelvic tissues. In some instances it will be necessary to tuck one or both arms to allow for ease of operation. This is particularly true in the case of pelvic surgery where the surgeon and assistant must stand alongside the patient's shoulders. It is important to note that adequate padding and proper positioning maneuvers will often avoid injuries to the neurovascular and musculoskeletal systems. It is also wise to apply alternating compression stockings to maintain the integrity of peripheral vascular flow to the lower extremities.

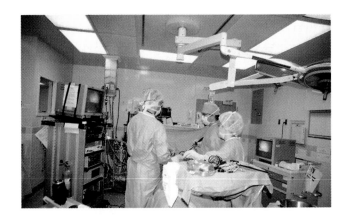

Fig. 8-2 Video setup with two monitors.

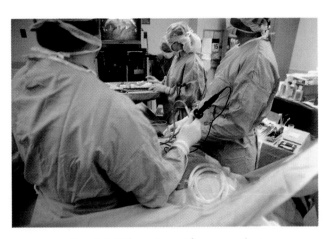

Fig. 8-1 Video setup with one monitor.

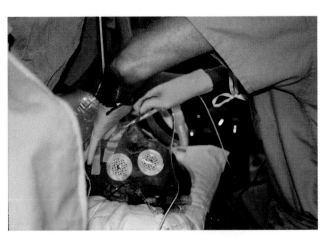

Fig. 8-3 Inserting nasogastric tube.

172

General anesthesia is most commonly chosen. Although laparoscopy has been performed under spinal or epidural block, or local infiltration with sedation, the applications are somewhat limited. The decision must be based on the expected duration of the procedure (less than 1 hour), the extent of the procedure, the patient's anesthetic risk, and the patient's willingness and ability to tolerate some discomfort. Studies have shown that general anesthesia affords better control of CO_2 absorption. The risk of absorption in the bloodstream is decreased by allowing respiratory elimination through assisted ventilation. Airway protection, greater muscle relaxation, and minimization of vagal responses may also be achieved with general anesthesia.

Anesthetic complications to be alert for with any laparoscopic intervention include regurgitation or aspiration of gastric contents, cardiac dysrhythmias, hypotension, hypertension, subcutaneous emphysema, venous CO_2 embolus, oliguria, hypoxemia, hypercapnia, pneumothorax, pneumomediastinum, pneumopericardium, and peripheral nerve damage. For the more extended procedures, such as nephrectomy, a central venous pressure (CVP) line and large bore intravenous (IV) lines will be inserted. The patient's respiratory status must be adequate to accommodate the increased arterial P_{CO_2} absorbed from the pneumoperitoneum (intraabdominal pressure could reach 20 mm Hg). The patient may have a type and crossmatch done or have autologous blood stored preoperatively.

Before laparoscopy, any coagulopathies and infection should be corrected. Active peritonitis is a contraindication to laparoscopy because of the high risk of sepsis. Additionally patients with uncorrectable coagulopathies and severe hiatal hernia are poor candidates for this approach.

The text and photographs in this chapter are intended to be generic for the specific laparoscopic interventions. Each is subject to alteration depending on the practice setting and the preference of the surgeon. Common surgical techniques and instrumentation are depicted and intended as an overview to enable the perioperative nurse to anticipate patient care needs. Instrumentation and actual equipment in practice will also vary according to physician preference and the procedural setting. It is important to focus on the principles involved in each procedure and consider the instrumentation as suggestions for the specialty of genitourinary laparoscopy.

NURSING CARE

Nursing diagnoses will vary according to the exact procedure performed and the patient's medical status. Nursing planning and care specific to each operative intervention are discussed under that procedure. General nursing diagnoses, preoperative planning, and perioperative interventions for a patient undergoing laparoscopy might include the following:

Nursing Diagnosis	Perioperative Planning and Intervention
Risk for viscus injury related to insufflation needle and trocar placement	Confirm proper placement of insufflation needle by syringe aspiration and saline instillation: there should no fluid return on aspiration, and saline injection should meet no resistance.
	Note baseline intraperitoneal pressure once insufflation needle is connected to CO_2 (<10 mm Hg).
	Observe for sudden rise in intraperitoneal pressure (>20 mm Hg) during instillation of gas. At one minute of instillation at 1L/min, there should be loss of liver dullness on percussion.
	Maintain insufflation at 1 to 6 L/min until pressure is 12 to 15 mm Hg before initiating trocar penetration.
	Elevate abdominal wall at the area of the umbilicus with towel clips or by finger grasp during trocar insertion.
	Observe for sudden drop in pressure and audible popping sound on insertion and escape of gas from cannula with trocar removal.
	Maintain pressure at 12 to 15 mm Hg on auto flow.
Anxiety related to knowledge deficit	Review purpose of planned procedure; ascertain level of comprehension.
	Document expressions of anxiety by the patient or family.
	Provide explanations and reassurance to the patient and family.
	Reinforce and review patient teaching; answer questions as necessary.
	Encourage participation in discharge planning; review discharge instructions.
	Keep family informed during intraoperative stage.
	Verify understanding of postoperative signs and symptoms to be reported.
	If patient controlled analgesia (PCA) is to be utilized, confirm that contact has been established with home care provider.
	Place follow-up call or make postoperative visit the day after surgery.
Risk for infection related to: Operative intervention Medical status	Maintain aseptic environment and properly sterilize instrumentation.
	Insert catheter aseptically and maintain closed urinary drainage system.
	Use appropriate technique during surgical prep.
	Drape patient according to aseptic standards.
	Observe for indications of fever, dysuria or pyuria, and reddened incisional sites.
	Provide adequate hydration through IV lines or fluid intake.
	Administer antibiotic therapies as ordered.

Nursing Diagnosis	Perioperative Planning and Intervention
Risk for altered tissue perfusion related to: Operative intervention Positioning	Assess bilateral pedal and radial pulses perioperatively. Apply alternating compression stockings. Adjust position as necessary to maintain peripheral circulation. Avoid leaning against or on patient during operative intervention. Observe and document status of capillary refill and extremity temperature. Encourage early ambulation postoperatively.

An essential part of the nursing care during laparoscopy includes maintenance of the equipment and instrumentation. The video unit, camera, operating lights, electrosurgery unit, suction unit, and the alternating compression machine should be checked for proper function before the patient enters the room. Instrumentation and endoscopes should be inspected for damage, debris or corrosion, and proper action before use.

Generally, monopolar electrofulguration is employed (Fig. 8-4). Most laparoscopic instrumentation is available with or without fulgurating capabilities (Fig. 8-5). The selection is dependent on the operating surgeon's preference. Until recently, bipolar instrumentation has been somewhat limited to Kleppinger forceps for tubal laparoscopy. Other bipolar instruments are now available, and the variety continues to expand. All laparoscopic genitourinary interventions should have an open setup and self-retaining retractors available in the event of uncontrolled bleeding or other operative difficulty. To remain cost effective, disposable items that will not be needed immediately or not routinely used should not be opened.

As perioperative patient care is implemented, the plan of care will be subject to adjustment on a continual basis based on data collected through the preoperative assessment and changing intraoperative circumstances. This ongoing evaluation and revision of care allows for an individualized approach. Once care has been implemented the postoperative assessment is completed. Often it will not be possible to determine long-term outcomes. Immediate postoperative assessment allows for a baseline determination of the effect of the nursing interventions provided. Priority postoperative assessment data appropriate for the continual evaluation of nursing care may include the following:

- Review of catheter care
- Understanding of the medication regimen
- Knowledge of reportable signs and symptoms
- Awareness of appointments for postoperative visit with physician
- Knowledge of the need for high fluid intake
- Readiness for discharge

An overview of the care provided and the subsequent evaluation is recorded to provide for the continuity of care throughout the recovery period. This documentation should be individualized according to the procedure and the needs of the patient. Surgical settings differ and perioperative documentation will have guidelines appropriate for the specific institution. A summary of the intraoperative activities designed to achieve certain outcome criteria should be reported to the perianesthesia nurse. Information to be recorded and reported will vary according to the procedure performed. Reports may differ

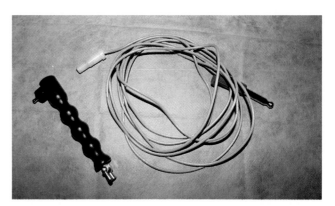

Fig. 8-4 Monopolar handle and electrocautery cable for reposable laparoscopic instruments.

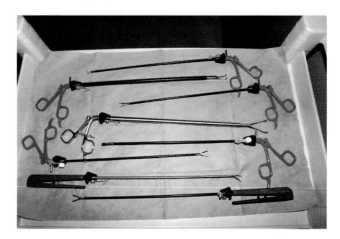

Fig. 8-5 Monopolar laparoscopic instrumentation, *top* to *bottom*:

1, Scissors with electrocautery ability; 2, Right angle, non-locking, with electrocautery ability; 3, Fine dissector, nonlocking, with electrocautery ability; 4, Grasper, locking; 5, Grasper, nonlocking with electrocautery ability; 6, Dissector, nonlocking, with electrocautery ability; 7, 8, Atraumatic locking graspers.

between an outpatient and inpatient setting depending on the amount of preoperative instruction afforded the patient and services available to meet each patient's requirements. Priority information for the genitourinary laparoscopy patient may include the following:

- Urethral catheter inserted (state type, size, method of securing, and collection device)
- Patency of catheter at discharge from the operating room

- Precautions pertinent to the patient's physical condition
- Fluid loss and replacement
- Status of peripheral vascular circulation preoperatively and postoperatively
- Skin integrity preoperatively and postoperatively
- Positions and positioning devices employed for surgery
- Level of comprehension during preoperative instruction
- Information taught to the patient preoperatively
- Nursing care provided

ROLE OF THE RN FIRST ASSISTANT (RNFA) IN LAPAROSCOPY

During genitourinary laparoscopy the RNFA functions in an expanded role of perioperative nursing. It has already been established that the RNFA has the benefit of increased didactic education as well as a background of perioperative experience to draw upon. The scope of practice will vary by each individual institution. However, as a perioperative nurse, the RNFA incorporates the nursing process while performing assistive behaviors. Ideally the RNFA has specialized education and training in the field of genitourinary surgery.

Although the majority of the time the focus of practice is during the intraoperative phase, the RNFA also functions preoperatively and postoperatively on the patient's and surgeon's behalf. The perioperative activities of the RNFA are interdependent and in collaboration with the operating surgeon.

Preoperatively, time may not allow for extended nurse-patient interaction. When the RNFA is part of the surgical team, he or she may augment the role of the perioperative RN (circulating nurse) through the assessment, planning, and implementation of patient care. With expanded experience and knowledge to utilize, the RNFA may plan the appropriate individualized nursing interventions and lead the surgical team during implementation, based on the assessment data collected and nursing diagnoses established. If the RNFA is privately employed by the operating surgeon, much of this data collection and patient care planning may have taken place during the preoperative interview and physical examination. These results can then be communicated to the perioperative genitourinary team.

The RNFA is expected to understand the theory behind positioning techniques and should not only lead the team toward optimal care, but also teach during the process. For example, bony prominences require adequate padding to protect them from pressure damage, which may lead to neurovascular compromise.

The RNFA is expected to know the various surgical approaches, potential alterations, and accompanying rationale, and he or she can assist the team in preparing for any given circumstance. For example, violation of the peritoneal or the pleural space during preperitoneal (extraperitoneal) laparoscopy will necessitate measures to facilitate a corrective repair.

The RNFA is expected to have a comprehensive awareness of the anatomy involved in a given procedure and should utilize this knowledge in the care provided. For example, care must be taken to protect the epigastric and other major vessels as well as the ureters from injury caused by dissection or electrofulguration. With a broad background to draw upon, the RNFA can incorporate the needs of each member of the surgical team to form a cohesive individualized approach.

Intraoperatively the RNFA generally will lead the implementation of patient positioning and padding, insert the Foley catheter, apply the alternating compression stockings, perform the surgical skin prep on the patient, and assist with draping. Additionally, during laparoscopy, the RNFA may assist with trocar incisions and insertion, will afford the surgeon a precise view of the operative area by skillfully maneuvering the laparoscope, will apply graspers and retract tissue, and, in some instances, will dissect with scissors and fulgurate bleeders. Once the intervention has concluded the RNFA will assist in evaluating the peritoneal cavity for hemostasis, instill irrigant, remove trocars, instill or inject local anesthetics, suture the puncture sites, insert vaginal packings, secure the Foley catheter and connect it to appropriate drainage as applicable, cleanse the patient of prep solution, evaluate skin integrity, and apply the surgical dressings.

Postoperatively the RNFA can evaluate patient outcomes based on the plan of care, enhance or reinforce patient teaching and evaluate the patient for other needs requiring follow-up management. Those that are privately employed have the advantage of seeing the patient after discharge and can more thoroughly evaluate patient outcomes in relation to the implementation of care. With communication between the private RNFA and the perioperative team, planning for future patient care and intervention can be dramatically improved, based on the follow-up information acquired.

LAPAROSCOPIC NEPHRECTOMY/ NEPHROURETERECTOMY

Compared to open nephrectomy, surgery time is much lengthier, averaging 5 hours. Postoperative recovery, analgesia requirements, and total hospital stay are, however, lessened dramatically with laparoscopic intervention. The use of postoperative patient-controlled analgesia (PCA) is generally appropriate and is usually replaced with oral analgesia by the first or second postoperative day. Historically, patients undergoing laparoscopic nephrectomy are discharged in 3 to 8 days. Most return to regular activity by the third postoperative week.

Preoperative patient preparation includes a chest x-ray, an ECG, serum electrolytes, CBC, PT, PTT, urinalysis and urine culture, type and crossmatch for 2 units of packed red blood cells or autologous blood donation, a full mechanical antibiotic bowel prep, and preoperative prophylactic IV antibiotics. Additionally those with malignancy may have tumor staging that includes CT scans of the abdomen, pelvis, and chest; bone scans; liver function studies; and Doppler ultrasound imaging of the renal vein. Pulmonary function and cardiac stress tests may also be done depending on the patient's medical status.

Description. The procedure always includes cystoscopy with placement of a renal balloon catheter, a ureteral catheter, and a Foley urethral catheter under C-arm fluoroscopy. A cystoscopy setup is needed. The laparoscopic instrument and equipment setup includes three 5 mm trocars, an insufflation needle, and two 10 to 12 mm trocars. There should always be an open setup available in the event laparoscopy is unsuccessful (Fig. 8-6).

After endoscopy, the patient is placed in the supine or semi-lateral position. The contralateral arm is padded from the shoulder to the fingertips to protect it during positioning. A CVP line and large-bore IV line are in place. After endotracheal intubation, a nasogastric tube and electrosurgical grounding pad are placed. The patient is prepped and draped in the usual manner for thoracoabdominal surgery (Figs. 8-7 to 8-10). Extra draping materials are utilized when the patient is repositioned from the supine position. If a beanbag positioner is desired, the patient is placed on the deflated device at the outset of the procedure (before the cystoscopy).

The approach chosen for laparoscopic nephrectomy or nephroureterectomy may be transabdominal or retroperitoneal, with transabdominal the most common choice. In the transabdominal approach, five trocar ports are positioned: a 10

mm lens site at the level of the umbilicus, a 12 mm trocar site at the upper midclavicular line, a 5 mm trocar in the lower midclavicular line, and two 5 mm trocar sites placed at the upper and lower anterior axillary line of the affected side. Additional or alternative ports may be placed depending on the situation.

Exposure of the renal vessels and ureter may depend on the identification of the ureter initially. This is facilitated by placing

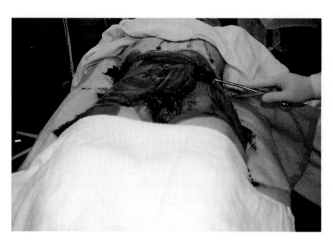

Fig. 8-8 Antiseptic prep application.

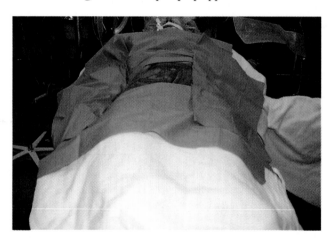

Fig. 8-9 Draping towels.

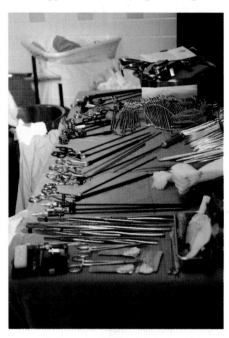

Fig. 8-6 Back table setup, laparoscopic nephrectomy

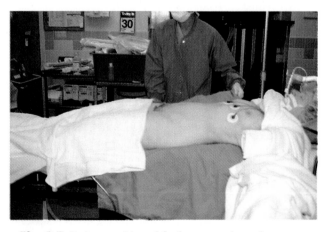

Fig. 8-7 Patient positioned for laparoscopic nephrectomy.

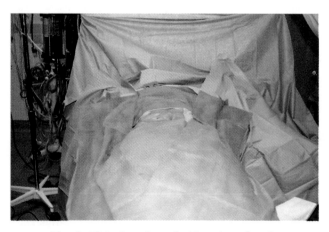

Fig. 8-10 Patient draped with universal pack.

a ureteral catheter during the cystoscopy. Traction on the ureter by the assistant through one of the laparoscopic ports allows elevation of the kidney for exposure of the renal vein and artery. These structures may then be occluded with endoscopic hemoclips, or clamped, ligated, and transected with an endoscopic vascular stapler.

Removal of the kidney may be accomplished by placement of the kidney into a specially designed entrapment bag (Lapsac) in which the kidney is morcellated (ground up and aspirated) and removed. As an alternative, the Lapsac may be drawn up to one of the port sites, which has been slightly enlarged, for removal. If the nephrectomy is being performed for a benign condition, placement into a Lapsac is not necessary, since spillage of malignant cells into the peritoneal cavity is not a concern.

If a nephroureterectomy is being performed for transitional cell carcinoma, the distal ureter must be transected along with a cuff of the bladder. This may be achieved by using an endoscopic vascular stapler after dissection to the ureterovesical junction has been accomplished.

Indications. Laparoscopic nephrectomy and nephroureterectomy are alternative procedures to open nephrectomy and nephroureterectomy, where a small solid renal mass has been demonstrated or a transitional cell carcinoma of the upper urinary tract is present. In the case of a solid renal mass the surrounding Gerota's fascia should be left intact to prevent contamination of the tissues surrounding the kidney from the seeding of tumor cells. The same surgical approach may be used for laparoscopic renal biopsy, partial nephrectomy, laparoscopic pyeloplasty, unroofing of a renal cyst, and tumor excision (Figs. 8-11 to 8-15).

Perioperative risks. In addition to the general laparoscopic risks, the risks inherent with laparoscopic nephrectomy/nephroureterectomy include congestive heart failure, pulmonary embolus, prolonged ileus, atrial fibrillation, hemorrhage, lymphocele, herniation at a trocar site, brachial plexus injury, and excessive blood loss.

The patient must be thoughtfully informed of these potential problems as well as of the potential benefits of laparoscopic

intervention by the operating surgeon and anesthesiologist. Although the perioperative genitourinary nurse should review more common untoward responses and the advantages of laparoscopic intervention, it is beyond the scope of perioperative nursing to detail the more unusual and potentially more

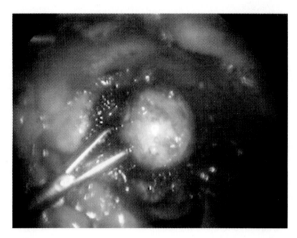
Fig. 8-12 Excision right renal mass, laparoscopically.

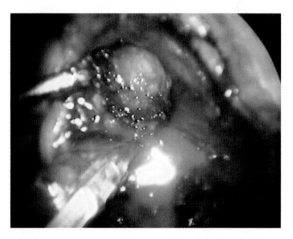
Fig. 8-13 Excision right renal mass, laparoscopically.

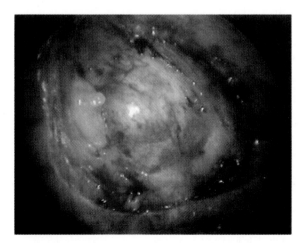
Fig. 8-11 Right renal mass seen through laparoscope.

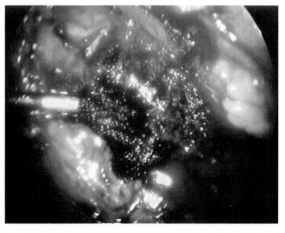
Fig. 8-14 Mass site, postexcision, covered with Surgicel.

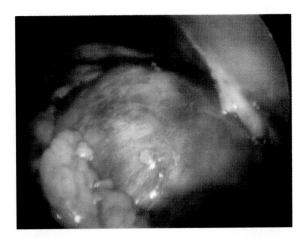

Fig. 8-15 Gerota's fascia replaced over mass site, post excision.

severe complications. This remains the domain of the surgeon and anesthesiologist, and questions posed by the patient should be directed to these individuals before proceeding with surgery.

Increased difficulty, necessitating lengthier surgery or conversion to open technique, may occur in patients with extensive adhesions or abdominal scarring, prior radiotherapy or chemotherapy, obesity, herniations, a history of bowel adhesions or intestinal obstruction, and a history of cardiopulmonary disease. These patients should be carefully evaluated preoperatively to ascertain if the laparoscopic approach may be contraindicated.

Equipment and instrumentation
Equipment
Video camera
Camera cable
Video monitor
CO_2 insufflator and spare tank
VCR and video printer
Electrosurgery digital unit with monopolar and bipolar ability
Alternating compression unit and thigh-length compression stockings
Beanbag or kidney braces, by surgeon preference
Allen stirrups (if frog-legged position is inadequate for cystoscopy)
Toboggan arm protectors
Allen lateral arm board
Pillows, 2
Small positioning pads, 6
Axillary roll
Padding for arm
Head and neck supports
Tape, 3 inch, and safety strap
Suction unit
Irrigant pump of choice
Pressure bag, 1 L, to pressurize irrigant to 250 mm Hg
Tissue morcellator
Absorbent towels for prep
Cystoscopy setup
Cystoscopy pack

Gowns, 2 or 3
Sterile gloves
Flexible cystoscope
Bentson guidewire, .035 inch
Occlusion balloon catheter, 7 Fr with 11.5 mm balloon
Stopcock, one way
Syringe, 1 ml
Hypodermic needle, 25 gauge
Amplatz stiff guidewire, .035 inch
Sidearm adapter
Sterile water, 3000 ml irrigant bag
Cystoscopy tubing
Methylene blue (optional)
Foley catheter, 16 Fr with 5 cc balloon
Urinary drainage bag
Laparoscopy instruments
Laparoscopes, 10 mm, 0- and 30-degree
Fiberoptic light cable
Insufflation needle
Insufflator tubing
Trocar and sheath, 10 to 12 mm, 2
Trocar and sheath, 5 mm, 3
Downsizers, 2
Metzenbaum scissors with fulgurating ability
Dissectors, locking and nonlocking, with blunt, tapered tip, 4 each
Right-angle hemostat, 2
Graspers, locking and nonlocking, 4 each
Allis clamps, 2
Babcock clamps, 2
Vein retractor
Needle holder
Fan retractor
Electrofulgurating spatula or J-hook
Electrofulgurating suction/irrigator
Electrofulgurating cables
Endoloops, Endostitch, Endoties
Endoscopic stapler, endoscopic hemoclips
GIA endoscopic vascular and tissue staplers
Entrapment sac
Miscellaneous supplies
Universal pack
Drape sheets, 2
Towel drapes, 4
Gowns, 6
Sterile towels, 8
Gloves, 2 pair each
Sterile basins
Knife blade, #11 or #15
Knife handle, #3
Towel clips, 2 to 4
Irrigant and pump tubing
Syringes, 20 ml and 60 ml
Syringe, 10 ml finger control
Hypodermic needle, #25 gauge at 1 1/4 inches
Prep solution and appliers
Absorbent prep drape
Sterile saline, 1 L bag

Nursing Care and Teaching Considerations for Laparoscopic Nephrectomy

1. Incorporate all general nursing diagnoses and interventions for laparoscopy.
2. Check equipment for proper function before patient's arrival.
3. Check all sterile supplies for package integrity and medications for dosage and expiration dates.
4. Check instrumentation for proper action and freedom from debris or damage.
5. Position video system appropriately for optimal visualization. Position electrosurgery unit according to room design and optimum location.
6. Assess patient for comprehension of planned surgical intervention and anxiety level. Review as needed, including postoperative expectations and common sequelae.
7. Assess patient for skin temperature and integrity, peripheral circulation (radial and pedal pulses), presence of implants, and general physical status (hearing, vision, numbness, etc.).
8. Assess patient for allergies and medical condition (asthma, COPD, obesity, past surgeries, etc.). Review pertinent preoperative studies (Hgb, HCT, PT, PTT, serum electrolytes, urine studies, type and crossmatch or availability of autologous blood, CT scan, etc.). Has preoperative bowel prep and IV antibiotic been given?
9. Document assessment findings.
10. Review postoperative expectations: coughing and deep breathing, presence of Foley catheter and IV lines, early ambulation, antibiotic therapies, oral intake and diet, anticipated date of hospital discharge, activity level, care of dressings and catheter, PCA, follow-up care.
11. Explain purpose of nursing interventions to patient as they are implemented.
12. Establish range of motion of extremities, neck and shoulders before induction of anesthesia so that patient may express comfort level.
13. Apply and begin operation of alternating compression stockings before induction of anesthesia and subsequent vasodilation. This allows patient awareness as well.
14. After cystoscopy, insert closed-system Foley catheter using aseptic technique.
15. Apply electrosurgery dispersive pad to nonbony, nonhairy site, away from any implants but as close to operative site as possible.
16. Position patient, in supine or lateral decubitus, under guidance of surgeon and anesthetist, utilizing proper body mechanics for both patient and personnel. Apply appropriate padding and safety straps for position chosen.
17. Reassess radial and pedal pulses after positioning; ensure that IV lines and Foley catheter are free of constriction. Confirm that linen beneath patient is smooth and wrinkle free to avoid skin breakdown.
18. Aseptically prep and drape patient according to institutional guidelines and AORN standards. Protect patient from pooling of prep solution by utilizing absorbent towels around prep sites and removing them after prep.
19. Turn on all video equipment. Connect and secure CO_2 tubing and turn on insufflator. Connect and secure light cable, camera cable, electrosurgery cable, and suction tubing. Turn on electrosurgery unit and suction unit.
20. Document nursing interventions.

Heparin, 5000 U

Ancef, 500 mg

Sterile water, 1000 ml bottle, 2

Sterile saline, 1000 ml bottle, 2

Marcaine plain 0.5% or Duranest 1%

Polypropylene (Prolene), #2 on cutting needle

Suture, 2-0 or 3-0, absorbable on small general closure (or gastrointestinal) needle

Suture, 4-0 absorbable on plastic cuticular needle

Umbilical tape

Steri-Strips

Nonadherent material (Telfa), 4, for specimens and dressings

Tegaderm, or comparable product, 4

Sterile gauze, 2 × 2s

Soft-tissue instrument set

Open nephrectomy setup

Procedural Steps

The technique of placing the patient in supine position to initiate the laparoscopy was the method used when laparoscopic nephrectomy was new. Some surgeons still use this approach while others place the patient in lateral decubitus position after endoscopic intervention. Assuring that the patient is adequately secured to the table is critical. Before prepping, the operating room bed is tilted laterally to afford a central abdominal access. The patient is prepped and draped, and access of the first three ports is achieved as described. Before insertion of the remaining trocars, the bed is returned to its normal configuration so that the patient is again in lateral decubitus position. The kidney rest is then elevated. The operation then continues as described.

When the procedure is initiated with the patient supine, the bed is in normal position. The patient is rolled to a lateral decubitus position after trocar placement. Appropriate precautions are taken to maintain integrity of the trocar sites and the operative field. The trocars are secured with polypropylene suture, and the operative field is covered with sterile drape sheets. The arm on the operative side is brought across the patient's chest and secured to the Allen arm support. The legs are checked for proper flexion, the beanbag is inflated, and the kidney rest elevated. If the beanbag is not employed, padding is placed against the back. Kidney braces may be placed. Padding should also be placed below all bony prominences, in the lower axilla, under the neck, and between the patient's legs and feet. The patient's hips and legs are properly secured (Figs. 8-16 to 8-20).

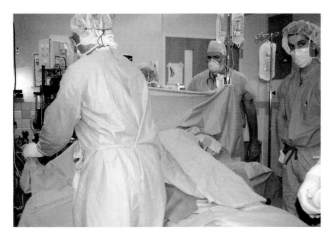

Fig. 8-16 Covering field with sterile drapes for repositioning.

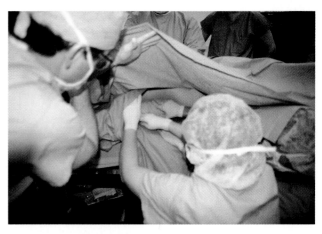

Fig. 8-19 Placing positioning pads.

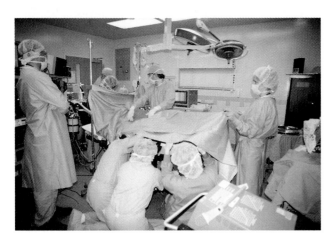

Fig. 8-17 Repositioning patient.

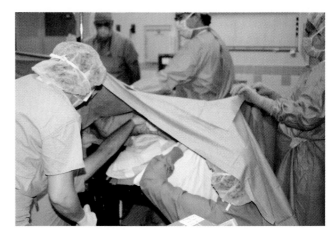

Fig. 8-20 Placing pillow between legs.

1. Access is gained to the peritoneal cavity through a 1 cm transverse subumbilical stab-wound incision, with the blade of choice.

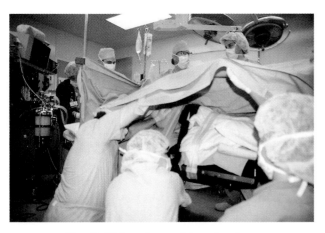

Fig. 8-18 Securing position of patient.

STEP **1-1**

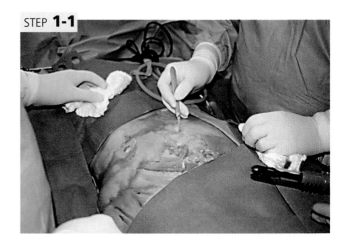

After elevating the anterior abdominal wall with towel clips, the insufflation needle is inserted with the stopcock valve control in the closed position.

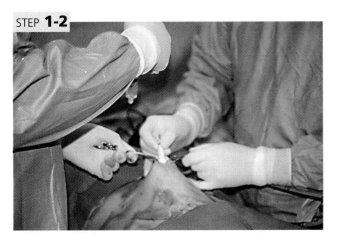

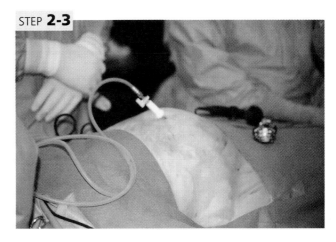

2. Once the insufflation needle is in place, sterile saline is dropped into the lumen of the needle, and the valve of the needle is opened.

If saline does not enter freely, it indicates improper placement of the needle.

3. A nick is made in the rectus fascia with the chosen blade, and the 10 mm trocar replaces the insufflation needle.

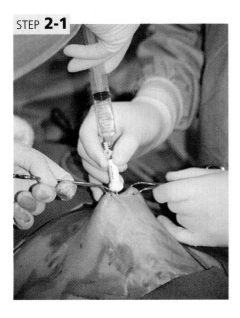

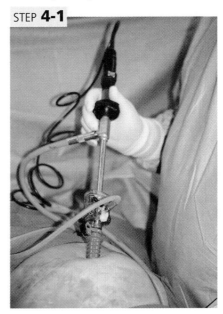

Towel clips are again used on each side of the incision to stabilize the abdominal wall during insertion.

4. The 10 mm laparoscope is inserted.

If the saline enters freely (a successful test), the abdominal cavity is inflated with CO_2 until a pressure of 15 to 20 mm of Hg is obtained.

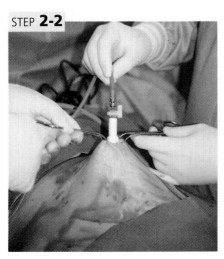

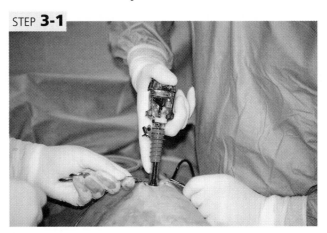

5. A second incision is made immediately below the costal margin in the mid-clavicular line, and a 10 mm trocar is inserted.

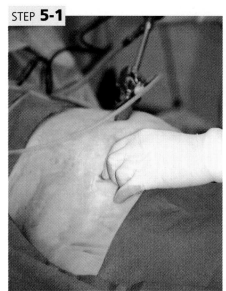

STEP **5-1**

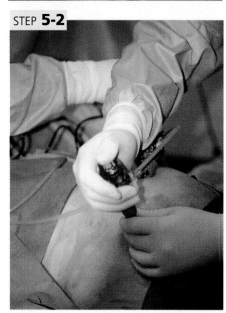

STEP **5-2**

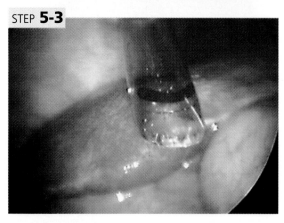

STEP **5-3**

Interior view of second trocar at subcostal, midclavicular line.

6. The third trocar, 5 mm, is inserted through a small incision 2 cm below the umbilicus in the midclavicular line.

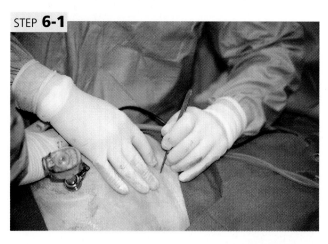

STEP **6-1**

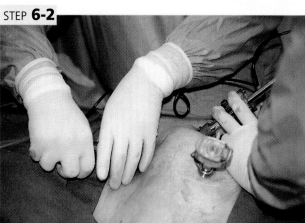

STEP **6-2**

7. The last two 5 mm trocars are placed, one in the anterior axillary line at a level with the umbilicus and one immediately subcostal in the anterior axillary line.

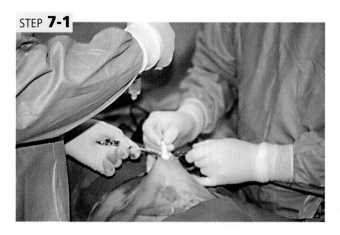

STEP **7-1**

STEP **7-2**

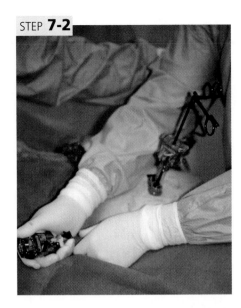

STEP **7-3**

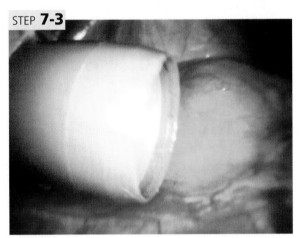

Interior view of fourth trocar at anterior axillary line after complete penetration.

STEP **7-4**

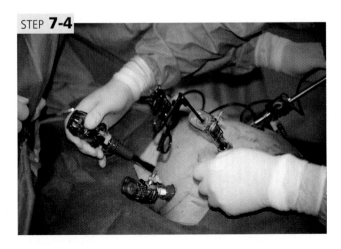

STEP **7-5**

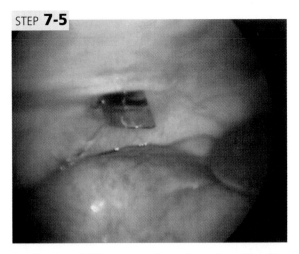

Interior view of fifth trocar at subcostal anterior axillary line.

All trocars are then withdrawn until 2 to 3 cm of each sheath protrude into the abdomen. The polypropylene suture may be used to secure the side arm ports to the patient's skin.

CONSIDERATIONS Each trocar site is laparoscopically inspected after trocar insertion to determine presence of bleeding or perforation. It may be necessary on occasion to extend the incision to allow trocar insertion.

CONSIDERATIONS

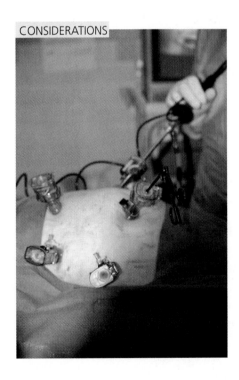

8. The ascending or descending colon is completely mobilized with fulguration scissors and deflected medially.

STEP 8-1

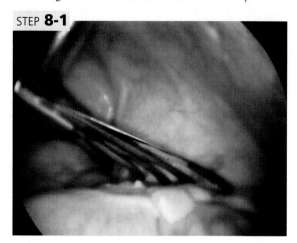

The retroperitoneum is opened.

STEP 8-2

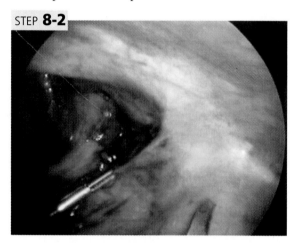

9. Through gentle motion of the ureteral catheter the ureter is identified and dissected. A babcock is clamped around the dissected ureter for retraction.

10. The ureter is dissected until the lower pole of the kidney is visualized. Any veins encountered are clipped twice proximally and twice distally. The kidney is cleared of surrounding tissue and freed laterally and superiorly. Gerota's fascia is entered to free the adrenal gland and exclude it from the dissection.

STEP 10-1

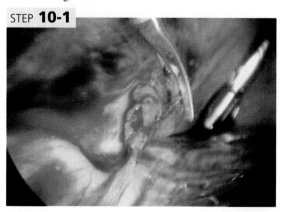

Interior view of incising left lower quadrant (LLQ) adhesion.

STEP 10-2

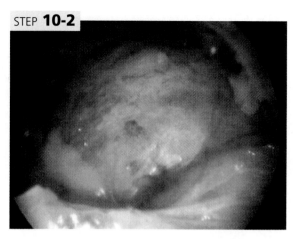

Interior view of exposing right kidney.

11. The renal artery and vein are identified and cleared to create a 360-degree window around each vessel. The clip applier is inserted through the 12 mm port. Two clips are placed on the specimen side, and three clips are clamped to the stump side of both vessels. The vessels are sharply incised.

12. Two pairs of clips are placed proximally and distally on the ureter, and it is sharply incised. The specimen end is grasped, and the kidney is moved into the upper abdominal quadrant.

13. The entrapment sac is introduced through the 12 mm port. The bottom of the sac is pulled into the abdomen with graspers until the neck of the sac clears the end of the port and is unfurled.

14. The sac is opened and the ureteral stump with attached kidney is placed inside. The drawstrings are pulled tight, closing the mouth of the sac.

15. The patient is returned to the supine position by tilting the OR bed, and the sac strings are extracted through the umbilical port. The port is removed under laporascopic observation and the neck of the sac is brought out to lie on the abdominal surface. The tissue morcellator is inserted into the sac, and the kidney is morcellated under suction in a clockwise fashion.

16. The abdominal cavity is exited with laparoscopic observation of each trocar site, during and after removal, to assure that hemostasis has been achieved. Fascial layers at the 12 mm trocar sites are closed with 2-0 or 3-0 absorbable suture in a figure-of-eight pattern.

STEP 16-1

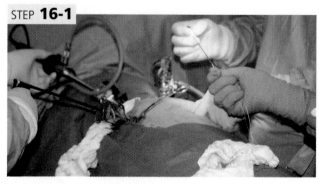

Endostitch for fascial closure.

STEP **16-2**

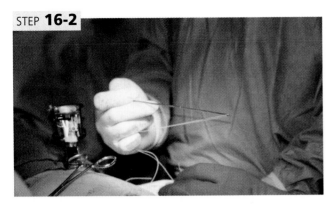

Endostitch readied for insertion.

STEP **16-3**

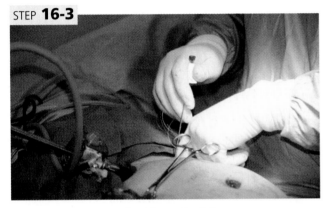

Inserting endostitch.

STEP **16-4**

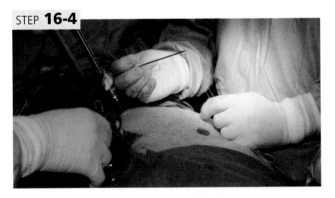

Removing endostitch after first pass.

17. Subcuticular closure of 4-0 absorbable suture is done on all port sites.

STEP **17-1**

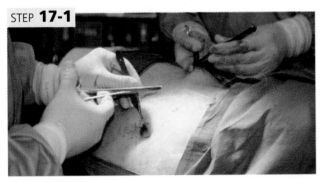

Steri-Strips, Telfa, and Tegaderm complete the dressings.

STEP **17-2**

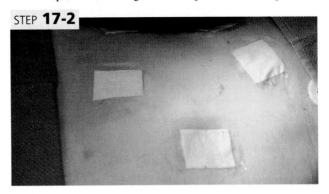

The nasogastric tube is removed in the operating room, and the Foley catheter is removed on the first postoperative day. Oral intake may begin 6 hours postoperatively. The compression stockings are removed when the patient is ambulatory. Most patients leave the hospital in 4 days, return to work in approximately 2 weeks with full convalescence in 3 weeks.

POSTOPERATIVE

Nursing Care and Discharge Planning for Laparoscopic Nephrectomy

1. Complete perioperative documentation including post-operative assessment.
2. Cleanse patient of prepping solutions before dressing application. Assess skin condition.
3. Evaluate status of peripheral vascular circulation.
4. Assess urinary output and secure Foley catheter.
5. Alternating compression stockings remain in place until patient is ambulatory, usually on the first postoperative day.
6. PCA for pain management is initiated in PACU.
7. Patient may resume diet as tolerated, starting slowly with clear liquids, 6 hours postoperatively.
8. Patient should drink 8 oz. liquid (half as fruit juice, half as water) q2h for 48 hours to assist voiding process, offset infection, ensure hydration, avoid potassium depletion, and accelerate healing process.
9. Prescribed medications should be taken as directed, antibiotics until gone. Aspirin and nonsteroidal anti-inflammatory agents should be avoided for 10 days unless advised by the surgeon as medically necessary.
10. Review symptoms of infection, herniation, lymphocele formation, delayed hemorrhage, transient sensory nerve deficit, and phlebitis (fever, warmth or redness at inci-sional sites, swelling or redness in groin, groin pain, lower abdominal ecchymosis, edema/redness/warmth in legs, tingling or numbness of anterior thigh or lateral abdominal or groin region, ache in lower extremities).
11. Review dressing care and bathing regimen. Patient may shower 24 hours postoperatively. Dressings should be kept clean and dry.
12. Review catheter care.

PELVIC LYMPH NODE DISSECTION (LYMPHADENECTOMY [LPLND])

Description. Access to lymph node packets is gained through four strategically placed laparoscopic trocars. This procedure is now successfully being done on an outpatient basis. A competent assistant is necessary in addition to the scrub nurse or technician. The patient will be in the supine position, and one or both arms are tucked at the patient's side. Both Trendelenburg and reverse Trendelenburg positions may be utilized intraoperatively. Rarely are shoulder braces required. In the event that they are, proper placement over the acromioclavicular process is mandatory to avoid brachial plexus injury and potential peripheral nerve damage.

The trocar sizes employed may vary depending on the preference of the individual operating surgeon. The procedure described is the common approach.

With the intraperitoneal approach the obliterated umbilical artery is identified, and an incision is made lateral to this structure to provide exposure to the pelvic sidewall. This allows for removal of obturator, hypogastric, and iliac lymph nodes, just as through a lower abdominal incision. The intraperitoneal approach provides for the spontaneous drainage of collections of lymphatic fluid into the peritoneal cavity. Lymphocele may still occur, however. Additionally there may be less chance of wound infection because of the protective effect of the omentum.

The preperitoneal method allows for a lower CO_2 pressure during the procedure and decreases the risk of injury to intraabdominal structures. There may be an increased risk of superficial wound infection because the protective infection-fighting properties of the omentum are absent in this approach. It is prudent to irrigate the area well with an antibiotic solution before closure.

Indications. Pelvic lymph node dissection may be performed laparoscopically to stage prostatic and bladder malignancies, before definitive therapy, by either the intraperitoneal or preperitoneal (extraperitoneal) approach. If definitive surgery is not performed during the same operative visit, because of metastatic extension into the pelvic lymph nodes, the patient may usually be discharged on the same or following day

Patients selected for laparoscopic pelvic lymph node dissection should exhibit no radiologic evidence of metastasis. Factors that increase the risk for disseminated disease include: PSA >20 ng/ml, an elevated prostatic acid phosphatase (PAP), a Gleason tumor grade >7, enlarged nodes on radiography, and a clinical stage B2/C lesion.

Perioperative risks. Inherent risks of laparoscopic lymph node dissection with either approach, in addition to the general operative and anesthetic risks of laparoscopy, include infection, hemorrhage, bowel injury, ureteral and bladder injury, herniation at a trocar site, transient sensory nerve loss in the anterior thigh, flank or lateral groin region, lymphocele or lymphedema, altered peripheral circulation, phlebitis or deep vein thrombosis, subcutaneous emphysema, and obturator injury.

The patient must be thoughtfully informed of these potential problems as well as of the potential benefits of laparoscopic intervention by the operating surgeon and anesthesiologist.

Although the perioperative genitourinary nurse should review more common untoward responses and the advantages of laparoscopic intervention, it is beyond the scope of perioperative nursing to detail the more unusual and potentially more severe complications. This remains the domain of the surgeon and anesthesiologist, and questions posed by the patient should be directed to these individuals before proceeding with surgery.

Increased difficulty, necessitating lengthier surgery or conversion to open technique, may occur in patients with extensive adhesions or abdominal scarring, prior radiotherapy or chemotherapy, obesity, herniations, a history of bowel adhesions, peritonitis, or intestinal obstruction, and uncorrectable coagulopathy. These patients should be carefully evaluated preoperatively to ascertain if the laparoscopic approach may be contraindicated.

Equipment and instrumentation

Equipment

Video camera

Camera cable

Video monitor

CO_2 insufflator and spare tank

VCR and video printer

Electrosurgery digital unit with monopolar and bipolar ability

Alternating compression unit and thigh-length compression stockings

Safety strap

Small positioning pads, 4

Bolster

Pillow

Toboggan arm protector, 2

Head and neck supports

Suction unit

Irrigant pump of choice

Absorbent towels for prep

Intraperitoneal trocars

Insufflation needle and insufflator tubing

Trocar and sheath, 10 to 12 mm, 2 (Fig. 8-21, *A*)

Trocar and sheath, 5 mm, 2

Downsizers, 2

Preperitoneal Trocars (Fig. 8-21, *B*)

Distention balloon system

Trocar balloon and sheath, 10 mm blunt tip

Trocar and sheath, 10 to 12 mm, 3 *or*

Trocar and sheath, 5 mm, 2 *and*

Trocar and sheath, 10 to 12 mm, 1, by surgeon preference

Endoscopy instruments

Laparoscopes, 10 mm, 0- and 30-degree

Fiberoptic light cable

Metzenbaum scissors with fulgurating ability

Dissectors, locking and nonlocking, with blunt, tapered tip, 2 each

Right-angle hemostat

Graspers, locking and nonlocking, 2 each

Allis or Babcock 2, optional

Vein retractor

Needle holder

Electrofulgurating spatula or J-hook and cable

Electrofulgurating suction and irrigator

Electrosurgery cables

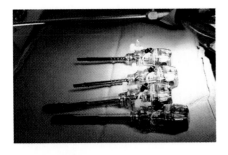

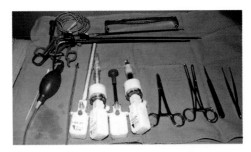

B

Fig. 8-21 **A,** Intraperitoneal trocars. **B,** Preperitoneal balloon system.

Endoloops, Endostitch, Endoties
Endoscopic hemoclips
Miscellaneous supplies
Laparotomy pack (or laparoscopy pack)
Drape towels, 4
Gowns, 3
Gloves, 2 pairs each
Sterile basins
Sterile towels, 8
Foley catheter, #16 Fr with 5 cc balloon
Urinary drainage bag
Knife blade, #11 or #15
Knife handle, #3
Towel clips, 2 to 4
Irrigant and pump tubing
Syringes, 10, 20, and 60 ml
Syringe, 10 ml, finger control

Hypodermic needle, #25 gauge $1^{1}/_{4}$ inches
Antiseptic prep solution
Absorbent prep drape
Antibiotic irrigant of choice
Saline irrigant bag, 1000 to 3000 ml by surgeon preference
Sterile water, 1000 ml bottle, 2
Sterile saline, 1000 ml bottle, 2
Marcaine plain 0.5% or Duranest 1%
Suture, 0 and 3-0 absorbable on small general closure or gastrointestinal needle
Suture, 4-0 absorbable on plastic cuticular needle
Steri-strips
Nonadherent material (Telfa), 4, for specimens and dressings
Tegaderm, 4
Sterile gauze, 2 × 2s
Soft-tissue instruments
Laparotomy instruments

PREOPERATIVE

Nursing Care and Teaching Considerations for LPLND

1. Incorporate all general nursing diagnoses and interventions for laparoscopy.
2. Check equipment for proper function before patient's arrival.
3. Check all sterile supplies for package integrity.
4. Check instrumentation for proper action and freedom from debris or damage.
5. Position video system appropriately for optimal visualization. Position electrosurgery unit according to room design and optimum location.
6. Assess patient for comprehension of planned surgical intervention and anxiety level. Review as needed, including postoperative expectations and common sequelae.
7. Assess patient for skin temperature and integrity, peripheral circulation (radial and pedal pulses), presence of implants, and general physical status (hearing, vision, numbness, etc.).
8. Assess patient for allergies and medical condition (asthma, COPD, obesity, past surgeries, etc.). Review pertinent laboratory studies (Hgb, PT, PTT, serum electrolytes, urine studies, type and crossmatch or availability of autologous blood, etc.).
9. Document assessment findings.
10. Review postoperative expectations: coughing and deep breathing, presence of Foley catheter and IV lines, early ambulation, antibiotic therapies, oral intake and diet, anticipated date of hospital discharge, activity level, care of dressings and catheter (if indicated), follow-up care.
11. Explain purpose of nursing interventions to patient as they are implemented.

12. Apply and begin operation of alternating compression stockings while patient is awake, prior to vasodilation, to afford awareness of how the stockings feel and explain purpose for them.
13. Establish range of motion of extremities and neck and shoulders before induction of anesthesia so that patient may express comfort level.
14. After intubation, insert closed system Foley catheter using aseptic technique.
15. Apply electrosurgery dispersive pad to nonbony, nonhairy site, away from any implants but as close to operative site as possible.
16. Position patient under guidance of surgeon and anesthetist, utilizing proper body mechanics for both patient and personnel. Tuck arm or arms and apply appropriate padding.
17. Reassess radial and pedal pulses after positioning, ensure that IV lines and Foley catheter are free of constriction. Confirm that linen beneath patient is smooth and wrinkle free to avoid skin breakdown.
18. Aseptically prep and drape patient according to institutional guidelines and AORN standards. Protect patient from pooling of prep solution by utilizing absorbent towels around torso and removing them after prep.
19. Turn on all video equipment. Connect and secure CO_2 tubing and turn on insufflator. Connect and secure light cable, camera cable, electrosurgery cable, and suction tubing. Turn on electrosurgery unit and suction unit.
20. Document nursing interventions.

Procedural Steps

1. The patient is placed in the supine position. The area of the umbilicus, just above the iliac crests, may be elevated slightly. This may be accomplished with a small bolster placed under the patient perpendicular to the line of the spinal column, or by elevating the kidney rest.

STEP 1-1

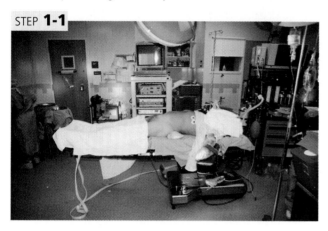

One or both arms are secured at the patient's side to afford better accessibility for the surgical team.

STEP 1-2

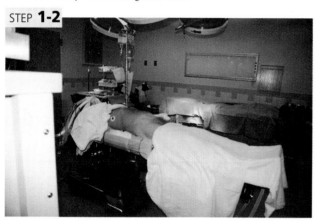

Pads are placed under the patient's heels and all other bony prominences subject to pressure intraoperatively. A pillow may be positioned under the knees to avoid the hyperextension that results from the subumbilical bolster or elevation of the heels.

CONSIDERATIONS Some surgeons may prefer modified lithotomy position if they plan to perform a perineal prostatectomy with the laparoscopic intervention.

CONSIDERATIONS

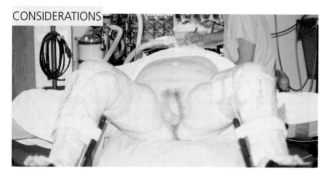

It can be difficult to achieve the recommended exaggerated lithotomy position when the patient is already draped, however.

Intraperitoneal Approach

2. The patient is draped as for laparotomy.

STEP 2-1

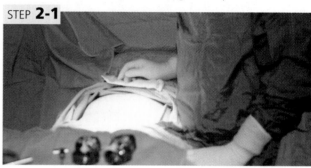

Access is gained to the peritoneal cavity through a 1 cm subumbilical stab-wound incision, with the blade of choice.

STEP 2-2

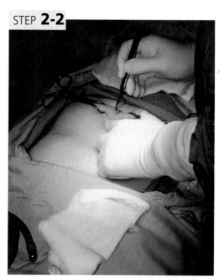

After elevating the anterior abdominal wall the insufflation needle is inserted with the stopcock valve control in the closed position.

STEP 2-3

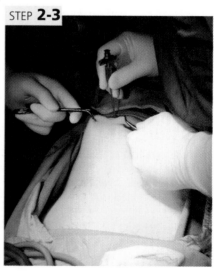

Once the insufflation needle is in place, sterile saline is dropped into the lumen of the needle, and the valve of the needle is opened.

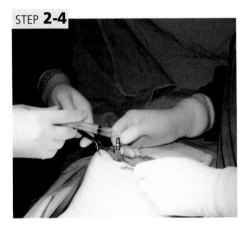

The drop test helps assure that the needle tip lies free within the peritoneal cavity. If saline enters freely, the drop test is successful, and 10 ml of saline is then instilled through the insufflation needle.

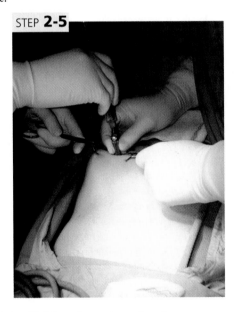

CO_2 is instilled into the peritoneal cavity to a pressure of 12 to 15 mm Hg.

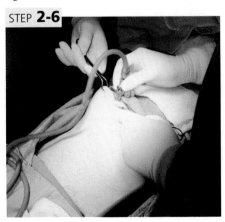

3. A 10 mm trocar is inserted, in place of the insufflation needle, at the subumbilical site.

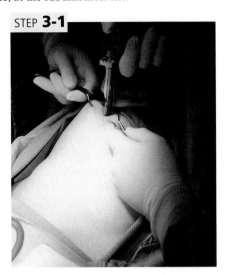

Additional trocars are then inserted under direct laparoscopic observation. One 5 mm trocar is placed in each lower quadrant, and a 10 mm trocar is inserted midline between the umbilicus and the symphysis pubis.

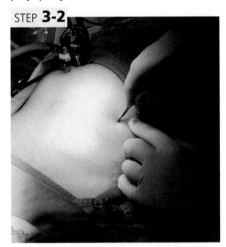

Incision left lower quadrant.

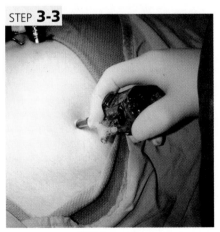

LLQ trocar, 5 mm.

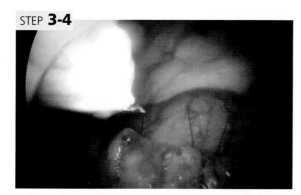

STEP **3-4**

Interior view, LLQ trocar.

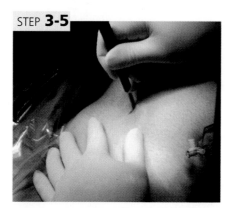

STEP **3-5**

Midline incision.

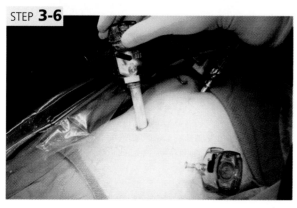

STEP **3-6**

Midline trocar, 10 mm.

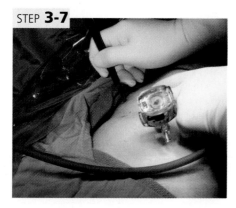

STEP **3-7**

Right lower quadrant (RLQ) incision.

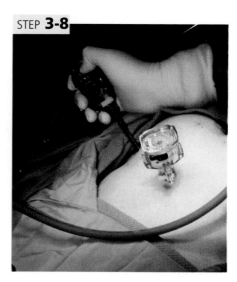

STEP **3-8**

RLQ trocar, 5 mm.

4. After access has been established, the peritoneum is grasped over the vas deferens, and an incision is made with scissors.

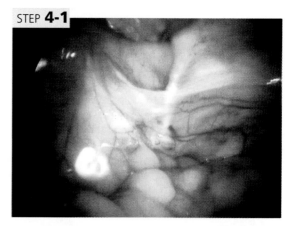

STEP **4-1**

Interior view, access to peritoneum established, vas deferens (white band on left), obliterated umbilical artery (narrow band in center).

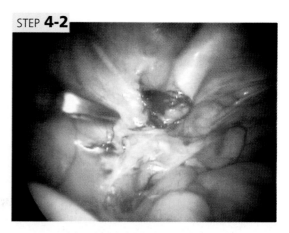

STEP **4-2**

Interior view, initial peritoneal incision.

5. The obliterated umbilical artery is grasped to stabilize tissue for dissection. The vas is identified, clipped or cauterized, and divided. The peritoneal dissection is continued lateral and cephalad to the sigmoid colon on the left and the ascending colon on the right.

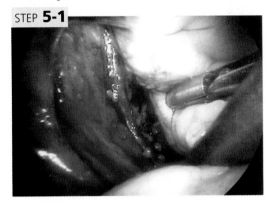

Interior view, obliterated umbilical artery retracted, external iliac vein along left with node pocket in center.

6. After identification of the spermatic cord structures, iliac vessels, ureters, and psoas muscle, the incision is developed to the pubic ramus.

7. Cloquet's node is identified and freed from under the external iliac vein at the level of the bifurcation of the common iliac vein.

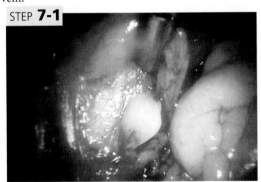

Interior view, left Cloquet's node (in center at tip of forcep).

This allows isolation of the obturator lymph node bundle, the obturator vessels, and the obturator nerve.

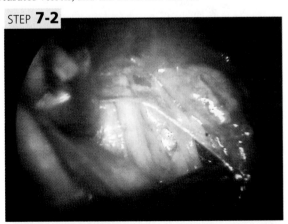

Interior view, left obturator vein (center) with obturator lymph packet to the right under forcep.

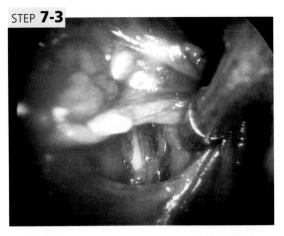

Interior view, left obturator nerve (white band in center cavity).

The lymph node bundle is carefully dissected away from its pelvic sidewall attachment, and the proximal and distal attachments are transected after electrofulguration or hemoclip application. The large lymph channel, once freed, is removed through one of the 10 mm trocars.

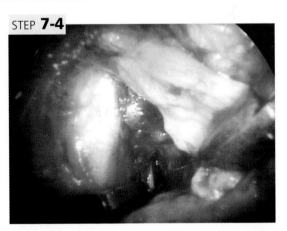

Interior view, left obturator/hypogastric node packet in forcep, obturator nerve in space to left/center at tip of scissor.

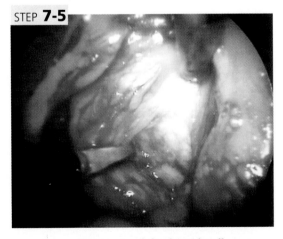

Interior view, left pelvic sidewall.

Endoclips or scissor coagulation may be employed. Clips offer a lower risk of postoperative lymphocele.

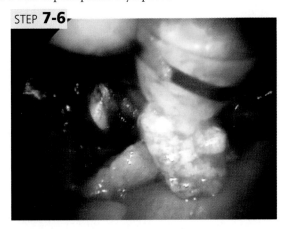

STEP 7-6

Interior view, left obturator/hypogastric node packet entering trocar.

8. Additional lymph node material is removed from the hypogastric and iliac areas by carefully dissecting these areas open, removing the tissue overlying the external iliac artery, and locating the nodes lying next to the vessels. Care must be taken to avoid vascular and ureteral injury.

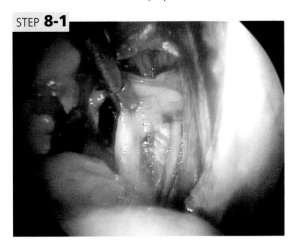

STEP 8-1

Interior view, right iliac node packet in forcep.

9. The procedure is repeated on the opposite side.

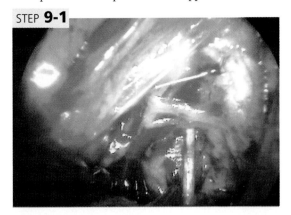

STEP 9-1

Interior view, right obturator vein (at tip of forcep) and nerve (narrow white tendonous band).

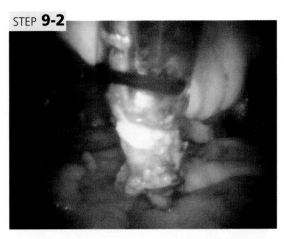

STEP 9-2

Interior view, right obturator/hypogastric node packet on forcep, entering trocar.

10. After completing the dissection, the operative sites are inspected for bleeding and hemostasis is achieved. Irrigant may be instilled to clear the field to allow for inspection of node cavities.

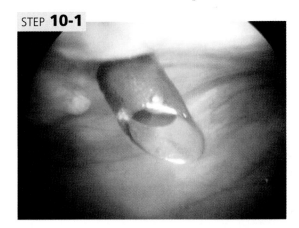

STEP 10-1

Interior view, irrigant being instilled.

Each trocar is removed under direct observation with the laparoscope to allow for identification of inner abdominal wall bleeding sites.

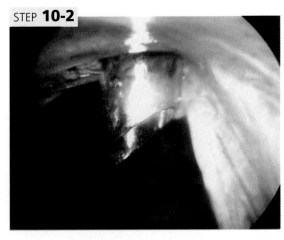

STEP 10-2

Interior view, umbilical trocar exiting.

11. After the gas has been evacuated from the abdomen, the 10 mm trocar sites are closed with 0 or 2-0 absorbable suture at the level of the fascia.

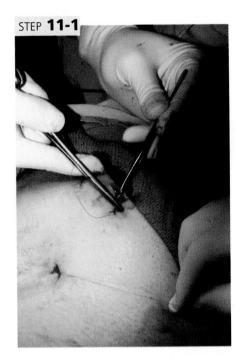

STEP **11-1**

12. All trocar sites are closed with a 4-0 absorbable subcuticular, interrupted or running, skin closure.

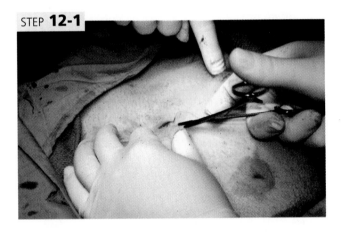

STEP **12-1**

Steri-Strips, Telfa, and Tegaderm are applied to the puncture sites after thorough cleansing of the abdomen. Local anesthetic may be instilled through the trocars before removal and injected subcutaneously before closure for postoperative comfort.

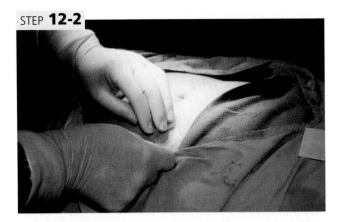

STEP **12-2**

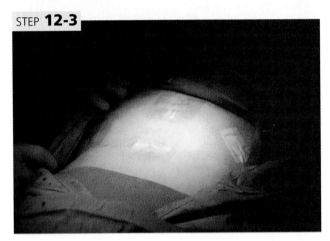

STEP **12-3**

13. If supine, the patient may be repositioned and prepared for radical perineal prostatectomy if the two procedures are combined.

CONSIDERATIONS Irrigation may be employed at any point intraoperatively to clear the viewing field or achieve hemostasis. The method utilized is dependent on the preference of the operating surgeon.

Preperitoneal Approach (Extraperitoneal)

2. After incision with the knife blade of choice, access is gained to the pelvic cavity by exposing the anterior rectus sheath, just below the umbilicus, and inserting a preperitoneal dilating trocar balloon.

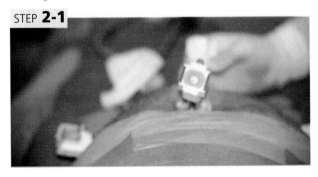

STEP **2-1**

This trocar is positioned with its tip just above the pubic bone. The space between the bladder and pubis is then dissected by inflating the balloon.

STEP **2-2**

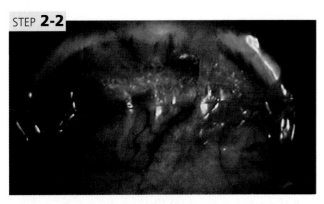

Interior view of preperitoneal dilating balloon fully inflated.

3. The dilating balloon is removed, and the specially designed 10 mm blunt-tip tissue-retracting balloon trocar is placed in the retroperitoneal space. The balloon is inflated with 30 to 35 cc of air. Three additional trocars are then inserted, as in the intraperitoneal approach, to allow removal of the pelvic nodes (refer to intraperitoneal approach, step 3).

STEP **3-1**

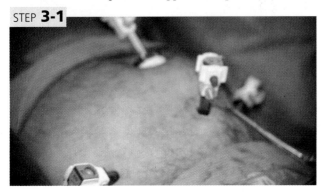

Exposure to the pelvic sidewall is gained by carefully dissecting off the peritoneum.

STEP **3-2**

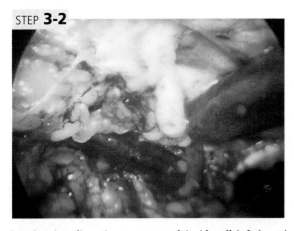

Interior view, dissection to expose pelvic sidewall, inferior epi-gastric artery (blue band over forcep near center), and umbilical trocar on right side with lymph node packet at its tip (white).

STEP **3-3**

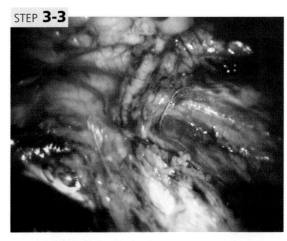

Interior view, dissection to expose left interior epigastric artery.

CONSIDERATIONS Violation of the peritoneum may be corrected by inflation with CO_2 to allow endoscopic peritoneal closure.

4. Cloquet's node is identified and freed from under the external iliac vein at the level of the bifurcation of the common iliac vein. This allows isolation of the obturator lymph node bundle, the obturator vessels, and the obturator nerve.

STEP **4-1**

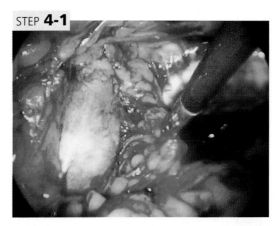

Interior view, left external iliac vein (white structure on left) and obturator lymph node packet in forcep with pubis behind forcep.

STEP **4-2**

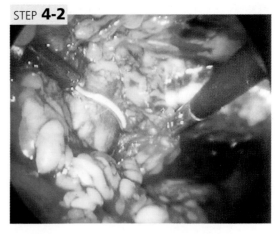

Interior view, dissection of left obturator lymph node packet (in forcep on right).

The lymph node bundle is carefully dissected away from its pelvic sidewall attachment, and the proximal and distal attachments are transected after electrofulguration or hemoclip application. The large lymph channel, once freed, is removed through one of the 10 mm trocars. Endoscopic hemoclips or scissor coagulation may be employed. Clips offer a lower risk of postoperative lymphocele.

STEP 4-3

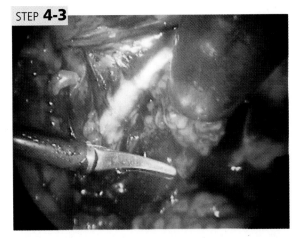

Interior view, left obturator packet entering trocar (forcep inside trocar).

STEP 4-4

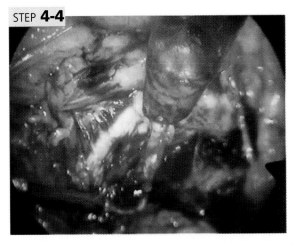

Interior view, left obturator nerve (small white horizontal spot) just above scirrors.

5. Additional lymph node material is removed from the hypogastric and iliac areas by carefully dissecting these areas open, removing the tissue overlying the external iliac artery, and locating the nodes lying next to the vessels. Care must be taken to avoid vascular and ureteral injury.

STEP 5-1

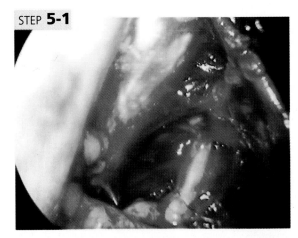

Interior view, external iliac artery/vein (large pink-white longitudinal band in left center) cavity after node packet removed with obturator nerve on right (small white band in right center).

6. The procedure is repeated on the opposite side.

STEP 6-1

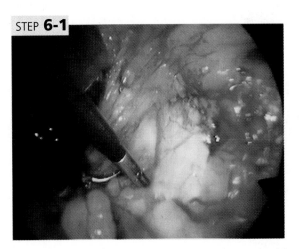

Interior view, right node dissection (node packet is behind forcep, pelvic bone is wide white band.)

STEP 6-2

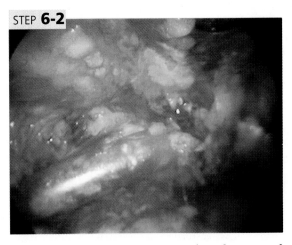

Interior view, right node packet exiting through trocar on the left.

7. After completing the dissection, the operative sites are inspected for bleeding, and hemostasis is achieved. Antibiotic irrigation may be instilled before trocar removal.

STEP 7-1

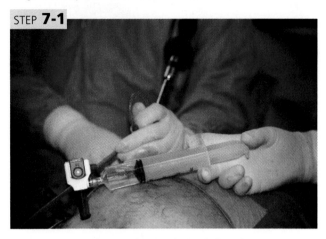

Instilling antibiotic solution before closure.

STEP 7-2

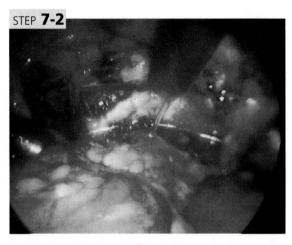

Interior view, irrigation of node site (narrow band perpendicular to forcep).

Each trocar is removed under direct observation with the laparoscope to allow for identification of inner abdominal wall bleeding sites.

8. After the gas has been evacuated from the abdomen, the 10 mm midline trocar site is closed with 3-0 absorbable suture at the level of the fascia. All trocar sites are closed with a 4-0 absorbable subcuticular, interrupted or running, skin closure. Local anesthetic may be instilled through the trocar sites before removal and injected subcutaneously before closure to afford postoperative pain control. Steri-Strips, Telfa, and Tegaderm are applied to the puncture sites after thorough cleansing of the abdomen.

CONSIDERATIONS The preperitoneal approach does not necessitate fascial closure of the umbilical site.

9. The patient may then be repositioned if in supine position and prepared for radical perineal prostatectomy if the two procedures are combined.

POSTOPERATIVE

Nursing Care and Discharge Planning for LPLND

1. Complete perioperative documentation including postoperative assessment.
2. Cleanse patient of prepping solutions before dressing application. Assess skin condition.
3. Evaluate status of peripheral vascular circulation.
4. Assess urinary output and secure Foley catheter.
5. Alternating compression stockings remain in place until discharge from outpatient facility or transfer to inhospital room.
6. If catheter is removed or no catheter is in place, patient must void before discharge.
7. Patient may resume diet as tolerated, starting slowly with clear liquids.
8. Patient should drink 8 oz liquids (half as fruit juice, half as water) q2h for 48 hours to assist voiding process, offset infection, ensure hydration, prevent potassium depletion, and accelerate healing process.
9. Prescribed medications should be taken as directed, antibiotics until gone. Aspirin and nonsteroidal anti-inflammatory agents should be avoided for 10 days unless advised by the surgeon as medically necessary.
10. Review symptoms of infection, herniation, lymphocele formation, delayed hemorrhage, transient sensory nerve deficit, and phlebitis (fever, warmth or redness at incisional sites, swelling or redness in groin, groin pain, lower abdominal ecchymosis, edema/redness/warmth in legs, tingling or numbness in anterior thigh or lateral abdominal or groin regions, ache in lower extremities).
11. Review dressing care and bathing regimen. Patient may shower 24 hours postoperatively. Dressings should be kept clean and dry.
12. Review catheter care if indicated.

LAPAROSCOPIC VARICOCELECTOMY

Description. A varicocelectomy is the high retroperitoneal ligation of the gonadal veins of the testis. When surgery for this condition was devised 70 years ago, the veins of the pampiniform plexus were ligated and divided individually.

The spermatic veins may be identified at a level just above the internal inguinal ring as seen through the laparoscope. At this location the testicular artery may be identified by careful separation of the artery and vein.

A Foley catheter is inserted to decrease the risk of bladder perforation. A nasogastric tube is still recommended but may or may not be employed. The patient is generally in the supine position with one or both arms tucked at the side. It is prudent to employ alternating compression stockings to avoid alterations in peripheral circulation to the lower extremities. The perineum and scrotum are surgically prepped along with the abdomen and draped into the sterile field. This allows for intraoperative manipulation and traction on the testicle to assist in identifying the cord structures during dissection.

PREOPERATIVE

Nursing Care and Teaching Considerations for Laparoscopic Varicocelectomy

1. Incorporate all general nursing diagnoses and interventions for laparoscopy.
2. Check equipment for proper function before patient's arrival.
3. Check all sterile supplies for package integrity.
4. Check instrumentation for proper action and freedom from debris or damage.
5. Position video system appropriately for optimal visualization. Position electrosurgery unit according to room design and optimum location.
6. Assess patient for comprehension of planned surgical intervention and anxiety level. Review as needed, including postoperative expectations and common sequelae.
7. Assess patient for skin temperature and integrity, peripheral circulation (radial and pedal pulses), presence of implants, and general physical status (hearing, vision, numbness, etc.).
8. Assess patient for allergies and medical condition (asthma, COPD, obesity, past surgeries, etc.). Review pertinent laboratory studies (Hgb, PT, PTT, electrolytes, urine studies, etc.).
9. Document assessment findings.
10. Review postoperative expectations: coughing and deep breathing, early ambulation, antibiotic therapies, oral intake, anticipated time of discharge from hospital or ambulatory care facility, care of dressings, postoperative activity level, and follow-up care.
11. Explain purpose of nursing interventions to patient as they are implemented.
12. Apply and begin operation of alternating compression stockings while patient is awake, before vasodilatior, to afford awareness of how the stockings feel and explain purpose for them.
13. Establish range of motion of extremities and neck and shoulders before induction of anesthesia so that patient may express comfort level.
14. After intubation, insert closed system Foley catheter using aseptic technique.
15. Apply electrosurgery dispersive pad to nonbony, nonhairy site, away from any implants but as close to operative site as possible.
16. Position patient in supine, under guidance of surgeon and anesthetist, utilizing proper body mechanics for both patient and personnel. Tuck arms and apply appropriate padding.
17. Reassess radial and pedal pulses after positioning, ensure that IV lines and Foley catheter are free of constriction. Confirm that linen beneath patient is smooth and wrinkle free to avoid skin breakdown.
18. Aseptically prep and drape patient according to institutional guidelines and AORN Standards. Protect patient from pooling of prep solution by utilizing absorbent towels around torso and under perineum, remove them after prep.
19. Turn on all video equipment. Connect and secure CO_2 tubing and turn on insufflator. Connect and secure light cable, camera cable, electrosurgery cable, and suction tubing. Turn on electrosurgery unit and suction unit.
20. Document nursing interventions.

This procedure is well suited for the outpatient setting, and most patients resume normal activity within 3 days postoperatively.

Indications. Laparoscopic varicocelectomy is performed to eliminate retrograde venous flow of blood through the spermatic veins into the venous plexus of the testis and improve spermatogenesis. A varicocele is the most common surgically treatable disorder in patients presenting with infertility. Other possible indications for varicocelectomy include long-term pain, generally increased with extended periods of standing, and testicular atrophy, particularly in the adolescent. Increase in size and improvement in the histologic appearance of the testicle frequently occurs after treatment.

Venous backflow may cause an aching sensation in the scrotum and have a detrimental effect on production of sperm cells by the testes. The condition occurs more frequently on the left side where the gonadal vein of the left testis unites retroperitoneally with the renal vein at a 90-degree angle and is consequently under greater backpressure. As a result of this unusual backpressure, the pampiniform plexus of the spermatic cord becomes tortuous and engorged, resembling a bag of worms. The procedure may be unilateral or bilateral depending on the operating surgeon's school of thought.

Perioperative risks. Inherent risks of laparoscopic varicocelectomy include infection, hemorrhage, herniation at a trocar site, transient sensory nerve loss in the anterior thigh, hydrocele, bowel aor bladder perforation, and pneumoscrotum. Additionally the overall risks associated with laparoscopy apply. To date, few complications have been documented.

The patient must be thoughtfully informed of these potential problems and of the potential benefits of laparoscopic intervention by the operating surgeon and anesthesiologist. Although the perioperative genitourinary nurse should review more common untoward responses and the advantages of laparoscopic intervention, it is beyond the scope of perioperative nursing to detail the more unusual and potentially more severe complications. This remains the domain of the surgeon and anesthesiologist, and questions posed by the patient should be directed to these individuals before proceeding with surgery.

Increased difficulty, necessitating lengthier surgery or conversion to open technique, may occur in patients with extensive adhesions or abdominal scarring, herniations, a history of bowel adhesions, peritonitis, or intestinal obstruction, and uncorrectable coagulopathy. These patients should be carefully evaluated preoperatively to ascertain if the laparoscopic approach may be contraindicated.

Equipment and instrumentation
Equipment
Video camera
Fiberoptic light cable
Video monitor

CO_2 insufflator and spare tank

VCR and video printer

Electrosurgery digital unit with monopolar and bipolar ability

Alternating compression unit and thigh-length compression stockings

Suction unit

Toboggan arm protectors, 2

Head and neck supports

Absorbent towels for prep

Safety strap

Endoscopy instruments

Laparoscope, 10 mm, 0- and 30-degree

Fiberoptic light cable

Laparoscope, 5 mm, 0- and 30-degree

Insufflation needle and insufflator tubing

Trocar and sheath, 10 to 12 mm, 1 or 2

Trocar and sheath, 5 mm, 2

Downsizer, 1 or 2

Metzenbaum scissors with fulgurating ability

Dissectors, locking and nonlocking, 2 each

Right-angle hemostat

Graspers, locking and nonlocking, 2 each

Vein retractor

Needle holder

Electrofulgurating spatula or J-hook

Electrofulgurating suction and irrigator

Electrosurgery cables

Endoloops, Endostitch, Endoties

Endoscopic hemoclips

Miscellaneous supplies

Laparotomy pack

Drape towels, 5

Gowns, 3

Gloves, 1 pair each

Sterile towels, 4

Sterile basins

Knife blade, no. 11 or 15

Knife handle, no. 3

Towel clips, 2 to 4

Syringe, 20 ml, 2

Syringe, 10 ml finger control

Hypodermic needle, #25 gauge, 1¼ inches

Papaverine HCl, 60 mg

Normal saline, 0.9%, 100 ml *or*

Lidocaine 1%, 60 ml

Marcaine plain 0.5% or Duranest 1%

Antiseptic prep solution

Absorbent prep drape

Antibiotic irrigant of choice

Sterile water, 1000 ml bottle

Sterile saline, 1000 ml bottle

Suture, 3-0 absorbable on small general closure or gastrointestinal needle

Suture, 4-0 absorbable on plastic cuticular needle

Steri-Strips

Nonadhesive material (Telfa), 2, for specimens and dressings

Tegaderm, 3 or 4

Soft-tissue instruments

Procedural Steps

1. The patient is placed in the supine position with arms tucked bilaterally and padded.

2. The pneumoperitoneum is established as for the intraperitoneal approach (refer to discussion of laparoscopic nephrectomy, steps 1 and 2).

STEP 2-1

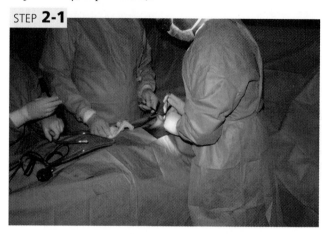

Establishing pneumoperitoneum.

STEP 2-2

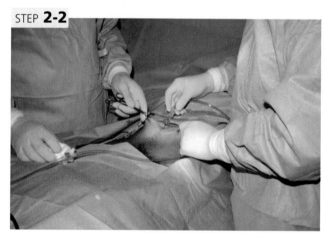

Instillation CO_2 through intraperitoneal Veress.

STEP 2-3

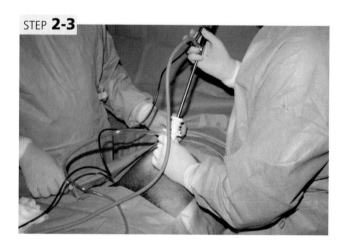

Insertion 10 mm laparoscope.

3. It is possible to perform varix ligation with a 5 mm trocar placed at each lower quadrant and a 10 to 12 mm trocar placed through the subumbilical site, instead of using four trocars. If four trocars are chosen, one 10 mm trocar may be placed suprapubically.

STEP 3-1

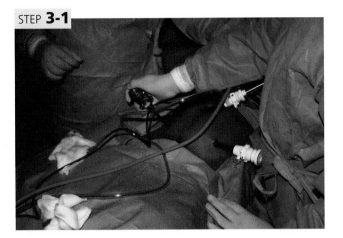

4. The peritoneum is entered laterally to the spermatic cord and incised in a T configuration across the cord.

STEP 4-1

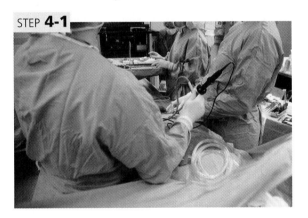

Interior view, entering peritoneum lateral to spermatic cord.

5. The spermatic cord is elevated, and its components are separated with blunt dissection after identification of the spermatic artery. Irrigation of the area with papaverine HCl (30 mg: 50 to 100 ml 0.9% saline) through one of the 5 mm ports facilitates dissection of the artery and veins. This promotes vessel dilation and causes the artery to pulsate, making identification easier. A similar effect may be achieved with 1% plain lidocaine.

6. Ligation of the veins is accomplished by applying vascular endoscopic hemoclips through the 10 mm trocar. This requires that a 5 mm laparoscope be utilized through one of the other ports.

STEP 6-1

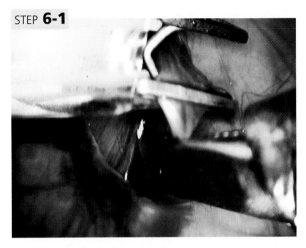

Interior view, applying second proximal clip to first vein.

STEP 6-2

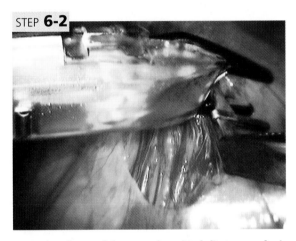

Interior view, applying second proximal clip to second vein.

STEP 6-3

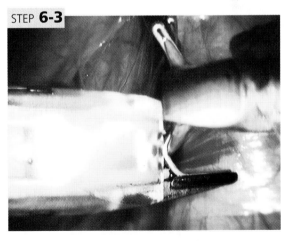

Interior view, applying distal clip to vein.

7. The ports are injected, closed, and dressed in the same manner as for laparoscopic node dissection after hemostasis and the integrity of the abdominal contents has been demonstrated.

POSTOPERATIVE

Nursing Care and Discharge Planning for Laporascopic Variocelectomy

1. Complete perioperative documentation including post-operative assessment.
2. Cleanse patient of prepping solutions before dressing application. Assess skin condition.
3. Evaluate status of peripheral vascular circulation and remove alternating compression stockings.
4. Assess urinary output and remove Foley catheter.
5. Patient must void before discharge.
6. Patient may resume diet as tolerated, starting slowly with clear liquids
7. Patient should drink 8 oz liquid (half as fruit juice, half as water) q2h for 48 hours to assist voiding process, offset infection, ensure hydration, prevent potassium depletion, and accelerate healing process.
8. Prescribed medications should be taken as directed, antibiotics until gone. Aspirin and nonsteroidal anti-inflammatory agents should be avoided for 10 days unless advised by the surgeon as medically necessary.
9. Patient may resume normal activity as tolerated but avoid heavy lifting for 3 days.
10. Review symptoms of infection, herniation, delayed hemorrhage, transient sensory nerve deficit, and pneumoscrotum (fever, warmth, redness, or swelling at incisional sites, groin pain, lower abdominal ecchymosis, tingling or numbness of anterior thigh, tissue-paper feel of scrotal cavity with swelling).
11. Review dressing care and bathing regimen. Patient may shower 24 hours postoperatively. Dressings should be kept clean and dry.

LAPAROSCOPIC (BURCH) BLADDER NECK SUSPENSION

Description. Bladder neck suspension by the Burch method is accomplished by attaching the endopelvic fascia (the supporting structure of the bladder neck) to Cooper's ligament. Actual approximation of the two structures is not necessary. Laparoscopic access is achieved by the intraperitoneal or extraperitoneal approach.

Indications. Bladder neck suspension procedures are indicated for genuine stress incontinence with a goal of 90% success at 5 years after surgery.

Perioperative risks. Inherent risks of any bladder neck suspension include infection, abscess, hemorrhage, hematoma, osteitis pubis, fistula, herniation at a trocar site, transient sensory nerve loss in the anterior thigh, adhesions, enterocele, bladder or bowel perforation, phlebitis, urinary retention, hematuria, detrusor instability, and sexual dysfunction. Additionally, the overall risks associated with laparoscopy apply. Prior bladder neck suspensions that have failed may make laparoscopy contraindicated. Documented laparoscopic complications have been few when compared with the open abdominal method. Long-term success rates are not yet available, however.

The patient must be thoughtfully informed of these potential problems and of the potential benefits of laparoscopic inter-

vention by the operating surgeon and anesthesiologist. Although the perioperative genitourinary nurse should review more common untoward responses and the advantages of laparoscopic intervention, it is beyond the scope of perioperative nursing to detail the more unusual and potentially more severe complications. This remains the domain of the surgeon and anesthesiologist, and questions posed by the patient should be directed to these individuals before proceeding with surgery.

Increased difficulty, necessitating lengthier surgery or conversion to open technique, may occur in patients with extensive adhesions or abdominal scarring, herniations, a history of bowel adhesions, peritonitis, or intestinal obstruction, prior radiotherapy or chemotherapy, total hip replacement that has been cemented, obesity, and uncorrectable coagulopathy. These patients should be carefully evaluated preoperatively to ascertain if the laparoscopic approach may be contraindicated.

Equipment and instrumentation

Equipment

Video camera
Camera cable
Video monitor
CO_2 insufflator and spare tank
VCR and video printer
Electrosurgery digital unit with monopolar and bipolar ability
Suction unit
Toboggan arm protectors, 2
Head and neck support
Allen stirrups
Safety strap
Alternating compression unit and thigh-length compression stockings
Absorbent towels for prep

Endoscopy instruments

Laparoscope, 10 mm, 0- and 30-degree
Laparoscope, 5 mm, 0- and 30-degree
Fiberoptic light cable
Preperitoneal trocar balloon system, 10 mm
Trocar and sheath, 10 mm, 2
Metzenbaum scissors with fulgurating ability
Dissectors, locking and nonlocking, 2 each
Right-angle hemostat
Graspers, locking and nonlocking, 2 each
Needle holder
Electrofulgurating spatula or J-hook
Electrofulgerating suction and irrigator
Electrosurgery cable
Endoloops, Endostitch, Endoties
Endoscopic hemoclip

Miscellaneous supplies

Laparoscopy pack
Drape towels, 5
Gowns, 3
Gloves, 2 pairs each
Sterile towels, 4
Sterile basins
Knife blade, no.11 or 15
Knife handle, no. 3

Towel clips, 2 to 4
Syringe, 20 ml Luer-Lok, 2
Syringe, 10 ml finger control
Hypodermic needle, #25 gauge 1¹/₂ inches
Normal saline, 30 ml, 0.9%
Methylene blue
Marcaine plain 0.5% or Duranest 1%
Antibiotic irrigant of choice
Antiseptic prep solution
Absorbent prep drape
Sterile water, 1000 ml bottle
Sterile saline, 1000 ml bottle
Saline, 0.9% bag, 1000 ml
Cystoscopy tubing
Suture, 4-0 absorbable on plastic cuticular needle
Foley, #20 Fr, 30 cc, 2- or 3-way (by surgeon preference)
Foley, #16 Fr, 5 cc *or*
Suprapubic catheter (surgeon preference)
Urinary drainage bag
Vaginal pack
Steri-Strips
Nonadherent material (Telfa), 2 for dressings
Tegaderm, 3
Soft-tissue instrument

Procedural Steps
Preperitoneal Approach

1. Three 10 mm trocars are inserted, one in each lower quadrant and one in the subumbilical position.

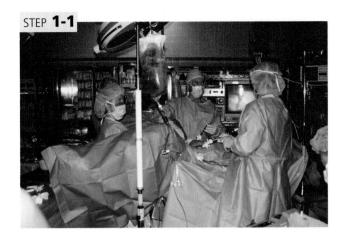

STEP **1-1**

The extraperitoneal approach necessitates the use of a balloon dilator mounted on a trocar to open the retropubic space. Identification of the urinary bladder may be facilitated by instil-

---

PREOPERATIVE

Nursing Care and Teaching Considerations for Laparoscopic Bladder Neck Suspension

1. Incorporate all general nursing diagnoses and interventions for laparoscopy.
2. Check equipment for proper function before patient's arrival.
3. Check all sterile supplies for package integrity.
4. Check instrumentation for proper action and freedom from debris or damage.
5. Position video system appropriately for optimal visualization. Position electrosurgery unit according to room design and optimum location.
6. Assess patient for comprehension of planned surgical intervention and anxiety level. Review as needed, including postoperative expectations and common sequelae.
7. Assess patient for skin temperature and integrity, peripheral circulation (radial and pedal pulses), presence of implants, and general physical status (hearing, vision, numbness, etc.).
8. Assess patient for allergies and medical condition (asthma, COPD, obesity, past surgeries, etc.). Review pertinent laboratory studies (Hgb, PT, PTT, electrolytes, urine studies, etc.).
9. Document assessment findings.
10. Review postoperative expectations: coughing and deep breathing, early ambulation, antibiotic therapies, oral intake, anticipated time of discharge from facility, care of dressings, presence of Foley or suprapubic catheter, presence of vaginal pack, catheter care, postoperative activity level, and follow-up care.
11. Explain purpose of nursing interventions to patient as they are implemented.
12. Apply and begin operation of alternating compression stockings while patient is awake to afford awareness of how the stockings feel and explain purpose for them.
13. Establish range of motion of extremities and neck or shoulders before induction of anesthesia so that patient may express comfort level.
14. Perform suprapubic shave prep.
15. Apply electrosurgery dispersive pad to nonbony, nonhairy site, away from any implants but as close to operative site as possible.
16. Position patient in dorsal lithotomy, under guidance of surgeon and anesthetist, utilizing proper body mechanics for both patient and personnel.
17. Reassess radial and pedal pulses after positioning; ensure that IV lines and Foley catheter are free of constriction. Confirm that linen beneath patient is smooth and wrinkle free to avoid skin breakdown.
18. Aseptically prep and drape patient according to institutional guidelines and AORN standards. Protect patient from pooling of prep solution by utilizing absorbent towels around torso and under perineum, remove them after prep. Aseptically insert and clamp Foley catheter after draping and maintain within sterile field.
19. Turn on all video equipment. Connect and secure CO_2 tubing and turn on insufflator. Connect and secure light cable, camera cable, electrosurgery cable, and suction tubing. Turn on electrosurgery unit and suction unit.
20. Document nursing interventions.

lation of 150 ml of saline containing one ampule of methylene blue dye into the bladder through a #20 Fr 30 cc Foley catheter.

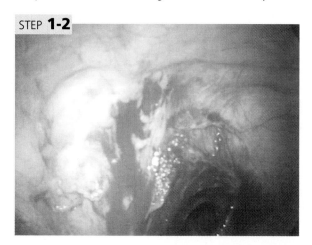

Interior view, bladder inflated with 150-200 ml saline.

2. Identifying the junction of the endopelvic fascia and bladder is aided by placing forward pressure on the anterior vaginal wall. This can be accomplished by an assistant who also places traction on the Foley catheter.

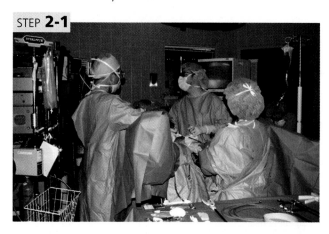

3. Dissection is carried out at 2.5 cm from the bladder reflection to the anterior abdominal wall, thus opening the paravaginal space.

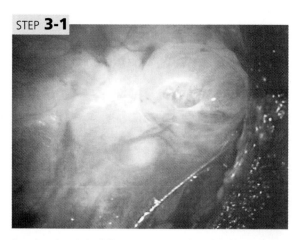

Interior view, initial dissection, 2.5 cm from bladder reflection.

CONSIDERATIONS   If the procedure is done intraperitoneally, the bladder must be dissected off the symphysis pubis to gain access to the endopelvic fascia on either side of the bladder neck.

4. Areolar tissue is cleared off the pelvic side wall to expose the obturator nerve and vessels, which can be used as landmarks for identifying the urethra located 2 to 3 cm toward the midline anteriorly.

5. Dissection between the pubis and bladder wall is then accomplished with endoscopic scissors.

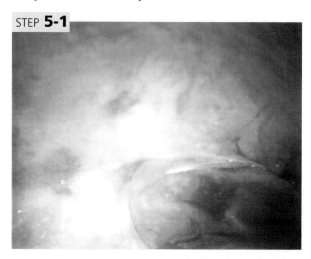

Interior view, dissection from pubis to bladder wall with endoshears.

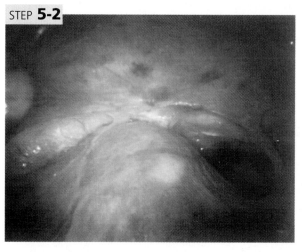

Interior view, exposure of medial bladder edge, lateral protrusions are paravaginal repair sites.

6. Sutures are placed laterally to the urethrovesical junction on each side, attaching tissues of the endopelvic fascia to Cooper's ligament.

STEP **6-1**

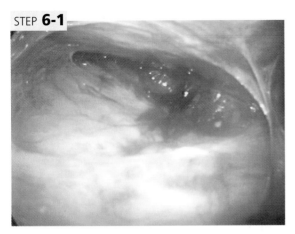

Interior view, left paravaginal space before suture repair.

Two to three sutures are placed on either side.

STEP **6-2**

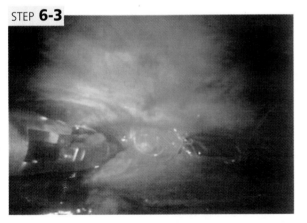

Placing endostitich.

STEP **6-3**

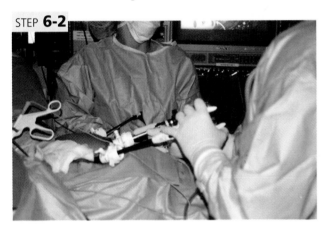

Interior view, placing first suture on left, first pass.

STEP **6-4**

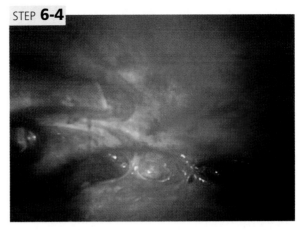

Interior view, first suture on left after first pass, traction applied.

STEP **6-5**

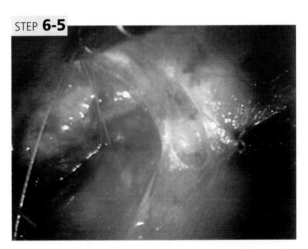

Interior view, tying first suture on left.

STEP **6-6**

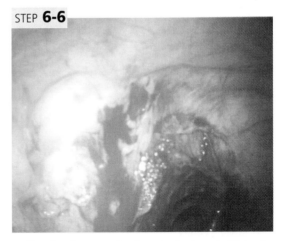

Interior view, completed paravaginal repair, bilateral.

CONSIDERATIONS When the procedure is performed laparoscopically, the increased predisposition to enterocele created by the Burch procedure can be eliminated by correcting the potential defect posterior to the urinary bladder in the pelvic floor.

7. The bladder may be drained through a Foley or suprapubic catheter postoperatively, but patients should be able to void after 6 to 8 hours.

POSTOPERATIVE

Nursing Care and Discharge Planning for Laparoscopic Bladder Neck Suspension

1. Complete perioperative documentation including postoperative assessment.
2. Cleanse patient of prepping solutions before dressing application. Assess skin condition.
3. Evaluate status of peripheral vascular circulation.
4. Assess urinary output and secure Foley catheter and suprapubic catheter.
5. Alternating compression stockings remain in place until discharge from outpatient facility or transfer to inhospital room.
6. Vaginal pack removed on the first postoperative day.
7. Patient may resume diet as tolerated, starting slowly with clear liquids.
8. Patient should drink 8 oz liquid (half as fruit juice, half as water) q2h for 48 hours to assist voiding process, offset infection, ensure hydration, prevent potassium depletion, and accelerate healing process.
9. Prescribed medications should be taken as directed, antibiotics until gone. Aspirin and nonsteroidal anti-inflammatory agents should be avoided for 48 hours unless advised by the surgeon as medically necessary.
10. Review symptoms of infection, herniation, lymphocele formation, delayed hemorrhage, transient sensory nerve deficit, and phlebitis (fever, warmth, or redness at incisional sites, swelling or redness in groin, groin pain, lower abdominal ecchymosis, edema, redness, or warmth in legs, tingling or numbness in anterior part of thigh or lateral abdominal or groin region, ache in lower extremities).
11. Review dressing care and bathing regimen. Patient may shower 24 hours postoperatively. Dressings should be kept clean and dry.
12. Review catheter care. Suprapubic catheter often allows same-day voiding trial with possible removal. Foley catheter may be left in place for 2 to 5 days.

Bibliography

1. Association of Operating Room Nurses, Inc: *Quality improvement in perioperative nursing*, Denver, 1992, AORN.
2. Association of Operating Room Nurses, Inc: *Standards and recommended practices*, Denver, 1995, AORN.
3. American Urologic Association Allied, Inc: *Standards of urologic nursing practice*, Richmond, Va., 1990, AUAA.
4. Benumof JL, Saidman LJ: *Anesthesia and perioperative complications*, St. Louis, 1992, Mosby.
5. Clayman RV et al:Laparoscopic nephroureterectomy, *J Laparoendosc Surg* 1:6, 1991.
6. Clayman RV, et al: Laparoscopic nephrectomy, *Surg Laparosc Endosc* 2:1, 29-34, 1992.
7. Das S, Crawford ED: *Urologic laparoscopy*, Philadelphia, 1994, WB Saunders.
8. Dorsey JH, Cundiff G: Laparoscopic procedures for incontinence and prolapse, *Obstet Gynecol* 5:223-230, 1994.
9. Droller MJ: *Surgical management of urologic disease*, St. Louis, 1992, Mosby.
10. Gershenson DM et al: *Operative gynecology*, Philadelphia, 1993, WB Saunders.
11. Gaur DD et al: Retroperitoneal laparoscopic nephrectomy, *J Urol* 149:103-105, 1993.
12. Goldstein M: *Surgery of male infertility*, Philadelphia, 1995, WB Saunders.
13. Gray M: *Genitourinary disorders*, St. Louis, 1992, Mosby.
14. Jordan GH, Winslow BH: Laparoendoscopic upper pole partial nephrectomy with ureterectomy, *J Urol* 150:940-943, 1993.
15. Kerbl K et al: Ligation of the renal pedicle during laparoscopic nephrectomy, *J Laparoendosc Surg* 3:1, 1993.
16. Litwack K: *Core curriculum for post anesthesia nursing practice*, ed 3, Philadelphia, 1995, WB Saunders.
17. Liu CY: Laparoscopic retropubic colposuspension (Burch procedure), *J Reprod Med* 38:7, 1993.
18. Meeker MH, Rothrock JC: *Alexander's care of the patient in surgery*, ed 10, St. Louis, 1995, Mosby.
19. Ono Y, et al: Laparoscopic nephrectomy without morcellation for renal cell carcinoma, *J Urol* 150:1222, 1993.
20. Ou CS, Presthus J, Beadle E: Laparoscopic bladder neck suspension using hernia mesh and surgical staples, *J Laparoendosc Surg*, 3:6, 1993.
21. Quilici PJ: *New developments in laparoscopy*, Norwalk, Conn., 1992, Auto Suture Company.
22. Resnick MI, Kursh ED: *Current therapy in genitourinary surgery*, ed 2, St. Louis, 1992, Mosby.
23. Resnick MI, Novick AC: *Urology secrets*, St. Louis, 1995, Mosby.
24. Rothrock JC: *Perioperative nursing care planning*, ed 2, St. Louis, 1996, Mosby.
25. Seidman EJ, Hanno PM: *Current urologic therapy three*, Philadelphia, 1994, WB Saunders.
26. Smith AD: *Controversies in endourology*, Philadelphia, 1995, WB Saunders.
27. Smith JA: *High tech urology*, Philadelphia, 1992, WB Saunders.
28. Tanagho EA, McAninch JW: *Smith's general urology*, ed 14, Norwalk, Conn., 1995, Appleton & Lange.
29. Tighe SM: *Instrumentation for the operating room*, ed 4, St. Louis, 1994, Mosby.
30. United States Surgical Corporation: *Laparoscopy in focus*, Ob/Gyn edition, 1:4.
31. Vaiden RE et al: *Core curriculum for the RN first assistant*, Denver, 1990, Association of Operating Room Nurses, Inc.
32. Walters MD, Karram MM: *Clinical urogynecology*, St. Louis, 1993, Mosby.
33. Whitehead ED, Nagler ED: *Management of impotence and infertility*, Philadelphia, 1994, Lippincott.

9

Open Interventions on the Genital System

New interventions, or new approaches to old methods, are being introduced on a continual basis. It is difficult to keep abreast of the rapid advancements being made. It is beyond the scope of this chapter to detail all the possibilities. If the genitourinary nurse is versed in the basics, adaptation to the unusual or infrequent procedure will not be difficult. Those interventions that are likely to be performed in the majority of settings are addressed.

For purposes of organization, surgical interventions for the genital system will include corrective measures for conditions of the scrotum, the testes and attached structures, minor conditions of the urethral meatus, and the penis.

The text and photographs to follow in this chapter are intended to be generic for the specific interventions. Each is subject to alteration depending on the practice setting and the preference of the surgeon. Common surgical techniques and instrumentation are depicted and intended as an overview to enable the perioperative nurse to anticipate patient care needs. Instrumentation and actual equipment in practice will also vary according to physician preference and the procedural setting. It is important to focus on the principles involved in each procedure and to consider the instrumentation as suggestions for the specialty of genitourinary surgery.

NURSING CARE

Nursing diagnoses will vary according to the exact procedure performed and the patient's medical status. Nursing planning and care specific to each operative intervention are discussed under that procedure. General nursing diagnoses, preoperative planning, and perioperative interventions for a patient undergoing open genitourinary intervention might include the following:

NURSING DIAGNOSIS	PERIOPERATIVE PLANNING AND INTERVENTION
Anxiety related to: Knowledge deficit Fear of recurrence or failure	Review purpose of planned procedure; ascertain level of comprehension. Document expressions of anxiety by the patient or family. Provide explanations and reassurance to the patient and family. Reinforce and review patient teaching; answer questions as necessary. Encourage participation in discharge planning; review discharge instructions. Keep family informed during intraoperative stage. Verify understanding of signs and symptoms to be reported. Place follow-up call the day after surgery.
Pain related to: Current medical status Extent of procedure	Provide adequate assistance when moving patient. Assess and maintain comfort during positioning. Provide positional explanations. Discuss postoperative expectations in light of preoperative conception and postoperative reality. Offer comfort measures to alleviate pain as appropriate. Collaborate with health care team to plan pain control management. Administer medication as ordered, explain side effects. If patient-controlled analgesic (PCA) is to be utilized, confirm that contact has been established with home care provider. Assist patient to utilize pain control strategies with emotional and informational support.
Risk for infection related to: Operative intervention Medical status Insertion of implant Hematoma formation	Maintain aseptic environment and properly sterilize instrumentation. Insert catheter aseptically and maintain closed urinary drainage system. Use appropriate technique during surgical prep. Drape patient according to aseptic standards. Observe for indications of fever, dysuria or pyuria, and reddened or warm incisional sites. Provide adequate hydration through intravenous lines (IV) or fluid intake. Administer antibiotic therapies as ordered. Apply ice to sites at risk for hematoma.

NURSING DIAGNOSIS	PERIOPERATIVE PLANNING AND INTERVENTION
Altered family process related to male subfertility	Discuss feelings relating to male subfertility. Teach appropriate coping strategies. Review options available: sperm banking, assisted reproductive techniques, corrective surgery, adoption. Collaborate with other health care professionals in planning care. Provide information on support groups.
Altered sexual function	Discuss possible causes of sexual dysfunction. Assist patient to verbalize concerns. Provide information regarding physiologic function during sexual activity. Discuss treatment options available. Provide information on support groups.
Risk for hemorrhage or hematocele related to: Vessel integrity Hematoma	Discuss signs and symptoms of bleeding. Reinforce importance of ice application. Review need to avoid aspirin and nonsteroidal medications for 10 days. Explain need for reduced activity level; review activity regimen. Discuss reasons for pressure dressings and scrotal support. Review bathing technique relating to wound status—shower after 24 hours; do not scrub wound but gently cleanse and pat dry.

The majority of the interventions involving the genital system may be successfully managed in an outpatient setting. The focus in patient education must be preparation for discharge shortly after the intervention. It is important to include significant others in the discharge planning and instruction. The pain encountered postoperatively will range from true discomfort to dull aching. Those that experience less discomfort are likely to discount the restrictions placed on their activity level. Delicate structures have been surgically manipulated, and it is important that all involved in the recovery period be aware of the need to curtail strenuous endeavors.

The patient will generally be in the supine or lithotomy position. It is easy to overlook the need to utilize certain comfort measures when the patient appears to be simply "lying down" or the planned procedure is not lengthy. Support should be provided beneath the knees, heels, and under the sacral area. Additionally, any pressure points (back of head, scapula, elbows, etc.) should be adequately protected. When lithotomy position is necessary, care must be taken to protect the popliteal space, Achilles tendon, calf region, tibial and peroneal nerves, and ilioinguinal nerves and avoid hyperextension of the hips. The Allen boot stirrups are considered the safest and most comfortable for the patient.

The anesthesia of choice for genital intervention may be general, spinal or epidural block, or local infiltration with sedation. The majority of the time, monitored anesthesia care (local infiltration with sedation) is employed unless the amount of dissection required necessitates another avenue. No matter what anesthetic is used, local anesthetic will likely be instilled to afford postoperative pain management. Table 9-1 is a guideline for suggested dosages of local anesthetic.

Anesthetic complications to be alert for include allergic response to the local anesthetic (tinnitus, agitation, urticaria, itching, blurred vision, drowsiness, respiratory depression, cardiac dysrhythmias, and seizure activity), hypotension or hypertension, peripheral nerve damage, regurgitation of gastric con-

Table 9-1 **Suggested Local Anesthetic Dose per Kilogram of Body Weight**

ANESTHETIC AGENT	MG/KG
Procaine	14-18
Lidocaine (Xylocaine)	7-9
Bupivacaine (Marcaine)	2-3

tents, spinal headache, and excessive bleeding. The patient is instructed to refrain from taking aspirin and nonsteroidal anti-inflammatory agents for 10 days preoperatively. If this was not complied with, excessive bleeding could occur and the use of spinal anesthesia may be contraindicated.

An essential part of the nursing care includes maintenance of the equipment and instrumentation. The operating lights, electrosurgery unit, and suction unit should be checked for proper function before the patient enters the room. Instrumentation should be inspected for damage, debris or corrosion, and proper action before use.

Monopolar and bipolar electrofulguration may be employed. The selection is dependent on the vessels involved and the operating surgeon's preference. To remain cost effective, disposable items that will not routinely be needed should not be opened.

As perioperative patient care is implemented, the plan of care will be subject to adjustment on a continual basis based on data collected through the preoperative assessment and changing intraoperative circumstances. This ongoing evaluation and revision of care allows for an individualized approach. Once care has been implemented the postoperative assessment is completed. Often it will not be possible to accurately determine long-term outcomes. Immediate postoperative assessment allows for a baseline determination of the effect of the nursing interventions provided. Priority postoperative assessment data appropriate for the continual evaluation of nursing care may include the following:

- Understanding the importance of ice applied to the scrotum for 24 hours
- Awareness of reportable signs and symptoms of hemorrhage or infection
- Discussion of dressing and wound care
- Knowledge of the need to curtail strenuous activity (time frame varies according to intervention)
- Awareness of diet or other restrictions related to the medication regimen
- Comprehension of the medication regimen ordered by the physician (aspirin and nonsteroidal antiinflammatory agents should not be used postoperatively unless cleared with the physician)
- Understanding the need for adequate fluid intake to accelerate healing and promote recovery from spinal anesthesia, if appropriate
- Awareness of follow-up requirements: physician visit as scheduled, semen analysis as applicable
- Review of catheter care when indicated
- Readiness for discharge

An overview of the care provided and the subsequent evaluation is recorded to provide for the continuity of care throughout the recovery period. This documentation should be individualized according to the procedure and the needs of the patient. Surgical settings differ and perioperative documentation will have guidelines appropriate for the specific institution. A summary of the intraoperative activities designed to achieve certain outcome criteria should be reported to the perianesthesia nurse. Information to be recorded and reported will vary according to the procedure performed. Reports may differ between surgical settings depending on the amount of preoperative instruction afforded the patient and services available to meet each patient's requirements. Priority information for the genitourinary patient may include the following:

- Wound status at the time of dressing application
- Patency of catheter or drains at discharge from the operating room
- Precautions pertinent to the patient's physical condition
- Fluid loss and replacement
- Status of peripheral vascular circulation preoperatively and postoperatively
- Skin integrity preoperatively and postoperatively
- Positions and positioning devices employed for surgery
- Level of comprehension during preoperative instruction
- Information taught to the patient preoperatively and intraoperatively
- Untoward reactions encountered intraoperatively
- Nursing care provided

THE ROLE OF THE RN FIRST ASSISTANT

The RNFA functions in an expanded role of perioperative nursing, incorporating the perioperative nursing process while performing assistive behaviors. The scope of practice will vary by each individual institution. Ideally the RNFA has specialized education and training in the field of genitourinary surgery.

Although most of the time, the focus of practice is during the intraoperative phase, the RNFA also functions preoperatively and postoperatively on the patient's and surgeon's behalf.

The perioperative activities of the RNFA are interdependent and in collaboration with the operating surgeon.

Preoperatively, time may not allow for extended nurse-patient interaction. When the RNFA is part of the surgical team, he or she may augment the role of the perioperative RN (circulating nurse) through the assessment, planning, and implementation of patient care. With expanded experience and knowledge to utilize, the RNFA may plan the appropriate individualized nursing interventions and lead the surgical team during implementation, based on the assessment data collected and nursing diagnoses established. If the RNFA is privately employed by the operating surgeon, much of this data collection and patient care planning may have taken place during the preoperative interview and physical examination. Collaborative effort can be successful when the information is communicated to the perioperative genitourinary team.

The RNFA is expected to understand the theory behind positioning techniques and should not only assist the surgeon to position the patient, leading the team toward optimal care, but also teach during the process. For example, bony prominences require adequate padding to protect them from pressure damage, which may lead to neurovascular compromise. The knees, heels, and sacrum are supported with padding to alleviate low back strain, protect pressure points, and provide a comfortable intraoperative course

The RNFA is expected to know the various surgical approaches, potential alterations, and accompanying rationale and can assist the team in preparing for any given circumstance. For example, uncontrolled bleeding will necessitate expanded instrumentation to allow for more extensive exploration so that hemostasis may be achieved. Identification of bleeding sites, aberrant and common vessels, and important reproductive structures is imperative for a good surgical outcome. Handling of tissue must be gentle and precise.

The RNFA is expected to have a comprehensive awareness of the anatomy involved in a given procedure and should utilize this knowledge in the care provided. For example, being cognizant of the need to assist the surgeon during surgical dissection or electrofulguration by retracting and protecting the spermatic artery from injury. With a broad background to draw upon, the RNFA can incorporate the needs of each member of the surgical team to form a cohesive individualized approach.

Intraoperatively the RNFA will assist the surgeon to lead the team in positioning and padding the patient, insert the Foley catheter, apply alternating compression stockings if warranted, perform the skin shave and antiseptic prep, and assist with draping. During the operative intervention the RNFA may retract tissue, irrigate and sponge the operative site, stabilize structures with tissue forceps, keep the field of vision clear, assist with evaluating the wound for hemostasis, identify bleeding sites, assist with electrocoagulation, irrigate the wound before closure, inject local anesthetics, and suture and dress the wound. Additionally the RNFA will insert vaginal packings, secure the Foley catheter and connect it to appropriate drainage as applicable, cleanse the patient of prep solution, evaluate skin integrity, and apply the surgical dressings and scrotal support.

Postoperatively the RNFA can evaluate patient outcomes based on the plan of care, enhance or reinforce patient teaching, and evaluate the patient for other needs requiring follow-up

Nursing Care and Teaching Considerations for Interventions on the Male Genital System

1. Incorporate all general nursing diagnoses and interventions.
2. Check overhead lights, operating room bed, suction unit, and electrosurgery unit for proper function before patient's arrival.
3. Check all sterile supplies for package integrity. Check all medications for dose and expiration dates.
4. Check instrumentation for proper action and freedom from debris or damage.
5. Assess patient for comprehension of planned surgical intervention and anxiety level. Review as needed, including postoperative expectations and common sequelae.
6. Assess patient for skin integrity, peripheral circulation, presence of implants, low back syndrome, and general physical status.
7. Assess patient for allergies and medical condition (asthma, obesity, diabetes, past surgeries, etc.). Review pertinent laboratory reports (hemoglobin [Hgb], prothrombin time [PT], partial thromboplastin time [PTT], urine studies, fertility studies, etc.).
8. Document assessment findings.
9. Review postoperative expectations: ice application to scrotum for 24 hours, ambulation, avoidance of strenuous activity for 4 weeks on average, antibiotic (if indicated) and pain regimens, anticipated time of discharge from the facility, care of dressings, signs and symptoms to report, oral intake and diet, follow-up visit with physician.
10. Explain purpose of nursing interventions as they are implemented.
11. Establish range of motion of extremities. Assess for low back stability.
12. Place patient in supine position with legs slightly separated and pad sacral area and under knees, heels, and other pressure sites. If lithotomy is employed, utilize Allen stirrups, placing legs to maintain hip alignment and simulation of normal extension with flexion. Assess calf for pressure points and place foot firmly in boot so that heel is touching the leg-foot juncture and bottom of foot is flat in the base.
13. If indicated, apply electrosurgery dispersive pad to non-hairy, nonbony site away from any implants but as close to the operative site as feasible.
14. Reassess peripheral circulation after positioning. Ensure that IV lines are free of constriction.
15. Confirm that linen beneath patient is smooth.
16. Perform shave prep as necessary.
17. Aseptically prep and drape patient according to Association of Operating Room Nurses (AORN) standards and institutional guidelines. Protect patient from pooling of prep solution with absorbent towels; remove after prep.
18. Position electrosurgery to afford maximum utilization.
19. Turn on electrical equipment.
20. Document nursing interventions.

management. Those that are privately employed have the advantage of seeing the patient after discharge and can more thoroughly evaluate patient outcomes in relation to the implementation of care. With communication between the private RNFA and the perioperative team, planning for future patient care and intervention can be dramatically improved, based on the follow-up information acquired.

HYDROCELECTOMY

Description. A hydrocelectomy is the excision of the tunica vaginalis of the testis to remove an enlarged, fluid-filled sac. A scrotal approach is generally chosen, but an inguinal incision may be required when tumor is a possibility or when transillumination during examination is not achievable. The hydrocele sac may be in communication with the peritoneal cavity, in which case the appropriate treatment is repair of the inguinal hernia. The hydrocele may be left undisturbed.

The procedure may be successfully accomplished with local anesthetic infiltration and sedation, or regional or general anesthesia, and is conducive to the outpatient setting. The patient will be in the supine position.

Indications. To correct an abnormally excessive accumulation of fluid between the visceral and parietal layers of the tunica vaginalis that causes pain, interferes with motion

because of its size, or is prone to infection. Hydrocele is often the result of infection or trauma. Less commonly, hydroceles may develop as a result of a testicular tumor. Of patients who have had an ipsilateral renal transplantation, it is estimated that 70% have developed hydroceles resulting from the division of the spermatic vessels and the vas deferens. Hydroceles under 2 years of age may be observed for a period of at least 1 year because in many cases these resolve spontaneously.

The patient will generally describe a feeling of heaviness, with accompanying scrotal enlargement. Occasionally, inguinal discomfort that radiates to the midportion of the back will be a presenting complaint.

Perioperative risks. Problems that may occur during or after a hydrocelectomy include bleeding, ischemia from the spermatic cord block, testicular artery injury, scrotal edema, allergic response to the local anesthetic, infection, postoperative hematoma, strangulation of the spermatic cord, and injury to the testis, epididymis, or vas deferens. The usual anesthetic risks, as previously discussed, exist in relation to patient age, size, and medical status. Constipation may result if the patient is prescribed narcotic pain management.

Avoiding the use of epinephrine in the local anesthetic and providing preoperative antibiotic prophylaxis are advisable. Epinephrine may prevent proper identification and hemostatic control of vessels because of its vasoconstrictive action. Additionally it may result in prolonged spermatic cord ischemic time.

Equipment and Instrumentation
Equipment
Electrosurgery unit with monopolar and bipolar ability
Safety strap
Head and neck support
Positioning pads as necessary
Suction unit
Instruments
Minor instrument set including the following:
Allis clamps, 8
Weitlaner retractor for inguinal approach
Miscellaneous supplies
Laparotomy pack *or*
Fenestrated drape and basic pack
Sterile gowns and gloves
Drape towels, adherent, 4
Sterile cloth towel
Electrosurgery pencil, hand control
Needle electrode
Electrosurgery dispersive pad *or*
Hand-held battery cautery
Knife blade, no. 10 or 15
Syringe, 10 ml finger-control
Hypodermic needle, 25 and 27 gauge, $1/4$ inch
Ties, absorbable, 3-0 and 4-0
Suture, absorbable, 3-0 and 4-0, on SH-1 or RB-1 needle
Suture, absorbable, 3-0 and 4-0, on small cuticular needle
Lidocaine plain, 1% (or anesthetic of choice)
Penrose drain, $1/4$ inch
Gauze sponges, plain and radiopaque
"Fluffs" dressings
Athletic supporter *or*
Mesh underwear
Antiseptic prep solution
Absorbent prep pad
Sterile water, 500 ml
Sterile saline, 500 ml

Procedural Steps
Scrotal Approach (Lord Procedure)

The patient is placed in the supine position. Preparation and draping of the patient include routine cleansing of the external genitals with an iodophor solution and draping of the patient with towels and a fenestrated sheet. Placing a sterile cloth towel beneath the scrotum assists in elevating the operative area and helps to absorb fluid. It may be necessary to shave the scrotum.

1. Local anesthetic is instilled by grasping the cord in one hand and placing the thumb and index finger of the other hand over the scrotum. The cord is infiltrated at the base of the scrotum with 10 to 15 ml of plain lidocaine 1%.

2. An anterolateral incision is made in the stretched skin of the scrotum over the hydrocele mass with a no. 10 or 15 blade. Bleeding is controlled with Crile hemostats, electrosurgery or vessel ligation with 3-0 absorbable ligatures.

CONSIDERATIONS Stretching the skin of the scrotum compresses the scrotal vessels. Incision is then made between the blood vessels.

3. The fascial layers are incised to expose the tunica vaginalis. The hydrocele is dissected free with fine scissors, forceps, and blunt dissection. The sac is opened, and Allis clamps are placed on each side incorporating the tissue adjacent to the tunica vaginalis and the skin. The incised edges are everted under tension with the Allis clamps.

CONSIDERATIONS The tension placed by the Allis clamp compresses the incised edge, controls bleeding, and prevents dissection between the tissue layers.

4. A pouch is created by dissecting between the tunica vaginalis and the dartos layer. Scrotal pressure is released. The tunica vaginalis is opened, and the fluid contents are aspirated or drained.

CONSIDERATIONS This pouch will hold the testis after the repair.

5. The testis is lifted, and the sac is inverted so that it surrounds the testicular attachments and epididymis. Excess tunica vaginalis may be excised. The tunica edges are sutured along the peritoneal surface with 3-0 absorbable suture in an interrupted fashion to the juncture of the testis. Six to eight sutures are placed around the circumference of the testis.

POSTOPERATIVE

Nursing Care and Discharge Planning for Hydrocelectomy

1. Application of ice for 24 to 48 hours reduces postoperative edema, pain, and bleeding.
2. Scrotal support and pressure dressings should be worn until the swelling is gone. The drain is usually removed at the first postoperative visit. Scrotal edema and swelling may last several weeks until lymphatic drainage occurs through newly established channels.
3. Avoid strenuous activity for approximately 2 weeks or until pain free to ensure proper healing. Most patients may return to work in 1 week.
4. Resume other activities as tolerated: if it hurts, don't do it!
5. Resume diet as tolerated beginning with clear liquids the first postoperative day. Increase fluid intake to assist healing and ward off infection.
6. Take medications as ordered: antibiotics until gone, pain medications before onset of discomfort (overlap dosage and gradually decrease use as discomfort subsides). If the pain medication is a narcotic, a stool softener should be taken daily to prevent constipation.
7. The patient should exercise safety precautions if the pain medication causes drowsiness or disequilibrium (do not drive, drink, or operate machinery).
8. Shower on first postoperative day: pat area dry; keep dressings clean and dry.
9. Ecchymosis of scrotum will be seen initially but will gradually fade.
10. Report any unresolved or increased pain, tenderness, redness, warmth, wound seepage, fever, edema, or bruising to rule out infection or hemorrhage.
11. Avoid aspirin and nonsteroidal antiinflammatory agents as advised by physician.

CONSIDERATIONS Some surgeons elect to sew the sac behind the spermatic cord in an interrupted fashion, and others may choose a continuous radial stitch around the posterior testis and epididymis. Theories differ regarding the approach.

6. The testis is replaced into the scrotum. A drain may be placed into the scrotum and brought out through a stab wound in its most dependent portion. The drain is loosely sutured to the external scrotal wall to prevent migration.

7. The scrotal incision may be closed with 3-0 absorbable sutures in a full-thickness, continuous manner, or in layers with 3-0 and 4-0 continuous absorbable sutures. A fluff compression dressing contained in a scrotal support or mesh underwear aids in reducing postoperative scrotal edema.

VASECTOMY

Description. A vasectomy is the excision of a section of the vas deferens. The vas is ligated high in the scrotum, and no more than a 2 cm section is excised. Various techniques for vasectomy have been developed and include the incisional approach, the no-scalpel method, and percutaneous injection. The last two approaches decrease the postoperative discomfort. Vasectomy requires only local anesthesia unless it is combined with another procedure such as transurethral prostatectomy (TURP) and is appropriate for the outpatient or office setting.

Indications. The operation may be performed electively as a permanent method of sterilization and also before prostatectomy to prevent possible postoperative epididymitis. Because of the serious implications of permanent sterilization, particular attention must be paid to acquiring informed consent. Recent studies have raised the question of a correlation between prostate cancer and vasectomy, but definitive causal relationships have not been established.

The patient having elective sterilization for birth control is encouraged to return to the office setting for a sperm count analysis. Generally two successive negative counts are sufficient to indicate that sterility has been achieved. Elective vasectomies are seen far less often in the operating room because more surgeons are performing the procedure in the office setting.

Perioperative risks. Early complications of vasectomy are less frequent in experienced hands and may include hematoma, infection, and sperm granuloma. Anesthetic complications are few and will generally be reactions to local anesthetics. It is not uncommon for the patient to exhibit a vagal response to the local anesthetic (hypotension, diaphoresis) at the initiation of the second side of the vasectomy.

Long-term complications include vasitis nodosa (recanalization, usually within 6 weeks), chronic testicular pain, alterations in testicular function, secondary epididymal obstruction, failure to induce sterilization, and ligation of structures other than the vas. Careful stripping of the vas from its sheath and preservation of vessels minimize bleeding and enhance the possibility for reversal in the future.

After vasectomy 60% to 80% develop an elevation of serum antisperm antibodies that very likely contributes to the success of sterilization. If azoospermia does not occur within 3 months after vasectomy, the procedure should be repeated. Drainage of sperm cells and testicular fluid is not necessarily halted by vasectomy. Many men will eventually experience an epididymal or efferent duct "blowout" leading to a sperm granuloma. This is the primary reason the success of vasectomy reversal decreases as the interval after vasectomy increases.

Equipment and instrumentation

Refer to hydrocelectomy for basic equipment and miscellaneous supplies

Specific instrumentation (Choice dependent on surgical approach)

Vasectomy ring clamp
Vasectomy hemostat
Towel clips, small, 1 or 2
Knife handle, no. 3
Suture scissors
Clip applier, small
Needle holder, 5 inches
Hemostat, straight Crile, 1 to 4
Allis clamp, 1 or 2
Adson tissue forceps
Hemoclips, small

Procedural Steps

The patient usually lies in the supine position, though the patient may be in the lithotomy position if vasectomy is performed before transurethral prostatectomy. The penis is retracted cephalad. A small area on the scrotum may need to be shaved. The entire groin is prepped with antiseptic solution, the area squared off, and a fenestrated drape applied. Adherent drape towels help to anchor the penis in the cephalad position. Placing a sterile cloth towel beneath the scrotum, before squaring off the area, assists in elevating it into the operative field.

Incisional Approach

1. The vas is located by digital palpation of the upper part of the scrotum. After injection of the local anesthetic, a small incision is made in the skin over the vas.

2. An Allis forceps, vas clamp, or small towel clamp, is inserted into the scrotal incision to mobilize the vas and deliver it to the surface of the wound. The vas is longitudinally denuded of its surrounding tunica. Once isolated, the vas is divided by electrosurgery, or hand-held battery cautery, and both segments are coagulated.

CONSIDERATIONS Hemostats may be placed before vasal division, the vas cut between the clamps, a section of tissue removed, and the segments cauterized. Alternatively the vasal ends may be folded back on themselves and ligatures or hemoclips applied instead of occlusion by electrocoagulation. Fascia should be placed between the severed ends by clipping or suturing one end in its sheath.

3. The severed ends of the vas are returned to the scrotum.

4. The skin incision is closed with 4-0 absorbable interrupted or continuous sutures. The patient is instructed to wear

a scrotal support of the appropriate size for approximately 3 to 4 days.

No-Scalpel Approach

The no-scalpel technique was devised in China and has five fundamental principles:

- Fixation of the vas deferens without entering the scrotal skin.
- Performance under direct vision to prevent damage from blind sharp scrotal penetration.
- Simplified instrumentation.
- Decreased operative time by simplification of the procedure.
- Elimination of an incision or use of a scalpel.

1. The right vas deferens is fixed under the scrotal skin with three fingers. A small wheal is raised in the median raphe of the scrotum with the anesthetic. The needle is advanced along the vas toward the external inguinal ring. Plain lidocaine 1% or 2%, 3 to 5 ml, is injected into the tissues around the vas.

2. The procedure is repeated on the left side. Pressure is applied to the wheal site to minimize edema.

3. Once adequate anesthesia is accomplished, the right vas is again fixed with three fingers. A vas ring clamp is applied over the scrotal skin, encircling the vas. Lifting the clamp upward, the skin over the vas is stretched as thin as possible leaving minimal tissue between the vas and the clamp.

4. The ring clamp is locked in place, and the scrotal skin cephalad to the clamp is stretched with an index finger. The skin is punctured, with the inner prong of the pointed dissecting hemostat, directly into the vas deferens.

POSTOPERATIVE

Nursing Care and Discharge Planning for Vasectomy

1. Ice to scrotum for 24 hours to reduce swelling and potential for bleeding.
2. Acetaminophen (Tylenol) for pain; avoid aspirin and non-steroidal antiinflammatory agents for 48 hours.
3. Avoid strenuous activity for 72 hours, and then resume activity as tolerated.
4. Wear scrotal support for 3 days postoperatively or until pain free. Wear during first postoperative week if strenuous activity is anticipated.
5. Shower on first postoperative day: pat wound dry; apply clean dressings. Change dressings as needed to keep them clean and dry.
6. Report any fever, swelling that increases after first postoperative day, unresolved or increased bleeding, pain that Tylenol does not resolve, or increased tenderness after 3 days. Dressings should not require changing more than twice after this time. Some spotting is normal for 2 or 3 days.
7. As healing occurs, a small lump may be noticed. This is normal and should resolve by 6 weeks.
8. Sexual activity may resume after first postoperative day as tolerated. A condom or other form of birth control must be employed until semen analysis confirms sterility.
9. Keep postoperative appointments: semen sample at 6 weeks or after 15 ejaculates, second semen sample at 4 weeks. Two consecutive negative analyses are necessary to confirm sterility.

5. Both prongs of the dissecting hemostat are placed into the puncture site and spread directly on top of the vas. When the surface of the vas is visualized, one prong is used to penetrate the vas itself. With a 180-degree skewering motion, the vas is brought out of the wound.

6. The ring clamp is moved to directly encircle the vasal tissue. The vas may then be divided and occluded by intraluminal electrocautery, clips, or suture ligation. Fascia should be placed between the severed ends of the vas.

7. The procedure is repeated on the left side. It is usually possible to place the ring clamp around the left vas through the initial entry site.

8. Sutures are not necessary. Ensuring that there is no bleeding, antibiotic ointment, pressure dressings, and a scrotal support are applied.

EPIDIDYMECTOMY

Description. An epididymectomy is the excision of the epididymis from the testis. As in vasectomy, local anesthesia with or without sedation is usually sufficient to render the patient pain free. The procedure is ideal for the outpatient setting. Operative loupes may be employed. The patient will be rendered sterile unless the opposite testis is functional and its vas has not been ligated.

Indications. Epididymectomy may be indicated to treat degenerative cystic disease, tuberculosis, unremitting pain, or infection of the epididymis. Lately it has been found that immunocompromised males (including those with AIDS) may develop cytomegalovirus infections of the epididymis that do not respond to antibiotics but may be resolved by surgical removal.

Perioperative risks. Complications that may result after epididymectomy include hemorrhage, hematoma, injury to spermatic vessels, infection, testicular damage or atrophy, and allergic reaction to the local anesthetic. Epididymal resection essentially eliminates drainage of sperm cells and testicular fluid from the testis. This may cause dull aching in the testis, which may require several months to resolve.

Equipment and instrumentation
Refer to hydrocelectomy in addition to the following:
Operative loupes
Bipolar forceps
Plastic instrument set

Procedural Steps

The patient is placed in the supine position and prepped and draped as described for hydrocelectomy.

1. After injection of the local anesthetic is accomplished, a vertical or transverse anterolateral incision is made over the testis in the scrotum to expose the tunica vaginalis. The tunica is incised to expose the testis and overlying epididymis.

CONSIDERATIONS When epididymectomy is performed for tuberculosis, the incision should be extended to the external inguinal ring to allow removal of the distal vas deferens.

2. A traction suture is placed in the globus major, and dissection begins at its apex. The rete tubules are ligated and divided close to the epididymis to avoid injury to the medial testicular vessels.

CONSIDERATIONS The efferent ducts are located superior to the testicular vascular pedicle. The testicular blood supply is medial to the epididymis at the juncture of the middle and upper third of the testis. Care must be taken to preserve these vessels. Bleeding is controlled by electrocoagulation and absorbable ligatures. If injury to the testicular vessels occurs, collateral circulation frequently compensates.

3. The globus major is freed under traction with sharp and blunt dissection. An incision is made along the superior head of the epididymis, which is then sharply dissected from the testis. The epididymal artery is divided and ligated with 3-0 absorbable ligatures.

4. The proximal vas deferens is located and ligated with 3-0 absorbable ties, along with the deferential vessels, close to the convoluted portion of the vas. The convoluted vas is dissected free.

5. The edges of the tunica vaginalis, along the base of the resected epididymis, are oversewn with a continuous 3-0 or 4-0 absorbable suture, or rendered hemostatically secure with bipolar cautery.

6. The dartos and skin is closed in layers with 3-0 and 4-0 absorbable sutures. A small drain may be left intrascrotally for 24 to 48 hours but is usually not necessary.

CONSIDERATIONS Meticulous fulguration or ligation of small vessels, particularly along the edge of the tunica vaginalis, and layered closure of the dartos and skin will assist in preventing the postoperative bleeding that is common to this procedure.

Infected fistulous tracts or obviously infected areas should be resected. Copious antibiotic irrigation should be administered, and a drain inserted in the scrotum. A drain is contraindicated in the presence of tuberculosis.

7. Gauze pressure dressings and a scrotal support are applied once the patient has been cleansed of prep solution. A hole may be made in the supporter for easy access to the penis for voiding purposes.

SPERMATOCELECTOMY

Description. Spermatocelectomy is removal of a cystic collection of spermatozoa usually located in the caput region of the epididymis or rete testis. The procedure may be performed satisfactorily in the outpatient setting with local anesthesia with or without sedation.

Indications. A spermatocele, a lobulated intrascrotal cystic mass, often multilocular, attached to the superior head of the epididymis, is usually caused by an obstruction of the tubular system that conveys the sperm. This is a not infrequent complication after vasectomy that does not present immediately. Unremitting pain or discomfort caused by increasing size of the spermatocele is the only valid indication for surgery.

Perioperative risks. Risks are as for epididymectomy as well as possible loss of fertility if the epididymis is transected. It has been reported that as many as 50% of patients undergoing spermatocelectomy have had a deterioration in spermatogenesis postoperatively. It is recommended that a preoperative semen analysis be performed for those concerned about maintaining fertility.

Equipment and instrumentation
Refer to epididymectomy.

Procedural Steps

The patient is positioned and prepared as described under hydrocelectomy.

1. After adequate instillation of local anesthetic at the base of the scrotum, the scrotum is held snugly, and its contents are forced against the skin. The mass is directly approached through a transverse scrotal incision

2. Allis clamps are placed on the skin and dartos layers as for hydrocelectomy. The tunica vaginalis is usually not incised. The cystic structure is dissected free by shelling it out to the thick

POSTOPERATIVE

Nursing Care and Discharge Planning for Epididymectomy or Spermatocelectomy

1. Persistent postoperative bleeding with interstitial fluid collections or hematoma is common. A drain may need to be inserted postoperatively, but most hematomas will eventually be resorbed.
2. Ecchymosis and swelling is common. The surgeon should be contacted if swelling continues to increase beyond 3 days, or if there is fever, increased warmth or redness, purulent drainage, excessive drainage or bleeding, or unremitting pain.
3. Medications should be taken as directed: antibiotics until gone, pain medications before onset of discomfort and reduced over time as pain level decreases, stool softener daily if a narcotic is ordered.
4. Apply ice to scrotum for 48 hours to reduce swelling, bleeding, and pain.
5. Avoid strenuous activity until pain free. Resume other activity as tolerated.
6. Wear scrotal support until swelling has subsided. If supporter has been cut for voiding purposes, the patient should be instructed to ensure that the penis is confined and protected to avoid trauma from friction and possible edema.
7. Shower first postoperative day: pat area dry; apply clean dressings. Keep wound clean and dry.
8. Exercise precautions if taking narcotics: do not drive, drink alcohol, or operate machinery.
9. Avoid aspirin and nonsteroidal antiinflammatory agents as directed by physician.
10. Resume diet as tolerated, maintaining adequate fluid intake.

base where it joins the epididymis. Bleeding is controlled with electrocoagulation or suture ligatures. Small epididymal vessels are fulgurated.

3. The areolar tissue is bluntly dissected with a gauze-covered finger or elevated and sharply dissected with scissors.

CONSIDERATIONS In some situations it may be necessary to open the spermatocele and allow approximately two thirds of the fluid to escape. A mosquito hemostat is employed to close the defect while dissection proceeds.

4. The spermatocele is ligated with 3-0 absorbable ties and divided at its attachment to the epididymis, ensuring hemostasis.

CONSIDERATIONS The base of a spermatocele is attached to the superior head of the epididymis. The base should be located and ligated to prevent local extravasation of sperm with resultant granuloma formation and to prevent recurrence. Small, curved arterial or right angle clamps are helpful.

5. The dartos is closed with 3-0 absorbable sutures in a figure-of-eight pattern. The skin is closed with an interrupted or continuous subcuticular stitch of 4-0 absorbable suture. Pressure dressings and a scrotal supporter or mesh underwear are applied.

VARICOCELECTOMY

Description. A varicocelectomy is the high ligation of the gonadal veins of the testes. The three open approaches for varicocelectomy are inguinal-subinguinal, retroperitoneal, and scrotal. Local anesthesia with sedation is frequently adequate for the inguinal or scrotal approach. The retroperitoneal approach requires regional or general anesthesia. The procedure may be easily performed in an outpatient setting.

Indications. Varicocelectomy is done to reduce venous backflow of blood into the venous plexus around the testes and therefore improve spermatogenesis. This condition has generally been considered more common on the left side where the gonadal vein unites retroperitoneally at a 90-degree angle with the renal vein and is under greater backpressure. The gonadal veins do not have valves to prevent retrograde blood flow. It is the increased heat of blood from the core of the body that apparently interferes with normal spermatogenesis. At the level of the scrotum, the pampiniform plexus of the spermatic cord becomes tortuous and engorged resembling a bag of worms. Progressive duration-dependent injury to the seminiferous epithelium results.

In 1889 Bennett provided one of the best descriptions of a varicocele as "a condition of the veins of the spermatic cord, of congenital origin, resulting in or associated with a deficient development or functional imperfection of the corresponding testis in the majority of cases."[27]

When surgery for this condition was devised 70 years ago, the veins of the pampiniform plexus were ligated and divided individually. Laparoscopic and microscopic varicocelectomy are variations to the standard open technique, and microscopic varicocelectomy may be the preferred method. Varicocele occurs in 10% to 15% of the general population and is considered a contributor in male factor infertility. Among infertile males, approximately one third are found to have varicoceles.

More recently sophisticated diagnostic techniques have revealed incompetence of the right spermatic vein in as many as 38% to 66% of infertile men with or without compromise on the left. Failure to appropriately diagnose and treat bilateral varicocele may result in an apparent left-sided failure when collateral channels between the left and right pampiniform plexis communicate, and fertility is not significantly altered.

Improvements in semen analysis after varicocelectomy range from 60% to 80%. Pregnancy rates that vary from 20% to 60% have been reported. Success of the intervention is related to the size of the varicocele and the age of patient. Generally the larger the varicocele and the younger the patient, the greater the improvement.

Perioperative risks. Complications related to varicocelectomy include hydrocele formation caused by lymphatic obstruction (7%), testicular atrophy caused by testicular artery damage or ligation, azoospermia, ilioinguinal nerve injury with sensory loss, epididymitis, infection, hemorrhage, hematoma, testicular injury, injury to the vas deferens, and recurrence caused by collateral or cremasteric vessels (9%, inguinal approach). The usual anesthetic risks apply in relation to the anesthesia of choice and the individual patient.

Equipment and instrumentation
Refer to hydrocelectomy in addition to:
Right-angle hemostats, 5 and 7 inches
Deaver retractors, narrow
Vascular forceps
Tenotomy scissors
Operative loupes
Doppler, portable scanner
Vascular transducer
Bipolar forceps
Vessel loops
Kittner dissectors
Syringe, 10 ml Luer-Lok
Papaverine, 80 mg
Sterile 0.9% IV saline, 60 ml

Procedural Steps

The patient is placed in the supine position and prepared as for hydrocelectomy.

Inguinal Approach (Modified Ivanissevich)

1. The incision may be made through a transverse or oblique inguinal incision over the external inguinal ring, with the medial edge about 2 finger breadths above the pubic symphysis at the lateral scrotal edge. A Weitlaner retractor is inserted.

CONSIDERATIONS The external inguinal ring is located by invaginating the scrotal skin.

2. Scarpa's fascia is bluntly divided, and the external oblique aponeurosis is incised with care taken to avoid injury to the

ilioinguinal nerve. Scissors are passed down to the external ring and rotated 90 degrees to create a groove between the blades. The fascia is incised along this groove from the external ring to the internal ring.

3. The spermatic cord is identified and mobilized at the level of the pubic tubercle by passing a Penrose drain beneath the cord and elevating it. The ilioinguinal nerve is retracted along with the cord.

4. The spermatic artery is identified and isolated with a vessel loop. The abnormal dilated veins in the inguinal canal are clamped and ligated with absorbable suture, and the redundant portions are excised. Small venous channels are coagulated with a bipolar cautery.

5. The vas deferens, along with its vasculature, is identified and preserved.

6. The three branches of the spermatic vein surrounding the spermatic artery are carefully dissected from the artery and the lymphatics for 2 to 3 cm in each direction.

CONSIDERATIONS Use of a vascular transducer and topical papaverine aids in preservation of the spermatic artery (papaverine will cause arterial dilation and increased pulsation).

7. Each branch is doubly clamped and ligated with 3-0 absorbable ties. The patient is placed in reverse Trendelenburg position to assist in identification of the veins.

8. The cord is elevated, and the external cremasteric veins are located and ligated.

9. The external oblique is closed with a continuous 2-0 absorbable suture, and the subcutaneous layer is closed with interrupted 3-0 absorbable suture.

10. The skin is closed with 4-0 absorbable suture in a subcuticular fashion. Local anesthetic infiltration at the end of the procedure helps to decrease the need for pain management. A small gauze dressing covers the wound. Fluffs and scrotal support are applied.

Retroperitoneal Approach *(Modified Palomo)*

1. A transverse abdominal incision is made medial to the anterior superior iliac spine at the level of the internal ring.

2. The external oblique fascia is incised, and then the internal oblique muscle is bluntly separated with a curved hemostat and retracted. The transversalis fascia is incised.

3. The retroperitoneal space is entered about 5 to 6 cm above and medial to the inguinal ligament.

4. The dilated internal spermatic vein is exposed where it exits the inguinal canal, dissected free of the spermatic artery and lymphatics, ligated into three branches, and divided.

CONSIDERATIONS It may be necessary to skeletonize the spermatic cord to visualize the artery. Topical papaverine and placing the patient in reverse Trendelenburg position will also help to identify the artery and vein.

5. Dissection continues toward the renal vein to isolate and eliminate collateral vessels.

CONSIDERATIONS Some believe that retroperitoneal ligation of the internal spermatic vein

reduces the number of veins contributing to the varicocele and lowers the risk of recurrence; others disagree with this theory. This approach has advantages for patients with previous inguinal surgery, minimizing potential injury to the testicular artery and ilioinguinal nerve. Identification and ligation of the external cremasteric veins is not possible, however.

5. Closure is done in layers with 2-0, 3-0, and 4-0 absorbable sutures for the muscle, fascia, subcutaneous tissue, and skin. A small dressing and scrotal support are applied.

Scrotal Approach

This method of varicocelectomy is not recommended for several reasons:

- Time consuming because of the complex network of the pampiniform plexus in the scrotum.
- Rate of failure high compared to other methods.
- Risk of testicular artery damage and testicular ischemia, as well as other complications, such as hydrocele formation, is higher when compared with other approaches.

POSTOPERATIVE

Nursing Care and Discharge Planning for Varicocelectomy

1. Normal nonstrenuous activity may resume after 2 days as tolerated. If it hurts, don't do it.
2. Strenuous activity should be deferred for 2 to 3 weeks.
3. Scrotal support may assist in decreasing postoperative scrotal edema.
4. Ice application may reduce postoperative scrotal edema.
5. Tortuosity of the vessels may not disappear, but no blood flow is occurring.
6. Ecchymosis is not uncommon. Excessive swelling of the scrotum or incisional site, redness or warmth at the incisional site, purulent or grossly bloody discharge from the wound, fever, and unremitting pain should be reported.
7. Absence of hydrocele formation or recurrence are not guaranteed. These are the highest risks.
8. Medications should be taken as directed: antibiotics until gone, pain medication before onset of discomfort and gradually decreased as comfort level rises; stool softener if pain medication is a narcotic substance.
9. Diet may resume as tolerated beginning with clear liquids. Fluid intake should be increased for 3 or 4 days.
10. Aspirin and nonsteroidal antiinflammatory agents should be avoided as directed by the physician.
11. Precautions surrounding narcotic use should be employed if appropriate (no alcohol; do not drive).

TESTICULAR BIOPSY

Description. A biopsy of the testicle is a wedge excision of suspicious tissue for diagnostic confirmation. Special fixatives, such as Bouin's or Zenker's solution, must be available. Formalin destroys the germinal epithelium and should not be used. Local anesthesia with sedation is commonly employed, but regional or general anesthesia may also be chosen. It is not necessary to infiltrate the spermatic cord. The procedure is conducive to the outpatient setting.

Generally, needle biopsy has not been widely accepted for several reasons. The amount of tissue obtained is frequently inadequate for histologic evaluation because too few round tubules are contained in the specimen. Second, the shearing force of the biopsy needle has caused significant trauma to the tissue being sampled as well as a higher incidence of histologic artifacts along the edges of the specimen. Finally, blind-needle biopsy has had a higher incidence of unrecognized vascular and epididymal injury.

Indications. There are two primary indications for a testicular biopsy. Men suffering from infertility, who are azoospermatic or oligospermatic with normal or minimally elevated follicle-stimulating hormone (FSH), may be evaluated through this means. Children with leukemia may also be evaluated to determine testicular relapse after chemotherapy. Although the method is controversial, in some circumstances a surgeon may choose to biopsy and evaluate a testicular lesion with a frozen section microscopic exam before standard treatment for testicular carcinoma.

Perioperative risks. Complications include testicular atrophy, hemorrhage, hematoma, inadvertent damage to the epididymis, hematocele, and infection, as well as the normal anesthetic risks previously discussed.

Equipment and instrumentation
Refer to hydrocelectomy in addition to the following:
Zenker's or Bouin's solution
Suture, 5-0 monofilament on cardiovascular needle

Procedural Steps

If required, hair may be removed from the scrotum, which is then aseptically cleansed. The patient is in the supine position and prepared as described under hydrocelectomy.

1. The testis is held firmly on its posterior aspect from the external scrotal surface. This causes the skin on the anterior aspect to stretch tightly over the incisional site, forcing the epididymis to remain posterior and allowing the scrotal skin to part without retraction.

2. The skin and dartos layer is infiltrated with local anesthetic for a distance of 3 cm. A 1 to 2 cm transverse incision is quickly made through the skin, dartos, and tunica vaginalis, with care taken to avoid injury to the epididymis. Hemostasis is achieved.

CONSIDERATIONS As the tunica vaginalis is incised, there should be a normal efflux of clear fluid. Absorbable 4-0 stay sutures may be placed in the tunica vaginalis.

3. The tunica albuginea is incised transversely for 4 to 7 mm, allowing for extrusion of a bead-sized portion of the testicular tubules.

CONSIDERATIONS Towels may be placed around the testis before opening the tunica albuginea and excising the tissue for biopsy.

4. A small ellipse of the tubules is resected with a scalpel in a shaving action with no-touch technique or with a small sharp scissors that have been moistened with sterile saline. The testis is held firmly throughout the biopsy.

CONSIDERATIONS Stay sutures of 4-0 absorbable suture or 5-0 monofilament suture may be placed in the tunica albuginea. This allows localization of the biopsy site should it slide from the incisional site. Some practitioners excise the specimen along with a small ellipse of tunica, rather than incising the tunica itself.

5. The specimen is placed in the fixative, and the tunica albuginea is closed with interrupted 4-0 absorbable or 5-0 monofilament suture.

CONSIDERATIONS Failure to close the tunica albuginea is likely to result in hematocele formation.

6. The tunica vaginalis is closed with 4-0 absorbable or 5-0 monofilament suture. Injection of Marcaine 0.5% plain at this point often decreases the need for postoperative analgesia.

7. The dartos and skin are closed as one, or in layers, with 4-0 interrupted absorbable suture.

CONSIDERATIONS Many practitioners will biopsy both testes and explore the epididymis at the same time.

8. Antibiotic ointment, gauze sponges, and fluffed dressings are placed over and around the scrotum. A suspensory support is applied to provide pressure and support.

POSTOPERATIVE

Nursing Care and Discharge Planning for Testicular Biopsy

1. Application of ice for 24 hours reduces edema, pain, and bleeding.
2. Mild oral analgesics will generally manage any postoperative discomfort, particularly if a local anesthetic was infiltrated at the end of the procedure.
3. Dressings may be removed after 24 hours, but scrotal support should be worn until swelling and pain has resolved.
4. Shower on first postoperative day: pat area dry, apply clean dressings, keep area clean and dry.
5. Ecchymosis and swelling is normal. Unresolved bleeding or increased swelling after 2 days should be reported. Hematoma and hematocele are the most frequent postoperative complaints.
6. Patient should report fever, unresolved pain, increased discharge from wound, and excessive warmth, redness, or discoloration.
7. Normal activity may resume after 2 or 3 days.
8. Normal diet may be resumed as tolerated.

TESTICULAR DETORSION

Description. Detorsion of the testicle involves manual manipulation and realignment of the spermatic cord and testis. If vascular flow returns, the testis is anchored in place. If vascular flow has been compromised for 24 to 48 hours, orchidectomy may be necessary. It is common practice to examine the contralateral testis and cord and anchor them in place to prevent future torsion from occurring.

Indications. Torsion causes the right testis to rotate clockwise and the left testis to rotate counterclockwise. Twisting of the vascular pedicle results, causing extreme pain. If the pain subsides, spontaneous detorsion may have occurred, or testicular compromise may have begun. Infarction usually occurs after 4 to 6 hours, but surgery performed within 12 hours has proved successful. After 12 to 24 hours preservation of the testis is still possible but very doubtful beyond this time. Testicular, spermatic cord, appendix testis, or epididymal torsion may be extravaginal or intravaginal in presentation. Intravaginal torsion is generally attributed to the abnormal attachment of the posterior aspect of the testes to the scrotal wall. In this instance the tunica covers the epididymis and testis.

Torsion of the appendices of the testis and epididymis may mimic testicular torsion, as can epididymitis. Careful examination of the involved side may reveal a blue dot under the skin of the testis, and it is the diagnostic sign of torsion of the appendix. Testicular ultrasonography with color flow imaging will be diagnostic in most cases.

This condition is more commonly found in pubescent boys and young adults. These patients generally present on an emergency basis. Surgery must occur as soon as possible, generally within 4 to 6 hours, to prevent histologic changes (infarction) ultimately leading to death and atrophy of the affected testicle. Current practice advises anchoring the testicle if the condition has been discovered within 24 hours, even when it does not appear viable. Interstitial cells may still be functional despite necrosis of the seminiferous tubules. Emotional support is important because the patient may fear loss of sexuality or disturbances in body image.

Perioperative risks. Complications may include hemorrhage, hematoma, infection, loss of fertility, recurrence, and testicular atrophy. The greatest risk is loss of the testicle when blood supply has been compromised for too long.

Equipment and instrumentation
Refer to hydrocelectomy.

Procedural Steps

1. The scrotum is grasped with the index finger and thumb pressing the testis forward. The cord is infiltrated with local anesthetic where it passes over the pubic symphysis. A transverse scrotal incision is made through the tunica vaginalis.

CONSIDERATIONS The scrotum may be edematous, and the tunica vaginalis may be discolored from the bloody serum contained within. A hydrocele is often present.

2. The tunica vaginalis is incised, the cord untwisted, and the testis wrapped in warm saline sponges. If normal color returns to the testis, interrupted sutures are placed in the severed edge of the tunica to approximate it behind the testicle and prevent a potential hydrocele sac.

CONSIDERATIONS The tunica albuginea may be incised for closer inspection. Excess tunica vaginalis may be trimmed. The testis is frequently preserved if the condition has been present for less than 24 hours, even if normal color does not fully return. If it is completely necrosed, it will generally be excised.

3. The testis is anchored with three nonabsorbable or synthetic 3-0 sutures through the tunica to the scrotal wall or median septum.

4. The contralateral scrotal compartment is always opened, and the other testicle and spermatic cord examined. To prevent a future torsion on the unaffected side, the testis is anchored to its surrounding structures.

5. Closure may be done in two or three layers with 3-0 and 4-0 absorbable interrupted sutures. A drain is often inserted in the dependent scrotum and loosely sutured to the scrotal skin. The incision may be sealed with a liquid dressing (collodion).

6. A support dressing of gauze sponges, fluffs, and a scrotal supporter is applied.

POSTOPERATIVE

Nursing Care and Discharge Planning for Testicular Detorsion

1. Ice application for 24 hours helps reduce swelling, bleeding, hematoma formation, and pain.
2. Strenuous activity should be eliminated for 2 to 4 weeks. Other activity may resume as tolerated, usually within 2 to 5 days.
3. Medications should be taken as directed: antibiotics until gone; pain medication before the onset of discomfort and decreased over time, stool softeners if a narcotic has been ordered.
4. Precautions surrounding antibiotics and narcotics should be exercised as indicated (avoid alcohol, driving, operating machinery). Report any medication reaction: rash, itching, nausea.
5. Diet may resume as tolerated beginning with clear liquids. Increase fluid intake for 2 or 3 days.
6. Wear scrotal support until pain free and swelling is gone.
7. Report any fever, excessive swelling, bleeding, excessive discoloration, redness, warmth, or purulent discharge. Ecchymosis and edema will occur postoperatively but should not increase after 2 to 3 days.
8. Shower on first postoperative day: pat area dry; apply clean dressings. Keep dressings clean and dry.
9. Drain may be removed at 1 week if swelling and hematoma are not pronounced.
10. Avoid aspirin and nonsteroidal anti-inflammatory agents as instructed by physician.

ORCHIECTOMY

Description. Orchiectomy (orchidectomy) is the removal of the testis or testes. Removal of both testes is castration. With bilateral orchiectomy the patient is rendered sterile and deficient of testosterone (the hormone responsible for secondary sexual characteristics and potency).

Radical inguinal orchiectomy is the usual approach for treatment of testicular cancer. Vascular and lymphatic channels are more easily controlled through an inguinal intervention. The scrotal approach is most commonly employed for testicular infarction, infection, trauma, or torsion, and when seeking hormonal control for prostate cancer. A transscrotal intracapsular orchiectomy is frequently chosen for the control of prostate cancer.

This procedure has recently been approached through laparoscopic techniques, usually with laparoscopic herniorrhaphy.

Indications. Bilateral orchiectomy is usually performed for the control of symptomatic metastatic carcinoma of the prostate gland. A unilateral orchiectomy may be indicated in cases of testicular cancer, trauma, torsion, intractable pain, or infection. This operation requires particular attention to acquiring informed consent for surgery because of potential legal implications.

Perioperative risks. Complications surrounding orchiectomy include hemorrhage, hematoma, infection, and wound rupture. Anesthetic risks include cardiac dysrhythmias from traction on the spermatic cord, hypothermia, third-space losses, and those general risks previously discussed.

Equipment and instrumentation
Refer to hydrocelectomy in addition to the following:
Statinsky clamps, 2, *or*
Rubber shod clamps, 2
Ties, 0, 2-0, and 3-0 absorbable synthetic
Ties, 0 and 2-0 nonabsorbable
Suture, 0 and 2-0 nonabsorbable or synthetic on SH-1 needle
Suture, 2-0 absorbable on SH-1 needle

Procedural Steps

The patient is placed in the supine position, prepped, and draped. Placing a sterile cloth towel beneath the scrotum, before squaring off with four towels, often allows adequate elevation of the scrotal contents.

Scrotal Approach

Simple orchiectomy
1. The testis is secured between the thumb and index finger of one hand, and the overlying skin is thinned. Local anesthetic is infiltrated into the spermatic cord and the scrotal skin.

2. The skin incision is made transversely over the anterolateral surface of the midportion of the scrotum and carried through the subcutaneous and fascial layers into the tunica vaginalis, exposing the testicle.

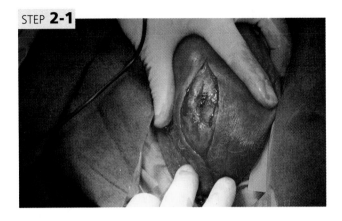

STEP 2-1

CONSIDERATIONS A long transverse incision may be made to expose both testes.

3. Bleeding vessels are clamped and tied with 3-0 synthetic absorbable suture or cauterized. The scrotal tissue is bluntly dissected with a sponge, and the testis and tunica vaginalis are displaced from the scrotum.

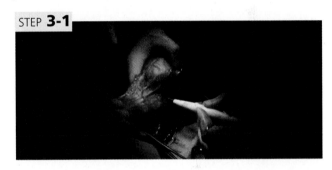

STEP 3-1

CONSIDERATIONS Some practitioners open the tunica vaginalis and extrude the testicle.

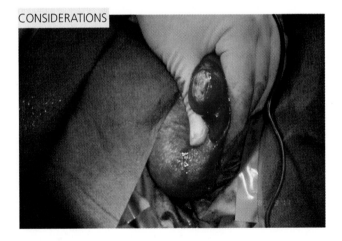

CONSIDERATIONS

4. The cord is dissected free, and the vas is separately ligated with a 2-0 absorbable tie.

CONSIDERATIONS Some practitioners will spare the epididymis by dissecting the testis free of the epididymis and ligating small vessels as they enter the hilum of the testis. The epididymis is sutured to itself with 3-0 figure-of-eight sutures, and a drain is placed in the dependent scrotum.

5. The spermatic cord is divided into two or three vascular bundles. Each vascular bundle is doubly clamped, cut, and ligated with 0 or 2-0 synthetic absorbable or nonabsorbable suture ligatures and then with a proximal free 0 or 2-0 synthetic absorbable or nonabsorbable tie.

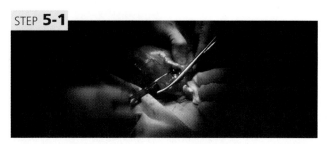

STEP **5-1**

Dividing spermatic structures.

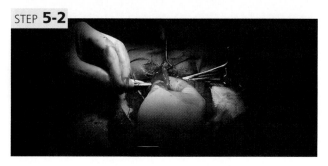

STEP **5-2**

Dividing spermatic structures.

CONSIDERATIONS If the vessels slip from the clamps, the incision should be extended into the groin and the inguinal canal opened.

6. The testis is removed.

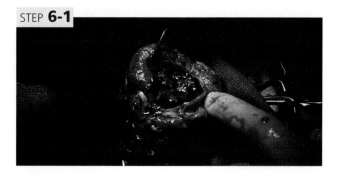

STEP **6-1**

7. Hemostasis is established with electrocoagulation or absorbable ties and sutures. A small Penrose drain may be placed in the empty hemiscrotum.

8. The scrotum is closed in two layers with 3-0 absorbable suture and 4-0 absorbable suture in a continuous or interrupted fashion.

9. Compression dressings of gauze sponges ("fluffs") are applied, followed by an athletic supporter or mesh underwear.

Intracapsular (subcapsular) orchiectomy

1. After exposure as described in steps 1 to 3 for simple orchiectomy, the tunica albuginea is incised along the entire length of the testis.

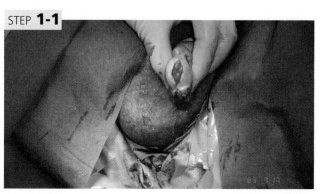

STEP **1-1**

2. The edges of the tunica are grasped with hemostats on three sides, and the tunica is everted.

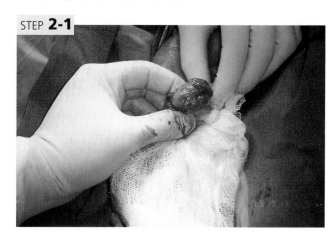

STEP **2-1**

With a gauze-covered finger the tubules are bluntly freed from the inner side and swept toward the center. Tunical vessels are fulgurated.

3. The hilum of the testis is ligated with 2-0 absorbable suture and divided with electrofulguration of the base to destroy interstitial cells.

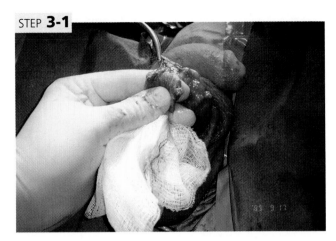

STEP **3-1**

4. The tunica is closed with a continuous 3-0 absorbable suture.

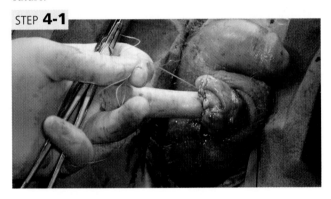

STEP **4-1**

The dartos and skin are closed individually with 3-0 and 4-0 absorbable sutures respectively. Support dressings are applied.

Inguinal Approach

Radical inguinal orchiectomy

1. The skin incision is begun just above the internal inguinal ring (above and parallel to the inguinal ligament), extending downward and inward over the inguinal canal to the external inguinal ring. Vessels are ligated with 3-0 absorbable ties.

2. The external oblique fascia is incised, and the spermatic cord is dissected free, cross-clamped, and divided into vascular bundles above the level of the pubic tubercle.

CONSIDERATIONS The ilioinguinal nerve is identified and preserved.

3. The lateral and medial edges of the external oblique are grasped. Gentle forward traction is applied to the cord, which is dissected from its bed inferiorly to expose the pubic tubercle and medially to expose all cord structures. A Penrose drain encircles the cord, its structures, and the cremaster muscle, near the inguinal ring.

4. The cord is lifted with the Penrose drain and freed to the internal inguinal ring. Perforating cremasteric vessels are ligated and divided.

5. The tunica vaginalis may be opened and the vas deferens ligated separately from the spermatic cord. This allows for possible future lymphadenectomy without needing to later mobilize the vas segment.

6. To prevent proximal drainage of tumor cells, the Penrose drain is adjusted to surround the cord approximately 1 inch below the internal inguinal ring and tightened. A clamp is applied to the Penrose drain for a tourniquet effect.

CONSIDERATIONS Noncrushing shodded clamps, or Statinsky clamps, may be utilized instead.

7. The testis is everted into the wound from the scrotum. The gubernacular attachments are clamped, divided, and ligated with 2-0 absorbable ligatures. The testis is excised along with the epididymis and the tunica vaginalis.

8. The cord is doubly clamped and ligated at the internal inguinal ring above the tourniquet with 0 or 2-0 nonabsorbable or synthetic absorbable sutures. The cord should lie retroperitoneally for identification during lymph node dissection.

CONSIDERATIONS Ligatures are cut long for identification at node dissection.

9. Hemostasis is established with electrocoagulation or absorbable ties and sutures. A small Penrose drain may be placed in the empty hemiscrotum and loosely sutured to the scrotal skin.

10. The conjoined tendon is sutured to the edge of the inguinal ligament. The external oblique fascia is imbricated and reapproximated with 2-0 absorbable interrupted or continuous sutures.

POSTOPERATIVE

Nursing Care and Discharge Planning for Orchiectomy

1. The patient should be assessed for fluid and electrolyte balance and cardiac stability. Electrocardiogram (ECG) changes should be immediately reported.
2. An enlarging scrotal hematoma should be reported immediately. This may indicate that a spermatic vessel is not secured and may require reexploration.
3. Report any wound separation, increased warmth or swelling, increased discoloration (some ecchymosis is normal), fever, excessive discharge, unremitting pain, or bleeding.
4. Ice application for 24 hours will assist in pain management, reduction of swelling, and hemostasis of scrotal cavity.
5. The drain may be removed after 2 or 3 days if the wound appears secure.
6. Scrotal support should be worn until swelling is gone.
7. Medications should be taken as ordered: antibiotics until gone; pain medications before onset of discomfort and reduced as tolerance increases; stool softener if a narcotic has been ordered. Comply with restrictions imposed by medication (alcohol, driving, etc.) and report any adverse effects of medication (itching, rash, nausea).
8. Avoid aspirin and nonsteroidal antiinflammatory agents as directed by physician.
9. Avoid strenuous activity for 2 to 3 weeks. Resume other activity as tolerated, usually in 2 or 3 days.
10. Resume diet as tolerated beginning with clear liquids.

11. Subcutaneous tissue, including Scarpa's fascia, is closed with 3-0 absorbable sutures in an interrupted or continuous fashion.

12. The skin is reapproximated with surgical staples or 4-0 subcuticular suture.

13. Compression dressings of gauze sponges ("fluffs") are applied, followed by an athletic supporter or mesh underwear.

CIRCUMCISION

Description. Circumcision is the excision of the foreskin (prepuce) of the glans penis. This is an ideal intervention for an outpatient setting.

Older children require general anesthesia. Adults may be offered the option of local, spinal, or general anesthesia. For older patients there is no need for the circumcision clamp, and only a plastic instrument set is used. Petrolatum gauze should be available to dress the area.

Indications. Circumcision is performed for the relief of phimosis, a condition in which the orifice of the prepuce is stenosed, or too narrow to permit easy retraction behind the glans. Another condition often requiring circumcision is balanoposthitis. This results in an inflamed glans and mucous membrane with purulent discharge. Circumcision may also be done to prevent recurrent paraphimosis, a condition in which the prepuce cannot be reduced easily from a retracted position. Associated abnormal diseases such as diabetes must be ruled out or controlled.

Circumcision may be done prophylactically in infancy or performed for religious reasons, as required in specific faiths. Provision should be made in a hospital to observe the religious needs and preferences of the parents.

Perioperative risks. The greatest risk with circumcision is to leave an inappropriate amount of foreskin for proper repair. If too much skin is left, it may reepithelialize or phimosis may occur. If too much inner preputial membrane remains, the penis may become buried. Additional risks include hemorrhage, skin necrosis, hematoma, infection, edema, injury to the glans penis with necrosis, chordee caused by delayed ventral healing, urethral penetration, urinary retention from dressings that are too constricting, injury to the dorsal penile nerves, and the anesthetic risks previously discussed.

Equipment and instrumentation
Refer to hydrocelectomy in addition to the following:
Bipolar forceps
Probe
Petrolatum gauze
Roller gauze such as Kling

Procedural Steps

1. The site of the corona of the glans is marked on the unretracted dorsal skin of the prepuce, and the site of the frenulum is marked on the ventral skin with a V.

PREOPERATIVE

Nursing Care and Teaching Considerations for Circumcision or Urethral Meatotomy

1. Ensure that associated infection has been treated preoperatively. If antibiotics are indicated, ensure they have been administered.
2. Incorporate general nursing diagnoses.
3. Review patient record for reports of preoperative studies: PT, PTT, complete blood count (CBC), urine culture. If indicated by patient age or medical status: chest x-ray, electrocardiogram (ECG), serum electrolytes, cardiac enzymes.
4. Check equipment, instrumentation, and sterile packages for function and integrity.
5. Assess patient for physical limitations, range of motion, skin integrity, allergies, other medical conditions (diabetes, asthma, chronic obstructive pulmonary disease [COPD]), cardiopulmonary status, peripheral vascular circulation, presence of implants.
6. Assess patient for comprehension of planned intervention and anxiety level.
7. Check medications for dosage and expiration dates.
8. Position patient under guidance of anesthetist and surgeon. Ensure that IV lines are unrestricted. Foley catheter and alternating compression stockings are generally not indicated.
9. Prep and drape patient according to AORN standards. Protect patient from pooling of solutions.
10. Document assessment findings and nursing interventions

STEP **1-1**

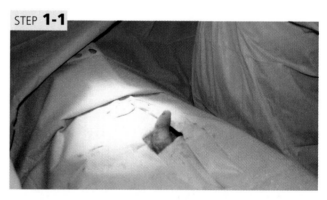

Patient with paraphimosis draped for circumcision.

STEP **1-2**

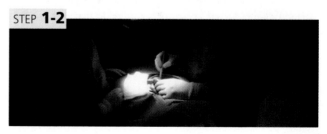

Marking incision lines.

2. Incision is made along the marks proximally and distally toward the coronal margin. Approximately 5 cm of coronal mucosa is left intact.

STEP **2-1**

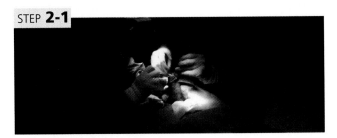

CONSIDERATIONS Placing a straight hemostat on the line of incision helps reduce incisional bleeding by crushing the small vessels present.

3. The prepuce is retracted using a mosquito clamp and traction with a gauze-covered finger and thumb, freeing it from the glans.

CONSIDERATIONS If the prepuce is adherent, a probe or hemostat may be used to break up adhesions.

4. Smegma is cleared, and the second incision is marked proximal to the sulcus across the base of the frenulum.

5. The dorsal skin is sharply divided with scissors; the edges are elevated and freed from the dartos fascia.

STEP **5-1**

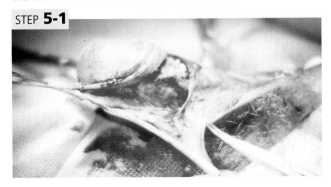

Bleeders are fulgurated with bipolar cautery or tied with 4-0 absorbable ligatures.

CONSIDERATIONS Alternatively the redundant skin may be undermined between the circumferential incisions and removed as a complete cuff.

CONSIDERATIONS

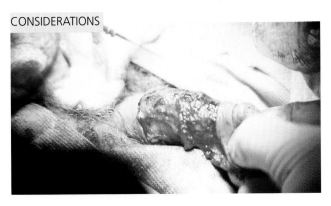

Before closure, the area may be cleansed with an appropriate antiseptic solution such as betadine or Hibiclens.

6. The raw edges of the skin incision are approximated to a coronal cuff of mucosal prepuce with 3-0 or 4-0 absorbable sutures on plastic cutting needles.

STEP **6-1**

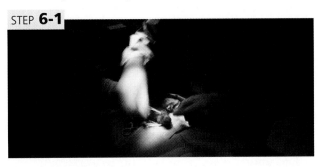

CONSIDERATIONS Sutures are placed through the skin of the shaft and corona in four quadrants and left long to serve as tractors.

CONSIDERATIONS

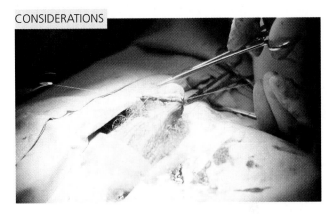

Two stitches are placed between each of the initial four, and two stitches are placed to approximate the V of the frenulum.

7. The tractor sutures are shortened, and the wound is dressed with petrolatum gauze. Roller gauze may be loosely wrapped around the Vaseline gauze.

STEP **7-1**

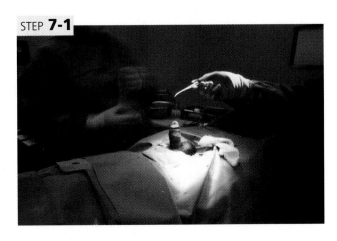

URETHRAL MEATOTOMY

Description. Urethral meatotomy is an incisional enlargement of the external urethral meatus. In more severe cases, a meatoplasty may be necessary.

Indications. To relieve congenital or acquired stenosis or stricture at the external meatus. Difficulty in directing the urinary stream and urinary infrequency are the chief presenting complaints. Dysuria and frequency may also be seen if a urinary tract infection exists. This condition is rarely seen in females. Some strictures of long duration involve the entire urethra necessitating urethroplasty, glanuloplasty, meatoplasty, or any combination of the three.

Perioperative risks. The primary risks are recurrence and continued inability to properly direct the urinary stream.

Equipment and instrumentation
Equipment
Safety strap
Head cradle
Stirrups
Positioning pads
Instruments
Crile hemostat, straight
Mosquito hemostat, curved, 4
Knife handle, #3
Needle holder, 5 inches
Suture scissors
Miscellaneous supplies
Basic pack
Fenestrated sheet *or*
Lithotomy sheet
Sterile gowns
Sterile gloves
Knife blade, #15
Ties, 4-0 absorbable
Suture, 4-0 absorbable on P-3 or PS-3 needle
Syringe, 10 ml finger control
Hypodermic needle, #30 gauge $1/2$ inch
Lidocaine 1%
Vaseline gauze *or*
Antibiotic ointment
Sterile water, 500 ml
Antiseptic prep solution
Absorbent prep drape

Procedural Steps

The patient is placed in the supine position. Local anesthesia is instilled through the meatus and directed at the frenulum. Some surgeons may prefer the lithotomy position.

1. A straight hemostat is placed on the ventral surface of the meatus.

2. An incision is made along the ventrum with sharp scissors or a small knife blade creating a V-shaped defect. A 30 Fr urethral dilator is used to calibrate the opening.

3. Bleeding vessels are clamped and fulgurated.

4. The mucosal layer is sutured to the skin with 4-0 absorbable sutures.

5. A dressing of petrolatum gauze or antibiotic ointment is applied.

CONSIDERATIONS A dorsal slit may be done before endoscopic instrumentation with a small knife blade. The knife is inserted cutting side up into the meatus to incise the roof of the fossa navicularis. This is repeated until a 30 Fr urethral dilator may be passed with ease.

POSTOPERATIVE

Nursing Care and Discharge Planning for Circumcision/Urtethral Meatotomy

1. Darkening of the glans penis should be reported immediately, and the dressings loosened or removed.
2. Application of ice for 24 hours helps reduce swelling and pain.
3. A scrotal support that holds the penis securely may help reduce pain during healing.
4. Normal acitivity may be resumed in 2 or 3 days as tolerated.
5. Aspirin and nonsteroidal antiinflammatory agents should be avoided as instructed by the physician.
6. Wound separation, excessive bleeding, increased warmth or redness, fever, and purulent discharge should be reported.
7. Pain may generally be managed with a mild oral analgesic. If it has a narcotic base, a stool softener should be used daily.
8. Burning on urination may occur. If it does not resolve in 2 to 3 days, medication may be ordered to relieve the discomfort.
9. Diet may be resumed as tolerated. Fluid intake should be increased for 2 to 3 days.

EXCISION OF URETHRAL CARUNCLE

Description. Excision of an urethral caruncle entails the removal of papillary or sessile tumors from the urethra. Local anesthesia with or without sedation is usually sufficient for a pain-free intervention in an outpatient setting.

Indications. A urethral caruncle or inflammatory prolapse of the external urinary meatus presenting in a female patient. It is important to differentiate between a urethral caruncle and a carcinoma. Less commonly, these have occurred in men.

Perioperative risks. Actual complications with this procedure have been minimal and related more to the patient's medical condition rather than to the intervention. Potential risks include infection, meatal stricture, dysuria, urgency, frequency, hematuria, reaction to local anesthesia, positional injury, wound hemorrhage, and hematoma.

Equipment and instrumentation
Equipment
Electrosurgery unit
Stirrups
Stool
Headlight
Safety strap
Head cradle

Positioning pads
Arm boards, padded
Fiberoptic light source
Instruments
Plastic instrument set
Flexible cystoscope
Miscellaneous supplies
Lithotomy pack *or*
Cystoscopy pack
Sterile gowns
Sterile gloves
Lubricating jelly
Knife blade, #15
Electrosurgery pencil, hand control
Electrosurgery needle tip
Gauze sponges
Kittner dissectors
Sterile applicators
Suture, 4-0 absorbable on P3 or PS-3 needle
Syringe, 10 ml finger control
Syringe, 10 ml Luer-Lok
Hypodermic needle, #27 gauge $1^1/_4$ inches
Local anesthetic of choice (lidocaine or bupivacaine)
Sterile water, 500 ml
Sterile saline, 500 ml
Antibiotic ointment
Foley catheter, #14 Fr, 5 cc balloon
Urine drainage bag
Antiseptic prep solution
Absorbent prep drape
Extra supplies for cystoscopy
Sterile water for irrigant, 1000 ml
Cystoscopy irrigation tubing

PREOPERATIVE

Nursing Care and Teaching Considerations for Urethral Caruncle

1. Review patient record for reports of pertinent studies such as urine culture, PT, PTT, CBC, ECG, chest x-ray, urethrogram, and cystogram.
2. Assess patient for physical, mental, and medical status, such as range of motion, presence of implants, COPD, cardiac history, allergies, anxiety, comprehension level, and physical impairments.
3. Discuss intraoperative course and postoperative expectations; explain and answer questions as necessary. For example, burning, urgency, frequency, and moderate hematuria are to be expected for a few days.
4. Check equipment, sterile supplies, and instrumentation for proper function and integrity.
5. Check medications for proper dosage and expiration dates.
6. Ensure adequate positioning devices are available for patient comfort and safety.
7. Document assessment findings and nursing interventions

Procedural Steps

1. The patient is placed in the lithotomy position. The area is prepped and draped. A urethral catheter of an appropriate size may be required if the distal urethral prolapse is severe.

CONSIDERATIONS Flexible cystoscopy may be performed before or after the intervention, or at both times.

2. The tumor is exposed and excised within a wedge of ventral urethral tissue with a small, fine-tipped, Metzenbaum or plastic scissors. Figure-of-eight 4-0 absorbable sutures are placed at the edge of the incision and are usually sufficient to achieve good hemostasis.

3. Antibiotic ointment may be applied. A Foley catheter assists hemostasis.

POSTOPERATIVE

Nursing Care and Discharge Planning for Urethral Caruncle

1. The Foley catheter assists hemostasis and is removed after 1 or 2 days.
2. Transient episodes of stress incontinence may occur. These will diminish with healing.
3. Urethral irritation may occur. Sitz baths and oral urinary analgesia should be provided.
4. Patient may be discharged the same day.
5. Fluids should be increased for 2 to 3 days to assist voiding and healing.
6. Diet may resume as tolerated.
7. Activity may resume as tolerated.

PENILE IMPLANT

Description. Insertion of a penile implant may be approached through a penoscrotal, suprapubic, or infrapubic incision. Penoscrotal, the currently favored approach, will be described. Regional or general anesthesia is generally required, though local infiltration has been met with some success. The patient is placed in either the supine or the lithotomy position. Routine skin prepping and draping are carried out. To prevent urethral injury and potential urinary retention, a 14 Fr Foley catheter may be inserted to allow identification of the urethra intraoperatively. Electrosurgery may be required. Often a penile block is instilled intraoperatively, before the incision, into the corpus cavernosa and the incisional sites. This enables the surgeon to evaluate erectile size and provides postoperative pain management. This also allows for the procedure to be done on an outpatient basis.

A separate sterile Mayo stand or small table covered with a plastic drape is set up for the implants. Cloth or paper may shed lint or fiber particles and should not contact the implant components.

It is advisable to have the implant representative present for the first few procedures until the nursing staff feels comfortable performing the intervention. The representative is a valuable asset to the team by providing instruction, rationale, procedural steps, and solutions to possible concerns or problems.

Indications. A penile prosthesis is implanted for treatment of organic sexual impotence. Sexual impotence may be caused by diabetes mellitus, priapism, Peyronie's disease, penile trauma, pelvic trauma, radical pelvic surgery, neurologic disease (in selected cases), cardiovascular disease, spinal cord injury, medication regimens, alcoholism, hypertension, hormonal deficiency, and idiopathic impotence (in carefully screened patients). The penile implant serves as a stent to enable vaginal penetration for sexual intercourse.

Data has revealed that 1 in 10 men, worldwide, is impotent. At least half of the cases have a physical cause. Most men have tried other avenues before implantation, such as vacuum devices and intracavernosal injection therapy.

Perioperative risks. A disastrous complication to a penile implant is infection of the prosthesis, occurring approximately 3% of the time. Delayed or immediate salvage attempts may be successful depending on the patient condition, degree of infection, and offending organism.

PREOPERATIVE

Nursing Care and Teaching Considerations for Penile Implant

1. The patient will have undergone intensive review that may include general and sexual history, psychologic testing, physical exam with chest x-ray and ECG if indicated, nocturnal penile tumescence monitoring, Doppler penile arterial flow studies (duplex Doppler), cavernosograms, laboratory serum analyses, FSH, luetinizing hormone (LH), testosterone (if libido is low), semen analysis, serum chemistries, prolactin, cardiac enzymes, prostate specific antigen (PSA). Review patient record for reports.
2. Assess patient for comprehension of planned intervention and postoperative expectations. Address anxieties and questions as necessary. Discuss risks of infection, erosion, mechanical failure, alteration or change in size and girth of erection (generally will be reduced).
3. Evaluate patient for skin integrity, presence of infection, range of motion, allergies (iodine), physical limitations, cardiac history, peripheral vascular circulation, presence of implants, past surgeries, pulmonary status, diabetes.
4. Determine if patient performed prophylactic hexachlorophene scrub to perineum daily for 1 week before operation.
5. Check equipment, packaging, and instrumentation for function and integrity.
6. Sales representative should be present until staff feels comfortable performing procedure.
7. Check medications for dosages and expiration dates. Prepare antibiotic irrigant and filling solution for implant.
8. Position patient under guidance of surgeon and anesthetist. Ensure that linen is smooth, IV lines are unrestricted, and padding is applied to pressure areas.
9. Apply alternating compression stockings and patient dispersive pad.
10. Prep and drape patient according to AORN standards. Protect patient from pooling of solutions. Perform 5-minute iodophor scrub to perineum.
11. Document assessment findings and nursing interventions.

Meticulous aseptic technique and careful draping are essential. The sterile team should be double gloved throughout the procedure. Some surgeons coat their hands with povidone-iodine solution just before donning sterile gloves. A 5-minute povidone-iodine scrub of the operative area is critical in reducing skin flora. Intraoperatively and before insertion of the implant components, a prophylactic antibiotic irrigant of bacitracin and kanamycin in normal saline is recommended for the implants and in the insertion sites. Systemic antibiotics may also be required. As with any implant, it is vital to maintain an environment conducive to infection prevention. Traffic in and out of the room should be minimized.

Additional complications include hematoma, implant erosion, implant malfunction, improper placement of implant, damage to implant integrity, hemorrhage, and persistent pain.

Equipment and instrumentation
Equipment
Electrosurgery unit with bipolar ability
Suction unit
Alternating compression unit
Positioning pads
Penile prosthesis of urologist's choice
Instruments
Minor set with fine instruments
Hegar dilators
Furlow inserter
Closing tool
Denis Browne or Lone-Star retractor (optional)
Assembly tool for clamping connectors
Implant sizing rod
Miscellaneous supplies
Connectors of choice
Implant prep kit
Lidocaine, 1%, 50 ml
Normal saline, 0.9%, 150 ml (2) injectable,150 ml
Methylene blue, 1 ml
Papaverine, 2 ml
Marcaine 0.5% or Duranest 1%
Normal saline
Bacitracin, 50,000 U
Kanamycin, 80 mg
Sterile saline, 1000 ml, 2
Sterile water, 1000 ml, 2
Laparotomy pack *or*
Lithotomy pack
Sterile gowns
Sterile gloves, 2 each
Adherent drape towels, 4
Sterile cloth towel
Plastic-coated drape sheet or Mayo cover
Syringe, 60 ml, 3
Syringe, 20 ml
Syringe, 10 ml
Syringe, 10 ml finger control
Hypodermic needle, #25 gauge, 1 1/4 inches
Butterfly needle, 21 gauge
Penrose drain, 1/2 inch

Sterile basins, medium round (2), large round (2-3), graduate, small round, small rectangular

Antiseptic prep solution

Absorbent prep drape

Procedural Steps
Implantation of Noninflatable (Semirigid-malleable) Prosthesis

The patient is placed in the supine position. The operative area should have been shaved in the preoperative area. A 5-minute p-i scrub of the intended operative site is performed, followed by antiseptic prep solution. The patient is draped with one cloth towel beneath the scrotum, four adherent towels around the site (one under the scrotum), and a laparotomy sheet. All scrubbed personnel are double gloved.

A penile block of 1% lidocaine 50 ml: Papaverine 80 mg: 0.9% NS 150 ml: methylene blue 0.5 ml may be administered before the incision. A Penrose drain is placed around the base of the penis and clamped as a tourniquet. The butterfly needle is attached to a 60 ml syringe containing the local anesthetic mixture. The corpora are injected bilaterally. This affords preoperative evaluation of the girth and length of the erect penis and allows for decreased pain immediately postoperatively. Additional local anesthetic, for postoperative pain management, commonly 0.5% Marcaine, may be instilled suprapubically along the intended incision line and subcutaneously after incision. Experience has demonstrated that patients receiving this protocol have exhibited decreased discomfort in the first postoperative day.

1. A midline incision is made from the base of the penis into the scrotum for approximately 3 cm.

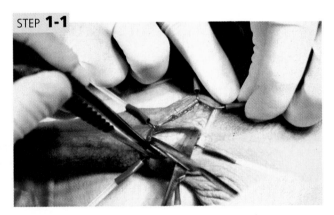

STEP 1-1

(Courtesy American Medical Systems, Minnetonka, Minn.)

Some surgeons may choose a suprapubic or dorsal penile approach.

2. The tunica albuginea is incised for about 2 cm over the most proximal portion of the corpora in a longitudinal manner

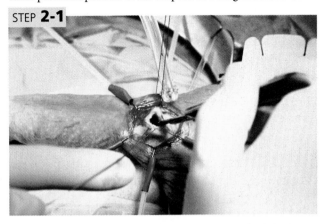

STEP 2-1

(Courtesy American Medical Systems, Minnetonka, Minn.)

and monofilament nonabsorbable stay sutures are placed. The corpora is dilated proximally and distally with 7 to 14 mm Hegar dilators.

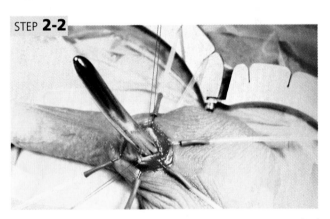

STEP 2-2

Dilating proximally with Hegar dilator. *(Courtesy American Medical Systems, Minnetonka, Minn.)*

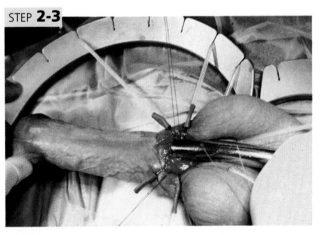

STEP 2-3

Dilating distally with Hegar dilator. *(Courtesy American Medical Systems, Minnetonka, Minn.)*

CONSIDERATIONS Care must be taken not to perforate the urethra. The curve of the dilator should follow the diagonal crus angle downward. When dilating distally, the Hegar dilator is held lateral and dorsal. Dilation is accomplished past the corona to the mid glans.

3. Measurements of the entire corporal length, distal and proximal, are taken with the Furlow inserter or sizing instrument.

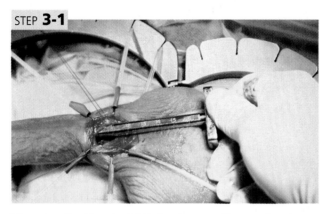

STEP **3-1**

Measuring distal length with Furlow inserter. *(Courtesy American Medical Systems, Minnetonka, Minn.)*

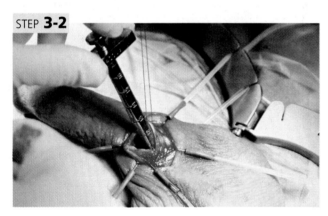

STEP **3-2**

Measuring proximal length with Furlow inserter. *(Courtesy American Medical Systems, Minnetonka, Minn.)*

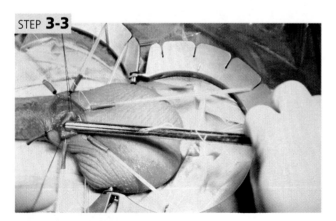

STEP **3-3**

Measuring distal length with sizing instrument. *(Courtesy American Medical Systems, Minnetonka, Minn.)*

CONSIDERATIONS Antibiotic irrigation should be used liberally throughout the procedure: after corporal entry, before and after dilating, before and after measuring, before and after sizing, before insertion of prosthesis, and before and during wound closure.

CONSIDERATIONS

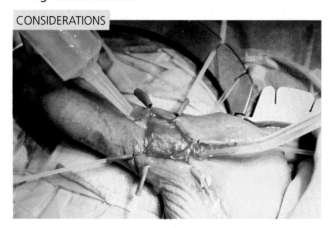

(Courtesy American Medical Systems, Minnetonka, Minn.)

The dilators, measuring and sizing instruments, and implant should be dipped in the solution before insertion as well. This helps reduce the risk of infection and also clears any particulate matter that may be on the items.

If the irrigant within the bulb syringe becomes bloody, it should be evacuated into an empty basin so that the irrigant container is not compromised. The Furlow inserter has a hollow channel that should be flushed with water into the empty basin after each use to clear blood and debris.

4. After placement of the closure sutures, the prosthesis is inserted in the corpora. Proper placement is evident immediately by a change in the configuration of the penis with no buckling of the glans.

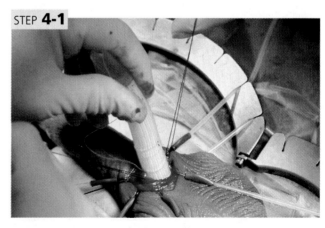

STEP **4-1**

Placing proximal end of implant. *(Courtesy American Medical Systems, Minnnetonka, Minn.)*

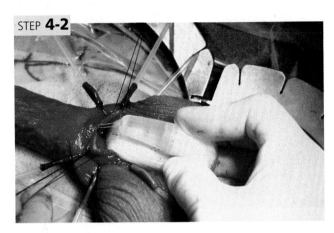

Placing distal end of implant. *(Courtesy American Medical Systems, Minnetonka, Minn.)*

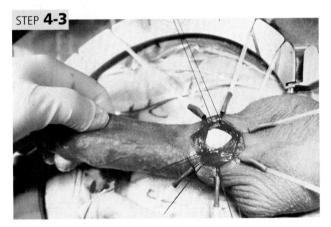

Implant in place. *(Courtesy American Medical Systems, Minnetonka, Minn.)*

CONSIDERATIONS Rear-tip extenders may be placed on the proximal end of the prosthesis to achieve the measured length. With certain implants, the diameter may be reduced by incising the silicone jacket that covers the implant. A vein retractor may prove helpful to lift the glans or distal end of the corpus over the distal tip of the prosthesis once the proximal end has been placed.

5. The tunica albuginea is then closed with the previously placed 2-0 or 3-0 absorbable suture.

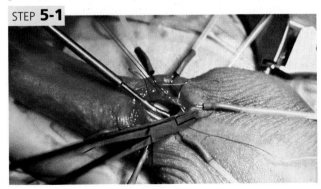

Closing tool protects implant during tunica closure. *(Courtesy American Medical Systems, Minnetonka, Minn.)*

Absorbable sutures of 3-0 or 4-0 are used for skin closure.

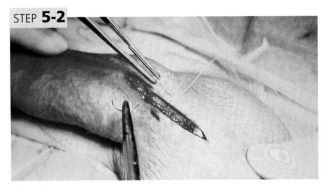

(Courtesy American Medical Systems, Minnetonka, Minn.)

6. Petrolatum gauze or 2-inch roller gauze may be used for the dressing.

7. A Foley catheter is inserted, and the amount and color of urine are noted. Some surgeons divert the urine intraoperatively. Mesh underwear or an athletic supporter may be applied to keep the penis cephalad and protected.

Implantation of Inflatable Prosthesis

The same patient preparation and intraoperative considerations apply as with the noninflatable implant.

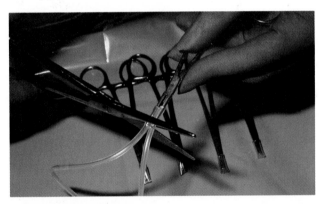

Preparing shodded hemostats. *(Courtesy American Medical Systems, Minnetonka, Minn.)*

1. A midline incision is made from the base of the penis into the scrotum for approximately 3 cm.

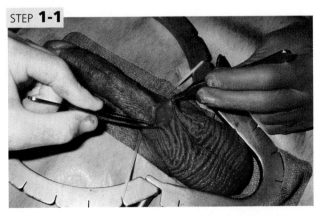

(Courtesy American Medical Systems, Minnetonka, Minn.)

A Foley catheter is inserted to identify and retract the urethra out of the operative field.

2. The tunica albuginea of each corpora is incised in the most proximal portion, and 2-0 or 3-0 nonabsorbable stay sutures are placed.

STEP **2-1**

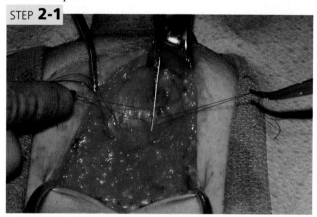

(Courtesy American Medical Systems, Minnetonka, Minn.)

The corpora are dilated distally and proximally with 7 to 14 mm Hegar dilators.

STEP **2-2**

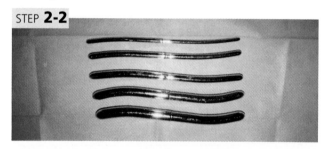

Hegar dilators.

STEP **2-3**

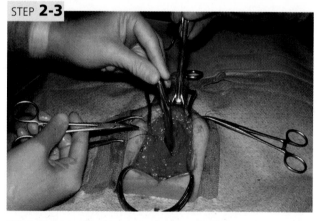

Dilating proximally. *(Courtesy American Medical Systems, Minnetonka, Minn.)*

The Furlow inserter is used for measuring the entire corporal length, proximal and distal.

STEP **2-4**

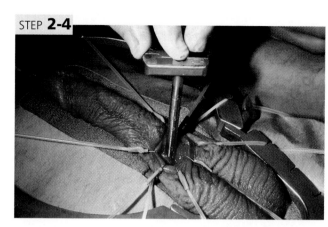

Measuring proximally with Furlow inserter. *(Courtesy American Medical Systems, Minnetonka, Minn.)*

STEP **2-5**

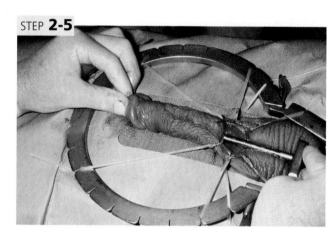

Measuring distally with Furlow inserter. *(Courtesy American Medical Systems, Minnetonka, Minn.)*

3. Corporal sutures of 2-0 absorbable material are placed along the tunica incision, left uncut with needle attached, and tagged.

4. The cylinders are packaged with attached traction sutures at the distal end.

STEP **4-1**

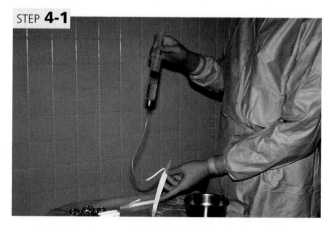

Preparing cylinders. *(Courtesy American Medical Systems, Minnetonka, Minn.)*

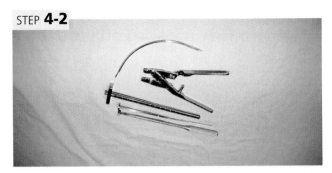

Top to bottom: **tubing passer, assembly tool, Furlow inserter, closing tool.**

These are placed through the eye of a Keith needle and slipped into the groove of the Furlow inserter.

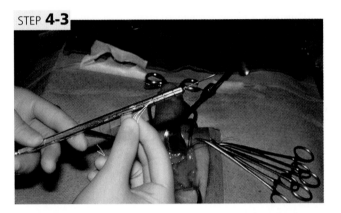

(Courtesy American Medical Systems, Minnetonka, Minn.)

The Furlow inserter is passed up the corporal tunnel, and the plunger is pushed to release the Keith needle, which punctures the glans. The needle is grasped with a Kelly hemostat and pulled through the glans, allowing the cylinders to slide to the channel opening.

5. The Furlow inserter is removed, and the cylinder is inserted and guided to the proper position beneath the glans penis.

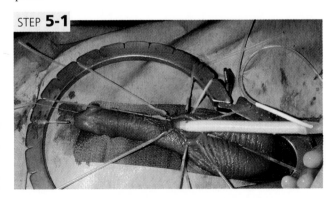

(Courtesy American Medical Systems, Minnetonka, Minn.)

If necessary, rear-tip extenders are added to the proximal cylinder end. The proximal end is positioned in the crus. The procedure is repeated on the other channel.

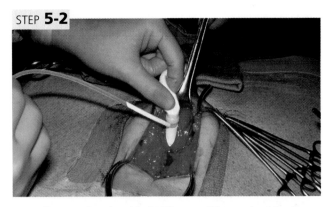

(Courtesy American Medical Systems, Minnetonka, Minn.)

6. The external inguinal ring is palpated, and a path is bluntly created.

7. Dissecting scissors are used to separate the transversalis fascia on the inguinal floor. The area is bluntly enlarged to allow palpation of Cooper's ligament.

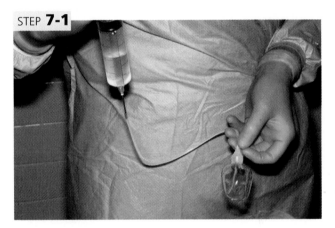

Preparing reservoir. *(Courtesy American Medical Systems, Minnetonka, Minn.)*

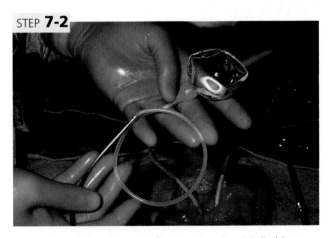

Reservoir ready for placement. *(Courtesy American Medical Systems, Minnetonka, Minn.)*

The reservoir is then positioned into the perivesical space.

STEP **7-3**

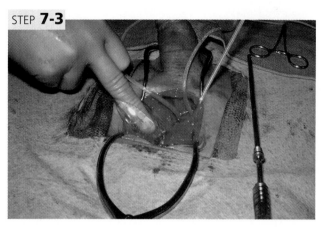

(Courtesy American Medical Systems, Minnetonka, Minn.)

8. The reservoir is filled with the appropriate amount of saline for its capacity (different sizes are available) and pulled against the floor of Hesselbach's triangle.

STEP **8-1**

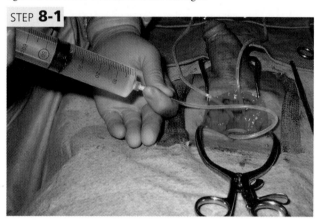

(Courtesy American Medical Systems, Minnetonka, Minn.)

It is not necessary to suture this site.

9. The pump is then placed in the most dependent portion of the scrotum.

STEP **9-1**

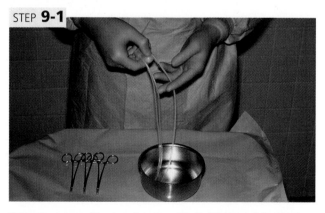

Preparing pump. *(Courtesy American Medical Systems, Minnetonka, Minn.)*

It is generally positioned on the patient's dominant side. The space is created by blunt dissection lateral to the testicle.

STEP **9-2**

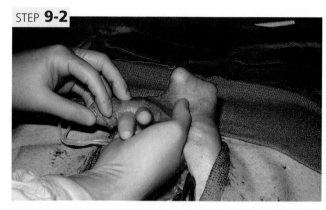

Creating scrotal pocket for pump. *(Courtesy American Medical Systems, Minnetonka, Minn.*

STEP **9-3**

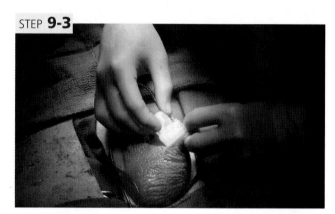

Placing pump into scrotal pocket. *(Courtesy American Medical Systems, Minnetonka, Minn.*

The tunica of the scrotum is closed over the pump with a running stitch of 3-0 absorbable suture. A Babcock clamp holds pump in place during closure.

STEP **9-4**

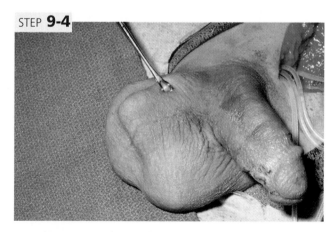

(Courtesy American Medical systems, Minnetonka, Minn.)

10. The cylinder and reservoir tubings are connected to the pump with the connectors of choice, using the assembly tool to clamp them in place. The cylinders are then tested for inflation and deflation.

STEP **10-1**

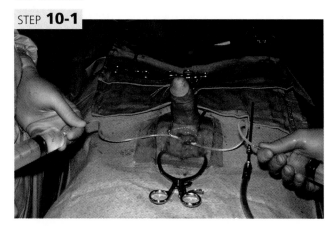

Testing cylanders before connecting them. *(Courtesy American Medical Systems, Minnetonka, Minn.)*

STEP **10-2**

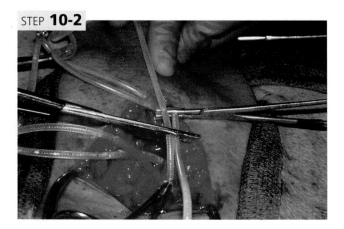

The tubings are cut to the desired length . *(Courtesy American Medical Systems, Minnetonka, Minn.*

STEP **10-3**

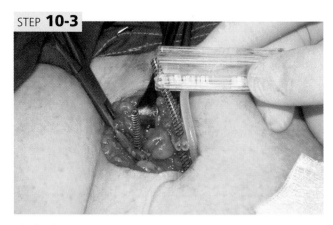

The "quik-connectors" are applied to the tubing ends. *(Courtesy American Medical Systems, Minnetonka, Minn.)*

STEP **10-4**

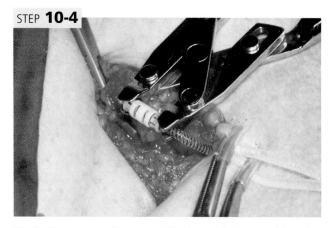

The "quik-connectors" are secured in place with the assembly tool. *(Courtesy American Medical Systems, Minnetonka, Minn.)*

STEP **10-5**

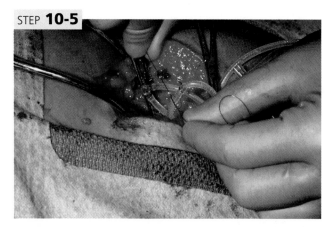

Alternatively, standard connectors and nonabsorbable ties are used to connect the tubings. *(Courtesy American Medical Systems, Minnetonka, Minn.)*

11. After generous antibiotic irrigation,

STEP **11-1**

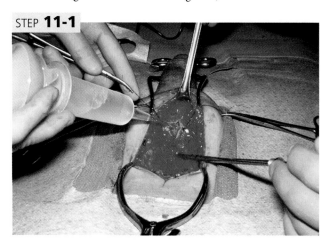

(Courtesy American Medical Systems, Minnetonka, Minn.)

the incision is closed in a subcuticular fashion, and a dressing is applied.

STEP **11-2**

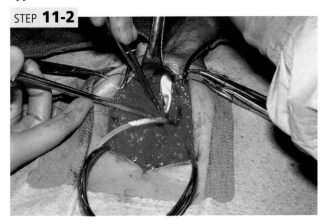

The corpora are closed. *(Courtesy American Medical Systems, Minnetonka, Minn.)*

STEP **11-3**

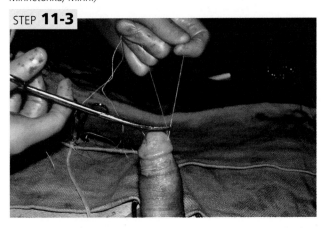

The cylinder traction sutures are cut *(Courtesy American Medical Systems, Minnetonka, Minn.)*

The penis is positioned flush with the lower abdomen for patient comfort. Mesh pants are useful as a nonadherent support dressing.

12. The prosthetic device is left in a partially inflated position to reduce bleeding and promote healing.

STEP **12-1**

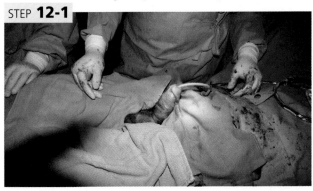

The Foley catheter is left in place and loosely secured to the lower abdomen over a gauze pad. Care should be taken to avoid pressure on the abdomen from the junction of the Foley catheter and the urinary drainage tubing.

POSTOPERATIVE

Nursing Care and Discharge Planning for Penile Implant

1. Frequent wound assessment is important to assess for hemorrhage.
2. Urethral catheter should be monitored for character and output. This is generally removed by the time the patient leaves the postanesthesia care unit (PACU).
3. Ecchymosis, pain, and swelling are common but transient and should resolve in 3 or 4 weeks. Patients with a malleable implant may have pain for a longer time period, since the device cannot be deflated.
4. Observe for signs of infection: warmth, redness, fever, increased pain, discharge from wound. Infection may be immediately apparent or manifest itself with chronic penile pain, depending on the offending organism.
5. Diet may be resumed as tolerated, beginning with clear liquids.
6. Antibiotic therapy is provided until tissues and incision appear well healed.
7. Pain is initially controlled with oral narcotic analgesia and then antiinflammatory agents, and finally acetaminophen. Stool softeners should be provided while receiving narcotic therapy. Instruct patient regarding precautions and side effects of narcotics and antibiotics.
8. Activity may resume as tolerated. Lifting over 20 lb should be avoided for 4 weeks. Sexual activity may resume after 6 weeks.
9. Appropriate device tracking documentation for the facility and the manufacturers use must be completed.
10. Patient may be discharged the same day or first postoperative day if pain is controlled orally. The use of a penile block intraoperatively aids this process.
11. Patient will be instructed in inflation and deflation techniques when pain level allows use of the device; average is 6 weeks.

LASER ABLATION OF CONDYLOMAS AND PENILE CARCINOMA

Description. Laser ablation of condyloma or penile cancer is the eradication of diseased tissue by means of a laser beam. Laser treatment may be performed successfully with a local infiltration of anesthetic in an outpatient or office setting. A U-shaped craterlike lesion of predetermined depth with a 2 mm radius can be created. A power setting ranging from 2 to 20 W on continuous or superpulse mode is generally used. With laser ablation, less edema and necrosis occur, fibrosis is minimized, and rapid healing is facilitated. The argon, CO_2, KTP-532, and Nd:YAG lasers are all suitable for this therapeutic application.

Indications. Laser therapy has been determined, through clinical trials, to be effective therapy for condylomas and penile cancers that are refractive to other treatments, but the tumor must be superficial.

PREOPERATIVE

Nursing Care and Teaching Considerations for Laser Ablations

1. Review patient record for reports of preoperative studies: PT, PTT, CBC, chest x-ray, ECG. Others may be indicated by medical condition.
2. Incorporate nursing diagnoses.
3. Comply with appropriate laser precautions. Both CO_2 and Nd:YAG or KTP could be used on the same patient. Perform preoperative laser checks.
4. Assess patient for allergies, physical impairments, diabetes, skin integrity, cardiopulmonary status, peripheral vascular circulation, range of motion.
5. Discuss perioperative course and postoperative precautions. Assess comprehension and anxiety level. A biopsy specimen will be sent for confirmation of disease entity.
6. Discuss condylomas if indicated: sexual transmission, latent viral disease associated with cervical dysplasia in women, need for condom until recurrence in both partners is ruled out (recurrence rate = 50% within 3 months).
7. Check equipment, instrumentation, and supplies for function and integrity.
8. Check medications for dosage and expiration dates.
9. Position patient under guidance of surgeon and anesthetist. Ensure that linen is smooth and IV lines are unrestricted. Electrosurgery should be available but not connected.
10. Document assessment findings and nursing interventions.

One of the major advantages of the laser is that heat is distributed evenly to the tissue underlying the lesion. Tissue loss and stricture is less than that with treatment by electrosurgery. Both CO_2 and Nd:YAG or KTP-532 may be used, depending on the character of the tumor. The recurrence rate after laser ablation has been extremely low, with cure rates ranging from 88% to 95%. When any laser is being used, guidelines appropriate to that system must be initiated.

Perioperative risks. The prime risk with laser surgery is damage to the eye. This can be avoided by ensuring that the proper glasses or goggles are utilized and that all other laser precautions are followed. Other risks include dysuria, infection, scarring, recurrence, and bleeding. Anesthetic risks may include hypotension or hypertension, inadequate pulmonary exchange, and reaction to local anesthetics or sedation.

Equipment and instrumentation
Equipment
Laser unit of choice
Laser goggles
Laser signs
Laser fiber or contact handpiece
Microscope by choice
Smoke evacuator
Electrosurgery unit
Fiberoptic light source
Instruments
Plastic instruments
Flexible cystoscope

Miscellaneous supplies
Basic pack *or*
Cystoscopy pack
Gowns
Gloves
Cloth towels
Gauze sponges
Cotton balls
Syringe, 10 ml, finger control
Hypodermic needle, #25 gauge or #27 gauge, 1 inch
Knife blade, #15
Acetic acid (vinegar)
Water
Suction tubing
Cystoscopy tubing
Cystoscopy water
Electrosurgery pencil, hand control
Suture, 4-0 absorbable on PS-3 needle
Antibiotic ointment
Local anesthetic

Procedural Steps

1. The operator moves the beam transversely across the tissue and then in a crosshatch matrix, thereby treating all perimeters of the lesion.

CONSIDERATIONS Periodically the area should be wiped with a sponge moistened in acetic acid (3% to 5% vinegar). This treatment causes diseased tissue to stand out and allows therapy to deeper layers.

2. The affected areas may be coated with antibiotic ointment. Wounds are generally left uncovered. A mild oral pain medication is usually adequate for postoperative discomfort.

POSTOPERATIVE

Nursing Care and Discharge Planning for Laser Abblations

1. Assess laser site for hemostasis.
2. Provide antibiotic ointment and oral pain medication.
3. Patient may resume activity and diet as tolerated.
4. Precautions should be taken (if condylomas) with sexual activity.
5. Dysuria is common. Urinary analgesia should be offered.
6. Wound site will display a thick eschar with a reddened border. Redness beyond this should be treated as an infection.
7. After healing, cosmetic result is good despite initial appearance of tissue.
8. Patient is discharged the same day.

PENECTOMY

Description. Penectomy is the partial or total removal of a cancerous penis. The procedure selected depends on the extent of involvement and disease stage. A 2 cm margin beyond the tumor should be excised for adequate local management. If the lesion is confined to the foreskin, a circumcision may achieve the desired result. If the lesion is invasive, an inguinal node dissection may be necessary. The procedure may be done under spinal, epidural, or general anesthesia.

Reconstruction is possible after penectomy. Evaluation must take into account sexual, urinary, and cosmetic factors. Extensive or proximally invasive lesions that include the scrotum, perineum, abdominal wall, or pubis generally necessitate emasculation as well as expanded resection of involved tissues. Under normal circumstances, the scrotum is left to help maintain lymphatic drainage.

Inguinal node enlargement without inflammation, or persistent inflammation of inguinal nodes, requires an ilioinguinal node dissection. If the patient has had previous inguinal surgery, the old incisions should be cultured preoperatively and completely excised during node dissection.

Indications. Invasive penile cancer not amenable to irradiation because of size, depth, or location is best dealt with by penectomy. At least 3 cm of viable proximal shaft is necessary in order to consider a partial penectomy. This affords a length sufficient for directable and upright urination. If the residual stump is inadequate in length, detachment and mobilization of the suspensory ligaments may be an option. A total penectomy is generally required when tumor margins are beyond a 2 cm retrievable length from the penoscrotal junction. The patient will then require a perineal urethrostomy. A patient presenting with unexplained urethral bleeding should be evaluated for urethral carcinoma.

Perioperative risks. Concerns surrounding penectomy, partial or total, include infection, hemorrhage, tumor spillage, urethral meatal stenosis, bleeding from the stump secondary to erections, urinary retention, incontinence, and inability to function sexually because of length. Anesthetic concerns may include hypotension or hypertension, cardiac dysrhythmias, pulmonary edema, and pulmonary embolus.

Equipment and instrumentation
Equipment
Electrosurgery unit
Suction unit
Alternating compression machine
Instruments
Minor instrument set
Miscellaneous supplies
Laparotomy pack
Sterile gowns
Sterile gloves
Drape towels
Sterile cloth towels
Suction tubing
Electrosurgery pencil, hand control
Alternating compression stockings, thigh length
Penrose drain, 1/2 inch
Raytec sponges
Kittner dissectors
Suture: 2-0, 3-0, 4-0 absorbable on SH-1, CT-2, RB-1, UR needles
Suture, 4-0 absorbable cuticular

Suture ligatures, 2-0 and 3-0
Gauze pressure dressings
Foley catheter, #14 Fr, 5 cc balloon
Urine drainage bag
Sterile water, 1000 ml
Sterile saline, 1000 ml
Syringe, 10 ml
Antiseptic prep solution
Absorbent prep drape

PREOPERATIVE

Nursing Care and Teaching Considerations for Penectomy

1. Review patient record for reports of preoperative studies: computed tomography (CT) scan, bone scan, PT, PTT, CBC, urine culture, tumor biopsy and culture, pelvic sonograms, intravenous pyelogram (IVP), chest x-ray, serum electrolytes and cardiac enzymes if indicated by medical state.
2. Most tumors are infected because of necrotic tissue. Ascertain that antibiotic coverage has been initiated.
3. Assess patient for allergies, obesity, diabetes, asthma, cardiopulmonary status, range of motion, physical impairments, skin integrity,
4. Evaluation for urethral carcinoma, if indicated, includes cystoscopy and retrograde pyelograms (RGP), urine cytologic evaluation or transurethral biopsy, tumor and urine cultures, diagnostics listed in step 1.
5. Discuss perioperative course with patient. Assess comprehension and anxiety level.
6. Review signs and symptoms to be reported: fever, purulent drainage, pyuria, increased pain or warmth at wound, redness.
7. Check equipment, instrumentation, and packaging for function and integrity.
8. Check medications for dosage and expiration dates.
9. Position patient under guidance of surgeon and anesthetist. Ensure that linen is smooth and IV lines unrestricted.
10. Apply alternating compression stockings and electrosurgery dispersive pad.
11. Prep and drape patient according to AORN standards.
12. Document assessment findings and nursing interventions.

Procedural Steps
Partial Penectomy

1. The lesion is excluded by a towel attached to the planned amputation line. A penile tourniquet is applied at the base.
2. After circumferential skin incision, the cavernous bodies are divided to the urethra with a 2 cm gross margin.
3. Dorsal vessels are ligated, margins of the tunica albuginea are approximated, and the urethra is dissected proximally and distally (spatulated) to obtain a 1 cm redundant flap.
4. The urethra is divided without sacrificing the tumor margin. Interrupted sutures are placed on the opposite margins of the tunica albuginea to secure the corpora.
5. The tourniquet is removed, and hemostasis is achieved.

6. After the dorsal urethrotomy, a skin-to-urethra anastomosis is performed. The redundant skin flap is then dorsally approximated.

7. A small urinary catheter is inserted, and a nonadherent dressing is applied. These are generally removed in 3 or 4 days.

Total Penectomy

1. A vertical elliptic incision is made around the penile base.

2. The distal urethra and its ventral traction are divided through an incision in Buck's fascia, mobilizing the urethra and aiding the dissection, which extends from the corpora to the bulbar region. The corpora are then separated and ligated.

3. The suspensory ligaments and dorsal vessels are divided as corporal dissection is carried out. The urethra is transected from the corpora.

4. An ellipse of skin approximately 1 cm in size is taken from the perineal area. A tunnel is fashioned in the perineal subcutaneous layer of tissue. A traction suture through the tunnel, at the penile base, aids dissection for transposition of the urethra to the perineum.

5. The urethra is grasped with a forceps and transferred to the perineum.

6. The urethra is spatulated and a skin-to-urethra anastomosis is performed through a buttonhole incision in the perineum.

7. The primary incision is closed horizontally, which elevates the scrotum away from the urethral opening.

8. A urinary catheter is inserted, and the wound is covered with a nonadherent dressing.

POSTOPERATIVE

Nursing Care and Discharge Planning for Penectomy

1. The patient will have a urethral catheter until fully ambulatory.
2. Antibiotics are continued as necessary. Pain management may include epidural catheter, PCA, IV, intramuscular (IM), or oral therapy. Stool softeners should be provided.
3. The patient may shower the first postoperative day.
4. Early ambulation is encouraged.
5. Activity may resume as tolerated. Lifting over 20 lb. should be avoided for several weeks.
6. Diet may resume as tolerated. Fluid intake should be increased.
7. Ecchymosis, swelling, and dysuria should subside after 2 to 3 weeks.
8. Patient is generally discharged in 2 to3 days

GLOSSARY

Areolar The colored ring around a vesicle, pustule, or nipple.

Caput A knoblike protuberance, such as bone or muscle; swelling.

Deferential Supplying the vas deferens.

Efferent Conducting outward from a part or organ.

Globus major Epididymal head.

Gubernaculum A fibrous cord that connects the fetal testis with the bottom of the scrotum; by failing to elongate with the rest of the fetus it causes descent of the testis.

Dartos A thin layer of vascular contractile tissue containing smooth muscle fibers but no fat; situated beneath the scrotal skin or labia majora.

Imbricate Overlap, as in successive layers of tissue in a surgical closure.

Invaginate To cover or enclose as within the body; to fold in so that an outer surface becomes an inner surface.

Multilocular Having or divided into many small chambers or vesicles.

Raphe Seamlike union of two lateral halves of a part or organ as the tongue, perineum, or scrotum, having an external ridge or furrow and an internal fibrous connective tissue septum.

Rete A network of blood vessels or nerves; a plexus; an anatomic part resembling or including a network.

Smegma The secretion of a sebaceous gland; cheesy sebaceous matter that collects between the glans penis and the foreskin, or around the clitoris and labia minora.

Sulcus A furrow or groove that separates a part into anterior and posterior.

Bibliography

1. American Urological Association Allied: *Standards of urologic nursing practice*, Richmond, Virg,1990, AUAA.
2. Association of Operating Room Nurses: *Quality improvement in perioperative nursing*, Denver, 1992, AORN.
3. Association of Operating Room Nurses: *Standards and recommended practices*, Denver, 1995, AORN.
4. Bennett AH: *Impotence*, Philadelphia, 1994, WB Saunders.
5. Benumof JL, Saidman LJ: *Anesthesia and perioperative complications*, St. Louis, 1992, Mosby.
6. Droller MJ: *Surgical management of urologic disease: an anatomic approach*, St. Louis, 1992, Mosby.
7. Gillenwater JT et al: *Adult and pediatric urology*, vols 1-3, St. Louis, 1996, Mosby.
8. Gray M: *Genitourinary disorders*, St. Louis, 1992, Mosby.
9. Hinman F:*Atlas of urologic surgery*, Philadelphia, 1989, WB Saunders.
10. Litwack K: *Core curriculum for post anesthesia nursing practice*, ed 3, Philadelphia, 1995, WB Saunders.
11. Meeker MH, Rothrock JC: *Alexander's care of the patient in surgery*, ed10, St. Louis, 1995, Mosby.
12. Resnick MI, Novick AC: *Urology secrets*, St. Louis, 1995, Mosby.
13. Resnick MI, Kursh ED: *Current therapy in genitourinary surgery*, ed 2, St. Louis, 1992, Mosby.
14. Rothrock JC: *Perioperative nursing care planning*, ed 2, St. Louis, 1996, Mosby.
15. Seidman EJ, Hanno PM: *Current urologic therapy*, ed 3, Philadelphia, 1994, WB Saunders.
16. Smith AD: *Controversies in endourology*, Philadelphia, 1995, WB Saunders.
17. Tanagho EA, McAninch JW: *Smith's general urology*, ed 14, Norwalk, Conn, 1995, Appleton & Lange.
18. Vaiden RE et al: *Core curriculum for the RN first assistant*, Denver, 1990, AORN.
19. Whitehead ED, Nagler HM: *Management of impotence and infertility*, Philadelphia, 1994, Lippincott.

10

Open Interventions on the Lower Urinary Tract

The lower urinary tract is composed of the urethra, bladder, and prostate gland. Interventions in this section will generally be more involved than those discussed in Chapter 9.

The patient may be placed in supine or lithotomy position. Anesthesia will usually be regional or general, augmented by local infiltration for pain management and hemostasis. Epinephrine will be used more frequently with these procedures, generally at a 1:200,000 concentration. It should not be used, however, when infection is present, because it may exacerbate the condition. Marcaine (bupivacaine Hcl) and Duranes Ft (etidocaine Hcl) are the most popular substances used because of their extended effect.

Bacterial endocarditis is of great concern during interventions on the lower urinary tract. Patients should be covered prophylactically with antibiotics for these procedures. Prophylactic therapy is usually intramuscular administration of gentamicin 1 hour preoperatively and repeated two more times at 8-hour intervals. If an indwelling Foley catheter is used, ampicillin IV may be added to the IV. After catheter removal, orally administered Bactrim (sulfamethoxazole and trimethoprim) may be ordered for several days postoperatively. If the patient is known to be at increased risk because of the presence of an implant or structural heart disease, as indicated by their cardiologic history or the presence of a heart murmur, antibiotic coverage may be aqueous penicillin, ampicillin and gentamicin, or streptomycin.

Stones may be removed from the bladder through a suprapubic incision (cystolithotomy). Bladder tumors, diverticula, congenital defects, or trauma may mandate an intraabdominal approach. A thorough diagnostic work-up and endoscopic examination help to determine the appropriate surgical approach to be employed. Radical procedures, such as total cystectomy, are performed for the treatment of invasive carcinoma of the bladder and require permanent urinary diversion.

The text and photographs to follow in this chapter are intended to be generic for the specific interventions. Each is subject to alteration depending on the practice setting and the preference of the surgeon. Common surgical techniques and instrumentation are depicted and intended as an overview to enable the perioperative nurse to anticipate patient care needs. Instrumentation and actual equipment in practice will also vary according to physician preference and the procedural setting. It is important to focus on the principles involved in each procedure and to consider the instrumentation as suggestions for the specialty of genitourinary surgery.

NURSING CARE

For most open-bladder surgery the patient is placed in the supine position with a bolster under the pelvis. The Trendelenburg position may be desired because this position allows the viscera to fall cephalad, providing excellent exposure of the pelvic organs.

Before vaginal procedures, an iodophor douche is commonly given. When interventions involve the genital region, a hexachlorophene or Hibiclens (chlorhexidine qluconate) shower is often ordered. Before procedures involving the bowel, an oral bowel prep or balanced lavage enema may be required.

Additional nursing diagnoses that may be appropriate for interventions involving the lower urinary tract are as follows:

NURSING DIAGNOSIS	PERIOPERATIVE PLANNING AND INTERVENTION
High risk for injury related to position	Correctly position patient in proper body alignment after adequate relaxation of leg and perineal muscles; avoid severe hip and arm flexion.
	Reduce pressure on sensitive neurovascular areas such as popliteal space, peroneal nerve, calf area, and acromioclavicular region by padding as necessary.
	Assess character and presence of bilateral pedal pulses perioperatively.
	Avoid pooling of surgical prep solutions under buttocks, sacrum, or back.
	Avoid hairy areas or areas where prosthetic joint implants are in place when placing electrocautery dispersive pad.
Fluid volume deficit related to blood loss	Assess nutritional status, skin turgor, and medications affecting fluid balance.
	Observe for and report significant blood loss intraoperatively.
	Record all solutions administered from the surgical field.

Nursing Diagnosis	Perioperative Planning and Intervention
Fluid volume deficit related to blood loss—cont'd	Maintain adequate hydration through IV solutions, blood products, or oral fluids. Observe for and report significant drainage. Evaluate electrolytes postoperatively compared with perioperative studies.
Urinary retention related to surgical intervention	Assess abdomen for distention. If no catheter is in place, straight catheterize as necessary, preferably after anesthetizing urethral meatus with topical anesthetic. Maintain patent, tension-free urinary catheter. Evaluate catheter position by determining length of catheter protruding from urethra; reposition catheter as necessary (one-half or less should extend from the male urethra and two-thirds from the female urethra). Determine status of gross sensory motor function, particularly after spinal anesthesia. Irrigate catheter as necessary; observe for clot formation; note amount and character of urinary output.
Altered pattern of urinary elimination related to: Instrumentation Type of procedure	Maintain patent, tension-free urinary catheter by securing to leg. Secure all connections. Keep collection device below bladder level. Assess and document return flow of urine, include character and color. Observe for and document signs of dysuria and excessive or diminished urinary output. Irrigate catheter as indicated. Observe and document any abdominal distention. Maintain adequate hydration.
Risk for hemorrhage/hematuria related to operative intervention	Discuss signs and symptoms of bleeding. Review need to avoid aspirin and nonsteroidal medications for 10 days. Explain need for reduced activity level; review activity regimen. Provide adequate hydration through IV solutions and oral fluid intake. Assess urinary output for signs of hematuria; report evidence of frank bleeding or clots. Review bathing techniques related to wound status.
Body image disturbance related to operative procedure	Discuss alteration in appearance and lifestyle. Reinforce realistic goals. Teach appropriate coping strategies. Instruct the patient in self-care of the altered body area. Emphasize the patient's strengths and roles within family relationships. Collaborate with other health care professionals when planning care and interventions. Provide information regarding support groups.

The interventions involving the lower urinary tract may be managed in an inpatient or outpatient setting, depending on the extent of the procedure and the patient's condition. Patient education must be individualized based on the data assessment and intervention. It is important to include significant others in the discharge planning and instruction. The pain encountered postoperatively will vary. Pain management and coping techniques will assist the patient toward an uneventful recovery. Local anesthetics are frequently instilled to provide comfort in the immediate postoperative period.

The patient will generally be in the supine or lithotomy position. Support should be provided beneath the knees, heels, and the sacral area. Additionally, any pressure points (back of head, scapula, elbows) should be adequately protected. When lithotomy position is necessary, care must be taken to protect the popliteal space, Achilles tendon, calf region, tibial and peroneal nerves, and ilioinguinal nerves and to avoid hyperextension of the hips. The Allen boot stirrups are considered the safest and most comfortable for the patient.

The anesthesia of choice for lower urinary tract intervention may be general, spinal, or epidural block. Anesthetic complications to be alert for include hypotension or hypertension, peripheral nerve damage, regurgitation of gastric contents, spinal headache, cardiopulmonary compromise, hypovolemia or hypervolemia, and excessive bleeding. The patient is instructed to refrain from taking aspirin and nonsteroidal anti-inflammatory agents for 10 days preoperatively, unless their cardiac status demands otherwise.

The operating lights, electrosurgery unit, and suction unit should be checked for proper function before the patient enters the room. Instrumentation should be inspected for damage, debris or corrosion, and proper action before use. Implants and grafts are employed during some of the procedures highlighted and must be handled according to the manufacturer's and Association of Operating Room Nurses (AORN) guidelines.

As perioperative patient care is implemented, the plan of care will be subject to adjustment on a continual basis based on data collected through the preoperative assessment and changing intraoperative circumstances. This ongoing evaluation and revision of care allows for an individualized approach. Once care has been implemented the postoperative assessment is completed. Often it will not be possible to properly determine long-term outcomes. Immediate postoperative assessment allows for a baseline determination of the effect of the nursing interventions provided. Priority postoperative assessment data appropriate for the continual evaluation of nursing care includes but is not limited to the following:

- Awareness of reportable signs and symptoms of hemorrhage or infection
- Discussion of dressing, wound, and stomal care
- Discussion of probable postoperative pain
- Review of coughing and deep-breathing techniques to assist pulmonary exchange
- Awareness of need to ambulate as soon as possible to prevent stasis and pneumonia and assist peristalsis
- Awareness of diet or other restrictions related to the medication regimen
- Comprehension of the medication regimen ordered by the physician (aspirin and nonsteroidal antiinflammatory agents should not be used postoperatively unless cleared with the physician)
- Understanding the need for adequate fluid intake to accelerate healing and promote recovery from spinal anesthesia, if appropriate
- Review of drain care
- Review of catheter care

An overview of the care provided and the subsequent evaluation is recorded to provide for the continuity of care throughout the recovery period. This documentation should be individualized according to the procedure and the needs of the patient. Surgical settings differ and perioperative documentation will have guidelines appropriate for the specific institution. A summary of the intraoperative activities designed to achieve certain outcome criteria should be reported to the perianesthesia nurse. Information to be recorded and reported will vary according to the procedure performed. Reports may differ between surgical settings depending on the amount of preoperative instruction afforded the patient and services available to meet each patient's requirements. Priority information for the genitourinary patient may include the following:

- Wound status at the time of dressing application
- Patency of catheters or drains at discharge from the operating room
- Precautions pertinent to the patient's physical condition
- Fluid loss and replacement
- Status of peripheral vascular circulation
- Skin integrity preoperatively and postoperatively
- Positions and positioning devices employed for surgery
- Level of comprehension during preoperative instruction
- Information taught to the patient preoperatively and intraoperatively
- Untoward reactions encountered intraoperatively
- Nursing care provided

THE ROLE OF THE RN FIRST ASSISTANT

As with the other interventions discussed, the RNFA may augment the role of the perioperative RN through the assessment, planning, and implementation of patient care. Appropriate individualized plans of care may be developed based on the assessment data collected.

Not infrequently, the patient is immunosuppressed, dehydrated, or otherwise compromised. The RNFA may be vital to the nursing process by evaluating the physiologic status of these patients and determining intraoperative nutritional and fluid needs. Many patients about to undergo cystectomy, for example, have been receiving chemotherapy, are deficient in vitamin C, and may be anemic or in a hypovolemic state. There may also be other effects of their disease that put them at increased risk for infection, cardiovascular or cardiopulmonary collapse, and hemorrhage. The perioperative nurses and the perianesthesia nurses, when working in collaboration with the surgeon, may assess and address the needs of each patient.

Many of these patients require extensive teaching as well as support measures to understand their disease, their unique needs, and postoperative course. The RNFA has the opportunity to influence the process through focused care preoperatively, intraoperatively, and postoperatively.

Intraoperatively the RNFA functions as previously discussed in the other chapters and must be attuned to changing needs in the course of the intervention. With knowledge of the anatomy and physiology, body mechanics and positioning needs, and varied surgical approaches, the RNFA may lead the perioperative team toward optimum patient care.

URETHROPLASTY

Description. Urethroplasty is reconstructive surgery of the urethra. Urethral grafts are generally required and may include free skin grafts and mobilized vascular flaps. There are many combinations of these procedures, and in all of them some type of temporary urinary diversion may be used, depending on the location and severity of the condition.

Indications. Strictures, urethral fractures, or narrowing of the urethral lumen, which are congenital, inflammatory, or traumatic in origin. Various surgical techniques are described in the surgical treatment of stricture disease.

Evaluation preoperatively is initiated from the patient's complaint of obstructive symptoms, frequently associated with a urinary tract infection. Techniques utilized to determine diagnosis include urodynamics (voiding pressures above and below the site of obstruction), urinary flow cytometry, intravenous urography (IVU) to rule out upper tract disease, cystoscopy, and urethrography. The length and density of the diseased urethra is determined to plan the appropriate reconstructive procedure. Any associated urinary tract infection must be treated and eradicated before surgical violation. Definitive repair should wait for 10 to 12 weeks after diagnostic instrumentation until the inflammatory reaction subsides.

Perioperative risks. Loss of flap viability because of ischemia from inadequate vascularity and urethrocutaneous fistula are the two most disasterous complications. Possible alterations in sexual function or continence may also occur postoperatively.

Other complications to guard against include infection, meatal stenosis, edema, hemorrhage, erections before healing, urethral diverticulum, recurrent stricture, retrusive meatus, chronic inflammation, and penile scarring. The anesthetic risks previously discussed apply.

Equipment and instrumentation
Equipment
Electrosurgery unit
Headlight
Suction unit
Alternating compression unit
Allen stirrups
Pillows, gel pads
Instruments
Minor instrument set
Plastic instrument set
Cystoscopy set
Van Buren urethral dilators
Bipolar forceps
Miscellaneous supplies
Cystoscopy pack *or*
Lithotomy pack
Sterile gowns and gloves
Drape towels, 5
Sterile cloth towels
Impervious rectal drape
Robinson catheter, #14 Fr
Knife blades, #15
Bipolar cable
Suction tubing
Electrosurgery pencil, hand control
Electrosurgery needle tip
Suprapubic catheter
Foley catheter, #14, 5 Fr balloon
Urine drainage bag
Syringes, 10 ml luerlock and finger control
Hypodermic needle, #27 gauge, 1 1/4 inches
Suture, absorbable 4-0 on SH-1 needle
Suture, absorbable 4-0 on PS-3 needle
Kittner dissectors
Radiopaque gauze sponges
Gauze dressings
Nonadherent dressing (petrolatum gauze, Adaptic)
Scrotal support *or*
Mesh underwear
Sterile saline, 500 ml
Sterile water, 500 ml
Alternating compression stockings, thigh length
Antiseptic prep solution
Absorbent prep drape

JOHANSON URETHROPLASTY

The Johanson urethroplasty is a two-stage procedure to repair and reconstruct the urethra affected by severe urethral stricture disease. Approximately 3 months after the first stage, if the

PREOPERATIVE

Nursing Care and Teaching Considerations for Urethroplasty

1. Review patient record for reports of preoperative studies intravenous pyelography (IVP), prothrombin time (PT), partial thromboplastin time (PTT), complete blood count (CBC), chest x-ray, electrocardiogram (ECG), urine culture, electrolytes and enzymes as determined by medical history.
2. Discuss possible alterations in sexual function or voiding pattern.
3. Discuss possibility of urinary diversion and care involved.
4. Review patient's understanding of intended procedure and postoperative expectations.
5. Assess patient for skin integrity, range of motion, physical limitations, allergies, anxiety level, presence of implants.
6. Check equipment, instrumentation, and packaging for proper function and integrity
7. Check medications for dosage and expiration dates.
8. Collect appropriate positioning devices. Position patient under direction of surgeon and anesthetist. Apply alternating compression stockings.
9. Ensure that linen is smooth and IV lines are not constricted.
10. Apply patient dispersive pad to nonhairy fleshy site close to perineum.
11. Prep and drape patient according to AORN guidelines. Protect patient from pooling of prep solutions.
12. Document assessment findings and nursing intervention.

operative site is healing and the patient is voiding adequately, a second-stage procedure is performed.

Procedural Steps
First Stage

The patient is placed in the exaggerated lithotomy position. Routine prepping and draping procedures are employed with precautions for protecting the anus (the use of an impervious plastic adherent drape).

1. An inverted **U** incision is made in the perineum from the inner borders of the ischial tuberosities up to and including the base of the scrotum. A Van Buren sound is passed into the urethra up to the stricture. The bulbocavernosus muscle is dissected and retracted laterally.

2. An incision is made in the urethra over the strictured area and is extended in each direction at least 1 cm beyond the diseased area.

3. The abnormal scar tissue is excised or simply incised, because scrotal skin ultimately increases the lumen. A #28 dilator is passed through both the proximal and the distal urethral lumens to rule out further stricture. The remaining urethral mucosa is sutured with 4-0 absorbable suture to the scrotal skin. A cystotomy tube to divert the urinary stream may be left indwelling and removed in 5 to 7 days.

Second Stage (Mobilized Vascular Flap)

1. A red rubber catheter is temporarily inserted into the bladder through the proximal urethral stoma. The penoscrotal skin is incised longitudinally, adjacent to the urethra. A new urethra is constructed by developing the ventral preputial skin, which is dissected free and fanned out.

2. The rectangle of skin is rolled into the neourethra and measured.

3. A channel is sharply created on the ventral aspect of the glans in a plane just above the corpora. The glans tissue is removed forming a groove approximately 14 Fr in diameter.

4. Layers of subcutaneous tissue are dissected free from the dorsal penile skin to create an island flap that is spiraled to the ventrum. The flaps are brought together in the midline and closed with a continuous or interrupted 4-0 absorbable suture.

5. The neourethra is anastomosed proximally to the urethra and carried to the tip of the glans.

6. The dorsal penile flaps are transposed laterally to the midline, and excess skin is excised.

7. Closure is with 4-0 absorbable interrupted mattress sutures around the glans and down the penile shaft.

8. A bulky pressure dressing is applied. Suprapubic cystostomy drainage is an option, but a urethral catheter usually suffices.

CONSIDERATIONS Vascularized flaps of preputial or penile skin may be mobilized to the ventrum by leaving them attached to the outer surface of the prepuce or as an island flap. One modification is the transverse preputial island flap neourethra with glans-channel positioning for the meatus. Preputial skin is preferred because of its rich reliable blood supply and non–hair-bearing characteristics.

HORTON-DEVINE URETHROPLASTY (URETHRAL PATCH GRAFT)

Urethral patch graft is a one-stage operative procedure that incorporates a free skin graft to correct a urethral stricture.

Procedural Steps

1. The patient is placed in the lithotomy position.

2. A 17 Fr panendoscope is passed into the posterior urethra followed by a #20 urethral dilator.

3. A perineal vertical midline incision is made into the urethral lumen. The panendoscope is reinserted, and the incision is examined to determine if it crossed the stricture.

4. The defect is measured.

5. A circumferential incision is made on the posterior penile shaft to harvest an oval piece of skin the size of the defect.

CONSIDERATIONS Free skin grafts should be full thickness grafts. Since the free graft must be revascularized, it is important that it have a perfect skin cover of dorsal, preputial, penile skin that is well vascularized. This type of graft is generally used with a one-stage repair.

6. The epidermal side of the graft is defatted, and absorbable sutures of 4-0 are placed at its apex and base.

7. The apex is sutured into position at the proximal and distal ends of the stricture with the epidermal side toward the urethral lumen.

8. The graft is anastomosed proximally to the urethra with the suture line of the graft next to the corpora. The middle glans dart is fixed to the corpora. The graft is formed into a neourethra over a Silastic stenting catheter.

9. The panendoscope is again inserted, and the urethra is irrigated to check for leaks along the suture line.

10. A Foley or fenestrated catheter is inserted to serve as a stent.

11. The corpora spongiosa is approximated and closed over the patched area as a separate layer with interrupted 3-0 absorbable sutures.

12. Subcutaneous 4-0 absorbable sutures are placed.

13. The skin and the graft site are closed with interrupted 4-0 sutures.

14. A suprapubic catheter is inserted to divert urine for healing.

15. Petrolatum gauze is wrapped around the penis and covered with gauze sponges and fluffed dressings. A scrotal supporter is applied to provide support and pressure.

POSTOPERATIVE

Nursing Care and Discharge Planning for Urethroplasty

1. Urinary catheter is removed in 3 to 7 days.
2. Urethral stent is removed after 1 to 2 weeks.
3. Antibiotics are taken according to physician's order until tissue is well healed.
4. Medication for pain and dysuria should be taken before onset of discomfort. Orally administered narcotics followed by antiinflammatory agents, Tylenol, and Pyridium usually are effective.
5. Stool softeners should be taken while the patient is receiving narcotic pain management.
6. Discuss signs and symptoms to be reported: prolonged bleeding, increased pain or edema, redness, purulent discharge from wound, pyuria, fever.
7. Some ecchymosis and swelling will occur but should resolve at about 3 weeks.
8. Diet may be resumed as tolerated. Fluid intake should be increased to 8 oz 4 to 6 times daily (half as fruit juice, half as water).
9. Activity may be resumed as tolerated. Lifting more than 20 lb. should be avoided for 4 weeks. Sexual activity may resume at the discretion of the surgeon, based on extent of disease and repair.
10. Patient may be discharged the same day.
11. Patient may shower the first postoperative day, using water-repellent covering over wound. Dressings should be kept clean and dry.

PROSTATECTOMY

Description. Prostatic enlargement may be benign or malignant. In benign prostatic hypertrophy, only the peri-urethral adenomatous portion of the gland is removed. Operable prostatic malignancy requires radical prostatectomy, which includes removal of the entire prostate gland and the seminal vesicles.

Three open surgical approaches are possible in removing the benign hyperplastic obstructive prostate gland: retropubic prostatectomy, suprapubic prostatectomy, and perineal prostatectomy. If the prostate gland is cancerous, a radical retropubic or radical perineal prostatectomy in conjunction with open or laparoscopic retroperitoneal lymph node dissection is performed. Many patients desire to retain sexual function. The surgeon may attempt to save the neurovascular bundles in what is termed a *nerve-sparing* approach. The site and size of the prostatic lesion, however, often determines if this can be achieved successfully and without undue risk to the patient.

Spinal, epidural, and general anesthesia may be equally acceptable types of anesthesia for patients undergoing open prostatectomy, depending on the medical condition of the patient. The patient is placed in a slight Trendelenburg position with the pelvis elevated at the level of the umbilicus.

Indications. Glandular hyperplasia of the prostatic urethra usually manifests itself after 55 years of age. Prostatic enlargement may occur in one or more lobes of the prostate but most frequently is encountered in the lateral or median lobes. Progressive growth of the hyperplastic gland compresses the remaining normal prostatic tissue, forming what is called a "surgical capsule." The growth of adenomatous tissue slowly encroaches on the prostatic urethral lumen, causing obstruction to the urinary outflow.

A blood sample is drawn to determine the prostate specific antigen (PSA) level, followed by a digital rectal examination (DRE). The blood should be drawn first because manipulation of the gland has been known to alter the efficacy of the PSA test. If this test is elevated, the patient is at risk for carcinoma of the prostate. Clinical evaluation and an elevated PSA level may indicate the need for a transrectal ultrasound needle biopsy to confirm the diagnosis. If the PSA is greater than 10, blood is again studied for the prostatic acid phosphatase (PAP) level. When the results of the biopsy indicate a malignancy, a bone scan and skeletal survey is necessary to rule out metastasis.

Several factors must be taken into account to determine the best route for removal of the prostatic obstruction: the age and medical condition of the patient, the size of the gland and location of the pathologic condition, and the presence of associated medical disease.

Perioperative risks. The most frequent complication with any prostatectomy is hemorrhage. Additionally, other risks pertinent to open prostatectomy include urinary retention, infection, wound dehiscence, incontinence, peripheral neurovascular compromise, deep vein thrombosis, pulmonary edema, pulmonary emboli, hypertension or hypotension, brachial plexus injury, ilioinguinal nerve injury, and cardiac dysrhythmias. Postoperative diuresis is a potential complication of prostatectomies performed for benign prostatic hyperplasia (BPH) as a result of the sudden release of obstruction. Excessive urinary output can lead to an abnormally high loss of water and sodium.

It is important that fluid and electrolyte balance be within range preoperatively and the presence of hypokalemia be ruled out or corrected. The patient should be evaluated for azotemia and the presence of any bleeding disorders.

Equipment and instrumentation
Equipment
Electrosurgery unit
Alternating compression machine
Suction unit
Allen stirrups (if perineal)
Positioning pads
Head cradle
Safety strap
Abdominal instruments
Laparotomy set
Bladder and prostatic instruments
Urethral suture guides
Bookwalter or US200 adjustable urology retractor
Deep, long-tipped right-angle clamps
Long Allis clamps
Straight and right-angle clip appliers and clips
Right-angle scissor
Perineal instruments *(additional)*
Straight and curved Lowsley tractors
Young prostatic tractor
Roux retractors
Jackson retractors, short and long blades
Doyen vaginal retractors
Perineal prostatic retractors
Sauerbruch retractors, narrow and wide
Self-retaining perineal retractor such as the UM150
Miscellaneous supplies
Alternating compression stockings, thigh length
Laparotomy pack
Drape towels, adherent, 4
Sterile cloth towels, 4 to 8
Sterile gowns
Sterile gloves
Suction tubing
Electrosurgery pencil, hand control
Electrosurgery spatula tip, long
Holster for electrosurgery pencil
Suture, absorbable 2-0 SH-1, CT-1, and UR-5 or
  UR-6 needle
Suture, absorbable 3-0 SH-1 needle
Ligaclips, medium, medium-large, large
Lubricant, water soluble
Toomey syringe
Urinary drainage system
Foley catheter, 20 Fr, 5 cc balloon

Foley catheter, 22 or 24 Fr, 30 cc balloon
Syringes, 10 and 30 ml
Penrose drain, medium or large
Jackson-Pratt drains
Antiseptic prep solution
Absorbent prep drape

PREOPERATIVE

Nursing Care and Teaching Considerations for Prostatectomy for BPH

1. Incorporate general nursing diagnoses.
2. Ascertain that prophylactic antibiotics were administered 1 hour preoperatively.
3. Confirm that enema or bowel prep was performed and results were obtained.
4. Review patient record for reports of preoperative studies: CBC, PT, PTT, PSA, serum electrolytes, serum chemistry survey, cardiac enzymes and blood gases (if indicated by patient history), urine analyses, chest x-ray, ECG.
5. Assess cardiovascular, pulmonary, and nutritional status.
6. Confirm that blood is available.
7. Establish that urinary or prostatic infection has been treated.
8. Assess patient for allergies, cardiovascular and pulmonary status, peripheral circulation, diabetes, range of motion, physical limitations, skin integrity.
9. Discuss patient's understanding of proposed procedure and postoperative course. Assess anxiety level. Reinforce teaching as necessary.
10. Check equipment, instrumentation, and packaging for function and integrity.
11. Check medications for dosages and expiration dates.
12. Position patient according to intended approach under the guidance of surgeon and anesthetist. Apply alternating compression stockings before induction of anesthesia and resultant vasodilation. Ensure that linen is smooth and IV lines are unrestricted.
13. Prep and drape patient according to AORN standards. Protect from pooling of solutions.
14. Document assessment findings and nursing interventions.

SIMPLE RETROPUBIC PROSTATECTOMY

Description. Simple retropubic prostatectomy is the enucleation of hypertrophic prostatic tissue through an incision in the anterior prostatic capsule by an extravesical approach. The retropubic approach offers ideal exposure of the prostate bed and vesical neck, excellent hemostasis is obtained, and intraoperative and postoperative bleeding is minimized.

Indications. The retropubic approach for benign prostatic hyperplasia is indicated when the prostate gland is too large for transurethral prostatic resection (TURP) to be completed in a reasonable length of time (no more than 1 to $1^1/_2$ hours).

Perioperative risks. Risks surrounding retropubic prostatectomy for BPH include hemorrhage, clot obstruction, deep venous thrombosis, pulmonary emboli, rectal injury, urethrorectal fistula, suprapubic fistula, residual obstructive tissue, ureteral obstruction demonstrated by flank pain, bladder neck contracture, urethral stricture, urinary incontinence, postoperative diuresis, urinary retention, bladder spasm, impotence, and retrograde ejaculation.

Procedural Steps

1. The patient is placed in a slight Trendelenburg position with the pelvis elevated and the legs slightly abducted. Routine skin preparation and draping is accomplished. The first towel, with a cuff, is placed under the scrotum. Three towels are placed around the lower abdominal incision site, followed by a sterile laparotomy sheet.

2. A #20, 5 cc Foley catheter to closed drainage is placed into the bladder through the urethra. A fifth towel, folded in half, is placed over the penis and scrotum below the retropubic incision site and secured with two towel clamps.

CONSIDERATIONS The catheter may later be cut and used as a tractor to reanastamose the bladder neck.

3. A low vertical midline or Pfannenstiel, incision is made, and the anterior rectus sheath, along with portions of the internal and external oblique muscles, is incised. The rectus abdominis muscles are retracted laterally to expose the space of Retzius. As dissection continues into the space of Retzius, the bladder and peritoneum are retracted cephalad.

4. The anterior surface of the prostate is exposed by sweeping the fat laterally with Kittner dissectors. Veins are ligated or fulgurated near the vesical neck, and a padded self-retaining retractor is placed.

5. Traction sutures of 0 or 2-0 absorbable material are placed deeply into the prostatic capsule, tied, left long, and tagged with hemostats. The anterior surface of the prostatic capsule is transversely incised into the adenoma with cutting current. Suction controls visualization, and vessels are ligated or fulgurated as they are encountered.

6. The prostatic adenoma is identified and sharply separated. It is then sharply dissected or finger enucleated from the "surgical capsule." When the apex is encountered, the junction with the urethra is carefully divided with scissors.

CONSIDERATIONS If a rectal tear occurs, it is closed in two layers and covered with an omental flap.

7. Hemostatic sutures of 2-0 absorbable material are placed at 5 and 7 o'clock positions, encompassing the vesical neck and prostatic capsule to obliterate the prostatic arteries. Other bleeding points within the capsule may be ligated with 2-0 absorbable sutures. Ureteral orifices are identified, and any bladder calculi are removed.

8. A wedge is excised from the posterior lip of the vesical neck, and the vesical mucosa is anastomosed to the prostatic capsule with 2-0 absorbable suture in a continuous fashion. A #22 or #24 Fr Foley catheter with 30 cc balloon is inserted in place of the original one. Frequently a three-way catheter is used to afford continuous bladder irrigation.

9. The capsular incision is closed with a continuous or interrupted 2-0 absorbable suture. The catheter is pulled into the fossa, and traction is applied to serve as a tamponade. A drain is placed in the space of Retzius and brought out through a separate stab wound. The abdominal incision is closed in layers, and the wound is dressed.

10. If continuous bladder irrigation (CBI) is to be used, normal saline is instilled through a 4000 ml closed irrigation system.

SUPRAPUBIC PROSTATECTOMY

Description. Suprapubic prostatectomy is the transvesical removal of benign periurethral glandular tissue obstructing the outlet of the urinary tract through a low midline, or Pfannenstiel, incision. The suprapubic approach allows access for surgical correction of any existing bladder condition such as vesical calculi or vesical diverticula.

Indications. Suprapubic prostatectomy is indicated for patients with BPH whose prostate glands are too large to permit a TURP to be accomplished within 1 ¹/₂ hours.

Perioperative risks. One disadvantage of the suprapubic approach is establishing hemostasis. Because the prostate is located beneath the symphysis pubis, ligation of bleeding capsular vessels is difficult. Excessive bleeding may occur if the internal urethral vessels below the bladder neck at 5 and 7 o'clock positions are not suture ligated. The deep dorsal venous complex is the other major source of potential hemorrhage. Prolonged venous leakage is usually controllable with catheter drainage. As previously indicated, postoperative diuresis may occur in the patient with BPH as a result of the sudden release of chronic obstruction.

Procedural Steps

1. Steps number 1 and 2 are identical to those in retropubic prostatectomy.

CONSIDERATIONS The bladder is inflated with a preferred irrigating fluid. This maneuver facilitates identification of the bladder.

3. A transverse or midline lower abdominal incision is made through the skin and the two layers of superficial fascia from the symphysis to the left side of the umbilicus. The external and internal oblique muscles are incised along the lines of the original incision. The rectus muscles are separated in the midline and retracted laterally, and investing fascia is incised. Bleeding vessels are clamped, coagulated, or tied with 3-0 absorbable ties.

4. A padded self-retaining retractor is placed. The peritoneal reflection is pushed bluntly upward, and the perivesical tissue is laterally separated to expose the bladder at the space of Retzius.

5. After the placement of traction sutures, the bladder is opened between them, at the dome, with a scalpel. Liquid contents are aspirated and the bladder incision is enlarged. The dome is packed and elevated with a retractor and the vesical neck is inspected. The bladder is manually explored for calculi, tumor, or diverticula. The trigone and ureteral orifices are located.

6. The mucosa is incised circumferentially, peripheral to the adenoma, with the coagulating current and the adenoma is separated with scissors or manually enucleated.

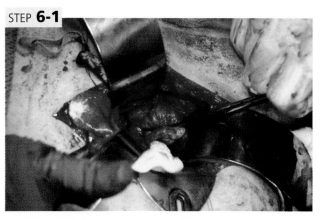

STEP 6-1

Prostate adenoma is enucleated.

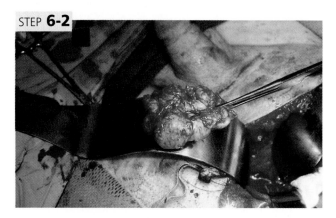

STEP 6-2

Adenoma excised.

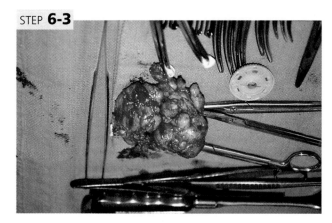

STEP 6-3

Prostatic adenoma.

CONSIDERATIONS If difficulty is experienced with the enucleation, a finger may be placed in the rectum to elevate the prostate gland. Aseptic technique is maintained during enucleation with the use of a sterile second glove on the hand used in the rectum.

7. After enucleation is completed, attention is directed to maintaining good hemostasis by packing the fossa with moist, narrow laparotomy sponges for 5 minutes. The vesical neck is suture ligated with 2-0 absorbable material at the 4 and 8 o'clock positions. Two additional sutures are placed at 11 and 1

o'clock positions to ligate anterior arteries. Other significant bleeding points may also be ligated with 3-0 absorbable suture.

CONSIDERATIONS As the pack is removed, the sutures are pulled downward.

8. A suprapubic catheter of the urologist's choice is placed into the bladder lumen through a small stab incision. A 22 or 24 Fr two- or three-way Foley catheter with a 30 cc balloon is inserted into the urethra, and the balloon is inflated to a size that prevents the catheter from migrating or being pulled into the prostatic fossa.

STEP **8-1**

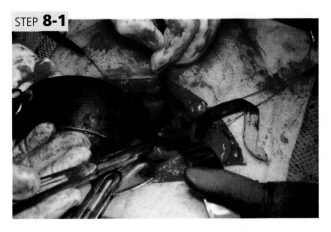

Foley entering bladder through urethra.

The cystotomy incision is then closed with interrupted 2-0 absorbable sutures. A drain is placed along the cystotomy incision, brought out through a separate stab wound, and secured to the skin with a 3-0 nonabsorbable suture. The muscles, fascia, and subcutaneous tissues are closed in layers, and a dressing is applied.

9. Normal saline irrigation solution may be connected to the Foley catheter to provide continuous irrigation to the bladder to reduce clot formation and maintain catheter patency. Continuous irrigation may be initiated during closure.

SIMPLE PERINEAL PROSTATECTOMY

Description. Perineal prostatectomy is the removal of a prostatic adenoma through a perineal approach. The instrument setup is as described for suprapubic prostatectomy, omitting abdominal self-retaining retractors.

Hugh Hampton Young, a strong proponent of the perineal approach, once remarked: "Why these gentlemen prefer darkness to light and object to a technique carried out under full visual control is incomprehensible. In my opinion, the near future will see the surgery of the prostate on the same rational basis of careful technique under visual inspection as that of other parts of the body. I may also add that the instrument which I have called my 'prostatic tractor' has transformed, for me, the operation of prostatectomy. Where before it was. . . an operation done somewhat haphazardly, depending largely on the sense of touch, and in the dark; now the entire operation is performed in a shallow wound, accurately under visual control, proper regard being paid to the urethra and to the ejaculatory ducts, so that they are preserved to continue their pleasant duties."[16]

Indications. When the prostate size is large enough to compromise a safe TURP, this approach may be the best alternative to minimize postoperative pain and morbidity. A perineal approach to the prostate gland is suitable when open prostatic biopsy is desired, and, after pathologic confirmation, radical excision may follow. Other advantages include preservation of the bladder neck and easier control of bleeding.

Perioperative risks. In the past, perineal prostatectomy was believed to hold a greater risk for loss of sexual potency, rectal perforation, and the formation of urethrorectal fistulas. This risk has lessened with the knowledge that incising Denonvillier's fascia vertically and carefully separating the prostate from the rectal wall decreases the chance for damage to these structures.

Despite the extreme positioning, this approach affords less interference with cardiovascular, pulmonary, and intestinal function, allowing surgery for those considered poor-risk. In the obese patient, particular care must be taken to avoid pressure on the ilioinguinal nerve as a result of lithotomy position. The risk of impotency has been reduced because of modifications in the technique that preserve the posterior fascial layer.

Procedural Steps

The patient is placed in an exaggerated lithotomy position with the legs above the level of the pelvis. A bolster beneath the sacrum allows the perineum to be as parallel to the operating room bed as possible, with the buttocks extending several inches over the table edge. Stirrups should be well padded to protect the popliteal fossa and peroneal nerve. The alternating compression device is recommended to assist peripheral vascular flow. Well-padded shoulder braces are placed over the acromial processes in a manner to prevent stretch or pressure injury to the brachial plexus. Routine skin preparation is carried out. Some surgeons may instill Iodophor solution into the rectum. Special draping includes a towel folded in half over the pubic area, two towels with a cuff on either side of the perineum, two leggings, with points down over the legs, an impervious drape over the anus, a large sheet fully opened with a large cuff placed across from one stirrup to the other and secured by towel clamps, and a laparotomy sheet with the short end to the floor. Two sheets are elevated on IV poles and clamped together midline to cover each arm board and the lateral abdominal areas.

1. A well-lubricated curved Lowsley tractor is placed through the urethra into the bladder and held back by the surgical assistant, causing the prostate to be pushed down toward the perineum.

STEP **1-1**

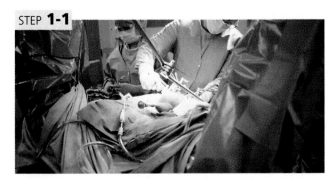

Lowsley tractor in place in male urethra.

CONSIDERATIONS The tractor is positioned so that the angle lies in the bulbous urethra allowing palpation of the prostatic apex.

2. An inverted U-shaped incision is made from just inside one ischial tuberosity to the other, curving anterior and equidistant to the anus. The incision is extended posteriorly opposite the dorsal anal margin.

CONSIDERATIONS This extension of the incision allows later mobilization of the rectum. Subcutaneous fat is preserved.

3. Three Allis clamps are secured to the posterior edge of the incision and retracted downward over the anal drape. The exposed superficial fascia is divided with electrosurgery, in the cutting mode, in the line of the incision.

4. Subcutaneous bleeders are clamped with hemostats and coagulated or tied with 3-0 absorbable ligatures.

5. The superficial perineal fascia is incised laterally, upward, and 3 to 4 cm into the ischial rectal fascia bilaterally.

STEP **5-1**

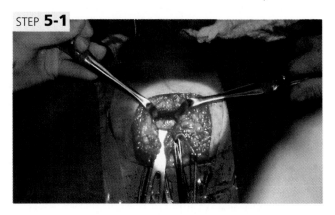

The superficial perineal fascia revealed.

6. The central tendon is isolated and clamped and cut distal to the external anal sphincter.

STEP **6-1**

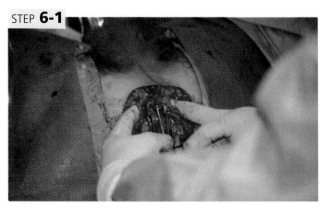

Central tendon exposed.

The levator ani muscle is exposed and retracted laterally. The prostate gland is then elevated with the Lowsley tractor, with the blades opened. The apex is identified, and the rectum is minimally displaced backward with blunt dissection.

CONSIDERATIONS The pelvic nerve plexus and cavernous nerves are contained within the lateral rectal and lateral pelvic fascia.

Biopsy of the prostate may be performed for pathologic confirmation. If the results are negative for carcinoma, the prostatic adenoma is removed. If the frozen section reveals malignancy, the urologist may choose to do a radical prostatectomy at this time.

7. The levator ani muscles are bluntly spread, and the rectourethral muscle is incised at its junction with the rectal wall and pushed downward from the central tendon.

8. The Lowsley tractor is tilted, and the apical portion of the ventral rectal fascia is exposed (Denonvillier's fascia, or the "pearly gates"). A superficial vertical incision is made into its posterior lamella over the body of the prostate.

CONSIDERATIONS A vertical incision protects the lateral cavernous nerves.

9. The rectum is retracted and the prostatic capsule is incised in a inverted U-shaped fashion, with the apex slightly proximal to the vermontanum. Incision is deepened to expose the cleavage plane of the adenoma.

10. The U flap is turned downward with an Allis clamp, and the capsule is bluntly freed from the adenoma. The dorsal urethra is divided to free the apex of the adenoma, and then the apex of the urethra is sharply dissected. The adenoma is manually enucleated from the "surgical capsule" while keeping it attached to the vesical neck.

11. The adenoma is grasped with a prostatic clamp and completely freed by blunt displacement of the circular fibers of the vesical neck. Vesical neck vessels are fulgurated or suture ligated with 2-0 absorbable material. A cone of bladder mucosa is formed and is then opened, grasped with an Allis clamp, and held in the wound. Excision is completed including all subtrigonal and subcervical lobes.

CONSIDERATIONS A large median lobe may require digital dilation of the bladder neck.

12. Bleeding in the bladder mucosa is controlled at the 5 o'clock and 7 o'clock positions with 3-0 figure-of-eight absorbable stitches and the sutures left long. The posterior vesical neck is drawn into the fossa and circumferentially sutured to the posterior flap of the capsule with 3-0 absorbable material.

13. The two long sutures are passed through the prostatic capsule on each side and tied to collapse the fossa created by the excised adenoma and provide hemostasis.

14. A 22 Fr Foley catheter with a 30 cc balloon is inserted through the urethra into the bladder, and the balloon is inflated. The catheter is irrigated to remove clots, and the position is checked.

\15. The urethra is reapproximated with 2-0 continuous absorbable sutures. A drain is left in place at the level of the capsulotomy incision. The subcutaneous layer is closed with a continuous 3-0 absorbable suture. The skin is closed with a continuous subcuticular stitch of 4-0 absorbable material.

16. The subcutaneous tissue is reapproximated with 3-0 absorbable suture. The skin incision is reapproximated with 4-0 absorbable subcutaneous sutures.

POSTOPERATIVE

Nursing Care and Discharge Planning for Prostatectomy for BPH

1. Monitor urinary output, urinary sodium and potassium, serum electrolytes, and blood pressure. Observe for diuresis (>100 ml/hr requires intervention) or for retention that requires treatment (<30 ml/hr). Irrigate for clots as necessary. Check catheter position, one third of length should be protruding. Assess for abdominal distention.

2. Observe for persistent bleeding and report. Surgical correction may be indicated.

3. Observe for signs and symptoms of infection: fever, redness or warmth at wound site, pyuria, increased pain, purulent discharge from wound.

4. Provide pain medication before onset of discomfort. Provide daily stool softener. Discuss medication regimen patient will be on after discharge. Antibiotics should be taken until gone. Aspirin and nonsteroidal antiinflammatory agents should only be taken under physician's guidance.

5. Patient may resume diet as tolerated, starting with clear liquids. Fluid intake should be increased to 8 oz q2h for several days and then 8 oz at least 4 times daily (half should be as fruit juice, half as water).

6. Patient should be encouraged to ambulate and resume activity to level of tolerance. Strenuous activity should be avoided for 4 to 6 weeks.

7. Sexual activity may be resumed in 1 month as tolerated or able. Patient may or may not be successful initially. Discuss alternative therapies for potency and retrograde ejaculation.

8. Foley will be removed in about 5 days. If a drain is in place, it will be removed in about 3 days or when swelling and significant drainage have subsided.

9. Ice may assist pain and swelling with the perineal approach. Perineal ecchymosis is common and should subside in about 3 days.

PREOPERATIVE

Nursing Care and Teaching Considerations for Radical (total) Prostatectomy

1. Review patient record for reports of preoperative studies: PSA, PAP, CT scan, bone scan, MRI, PT, PTT, CBC, serum chemistry survey, serum electrolytes, cardiac enzymes, blood gases, urine analyses, chest x-ray, ECG.

2. Determine that blood is available (2 to 3 units).

3. Ensure that prophylactic antibiotics were administered 1 hour preoperatively.

4. Confirm that enema or bowel prep was successfully accomplished.

5. Assess cardiovascular and pulmonary status. Confirm if a central venous pressure (CVP) line, an A-line, or an epidural catheter is to be inserted.

6. Assess patient for medical and surgical history. Determine presence of allergies, other physical impairments, skin integrity, and implants.

7. Review postoperative course and anticipated sequelae. Establish comprehension and anxiety level and answer questions as necessary.

8. Check equipment, instrumentation, and sterile packaging for function and integrity.

9. Check medications for dosage and expiration dates.

10. Apply alternating compression stockings.

11. Position patient according to planned procedure under guidance of surgeon and anesthetist. Utilize positioning devices and padding appropriately.

12. Ensure that linen beneath patient is free of wrinkles and that IV lines are unrestricted.

13. Prep and drape patient according to AORN guidelines. Protect patient from pooling of prep solutions.

14. Apply electrosurgery dispersive pad to nonhairy fleshy site close to area of interest.

15. Document assessment findings and nursing care provided.

17. The wound is dressed according to the surgeon's preference and taped or held with mesh pants.

18. A vasectomy may be performed.

NERVE SPARING RADICAL RETROPUBIC PROSTATECTOMY

Description. This procedure involves removal of the entire gland, its capsule, and the seminal vesicles. Often, in the presence of more advanced tumor extension, one of the neurovascular bundles may still be spared, potentially allowing potency.

Indications. Radical prostatectomy is the treatment preferred for patients with organ-confined (within the prostatic capsule) carcinoma of the prostate.

Perioperative risks. Until recently, the risk of impotence with this approach was extremely high. Now, with careful anatomic dissection, the posterolateral neurovascular bundles, supplying the corpora cavernosa, may be spared for erectile potency in most patients who are potent preoperatively. Urinary incontinence is generally not the threat it used to be.

Urinary extravasation, postoperative hemorrhage, pelvic hematoma, and wound infection occur in a small percentage of patients. Ureteral obstruction has occurred as a result of edema of the bladder floor necessitating a percutaneous nephrostomy. Lymphoceles have occurred from inadequate obliteration of lymph channels during node dissection. Total urinary incontinence occurs in approximately 5% of patients and moderate incontinence in 20%. This often decreases over time with the assistance of perineal exercises and medication regimens. Rectal injury, deep venous thrombosis, pulmonary edema, and pulmonary emboli, though not common, are risks inherent with the procedure. Hemorrhage is a risk with any prostatectomy. Average blood loss with this approach is 600 to 1000 ml. Bleeding disorders should be ruled out or treated, and blood should be available.

Procedural Steps

Patient preparation and basic surgical instrumentation is as for the simple retropubic approach.

1. After insertion of a 20 or 22 Fr Foley catheter, a vertical midline, extraperitoneal incision is made from the symphysis to the umbilicus.

2. The rectus muscle is split in the midline, and the peritoneum and fascia are dissected off the posterior abdominal wall, beneath the level of the transversalis fascia.

CONSIDERATIONS This technique prevents injury to the inferior epigastric vessels.

3. The peritoneum is freed from the internal inguinal rings, and the vas deferens is ligated bilaterally.

CONSIDERATIONS A bilateral pelvic lymphadenectomy is performed by removing the external iliac, obturator, and hypogastric nodes en bloc. This is done primarily for tumor staging before postoperative radiation or chemotherapy. Theories differ on whether to proceed with surgery if nodal packets reveal metastatic disease. Current thought leans toward going ahead.

4. The pelvic sidewall is entered; the puboprostatic ligaments are exposed and bluntly dissected off the pubis.

STEP **4-1**

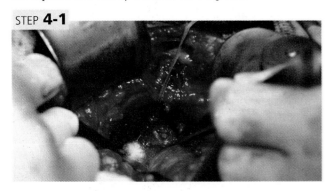

The levator ani muscles are identified and dissected laterally to the level of the urogenital diaphragm.

CONSIDERATIONS Care is taken to avoid injury to the dorsal vein.

5. Large veins, lateral to the ligaments, are ligated and divided to free the apex of the prostate. The dorsal venous complex, supplying the penis, is carefully retracted medially. The venous complex is separated from the urethra with a long-tipped right-angle clamp, doubly ligated with 0 or 2-0 absorbable or nonabsorbable ligatures, or a TA-30 stapler, and transected with a #15 scalpel.

STEP **5-1**

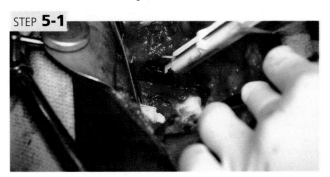

6. Back bleeding, from the vessels on the anterior surface of the prostate, is suture ligated.

7. The rectourethralis fibers are dissected free of and medial to the neurovascular bundles. The neurovascular bundles are gently pushed off the surface of the prostate.

STEP **7-1**

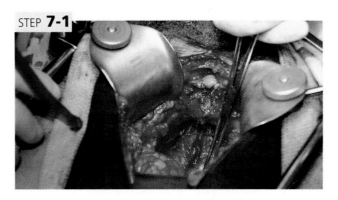

8. The right-angle scissors mobilizes the urethra from the rectourethralis muscle and a penrose drain, or vessel, loop is passed around it as a tractor.

STEP **8-1**

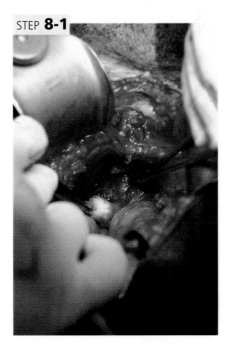

The urethra is elevated and divided and two traction sutures of 2-0 absorbable material are placed on the distal segment.

9. The catheter is clamped proximally and pulled upward through the urethral incision where it is cut and held cephalad. The posterior urethra is transected.

CONSIDERATIONS A section of the prostatic apex is excised and sent for frozen section to determine tumor margins.

10. The rectourethralis muscle is sharply transected. The anterior wall of the rectum is separated manually from Denonvillier's fascia. The prostatic fascia with its neurovascular bundle is freed laterally, from the prostate to the lateral pedicle.

Vessels on the lateral surface of the seminal vesicles are ligated and divided.

11. Traction is placed on the catheter, and the prostate is pulled upward to reveal the vesical neck.

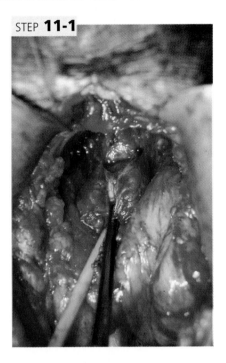

STEP **11-1**

The neck is transected anteriorly, the ureteral orifices are located, and the posterior neck is divided.

CONSIDERATIONS Indigo carmine and ureteral catheters may be employed to ensure identification of the ureteral orifices.

12. The bladder is held cephalad, and the prostate is freed from the rectum.

13. The vas deferens is dissected, clipped, and divided bilaterally in the midline behind the bladder neck. The seminal vesicles are clipped, and the prostate is removed.

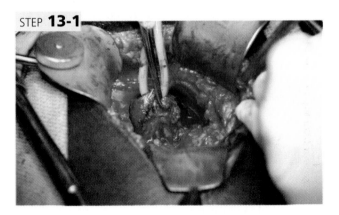

STEP **13-1**

14. Once bleeding is controlled the urethral suture guide is inserted in place of the Foley catheter and 6 sutures of 2-0 chromic on a $^5/_8$ needle are placed inside to outside on the distal urethral segment.

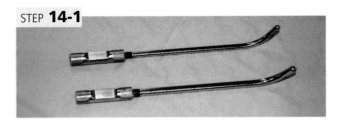

STEP **14-1**

Urethral suture guides.

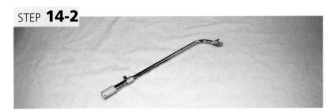

STEP **14-2**

Roth "grip-tip" urethral suture guide.

These are tagged and left uncut to be anastomosed to the bladder neck.

15. The bladder neck is trimmed and everted, and a rosebud stoma is fashioned. The sutures are placed from the urethra to a corresponding position on the bladder neck. A 22 Fr 30 cc Foley catheter is inserted through the urethra into the bladder. The sutures are brought together in single fashion and tied.

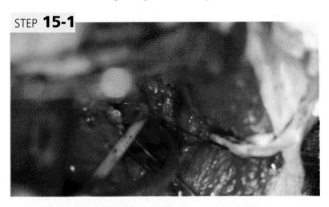

STEP **15-1**

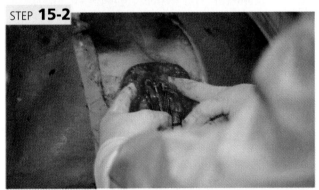

STEP **15-2**

16. Closure is as for simple retropubic prostatectomy. Continuous postoperative irrigation is rarely used. The Foley catheter is placed to gentle traction. Dressings follow simple routine.

TOTAL PERINEAL PROSTATECTOMY

Description. Total removal of the prostate gland and seminal vesicles through an incision between the scrotum and anus.

Indications. The treatment of localized adenocarcinoma of the prostate, offering a potential cure of deep visceral cancer with minimal morbidity and loss of body function.

Perioperative risks. Hemorrhage generally resulting from dissection of the bulbous urethra and ureteral injury usually resulting from dissection behind the trigone or high division of the bladder neck are the two major intraoperative problems encountered. Other potential problems include rectal injury, urethrorectal fistula, constipation, diarrhea, ureteral occlusion, perineal bleeding, catheter clot obstruction, perineal urinary leakage, urinary incontinence, impotence, and urethrovesical stricture.

Procedural Steps

Patient preparation and instrumentation is identical to simple perineal prostatectomy.

1. Surgical approach is as for simple perineal prostatectomy, steps 1 through 8.

9. The posterior layer of the ventral rectal fascia is separated from the true Denonvillier's fascia on the prostate.

> **CONSIDERATIONS** Adhesions are sharply divided against Denonvillier's fascia to protect the nerves located within the reflected ventral rectal fascia.

10. Dissection continues posteriorly and laterally to the base of the seminal vesicles where the true prostatic capsule is exposed by transverse incision into Denonvillier's fascia.

> **CONSIDERATIONS** This approach allows access to the seminal vesicles and ampullae. Lateral vascular pedicles may be identified and ligated at this point.

11. The prostate is freed laterally by blunt dissection, inside the fascia, and on each side of the apex.

12. The pelvic fascia over the proximal membranous urethra is incised. A right-angle clamp is employed to shell the membranous urethra from the fascia containing the cavernous nerves and is sharply incised.

STEP **12-1**

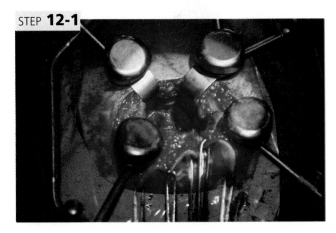

Urethra exposed.

STEP **12-2**

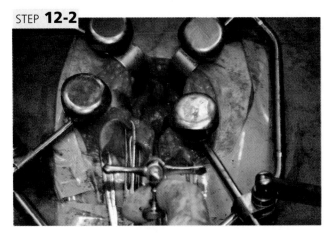

Urethra dissected, tagging sutures in place.

13. The posterior bladder neck is severed, and the bladder is retracted superiorly. A plane is then developed between the anterior bladder and the posterior prostate and seminal vesicles.

14. The vascular pedicles are identified at 5 and 7 o'clock positions, incised, and divided. The prostate is excised.

STEP **14-1**

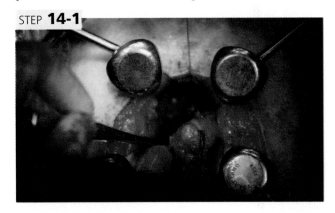

15. Before closure of the bladder neck, vest sutures of 0 or 2-0 chromic are placed in a mattress fashion in the open bladder neck at 2 o'clock and 10 o'clock positions. These are left long for later lateral perineal placement.

16. After placement of the Foley catheter, the urethra is reanastomosed to the bladder neck with four to six 2-0 chromic sutures, placed at 2, 4, 8, and 10 o'clock positions.

STEP **16-1**

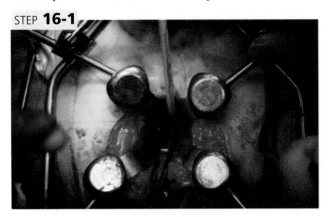

Foley catheter exiting urethra.

STEP**16-2**

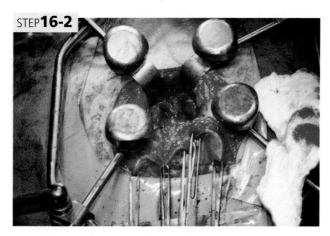

Urethral anastomosis completed.

CONSIDERATIONS Some surgeons opt to place sutures at 6 and 12 o'clock positions as well.

17. Once reanastomosis is accomplished the vest sutures are crossed and brought through the perineal body laterally and parallel to the urethra, anterior to the incision. These are secured just beneath the skin or to the skin with suture buttons.

18. A drain of the surgeon's preference is placed anterior to the rectal surface and drawn out through a separate stab wound.

STEP**18-1**

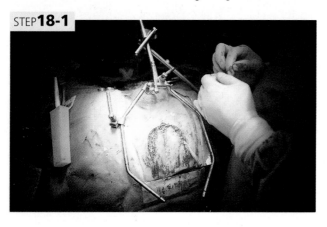

19. Final closure and dressings are as described in the simple procedure.

PELVIC LYMPH NODE DISSECTION

Description. Nodal dissection incorporates the primary, secondary, and tertiary levels of lymphatic drainage. Frequently an epidural anesthetic will be employed, allowing postoperative pain control.

Indications. For staging of metastatic disease before radical prostatectomy or cystectomy.

Perioperative risks. The most common problem encountered is postoperative lymphocele formation resulting from failure to clip all afferent lymphatics. Other complications encountered include thrombosis of the pelvic veins, pulmonary emboli, and

Nursing Care and Discharge Planning for Radical (Total) Prostatectomy

1. Enemas are contraindicated postoperatively. Ensure that stool softeners are administered.
2. Drain is removed in approximately 3 days.
3. Irrigate catheter as indicated to clear clots and prevent retention.
4. Review catheter and dressing care. Teach patient to irrigate catheter.
5. Catheter will be removed in approximately 1 to 2 weeks. Patient should be instructed about probability of temporary or transient incontinence that could persist for up to 1 year.
6. Patient may shower or bathe the first postoperative day, using water repellent protection over the dressings (e.g., cellophane). Dressings should be kept clean and dry.
7. Encourage early ambulation and nonstrenuous activity to the level of pain tolerance.
8. Lifting should be restricted to less than 20 lb. for 4 to 6 weeks.
9. Review signs and symptoms to be reported: urinary retention, pyuria, distention, fever, hemorrhage, increased pain or edema, edema in extremities, redness or warmth at incisional site, alteration in sensation in arms or legs.
10. Aspirin and nonsteroidal antiinflammatory agents should not be taken unless approved by the physician.
11. Patient will be discharged in 3 to 5 days.

lymphedema of the genitalia and legs. Phlebitis, deep vein occlusion, edema, and inguinal hernia may develop postoperatively.

Equipment and instrumentation
Equipment
Electrosurgery unit
Alternating compression unit
Headlight (optional)
Suction unit
Instrumentation
Laparotomy instrument set
Self-retaining retractor
Large hand-held retractors
Long vascular instruments
Clip appliers
Miscellaneous supplies
Laparotomy pack
Sterile gowns
Sterile gloves
Drape towels, adherent
Sterile cloth towels
Suction tubing
Electrosurgery pencil, hand control
Electrosurgery spatula, 6 inches long
Holster
Ligaclips: medium, medium large, large
Suture: 2-0, 3-0, absorbable on SH-1 needle
Suture: 0, 2-0, 3-0 ties, absorbable and nonabsorbable by preference

Suture: 0, 2-0, 3-0 on CT (general closure) needle
Skin clips *or*
4-0 monofilament, cuticular on FS needle *or*
4-0 subcuticular, absorbable on plastic needles
Steri-Strips
Antiseptic prep solution
Absorbent prep drape
Sterile water, 1000 ml
Sterile saline, 1000 ml

PREOPERATIVE

Nursing Care and Teaching Considerations for Pelvic Lymph Node Dissection

1. Review patient record for preoperative studies: PT, PTT, bleeding time, CBC, serum electrolytes, cardiac enzymes, urine culture, serum chemistry survey, chest x-ray, CT scan, serum alphafetoprotein, beta-HCG (tumor marker).
2. Ascertain that preoperative orders have been accomplished: CVP line, bowel prep, antibiotics if indicated, NPO (no oral intake).
3. Assess patient for skin integrity, peripheral vascular circulation, cardiovascular and pulmonary status, allergies, range of motion, physical limitations, medical and surgical history.
4. Discuss patient expectations and assess comprehension of intended procedure and anxiety level.
5. Check equipment, packaging, and instrumentation for function and integrity.
6. Check medications for dosage and expiration dates.
7. Position patient in supine. Ensure that IV lines are unrestricted and linen smooth.
8. Apply alternating compression stockings and patient dispersive pad appropriately.
9. Aseptically insert Foley catheter to closed drainage system and maintain kink free below bladder level.
10. Prep and drape patient according to AORN standards.
11. Document assessment findings and nursing interventions.

Procedural Steps

1. The patient is placed in the supine position with the pelvis slightly elevated. A Foley catheter to closed drainage is aseptically inserted. The patient is prepped and draped as for laparotomy.

2. After a low midline incision, the perivesical space is entered, and a defect is bluntly created between the bladder and the iliac vessels.

3. The peritoneum is sharply dissected from the anterior abdominal wall, the iliopsoas region, and the internal inguinal ring. The spermatic cord is freed and retracted with a Penrose drain.

4. The bladder is retracted medially, and the colon and peritoneal casing are retracted superiorly. Fibrofatty tissue over the external iliac vein is divided, and the dissection is carried distally to reach and resect the medial lymph node of Cloquet. Fibrofatty tissue is cleared from the bony pelvis and over Cooper's ligament.

5. The tissue between the iliac artery and vein is separated to expose the medial and anterior surface of the artery. The tissue

is then passed under the iliac vein and freed at its inferior margin to expose the obturator nerve.

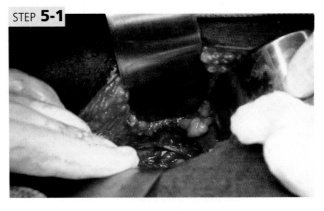

STEP **5-1**

Obturator nodal tissue is grasped and dissected to the obturator canal.

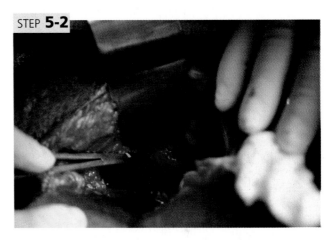

STEP **5-2**

6. The lymphatics are doubly clipped.

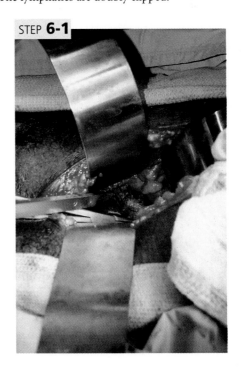

STEP **6-1**

Tissue dorsal to the obturator nerve is bluntly cleared. Tissue packets are removed.

STEP **6-2**

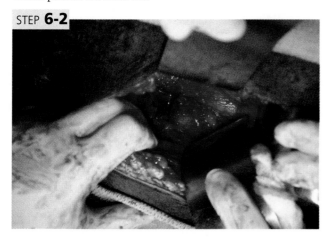

7. The internal iliac artery and its branches are freed of fibrofatty tissue to the level of the pelvis. The obliterated umbilical artery may be ligated and divided. The procedure is repeated on the opposite side.

POSTOPERATIVE

Nursing Care and Discharge Planning for Pelvic Lymph Node Dissection

1. Patient may bathe the first postoperative day with water-repellent material over dressings (e.g., cellophane).
2. Antibiotics are used when indicated. PCA or epidural analgesia is frequently employed initially. Ensure that stool softener is provided daily.
3. Encourage activity to the level of tolerance.
4. Lifting should be restricted to less than 20 lb. for 4 to 6 weeks.
5. Diet may slowly resume as tolerated. Fluid intake should be increased.
6. Foley catheter is removed when patient is ambulating.
7. Pelvic pain, swelling in the lower abdominal quadrants, or edema of the lower extremities may herald the development of a lymphocele.
8. Discharge is in 2 to 4 days
9. Signs and symptoms to be reported include fever, edema of legs and groin, redness or heat at incisional site, purulent drainage from wound, pyuria, dysuria. Transient loss of sensation in the thigh is not uncommon.

RETROPERITONEAL LYMPH NODE DISSECTION (RADICAL LYMPHADENECTOMY)

Description. Radical lymphadenectomy is the bilateral resection of retroperitoneal lymph nodes that includes the nodes, lymph channels, and fat around both renal pedicles, the aorta, the aortal bifurcation, and the vena cava. A thoracoabdominal or transabdominal approach may be used, and general anesthesia is employed. The patient will be hospitalized for 3 to 5 days.

In the thoracoabdominal approach the patient is positioned supine with the chest and upper abdomen rotated 45 degrees. With the transabdominal approach the patient is supine and a midline, xiphoid to suprapubic incision is made. One side may be elevated if the dissection is unilateral. More commonly the transabdominal approach is chosen, and this is what will be addressed.

Indications. The procedure is performed to treat nonseminomatous testicular tumors. These patients are subfertile 60% of the time. Many times, the diagnosis of testicular carcinoma is made after testicular biopsy and before they have decided to start a family. These patients do have an option, before orchiectomy and chemotherapy. Assisted reproductive techniques and sperm banking may allow them to have children in the future. Sperm banking may be done preoperatively on the chance that the patient may not produce ejaculate after the intervention. Although the sperm count motility and morphology may not be optimal, intercytoplasmic sperm injection may assist the patient and his wife to achieve a pregnancy.

Perioperative risks. Risks surrounding retroperitoneal lymph node dissection include vascular injuries, spinal cord injuries, bowel adhesions, pulmonary edema, loss of ejaculation, lymphocele, neurovascular compromise, pressure injury to bony prominences, brachial plexus injury, hemorrhage, and infection. A lower incidence of anejaculate has been reported after unilateral dissection.

Equipment and instrumentation
Equipment
Electrosurgery unit
Suction unit
Alternating compression machine
Headlights
Loupes (surgeon preference)
Positioning pads, pillows
Safety straps
Instruments
Laparotomy instrument set
Long fine dissection instruments
Vascular instruments
Ligaclip appliers
Bookwalter retractor
Long-hand held retractors
Miscellaneous supplies
Laparotomy pack *or*
Universal pack
Sterile gowns
Sterile gloves
Drape towels, adherent, 6
Sterile cloth towels, 6 to 8
Suction tubing
Electrosurgery pencil with hand control
Electrosurgery spatula tip, 6 inch
Holster for electrosurgery pencil
Alternating compression stockings, thigh length
Vessel loops
Umbilical tapes
Sutures, 0, 2-0 silk, 30 inches
Ligaclips

PREOPERATIVE

Nursing Care and Teaching Considerations for Radical Lymphadenectomy

1. Incorporate all nursing diagnoses for the genital system.
2. Review laboratory and other reports of preoperative studies: chest x-ray, ECG, abdominal and pelvic CT scans, tomograms of lung, IVP, serum blood chemistry survey, cardiac enzymes, urine analyses, alpha-fetoprotein, beta-HCG, CBC, PT, PTT. Take note of serum albumin, lymphocyte count, and serum sodium and creatinine levels.
3. Assess patient for peripheral circulation, presence of implants, range of motion, allergies, medical status (diabetes, obesity, asthma), cardiopulmonary status, anemia, skin integrity, physical impairments.
4. Ascertain that 6 units of blood are available.
5. Determine that chemical bowel prep was performed.
6. Explain to patient that CVP line, nasogastric tube, Foley catheter, and possible Swan-Ganz catheter will be present postoperatively.
7. Establish patient's comprehension of surgical procedure and anxiety level. Review as necessary including postoperative expectations and common sequelae (coughing and deep breathing, ambulation, pain management, nausea, dressing and catheter care).
8. Document assessment findings.
9. Check electrosurgery unit, operating room lights, suction unit, alternating compression machine, operating room bed for proper functioning.
10. Check sterile packaging for integrity. Check medications for dosage and expiration dates.
11. Check instrumentation for proper action and freedom from debris or damage.
12. Collect and provide appropriate positioning devices: head cradle, pads for heels, sacrum, elbows, wrists, low back. Position patient supine with legs slightly separated. Utilize safety strap and arm restraints.
13. Place electrosurgery dispersive pad in nonhairy location close to the operative site.
14. Apply alternating compression stockings while patient is awake.
15. Explain purpose of nursing interventions to patient as they are performed.
16. Aseptically insert closed system Foley catheter before prepping and draping the patient.
17. Ensure that linen beneath patient is smooth. Determine that IV lines and catheter are free of constriction.
18. Aseptically prep the operative site according to AORN standards and institutional guidelines. Protect patient from pooling of solutions.
19. Drape patient according to established protocol.
20. Document nursing care provided.

Kittner dissectors
Laparotomy sponges
Radiopaque gauze sponges
Intestinal bag, 2
Knife blades, #10 and #15, 4 each
Syringe, 10 ml finger control
Hypodermic needle, #25 gauge 1 1/4 inches
Foley catheter, #16 Fr, 5 cc balloon
Urinary drainage bag
Leg strap
Gauze dressings
Combine dressings
Nonallergic adhesive tape
Bupivacaine Hcl 0.5% (or choice)
Antiseptic prep solution
Sterile water, 1000 ml, warmed, 4
Sterile saline, 1000 ml, warmed, 2
Absorbent prep drape

Procedural Steps (Left Unilateral)

1. The patient is placed in the supine position. If the dissection is unilateral, the patient is supine with the operative side tilted upward. Routine skin preparation from nipples to midthigh and draping procedures are carried out. A Foley catheter will be inserted before prepping and draping. A nasogastric tube is inserted.

2. A midline abdominal incision is made from the xiphoid process to the symphysis pubis. Wound protectors and self-retaining retractors are placed. The falciform ligament is divided to afford upward displacement of the liver. Abdominal

contents including the liver, spleen, pancreas, bowel, and retroperitoneal lymph nodes are explored to determine the degree of gross nodal involvement. The omentum is reflected and the colon is either packed within the abdominal cavity or mobilized and kept in moist warm packs outside the abdomen.

CONSIDERATIONS An intestinal bag serves this purpose well.

3. The small bowel is packed off to the right side or exteriorized. The retroperitoneal attachment is freed from the cecum to the base of the foramen of Winslow. Dissection is extended medially and superiorly over the vena cava to the duodenojejunal flexure allowing cephalad mobilization of the pancreas and duodenum.

4. Dissection continues obliquely to the left around the cecum to the ligament of Treitz. The inferior mesenteric vein is divided, ligated, and dissected free from the base of the mesentery, where it ascends to enter the portal system. Proximal and distal lymphatic trunks are obliterated with hemoclips.

5. The underside of the bowel is separated from Gerota's fascia, and the balance of the cecum and duodenum are freed. The pancreas is bluntly dissected away from the anterior surface of Gerota's fascia. The small bowel, cecum, and ascending colon are exteriorized and placed in an intestinal bag. The bag and its contents are held on the chest against the trunk of the superior mesenteric artery.

CONSIDERATIONS The pancreas may be covered with moist laparotomy sponges and elevated with a retractor. The superior mesenteric artery should be identified at its origin and handled carefully.

6. The ureters and renal vessels are located to determine safe limits for dissection.

7. The posterior peritoneum is opened between the aorta and the vena cava, on the anterior vena cava at the level of the left renal vein, and dissection is begun.

8. The adrenal vein is exposed, doubly ligated, and divided.

CONSIDERATIONS This step has been determined unnecessary in low-stage disease.

4. By blunt and sharp dissection, the perivascular lymphatic structures are freed inferiorly from the left renal vein. Spermatic and lumbar tributary veins are clipped and divided.

CONSIDERATIONS The short lumbar vein, coursing through the perivascular lymphatic tissue to the left renal vein, is clipped or ligated close to the medial edge of the psoas muscle, exposing the left renal artery.

5. The left renal artery is skeletonized.

6. The adventitial plane over the infrarenal aorta is entered, and the aorta is cleared of tissue. Spermatic arteries are ligated and divided as they are encountered.

CONSIDERATIONS Clips on the aorta or vena cava will generally avulse. Placement in these sites is not recommended.

7. The left renal vein is lifted with a retractor, and the lymphatic tissue is pulled downward to reach the posterior superior portion of the hilar lymphatics behind the posterior layer of Gerota's fascia. Dissection continues laterally until the pelviureteric junction is seen.

8. Hilar lymphatics are dissected from the psoas fascia toward the aorta, and the posterior layer of Gerota's fascia is incised where it attaches to the spine. Lateral retroaortic tissue is freed.

9. The lumbar vessels and lumbar sympathetic trunk are inspected, and small connecting branches entering the lymphatic mass are sacrificed.

CONSIDERATIONS The anterior and posterior branches of the sympathetic nerve chain are retracted in vessel loops and spared in the patient with negative findings. A block dissection is performed if node findings are positive. In cases of extensive disease, the lumbar vessels are divided and ligated to better mobilize and retract major vessels allowing a full dissection.

10. The anterior and lateral aspects of the aorta are cleared, preserving preaortic and periaortic tissue beneath the inferior mesenteric artery. Care must be taken to identify aberrant vessels to the lower pole of the kidney.

11. Dissection continues down the aorta on the psoas fascia to the bifurcation of the left external and internal iliac arteries.

12. Freed tissue is passed under the aorta below the renal artery. Lumbar arteries in this area are ligated and divided as necessary (L2-3 commonly).

CONSIDERATIONS This technique affords improved hemostasis, aortal retraction, and exposure of paraaortic lymph nodes.

13. Continuing in a caudad direction, lumbar veins are ligated and divided allowing a 360-degree dissection around the vena cava and aorta.

14. Tissue surrounding the right renal vein and vena cava is cleared beginning on the anterior surface. The right spermatic vein is ligated at the vena cava. Vascular connections from the right ureter to the right spermatic vessels are clipped and ligated.

15. Dissection continues down the vena cava to the right common iliac and the beginning of the right external iliac artery. Tissue is passed to the midline.

CONSIDERATIONS The right common iliac artery should be retracted to allow ligation of veins entering the left common iliac vein and prevent bleeding caused by avulsion.

16. The aorta and vena cava are retracted to the left with vein retractors. The right renal artery is isolated and cleared of tissue, which is passed beneath the vena cava to the midline. All proximal lymphatic channels are obliterated with hemoclips.

17. Working in a caudad direction, dissection is performed along the anterior spinal ligament clearing all interaorto caval, medial retrocaval, and retroaortic lymph tissue. The point of fixation and posterior attachment are clipped and divided. Tissue division around the iliac artery is completed and the tissue is removed.

18. Spermatic vessels on the affected side are dissected to the external inguinal ring, including the stump from the previous orchiectomy and a section of peritoneum, and removed.

19. The wound is inspected for hemostasis and irrigated with warm sterile water. The parietal peritoneum is attached to the mesentery at its root with 3-0 interrupted silk sutures as the bowel is replaced into the wound.

20. Each renal artery is elevated with a vein retractor and the suprahilar nodal areas are inspected.

21. If reperitonealization is desired, the posterior peritoneum is closed with a 2-0 absorbable continuous suture. The viscera are repositioned in the abdominal cavity and the wound is closed, usually without placement of a drain.

INCONTINENCE PROCEDURES

VESICOURETHRAL SUSPENSION (MARSHALL-MARCHETTI-KRANTZ)

Description. The intent of the Marshall-Marchetti-Krantz (MMK) operation is to bring the bladder and urethra into the pelvis by suturing paraurethral vaginal tissue to the back of the symphysis pubis.

A recent modification of this technique is the Burch procedure. The approach mimics the MMK until placement of the buttressing sutures. Instead of attempting difficult periosteal sutures, nonabsorbable size 0 sutures are placed into Cooper's ligament from each side of the bladder neck. The Burch proce-

POSTOPERATIVE

Nursing Care and Discharge Planning for Radical Lymphadenectomy

1. Patient is at risk for third-space losses and ileus. Monitor urine osmolarity, serum sodium levels. Replace with sodium chloride solutions as appropriate.
2. Assess patient for cardiovascular status and respiratory excursion. Assist with coughing and deep breathing. IPPB (Intermittent positive-pressure breathing) may be indicated.
3. CVP line or Swan-Ganz catheter is removed when blood pressure, pulse, and Hgb and HCT levels are stable.
4. Foley catheter and alternating compression stockings are removed when patient is ambulating. Nasogastric tube is removed in 3 to 5 days, or when peristalsis has returned and patient is able to pass flatus.
5. Early ambulation is encouraged. Normal activity may slowly resume after 1-2 weeks. Lifting >20 lbs. and strenuous activity should be avoided for one month.
6. Antibiotics are not routine. Pain may usually be controlled with epidural catheter, PCA, IV, or IM therapy. Morphine or Demerol are usually adequate for control. Stool softeners should be provided.
7. Hydration is provided with IV therapy initially. Patient should increase fluid intake when able and slowly resume diet with frequent small meals. If bloating occurs, physician should be contacted. This could indicate the onset of a bowel obstruction.
8. Patient may shower on first postoperative day if tolerated.
9. Patient may be discharged after 6 to 10 days (when bowel function has returned and oral analgesia is effective).
10. Patient should be instructed to keep postoperative visits. Tumor markers (alpha fetoprotein, beta-HCG) and CT scan of the abdomen will be repeated at 3-month intervals if markers were elevated preoperatively or nodes were positive. If nodes were positive or markers become elevated postoperatively, referral to an oncologist for chemotherapy is indicated.
11. Opposite testis is inspected at monthly intervals to determine tumor recurrence.

dure is technically easier, and long-term results are fairly equivalent.

The patient will commonly have a vaginal pack and a urethral or suprapubic catheter, or both, and possibly a wound drain postoperatively.

Indications. An MMK is performed for the correction of stress incontinence caused by an abnormal urethrovesical angle.

Perioperative risks. Inability to void is the most common problem encountered after repair. This is usually a result of sutures placed too close to the urethra or to periurethral scarring. Additional difficulties include persistent detrusor instability, enterocele, urinary tract infection, stone formation, hemorrhage, hematoma, urinary drainage from inadvertent cystotomy, ureteral obstruction, vesicovaginal fistula, osteitis pubis, enterocele, and vaginal tears.

PREOPERATIVE

Nursing Care and Teaching Considerations for Bladder Neck Suspensions

1. Incorporate general nursing diagnoses.
2. Review patient record for preoperative studies: PT, PTT, CBC, ECG, cardiac enzymes and blood gases if indicated, urine culture, cystoscopy, cystogram, VUD, IVP, chest x-ray.
3. Review patient's medical and surgical history: obesity, diabetes, COPD, allergies, cardiovascular and pulmonary status, neurologic history, peripheral circulation.
4. Determine that preoperative antibiotics and enema were provided.
5. Assess patient for range of motion, physical limitations, skin integrity.
6. Establish comprehension of planned procedure and anxiety level, respond to questions as necessary. Spontaneous voiding may never return, requiring the patient to learn and accept intermittent self-catheterization. This is particularly true after a suburethral sling procedure.
7. Check equipment, packaging, and instrumentation for proper function and integrity.
8. Check medications for dosage and expiration dates.
9. Position patient under the guidance of the anesthetist. Ensure that IV lines are free of constriction and that linen beneath patient is smooth. Provide appropriate padding for position chosen.
10. Apply patient dispersive pad to nonhairy fleshy site near abdomen. Apply alternating compression stockings.
11. Prep and drape patient according to AORN standards. Protect patient from pooling of solutions.
12. Document nursing assessment and interventions.

The usual anesthetic and positioning risks apply in relation to patient age, size, and health status. A large percentage of patients with stress incontinence suffer from obesity and diabetes. It is important to evaluate for these conditions and prepare for proper patient management (positioning concerns relating to peripheral vascular circulation and pressure points, skin breakdown, risk for infection, and wound healing).

Equipment and instrumentation
Equipment
Electrosurgery unit
Alternating compression unit
Headlight
Allen stirrups
Positioning aides
Instrumentation
Laparotomy instrument set
Heaney instruments
Long instruments
Vaginal instruments (optional)
Miscellaneous supplies
Laparotomy pack *or*
Laparoscopy pack

Drape sheets
Drape towels
Sterile cloth towels
Sterile gowns
Sterile gloves
Laparotomy sponges
Radiopaque gauze sponges
Kittner dissectors
Foley catheter, #16 Fr, 5 cc balloon
Urine drainage bag
Suprapubic catheter
Vaginal pack
Syringe, 10 ml
Syringe, 10 ml finger control
Hypodermic needle, #25 gauge, 1 1/4 inches
Suture, 2-0 absorbable on UR needle
Sutures, 0, 2-0, 3-0 absorbable on CT-1 needle
Suture, 4-0 absorbable on cuticular needle *or*
Skin staples
Gauze dressings
Sterile saline, 1000 ml
Sterile water, 1000 ml
Local anesthetic

Procedural Steps

The patient is usually placed in a moderate Trendelenburg position. Legs are placed in stirrups or frog-legged position with supports under each knee to allow for intraoperative vaginal manipulation. Abdominal and vaginal preps are required. The perineum and abdomen are draped out. A Foley catheter is inserted into the urethra at the beginning of surgery.

1. A Foley catheter is inserted in the bladder through the urethra and clamped. A suprapubic transverse incision is made to expose the prevesical space of Retzius. The bladder retractor is positioned with small, moist laparotomy pads in place.

2. The bladder and urethra are freed from the posterior surface of the rectus muscle and symphysis pubis by gentle blunt manipulation.

3. The assistant places two fingers into the vagina and lifts the urethra upward against the symphysis pubis so that the periurethral musculofascial structures are more easily repaired by the surgeon.

4. Mattress sutures of 2-0 absorbable material on a Heaney needle holder are placed through the paraurethral tissue and the vaginal wall on each side of the urethra and tagged.

5. Two rows of absorbable sutures are placed on each side of the urethra, the most proximal are located at the urethrovesical junction, and tagged.

6. The sutures are then passed through the pubic periosteum, providing support to the urethra and bladder neck. After all sutures have been placed, they are individually tied as the assistant elevates the vagina to prevent tearing of the periosteum.

7. A fourth pair of sutures are placed laterally above the vesical neck and fastened to the upper symphysis or the insertion of the rectus muscle.

8. The area is drained, and the wound is closed in layers and dressed.

9. The vagina may be packed with 2-inch packing, which should be removed after 24 to 36 hours. The Foley catheter is connected to a closed urinary drainage system.

VAGINAL NEEDLE SUSPENSION

Description. The incision is superficial, the bladder and bladder neck are not dissected, and the paraurethral tissues that suspend the vesical neck are buttressed vaginally. Stamey was the first to use the cystoscope to place sutures exactly at the vesical neck. Urethrovesical needle suspensions include the modified Pereyra, the Stamey, the Pereyra-Raz, the Gittes cystourethropexy, and the Muzsnai culposuspension. Modifications are still occurring, many too recent to be found in textbooks but documented in technical articles and reports. One such adaptation utilizes the Mitek orthopedic suture anchor to facilitate suture placement. A similar product is commercially available in a prepackaged kit, designed for urethrovesical suspension.

The Gittes method, as well as some of the newer approaches, does not violate the anterior vaginal wall. For those who believe in the presence of the G spot, this is important anatomic architecture to preserve. Long-term results are about equal for all methods.

The procedure is ideal for the outpatient setting provided that the patient has adequate home support during the initial recovery period and is able to perform self-care. Anesthesia may be regional or general.

Indications. The primary reason for vaginal needle suspension is anatomic stress incontinence with urethral and bladder neck hypermobility. Endoscopic suspension of the vesical neck for stress incontinence, originally developed by Stamey, has distinct advantages over open retropubic urethrovesical suspensions.

Contraindications include intrinsic sphincter damage, moderate to severe cystocele without an ancillary corrective procedure, and detrusor instability without genuine stress incontinence.

Perioperative risks. Urethral bleeding, injury to periurethral fascia, retropubic bleeding, and bladder or trigone perforation are the major surgical intraoperative concerns. Voiding dysfunction (inability to void requiring short-term intermittent catheterization); wound infection; injury to the common peroneal, sciatic, obturator, tibial, femoral, saphenous, or ilioinguinal nerves; detrusor instability; and persistent incontinence (less than 10%) have been encountered postoperatively. Continence rates postoperatively average 80%.

Equipment and instrumentation
Equipment
Electrosurgery unit
Suction unit
Alternating compression unit
Allen stirrups
Rolling stool
Headlight (optional)
Instruments
Vaginal instrument set
Cystoscopy setup
Stamey needles, straight, 15-degree, and 30-degree *or*
Pereyra needle

Miscellaneous supplies

Martin needles, # 7 (optional)
Foley catheter, 14 Fr, 5 cc balloon
Suprapubic catheter, 12 Fr
Introducer for suprapubic catheter
Urine drainage bag
Syringe, Asepto
Vaginal packing
Nylon or Prolene suture ties, # 2
Gore-Tex bolsters, 4 mm
Antibiotic irrigation (often gentamicin)
Indigo carmine (for IV administration)
Triple sulfa vaginal cream
Local anesthetic with epinephrine
Syringe, 10 ml finger control
Hypodermic needle, #25 gauge, 1 1/4 inches, 2
Suture, 3-0 absorbable on CT-2 and SH-1 needle
Suture, 3-0 and 4-0 absorbable on PS-3 needle
Antiseptic prep solution
Absorbent prep drape

Procedural Steps

The patient is placed in the lithotomy position. Although the procedure is not lengthy, care must be taken to ensure proper body alignment and avoid pressure areas when positioning the patient. The legs, positioned in stirrups, are extended to promote a flat lower abdomen. The buttocks must be at the edge of the lower hinge of the operating room bed for placement of the weighted vaginal retractor. A lumbar support may assist to alleviate undue stress on the lower back and sacrum. After preoperative hair removal, the entire perineum, vagina, and suprapubic area are prepped. A drape is placed across the rectum to isolate it from the surgical field. Local anesthetic may be instilled for hemostasis and pain management.

1. The labia minora are sutured laterally with 3-0 silk to expose the vaginal introitus.

2. Two symmetrical transverse incisions are made to the left and right of the midline at the upper border of the symphysis pubis.

3. The tissue is spread bluntly to the anterior rectus muscle.

4. Antibiotic-soaked gauze sponges are packed into each incision while the vaginal portion of the procedure is carried out.

5. The urethral length is measured with a Foley catheter by positioning the inflated balloon at the internal vesical neck. The point of the urethral meatus is marked on the catheter, and the Foley is deflated and withdrawn. The catheter is then reinflated, and the length from meatal mark to the balloon is measured.

6. The Foley catheter is reinserted and inflated. The weighted speculum is placed in the vagina, and the anterior vaginal mucosa is incised in a U or T shape about 2 to 2.5 cm in length.

CONSIDERATIONS The Gittes technique requires no vaginal incision; one modification involves bilateral 2 cm incisions lateral to the midline.

7. The vaginal tissue is separated from the urethra by spreading the scissors in the plane between the tissues. The incision is complete when the tip of the index finger can rest against the bladder neck.

8. The needle of choice is inserted into the medial edge of one of the suprapubic incisions and through the rectus fascia just above the symphysis pubis.

CONSIDERATIONS The modification utilizing the Mitek requires a power drill to create a small crater in the pubic bone. The Mitek suture is then anchored in this defect.

9. The superior edge of the symphysis is probed with the needle tip, and the needle is passed 1 to 2 cm parallel to the posterior symphysis.

10. One index finger is inserted into the vagina at the bladder neck as the other maneuvers the needle along the bladder neck and through the fascia and periurethral tissues.

CONSIDERATIONS With the Mitek modification, the Stamey needle is passed from the vaginal wound to the suprapubic wound, and the suture is placed through the eye and carried back down to be sutured through the fascia and periurethral tissue. It is then returned to the suprapubic location where it will be tied in place.

11. The Foley catheter is removed and the cystoscope inserted to check the needle position.

12. Heavy no. 2 suture material is threaded into the needle eye and the needle is pulled suprapubically. Hemostats are placed on each suture end.

13. If a Stamey needle is used, it is passed a second time about 1 cm lateral to the first puncture and the suture is placed under tension. Position is again checked cystoscopically. The Pereyra needle is a double-pronged needle and need be passed only one time.

CONSIDERATIONS With the Stamey approach the vaginal end of the suture is buttressed with the Gore-Tex material and placed through the needle's eye. The Gore-Tex is guided into the urethrovesical junction.

14. The entire procedure is repeated on the other side.

15. The cystoscope is reinserted and the bladder filled. Under direct visualization, the sutures are pulled upward so that the flow of fluid is alternately released and stopped.

16. The Foley catheter is reinserted, and the sutures are tied into position in the suprapubic incisions. The incisions are then closed with absorbable sutures.

17. The vaginal mucosa is closed with 3-0 absorbable suture and the vaginal pack coated with triple sulfa cream is inserted. The Foley catheter may be removed.

18. A stab wound can be made in the lower abdomen for placement of a suprapubic catheter while the bladder is still full.

19. A small gauze dressing is placed over the abdominal wounds and the catheter secured and connected to drainage.

SUBURETHRAL SLING

Description. The pubovaginal (pubofascial) sling procedure utilizes an autograft strip of fascia lata, synthetic material (Gore-tex), or a freeze-dried or fresh-frozen strip of cadaver fascia lata. The graft is placed between the urethra and anterior vaginal wall and anchored to the anterior rectus fascia or pectineal ligament.

When the allograft material is used, the procedure lends itself to the outpatient setting. If an autograft is chosen, a 3-day hospital stay might be more advisable because of the potential for increased postoperative pain. The patient is in lithotomy position under regional or general anesthesia.

When fascia lata autograft is chosen, separate draping materials and instruments are needed for the operative leg. The graft may be harvested with the legs in stirrups. Compression dressings should be applied before proceeding with the balance of the procedure.

Indications. Some women display severe stress incontinence with little or no urethral mobility as intraabdominal pressures change. Frequently, they have had prior corrective surgery, neurologic injury, radiation therapy, poor urethral resistance, or pelvic trauma. Urine is lost with minimal exertion, and low urethral closing pressures are apparent during diagnostic examination. They have what is termed *type III stress incontinence* with a partially or totally opened urethral sphincter at rest.

This approach is indicated when it is believed that simple elevation and stabilization will not improve continence. Some practitioners advocate that patients with resting urethral closing pressures less than 20 cm H_2O are candidates. Others considered as candidates are patients with chronic pulmonary disease, obesity, athleticism, and congenital tissue weakness.

Fascia lata tends to be stronger, and less abdominal dissection is necessary. The strength of this tissue has lent itself to the allograft method using freeze-dried or fresh-frozen fascia lata. This accomplishes a good repair with minimal dissection and faster recovery time. The intervention to be described is the newer technique utilizing fresh frozen fascia lata graft. The traditional methods are discussed under considerations.

Perioperative risks. Urethral outlet resistance is increased, frequently resulting in obstruction as demonstrated by voiding difficulties. Postoperative problems that have been encountered include sudden nonpainful urgency, urge incontinence, urinary retention, ilioinguinal nerve injury, detrusor instability, synthetic graft erosion, wound infection, persistent urinary tract infection, sinus tract formation, persistent urgency and frequency, bladder or urethral injury, and fistula formation.

Equipment and instrumentation

Setup for vaginal needle suspension in addition to the following:

Power drill
Drill bit and guide
Mitek system (or equivalent)
Allograft material

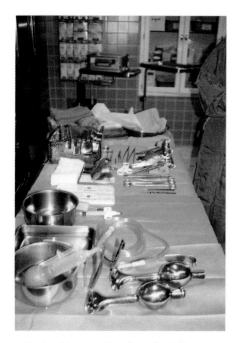

Back table setup for suburethral sling.

Procedural Steps

The patient is placed in lithotomy position and prepped and draped in a routine fashion. Alternating compression stockings and Allen stirrups are employed.

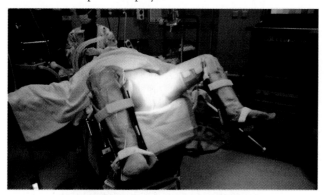

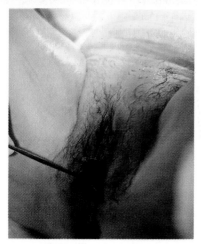

Lower abdomen, inner thighs, perineum, and vagina are prepped with Iodophor.

A Foley catheter is placed after cystoscopy. The labia minora are sutured back laterally with 3-0 silk. The vaginal speculum is placed, and local anesthetic with a vasopressive agent is injected into the vaginal mucosa to aid hemostasis.

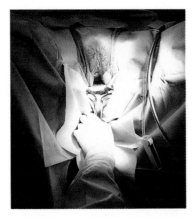

Weighted speculum is placed and vaginal vault inspected.

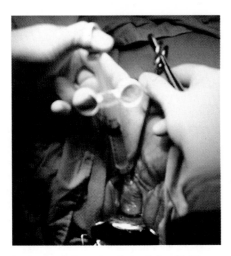

Local anesthetic containing epinephrine is instilled into vaginal mucosa to assist hemostasis.

Local anesthetic is injected deeply and laterally into the suprapubic incision site.

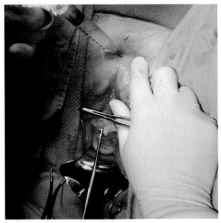

Local anesthetic is instilled deeply into low abdominal incisional site.

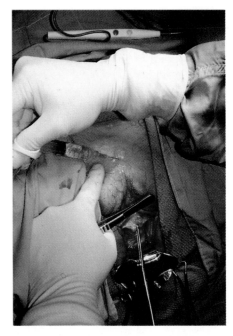

Local anesthetic is instilled laterally into low abdominal incision site.

1. A transverse midline abdominal incision is made at the upper border of the symphysis pubis.

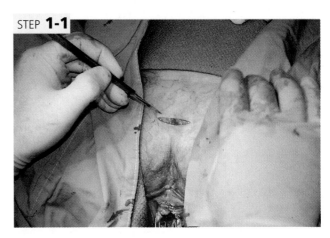

STEP **1-1**

CONSIDERATIONS When the rectus fascia is used, a Pfannenstiel incision is made, extending from one iliac crest to the other, exposing the anterior abdominal wall rectus fascia. Two incisions are made in the fascia, and it is dissected free. Each end is oversewn with no. 2 nylon suture. The margins from the excised graft are closed with interrupted absorbable 2-0 sutures.

Fascia lata from the lateral thigh is retrieved through two vertical incisions, one at the midthigh level and one approximately 3 cm above the knee. The fascia is incised twice at 3 cm intervals proximally. Dissection is carried bilaterally in a tunnel fashion to the knee wound. A Penrose drain is placed under the fascia at the knee wound and the fascia is detached, passed to the thigh wound, and removed. The graft margins are closed with interrupted 2-0 absorbable sutures. A drain is inserted, and the leg wound is closed in layers. A compression dressing is applied.

2. The tissue is spread bluntly to the anterior rectus muscle.

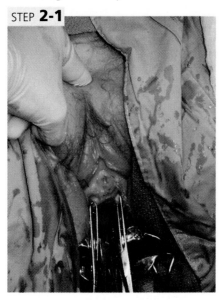

STEP **2-1**

Incision is carried bluntly to the rectus fascia. Note stream of urine as pressure is exerted.

3. Antibiotic-soaked gauze sponges are packed into the incision while the vaginal portion of the procedure is carried out.

4. The urethral length is measured with a Foley catheter by positioning the inflated balloon at the internal vesical neck. The point of the urethral meatus is marked on the catheter, and the Foley is deflated and withdrawn. The catheter is then reinflated, and the length from meatal mark to the balloon is measured.

5. The Foley catheter is reinserted and the weighted speculum is placed in the vagina, and the anterior vaginal mucosa is incised, lateral to the urethra, bilaterally.

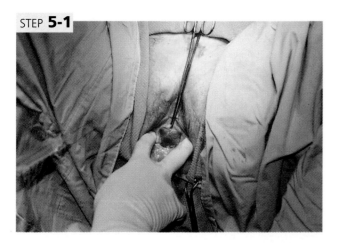

STEP **5-1**

CONSIDERATIONS The traditional approach utilizes an inverted U incision about 2 to 2.5 cm in length.

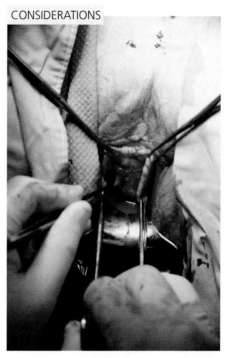

CONSIDERATIONS

An anterior vaginal wall flap is raised and dissection is carried to the pubic bone bilaterally. The endopelvic fascia is perforated and the retropubic space is entered.

6. Dissection is carried across the urethra, beneath the anterior vaginal mucosa, to create a space for the sling. Dissection is carried laterally to the pubic bone, the endopelvic fascia perforated, and the retropubic space entered.

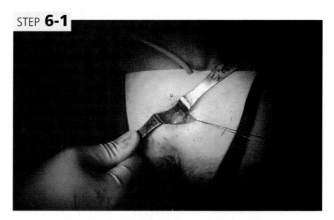

STEP **6-1**

Pubic bone exposed.

7. A power drill is used to create bilateral small defects in the pubic bone.

STEP **7-1**

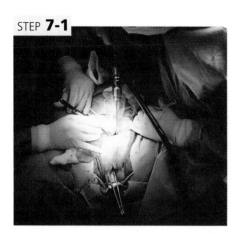

Creating defect with power drill.

The Mitek suture is anchored in the defect immediately after each one is established.

STEP **7-2**

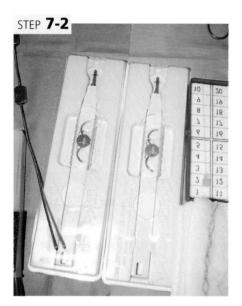

Mitek suture anchor system.

STEP **7-3**

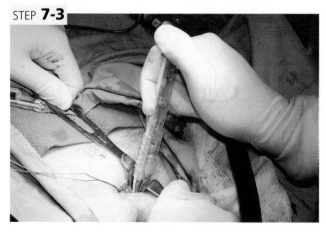

Placing first Mitek suture anchor.

STEP **7-4**

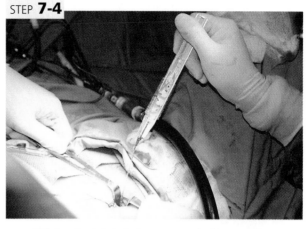

Withdrawing Mitek device, suture imbedded in pubic bone.

STEP **7-5**

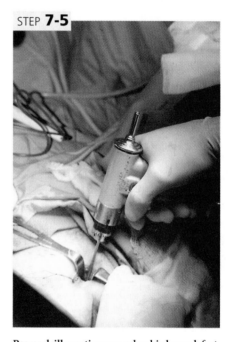

Power drill creating second pubic bone defect.

STEP **7-6**

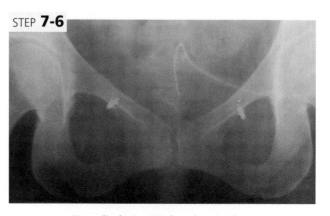

X-ray displaying Mitek anchors in place.

8. A Stamey needle is passed cephalad from one of the vaginal incisions to the ipsilateral pubic bone.

STEP **8-1**

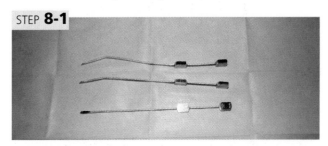

Stamey needles, 0 to 15 and 30 degrees.

STEP **8-2**

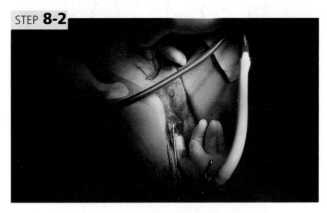

Stamey needle passing suture to vaginal introitus.

The free end of the Mitek suture is threaded through the eye of the needle.

9. The superior edge of the symphysis is probed with the needle tip, and the needle is passed 1 to 2 cm parallel to the posterior symphysis.

10. One index finger is inserted into the vagina at the bladder neck as the other maneuvers the needle along the bladder neck and through the fascia and periurethral tissues. The Foley is removed and the cystoscope is inserted to check the needle position.

STEP **10-1**

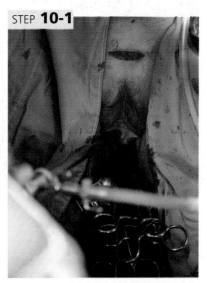

Cystoscopy is performed and bladder refilled.

The Foley is reinserted.

11. Steps 8 to 10 are repeated on the opposite side.

12. The free end of the Mitek is sutured and tied, but not cut, to the graft at one end.

STEP **12-1**

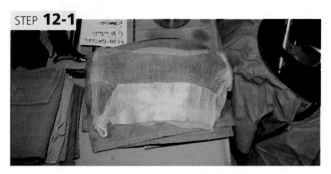

Fresh frozen fascia lata graft.

STEP **12-2**

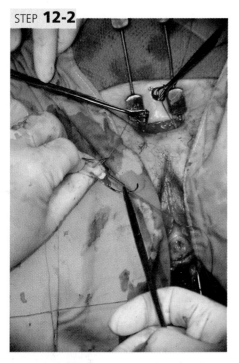

Attaching suture to graft material.

The graft is passed to the pubic site by threading the free end through the Stamey needle and passing the needle cephalad. The Stamey is removed, and the graft is retained by placing a hemostat on the suture. The second Mitek suture is threaded into the free end of the graft.

STEP **12-3**

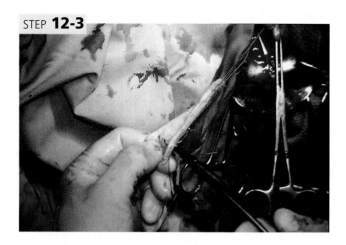

Cystoscopic examination is again performed.

CONSIDERATIONS The traditional approach sutures the graft on each end and passes a long curved clamp proximally to distally to grasp the sutured tissue. The graft is sutured in place to the pubic tubercle or paraurethral fascia after each pass.

CONSIDERATIONS

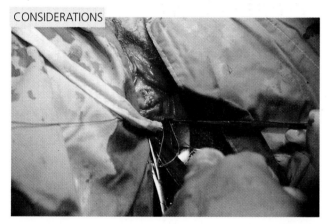

13. The free end of the graft is passed between the urethra and vaginal mucosa.

STEP **13-1**

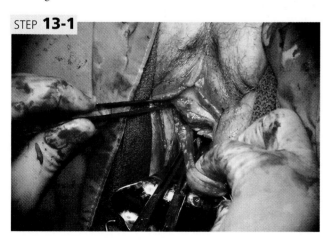

The length is measured by having the assistant secure the abdominal end of the graft as the surgeon temporarily places the free end into the opposite vaginal wound.

STEP **13-2**

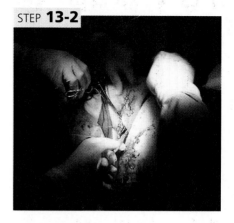

Excess graft material is excised and step 12 is repeated.
14. Tension is checked before suturing the sling in place.

STEP **14-1**

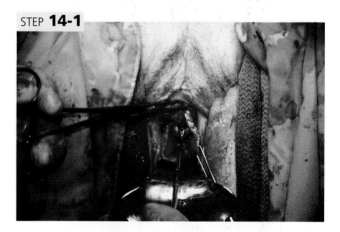

Testing graft tension from below.

STEP **14-2**

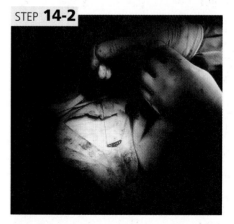

Testing graft tension and ability to stop urinary stream from above.

The cystoscope is reinserted, and the bladder is filled. Under direct visualization, the sutures are pulled upward so that the flow of fluid is alternately released and stopped.

15. One side of the graft is sutured in place suprapubically with a free Mayo needle.

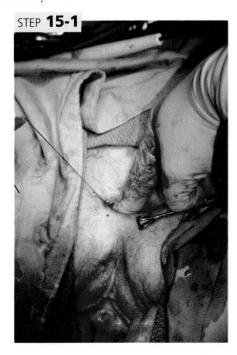

STEP **15-1**

Position and tension is again checked cystoscopically, and the second side is secured. The sutures are then cut.

16. A stab wound can be made in the lower abdomen for placement of a suprapubic catheter while the bladder is still full.

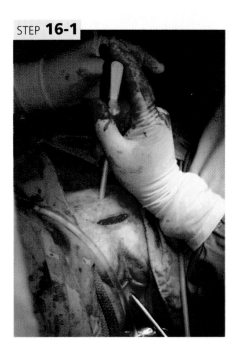

STEP **16-1**

17. The Foley catheter is reinserted, and the incisions are closed with absorbable sutures.

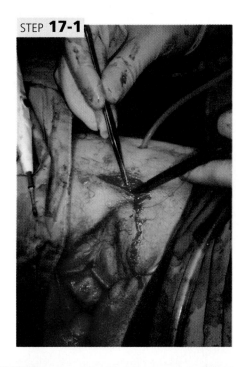

STEP **17-1**

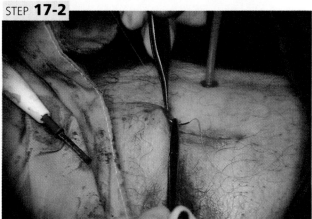

STEP **17-2**

18. The vaginal mucosa is closed with 3-0 absorbable suture, and a vaginal pack that has been coated with triple sulfa cream is inserted.

The Foley may be removed.

POSTOPERATIVE

Nursing Care and Discharge Planning for Bladder Neck Suspensions

1. Vaginal pack is removed the first postoperative day.
2. Suprapubic catheter is removed at 2 to 15 days, after successful voiding trials and confirmation that residual urine volume is less than 60 to 150 ml (time frame and acceptable residual dependent on specific intervention). Urethral catheter is removed 1 to 2 days postoperatively. Transient urge incontinence is common immediately postoperatively. Anticholinergic therapy can usually control it but may cause delayed voiding.
3. Review catheter care and instruct patient that it is not uncommon to have difficulty voiding at first. Intermittent catheterization may be required.
4. If fascia lata autograft was used, the leg dressings are removed on the second postoperative day. Until that time pressure dressings and ice should be applied.
5. Patient should be instructed to take antibiotics as ordered until gone (commonly while catheter is in place).
6. Pain medication should be taken before the onset of discomfort. If PCA has been instituted, patient should be properly coached in its use, and home care provider should be contacted, if applicable.
7. Encourage early ambulation and return to normal nonstrenuous activity as soon as possible. Strenuous activities should be avoided for 4 weeks.
8. Sexual activity may resume after 1 month.
9. Patient may be discharged the same day or on the second postoperative day if autograph was employed.

19. A small gauze dressing is placed over the abdominal wounds, and the catheter is secured and connected to drainage.

BLADDER AUGMENTATION

Description. Augmentation enterocystoplasty is the surgical procedure employed to enlarge the bladder capacity. A segment of bowel is reformed into a semispherical shape to decrease peristaltic contractions and anastomosed to the opened bladder dome. The result is a low-pressure reservoir that provides improved bladder capacity and urinary compliance.

Almost all segments of bowel as well as the stomach have been employed for bladder augmentation. Selection depends on anatomic factors, functional characteristics, and surgeon's preference. In some cases, ureteral reimplantation or associated bladder outlet procedures are deemed necessary. They should be incorporated to achieve a one-stage procedure.

Intermittent catheterization and bladder irrigations may be necessary postoperatively. The patient must be able and willing to learn and perform these and be accepting of this alteration in lifestyle.

Indications. A wide range of conditions that were previously treated with urinary diversion may now be successfully managed with this technique. Indications include reflex incontinence unresponsive to medical management, detrusor hyperactivity with compromised bladder function, chronically con-

PREOPERATIVE

Nursing Care and Teaching Considerations for Bladder Augmentation

1. Incorporate general nursing diagnoses.
2. Ensure that antibiotic therapy and mechanical and antimicrobial bowel preps have been successfully accomplished.
3. Discuss postoperative course with patient. Prolonged use of a urethral or suprapubic catheter will be necessary during healing to prevent bladder distention. Nasogastric tube will be in place postoperatively.
4. Review catheter care and wound care.
5. Assess patient for comprehension level and anxiety level.
6. Review patient record for reports of preoperative studies: VUD, cystoscopy, chest x-ray, ECG, PT, PTT, CBC, cardiac enzymes, serum electrolytes, serum chemistry survey, urine culture, creatinine clearance.
7. Assess patient health status and history: allergies, obesity, diabetes, malnutrition, anemia, nutritional level, presence of implants, skin integrity, range of motion, physical limitations, cardiovascular and pulmonary function, peripheral circulation.
8. Do appropriate equipment and supply checks for integrity and function. Apply alternating compression stockings.
9. Position patient under guidance of surgeon and anesthetist. Ensure that IV lines are not constricted and that linen is smooth.
10. Assist with insertion of CVP or A-line and epidural catheter, if indicated.
11. Apply patient dispersive pad to nonhairy fleshy site close to abdomen.
12. Prep and drape patient according to AORN standards. Protect from pooling of solutions.
13. Document assessment findings and nursing interventions.

tracted bladder as a result of radiation or repeated infections, and neuropathic bladder combined with recurrent urinary tract infections or compromised renal function.

Perioperative risks. Problems encountered with augmentation cytoplasty include obstruction or retention of urinary flow because of a mucous plug, bowel obstruction, urinary fistula, anastomosis leak or ischemia, wound infection, urinary tract infection, bladder rupture, intestinal colic, ileus, adhesions, metabolic disorders, hyperchloremic acidosis, and vitamin B_{12} deficiency. Intraoperatively, fluid and electrolyte balance and control of gastric contents must be maintained. Fecal spills during the procedure increase the risk of postoperative infection.

Equipment and instrumentation

Equipment

Electrosurgery unit
Alternating compression unit
Suction unit

Instruments

Laparotomy instrument set
Cystoscopy set
Intestinal instruments

Miscellaneous supplies

Laparotomy pack
Sterile gowns
Sterile gloves
Drape towels
Sterile cloth towels
Alternating compression stockings, thigh-length
Foley catheter, #16 Fr, 5 cc balloon
Suprapubic catheter
Urine drainage bag
Syringe, 60 and 10 ml
Syringe 10 ml finger control
Hypodermic needle, #25 gauge, $1^1/_4$ inches
Syringe, Asepto
Antibiotic irrigant
Sterile saline, 1000 ml
Sterile water, 1000 ml
Cystoscopy water
Cystoscopy tubing
Suction tubing
Electrosurgery pencil with hand control
Suture, 2-0 and 3-0 absorbable on UR, SH-1, and
    CT-1 needles
Suture, 4-0 absorbable on cuticular needle
Skin staples
Silk, 3-0 on SH-1 needle
Antiseptic prep solution
Absorbent prep drape

Procedural Steps

The patient is in the supine position and under general anesthesia. The female patient may be frog-legged or in lithotomy position, particularly if an outlet procedure is to be performed. A nasogastric tube is inserted after induction. The entire abdomen and genitalia are prepped and draped into the operating field.

A Foley catheter connected to closed drainage is inserted in the sterile field. The bladder is filled to capacity through the catheter once the abdomen has been entered. Instrumentation required includes basic laparotomy instruments and intestinal instruments.

1. A supraumbilical-to-symphysis midline abdominal incision is made. The peritoneal cavity is exposed with the aid of a large, self-retaining retractor.

2. The intestines and stomach are examined, and the appropriate segment for reconstruction is chosen.

3. A sagittal bladder incision is made from 2 cm cephalad to the bladder neck anteriorly across the anterior bladder wall, the peritonealized dome surface, and the posterior bladder wall to 2 cm above the posterior interureteric ridge. This causes the bladder to be bivalved in a clam-shaped design.

4. Traction sutures are placed bilaterally along the bladder incision. The length of the incision is measured to correlate with the corresponding segment of bowel or stomach. Average length required is 25 cm.

5. The segment to be used is mobilized, and the mesentery is closed cephalad so that the segment is on the retroperitoneum. The segment is left attached to its mesentery to maintain blood supply.

6. The isolated segment is opened, trimmed, and detubularized. It is then doubly folded and sutured to form a cup patch.

7. Anastomosis is accomplished with a running, intermittently locking, absorbable suture, beginning at the posterior apex and running up each side. With one third of the attachment complete, sutures are then placed at the anterior apex and placed in a continuous fashion to meet cephalad.

8. Integrity of the anastomosis is evaluated by again filling the bladder and observing for leaks.

POSTOPERATIVE

Nursing Care and Discharge Planning for Bladder Augmentation

1. Reinforce catheter care. Intermittent irrigation is often necessary to prevent obstruction from mucous buildup resulting from the intestinal segment. Hourly output measurements are generally ordered. The catheter is maintained for 10 to 14 days and removed after cystography excludes any leaks.

2. Long-term intermittent catheterization may be indicated. Teach patient proper technique and cleansing protocols.

3. Review medication regimen: antibiotics until cleared by physician (avg. 5 days), pain medication before onset of discomfort. PCA may be instituted. Stool softeners to prevent straining and constipation.

4. Reinforce need for high fluid intake (half as water, half as fruit juice) to keep urine draining without obstruction. Fluid and electrolyte balance must be closely monitored to prevent critical deficiencies (sodium, potassium, vitamin B_{12}). Hyperalimentation may be necessary if alimentation is delayed beyond 1 week.

5. Maintain nasogastric tube to drainage; ensure that it is not kinked or pulling on the nares. The tube may be removed before discharge from the OR. Reglan is provided intravenously. Occasional reinsertion of the nasogastric tube may be necessary for the first few days.

6. If a wound drain was inserted, it is removed after 4 or 5 days.

7. Encourage early ambulation. This will assist pulmonary perfusion and peripheral vascular circulation. Before ambulation, coughing and deep breathing and passive range of motion exercises should be performed. Provide a pillow or similar device for patient to splint abdomen. Alternating compression stockings should remain in place until patient is ambulating.

8. Patient must avoid strenuous activity for 6 weeks.

9. Diet resumed slowly; vitamin supplements may be indicated.

10. Patient may shower first postoperative day, keeping wound covered.

11. Reinforce dressing care.

12. Discharge approximately 5 to 10 days postoperatively.

9. A routine abdominal closure is performed, and dressings are applied.

10. The nasogastric tube stays in place for 3 postoperative days. The Foley catheter will remain for 7 to 14 days. Some surgeons may chose to place a suprapubic catheter instead of a Foley.

IMPLANTATION OF A PROSTHETIC URETHRAL SPHINCTER

Description. The artificial sphincter unit has an abdominally placed, pressure-regulated reservoir that maintains a constant, predetermined pressure on the periurethral cuff. Because of the connection between the reservoir and the cuff, any increase in intraabdominal pressure transmits more fluid into the cuff. This connection allows for a compensatory increase in urethral resistance during coughing or straining. The reservoir pressure needs to be between the systolic and diastolic blood pressures so that arterial blood may supply the urethra.

The scrotal or labial pump shifts the fluid in the cuff to the reservoir to allow bladder emptying. The fluid reenters the cuff through a resistor in about 60 to 120 seconds. The locking button in the AMS 800 artificial sphincter unit traps fluid in the reservoir to allow deactivation of the cuff.

The cuff may be placed around the bladder neck or bulbar urethra. Bladder neck placement is generally chosen for women, children, and men who wish to maintain antegrade ejaculation. Advantages to this placement include decreased tendency for erosion, functionally more physiologic, suitable when the bulbar urethra is small, less irritation with intermittent catheterization.

The patient will generally be in the lithotomy position under regional or general anesthesia. Local anesthetic may be used to assist in postoperative pain management. These procedures are being done more frequently on an outpatient basis.

Indications. This procedure is usually done as a last measure in patients with stress incontinence where other modalities have failed. Urodynamic studies are performed preoperatively to determine the resting pressure inside the bladder up to the functional capacity (volume at which patient voids) and intravesical voiding pressure.

Perioperative risks. Maintenance of patient body temperature and adherence to strict aseptic practice are key areas of focus intraoperatively. Problems with the device have included foreign-body reaction, persistent urethral pressure, and fluid hydraulic failure. Additional problems include infection, urethral damage, urinary retention, persistent incontinence, and cuff erosion. Over time tissue atrophy under the cuff may alter the fit causing the device to be less effective and necessitating a change in the cuff size.

Equipment and instrumentation
Equipment
Electrosurgery unit
Suction unit
Alternating compression machine
Allen stirrups
Stool, sitting

PREOPERATIVE

Nursing Care and Teaching Considerations for Prosthetic Urethral Sphincter

1. Patient must be free of infection. Urethral obstruction such as stricture disease must be corrected before implantation.
2. Incorporate general nursing diagnoses.
3. Review reports of preoperative studies in patient record: chest x-ray, urine culture, CBC, PT, PTT, serum electrolytes, IVP, VUD, EMG, cystoscopy, cystometrogram, urinary flow studies, residual volume studies, and psychologic evaluation.
4. Assess patient for allergies (especially iodine), peripheral circulation, cardiovascular and pulmonary function, skin integrity (perineum is often irritated from persistent urinary leakage), presence of any other infection (URI), range of motion, physical impairments, presence of other implants
5. Review perioperative course with patient. Assess comprehension and anxiety level. Address concerns appropriately. The patient must be manually dextrous enough to operate the device and be familiar with the activation-deactivation function.
6. Check equipment, packaging, and instrumentation for proper function and integrity.
7. Check medications for dosage and expiration dates.
8. Sales representative should be present for the first several procedures until staff feels comfortable with product.
9. Apply alternating compression stockings and patient dispersive pad according to protocol.
10. Position patient in lithotomy under guidance of surgeon and anesthetist.
11. Prep and drape patient according to AORN guidelines. Perform 5-minute iodophor scrub of low abdomen and perineum.
12. Document assessment findings and nursing interventions.

Instruments
Minor instrument set
Plastic instruments
Cystoscopy set
Tubing passer
Assembly tool
Miscellaneous supplies
Laparoscopy pack
Sterile gowns
Sterile gloves
Drape towels, 5
Sterile cloth towels
Cystoscopy tubing
Suction tubing
Electrosurgery pencil, hand control
Syringe, 10 ml finger control
Syringe, 20 ml, 2
Syringe, 60 ml
Syringe, 10 ml Luer-Lok

Hypodermic needle, #25 gauge, 1¼ inches
Knife blades, #15
Hypaque, 25% or similar contrast solution
Water for drug diluent
Sterile saline, 1000 ml
Sterile water, 1000 ml
Antibiotic irrigant
Suture, 3-0 absorbable on SH-1 and RB needles
Suture, 4-0 absorbable on PS-3 needle
Suture, Prolene 2-0 ties
Foley catheter, #14 Fr, 5 cc balloon
Urine drainage bag
Radiopaque gauze sponges
Gauze dressings
Mesh underwear
Artificial sphincter kit:
    Reservoir, cuff , pump, measuring strip, connectors
Antiseptic prep solution
Absorbent prep drape

Procedural Steps

The patient is placed in the supine, frog-legged, or lithotomy position. Antiseptic prep solution is applied after a 5-minute iodophor scrub of the operative site. Standard draping for the chosen position ensues. All scrubbed personnel remove any powder residue from their gloves.

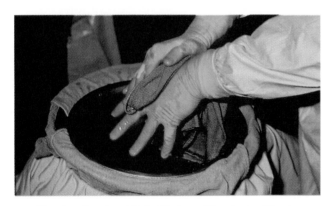

(Courtesy American Medical Systems, Minnetonka, Minn.)

The implant components are prepared before the start of the procedure by the scrub nurse.

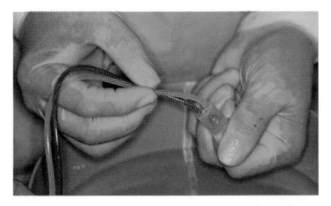

Preparing pump. *(Courtesy American Medical Systems, Minnetonka, Minn.)*

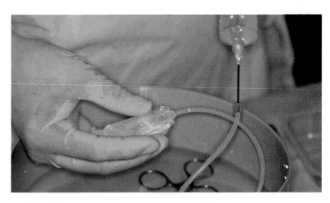

Preparing reservoir. *(Courtesy American Medical Systems, Minnetonka, Minn.)*

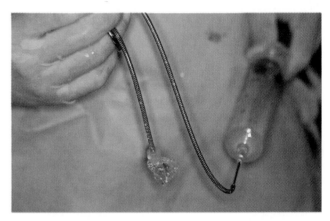

Reservoir prepared for insertion. *(Courtesy American Medical Systems, Minnetonka, Minn.)*

1. A perineal and a low abdominal or inguinal incision are made for placement of reservoir and cuff.

STEP **1-1**

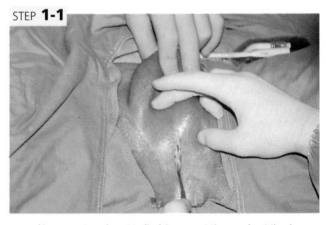

(Courtesy American Medical Systems, Minnetonka, Minn.)

STEP **1-2**

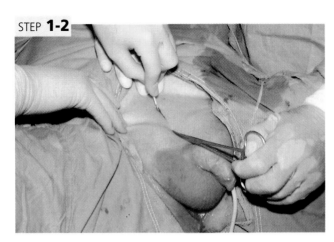

Abdominal incision is made. (*Courtesy American Medical Systems, Minnetonka, Minn.*)

2. The bulbar urethra is mobilized through a vertical incision behind the scrotum.

STEP **2-1**

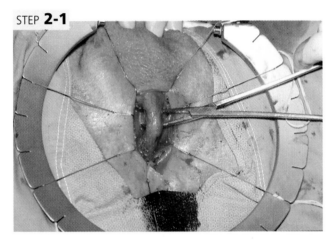

(*Courtesy American Medical Systems, Minnetonka, Minn.*)

The measuring strip is placed around the urethra.

STEP **2-2**

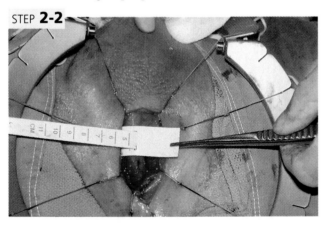

(*Courtesy American Medical Systems, Minnetonka, Minn.*)

The cuff is then placed and secured with the locking tab.

STEP **2-3**

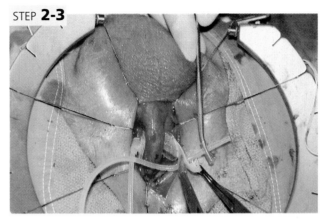

(*Courtesy American Medical Systems, Minnetonka, Minn.*)

STEP **2-4**

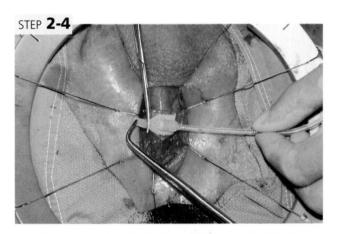

(*Courtesy American Medical Systems, Minnetonka, Minn.*)

CONSIDERATIONS If the cuff is to be around the bladder neck, the patient is supine and a lower abdominal incision is made to expose the bladder neck.

CONSIDERATIONS

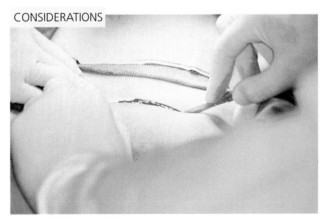

Low midline incision for bladder neck placement. (*Courtesy American Medical Systems, Minnetonka, Minn.*)

CONSIDERATIONS

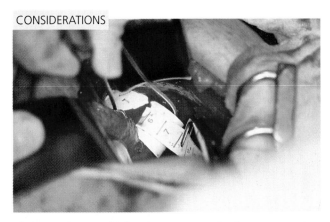

Bladder neck is measured with measuring strip. (*Courtesy American Medical Systems, Minnetonka, Minn.*)

CONSIDERATIONS

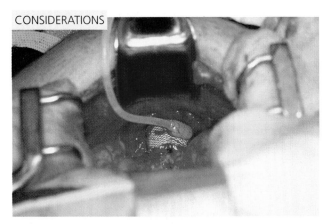

Cuff is placed around bladder neck. (*Courtesy American Medical Systems, Minnetonka, Minn.*)

4. The abdominal wound is generously irrigated with antibiotic solution.

STEP **4-1**

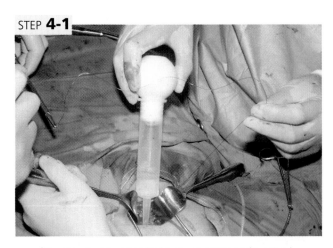

(*Courtesy American Medical Systems, Minnetonka, Minn.*)

A pocket is created for placement of the reservoir.

STEP **4-2**

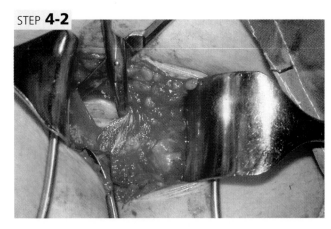

(*Courtesy American Medical Systems, Minnetonka, Minn.*)

The reservoir is placed in the prevesical space and tested for proper position.

STEP **4-3**

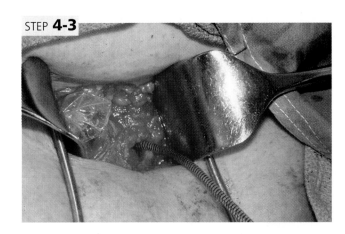

(*Courtesy American Medical Systems, Minnetonka, Minn.*)

STEP **4-4**

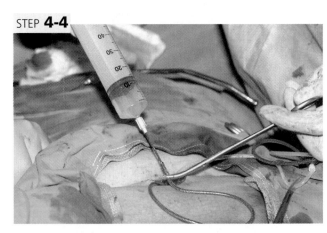

(*Courtesy American Medical Systems, Minnetonka, Minn.*)

The tubing from the cuff is tunneled into the abdominal wound.

STEP 4-5

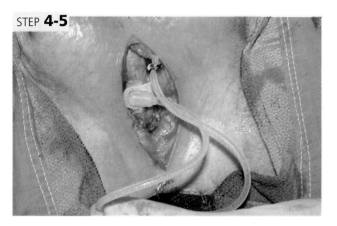

(Courtesy American Medical Systems, Minnetonka, Minn.)

5. The pump is introduced through the abdominal incision and transferred to the scrotum or labia through a subcutaneous tunnel.

STEP 5-1

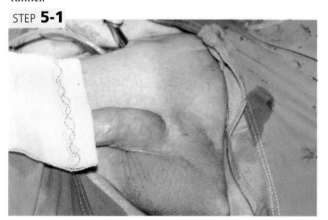

(Courtesy American Medical Systems, Minnetonka, Minn.)

STEP 5-2

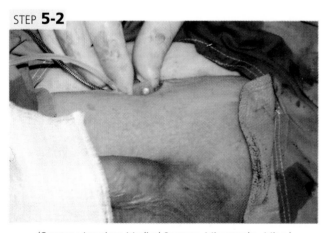

(Courtesy American Medical Systems, Minnetonka, Minn.)

6. The reservoir, cuff, and pump are filled with 12.5% Hypaque to the appropriate volume.

STEP 6-1

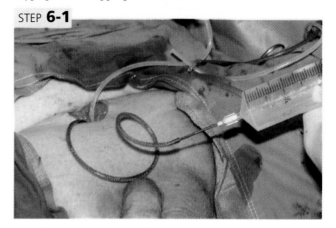

(Courtesy American Medical Systems, Minnetonka, Minn.)

The tubings are cut with a fresh pair of scissors ("virgin scissors") and connectors attached.

STEP 6-2

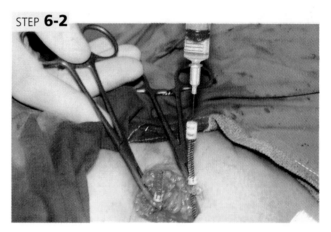

(Courtesy American Medical Systems, Minnetonka, Minn.)

The tubings are connected and secured with the assembly tool.

STEP 6-3

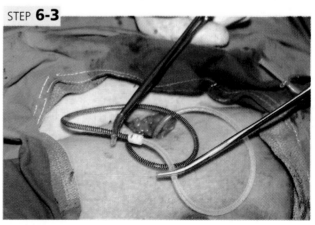

(Courtesy American Medical Systems, Minnetonka, Minn.)

STEP **6-4**

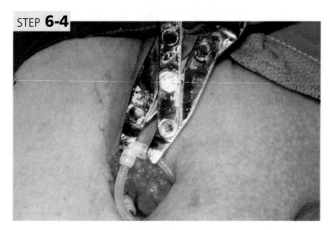

(Courtesy American Medical Systems, Minnetonka, Minn.)

7. The pump is activated and deactivated to determine integrity.

STEP **7-1**

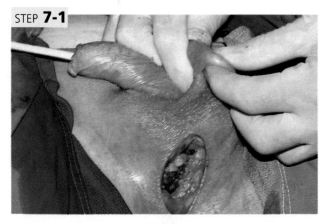

(Courtesy American Medical Systems, Minnetonka, Minn.)

8. The wounds are closed and dressed with gauze sponges.

STEP **8-1**

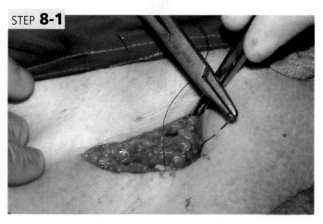

(Courtesy American Medical Systems, Minnetonka, Minn.)

STEP **8-2**

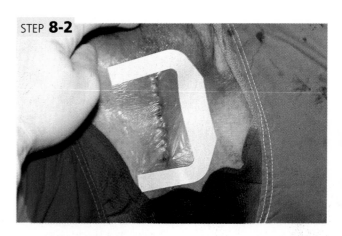

(Courtesy American Medical Systems, Minnetonka, Minn.)

A urethral catheter may or may not be inserted.

POSTOPERATIVE

Nursing Care and Discharge Planning for Prosthetic Urethral Sphincter

1. Ensure that cuff is deactivated. The device is left deactivated for 6 weeks after placement. Activation is accomplished after wounds are healed satisfactorily and sterile urine is demonstrated.
2. If urethral catheter is in place, maintain closed drainage system and monitor output.
3. Assess wound and urine for signs of infection. Perineal skin care should be routinely performed to assist healing; avoid lotions and powders.
4. Review signs and symptoms to be reported: fever, increased wound drainage, redness or warmth of incisional sites, pyuria, increased pain, abdominal distention.
5. Discuss wound and catheter care.
6. Discuss device management. Patient will be instructed by physician, after approximately 6 weeks, in deflation and inflation techniques.
7. Early ambulation is encouraged. Some modifications in lifestyle will be necessary (e.g., sports, bicycling). Patient should not lift more than 20 lb. until cleared by physician.
8. Encourage increased fluid intake to maintain fluid and electrolyte balance (half should be as fruit juice, half as water). Diet may resume slowly as tolerated.
9. Antibiotics should be taken until gone. Pain medication is generally mild and should be taken before onset of discomfort.
10. Complete tracking records for institution and manufacturer.

REPAIR OF VESICAL FISTULAS

Description. If a vesicovaginal fistula is in the trigone of the bladder, a vaginal approach may be employed. If the fistula is at the dome of the bladder, the approach will be transperitoneal or transvesical, or a combined approach. Vesicointestinal fistulas are more common than vesicovaginal fistulas. Of the intestinal fistulas, the sigmoid colon is most often involved. A colostomy proximal to the fistula may be performed to protect the repaired segment of bowel. The communicating area of bladder and bowel is totally resected. Generally, an end-to-end bowel resection is performed after excision of the involved intestinal segment. The bladder is then repaired in three layers. A suprapubic catheter is generally placed in the bladder for postoperative diversion of urine during healing. The instrument setup includes open-bladder instrumentation and an intestinal resection setup for vesicointestinal fistulas. For vesicovaginal fistulas, vaginal preparation and a colporrhaphy set with colostomy or ileostomy instruments are used.

Indications. Vesical fistulas occurring between the bladder and the intestines or vagina may be repaired surgically. Vesicointestinal fistula may be caused by ulcerative colitis, diverticulitis, radiation therapy, or neoplasms of the colon or rectum. Less commonly the fistula may involve the kidney: a colorenal fistula. Vesicovaginal fistula may be a complication of radiotherapy for cervical cancer, hysterectomy, or endoscopic procedures involving surgery of the trigone or vesical neck. Such fistulas are also caused by obstetrical injuries. Less commonly, the condition may actually be a ureterovaginal fistula.

Perioperative risks. Risks common to vesical fistula repairs include urinary reflux that usually subsides spontaneously, obstruction of the ureteral orifice (particularly larger defects) that may require reimplantation, wound infection, abscess formation, bladder infection, delayed healing, recurrence, pulmonary or cardiac complications, hyponatremia, and anemia. Patients with vesicointestinal fistulas may suffer malnutrition. This should be treated preoperatively, ideally until the serum albumin level and lymphocyte count is within acceptable range. The goal is to achieve weight gain and an anabolic state through nutritional supplements, as determined by serum albumin and lymphocyte levels, as well as Hgb and HCT. This is not always possible, however. Patients with extremely low lymphocyte levels that do not readily respond to treatment do not have a promising prognosis.

Equipment and instrumentation

Equipment
Electrosurgery unit
Alternating compression machine
Suction unit
Headlight
Fiberoptic light source
Stool, sitting
Allen stirrups
Armboards, padded
Positioning devices (pads, pillows, blankets, rolls)

Nursing Care and Teaching Considerations for Repair of Vesical Fistulas

1. Review reports of preoperative studies, which may include some or all of the following: IVP, retrograde ureterogram, cystoscopy, voiding cystogram, colorometric test, urine culture, PT, PTT, CBC, serum electrolytes, serum chemistry survey (especially serum albumin, lymphocytes), cardiac enzymes, ECG, chest x-ray.
2. Ascertain that preoperative orders have been accomplished: antibiotic therapy, enema, vaginal douche, NPO.
3. Ascertain patient's comprehension level of condition and anticipated procedure.
4. Determine anxiety level and ensure that concerns are addressed.
5. Review postoperative course, expectations, sequelae.
6. Assess patient for other physical limitations (range of motion, skin condition, allergies, cardiovascular status, sensory deficits).
7. Provide adequate positioning devices and personnel to ensure patient comfort and safety. Ensure that bed linen is wrinkle free and IV lines are free of constriction after positioning.
8. Apply alternating compression stockings. Insert Foley catheter if applicable to approach.
9. Confirm that all equipment, packaging, and instrumentation is functioning properly and free of damage. Inspect medications for dosage and expiration dates.
10. Protect patient form pooling of prep solutions. Place dispersive pad on fleshy, hair-free area close to operative site.
11. Document assessment findings and nursing interventions.

Instruments (dependent on approach)
Cystoscopy set
Minor instrument set
Laparotomy instruments
Long vascular instruments
Intestinal instruments
Weighted vaginal speculum
Right-angle vaginal retractors
Lowsley prostatic tractor
Heaney needle holder
Self-retaining retractor

Miscellaneous supplies
Laparotomy, lithotomy, or laparoscopy pack
Sterile gowns and gloves
Drape towels, adherent, 4 to 8
Sterile cloth towels, 2 to 8
Foley catheter: #16, #20, #22, #24 Fr, 5 cc balloon
Foley catheter, 8 Fr, 3 cc,
Malecot catheter, #22
Suprapubic catheter of choice

Urine drainage bag, 2
Leg strap
Ureteral catheter, #4 whistle tipped
Electrosurgery pencil with hand control
Electrosurgery spatula tip, 6 inch
Electrosurgery holster
Suction tubing
Jackson-Pratt or similar drain
Sump drain
Penrose drain, $1/2$ inch
Colostomy appliance
Suture, 4-0 silk multi-pack on SH-1 needle
Suture, 0, 2-0, 3-0 absorbable on SH-1 needle
Suture, 0, 2-0, 3-0 absorbable on CT-2 needle
Suture, 3-0 nonabsorbable on cuticular needle *or*
Suture, 4-0 absorbable on cuticular needle
Skin clips
Vaginal pack, 2
Hemoclips, medium, medium large
Rubber ball
Kittner dissectors
Laparotomy sponges
Radiopaque gauze sponges
Sterile water, 1000 ml, 2
Sterile saline, 1000 ml, 2 to 4
Epinephrine 1:1000, 1 ml
Normal saline, 0.9%, 200 ml
Local anesthetic
Syringes, 10 ml finger control and luer-lock
Syringe, Asepto
Hypodermic needle, #25 gauge, 1 $1/4$ inches
Water for cystoscopy irrigant, 3000 ml
Cystoscopy tubing
Alternating compression stockings, thigh length
Antiseptic prep solution
Absorbent prep drape
Montgomery straps *or*
Nonallergic adhesive tape, 3 inches

VESICOVAGINAL FISTULA REPAIR
Procedural Steps
Vaginal Approach

1. Alternating compression stockings are applied. With the patient in lithotomy or supine position, a suprapubic catheter is inserted, clamped, and connected to closed drainage. The patient is placed in hyperflexed lithotomy position or Kraske position (prone). The vagina and external genitalia are prepped with provodine-iodine solution. The area is draped with four adherent drape towels and a lithotomy or laparotomy sheet.

CONSIDERATIONS If the intended position is Kraske, separate draping material and instrumentation are set up for the suprapubic catheter insertion with the patient supine. The catheter is secured, and the patient is turned for the procedure.

2. The labia are sutured to the outer groin or inner thigh for retraction and visualization.

3. A weighted vaginal retractor is placed posteriorly, and the defect is examined. A relaxing vaginal incision may be necessary at 5 or 7 o'clock position.

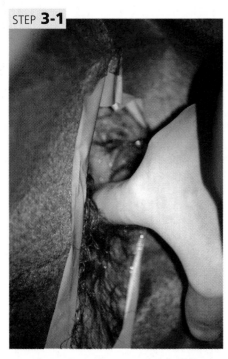

STEP **3-1**

Vagina is examined; note copious urine leakage.

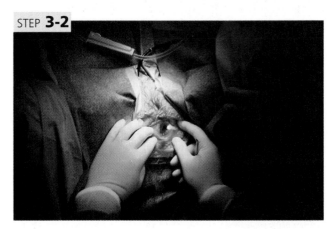

STEP **3-2**

Fistula is exposed, light is from flexible cystoscope entering from suprapubic bladder stab wound.

4. A 4 Fr ureteral catheter is inserted through the fistula, and the tract is dilated to admit the 8 Fr Foley catheter.

STEP **4-1**

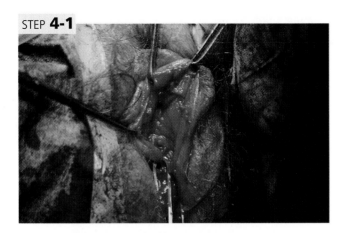

The balloon is inflated, and the catheter is used as a tractor.

5. The area is infiltrated with epinephrine solution 1:200,000.

STEP **5-1**

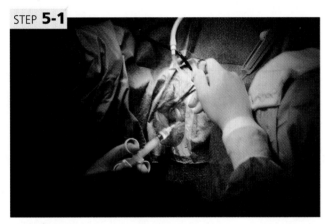

The vaginal mucosa and perivesical fascia around the defect is incised, well outside the scarred tissue.

STEP **5-2**

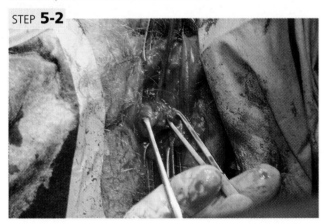

6. Two planes are developed: one between the mucosa and fascia and one between the fascia and the bladder wall with fine scissors, forceps, and Kittner dissectors. The bladder wall is freed from the vaginal wall.

7. The vesical defect is grasped with Allis clamps, and the scarred edges are everted. It is then closed vertically with inter-

rupted 3-0 absorbable sutures after removal of the catheter previously placed.

STEP **7-1**

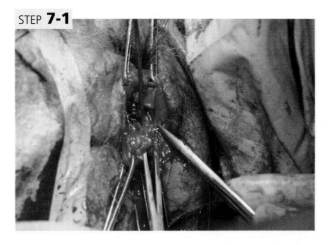

CONSIDERATIONS In some instances, a labial pedicle or full-thickness flap (Martius flap) may be placed between the vesical closure and the vaginal closure.

CONSIDERATIONS

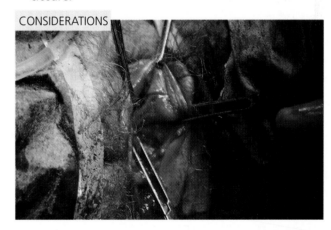

This prevents suture line stress and overlay and removes the need for a relaxing incision. Larger fistulas that do not adequately reapproximate may necessitate a vascularized muscle flap to reinforce closure.

8. The perivesical fascia and vaginal mucosa are approximated separately with transverse, interrupted 3-0 absorbable sutures.

STEP **8-1**

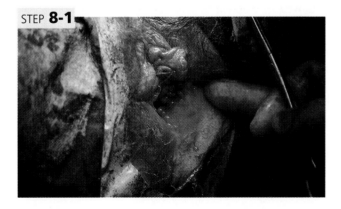

CONSIDERATIONS A one-sided ellipse of vaginal mucosa may be excised to offset the closure.

9. Alternatively, an inverted **U** incision may provide more exposure and result in a posterior flap that completely covers the site of the defect.

10. The suprapubic catheter is unclamped, the labial stitches are removed, and the vagina is loosely packed.

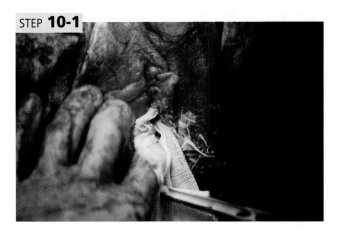

STEP **10-1**

Transperitoneal-Transvesical Approach

1. Alternating compression stockings are applied. The patient is placed in low lithotomy and moderate Trendelenburg position. The perineum and the abdomen are prepped and draped appropriately. A laparoscopy pack works well for this approach.

2. Ureteral catheters are inserted endoscopically and a no. 16 Fr Foley catheter is placed in the bladder and clamped. A rubber ball or tight gauze pack is placed in the vagina.

3. A vertical midline, or Pfannenstiel, incision is made. The peritoneum is incised and bluntly dissected from the dome of the bladder. The small bowel is packed cephalad.

4. Stay sutures of 2-0 absorbable suture are placed in the bladder dome, and the bladder is opened. The bladder wall and overlying peritoneum are divided down to the fistula. Stay sutures are placed periodically to serve as tractors for bladder elevation.

5. The peritoneum is incised transversely at the level of the fistula forming a pedicle flap. The vagina and bladder are separated widely on each side of the fistula. An assistant places upward pressure on the vaginal ball or pack to facilitate dissection.

6. As the fistula is exposed, it is excised until completely removed. A probe may be used to localize it, if small, or the 8 Fr balloon catheter may be inserted and used for traction during dissection.

7. The bladder and vagina are freed from each other until there is enough mobility for separate closures. The vagina is then closed, without tension, with inverting 2-0 or 3-0 interrupted sutures in two layers.

8. The peritoneal flap is swung into the defect and sutured in place for retroperitonealization. A 22 Fr Malecot catheter and a wound drain are inserted and pulled through separate stab wounds in the abdomen.

CONSIDERATIONS A long attached peritoneal or free peritoneal pedicle flap may be needed for reperitonealization. Alternatively the omentum may be brought from behind the right colon for an omental graft, or a vascularized muscle flap may be placed. Fistulas resulting from radiation necrosis may best be managed with the latter option.

9. The ureteral catheters are removed, and the bladder mucosa and submucosa are closed in separate layers with 2-0 or 3-0 absorbable suture in a running fashion. The muscularis and adventitia are externally approximated with interrupted 3-0 suture. The wound is closed in layers in the standard fashion with 2-0, 3-0, and 4-0 sutures or skin clips.

10. Dressings are applied, the Foley catheter is unclamped, the rubber ball or gauze roll are removed, and the vagina is loosely repacked.

VESICOSIGMOID FISTULA REPAIR
Procedural Steps
Abdominal Approach

1. With the patient in supine and Trendelenburg position a #20 or #22, 5 cc Foley catheter is inserted into the bladder, and the bladder is filled with 100 ml of sterile water. Once prepped and draped as for laparotomy a midline, or paramedian, and transperitoneal incisions are made.

2. The abdomen is explored, and the contents are examined. The descending and sigmoid colon are mobilized by incising along the fascia fusion line of Toldt. The involved loop of colon is identified.

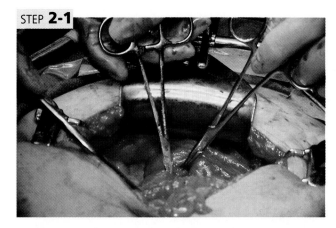

STEP **2-1**

CONSIDERATIONS If a walled-off inflammatory mass is found, a transverse colostomy should be performed and a two-stage intervention considered.

3. The fistulous tract is separated by blunt finger dissection. A probe is inserted to determine the extent of involvement.

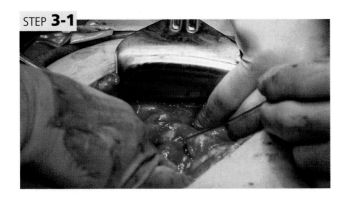

STEP **3-1**

The defects in the bladder and bowel are debrided to obtain healthy tissue.

CONSIDERATIONS Large inflammatory masses require a colon resection.

4. The bladder is closed in two layers with a 3-0 absorbable, submucosal running stitch, and a 2-0 absorbable, interrupted muscularis-adventitial stitch.

5. The edges of the bowel defect are trimmed to reach normal tissue, and stay sutures are placed on each side. The cavity is pulled transversely, and the mucosa and submucosa are closed in one pass with a Connell stitch of 3-0 chromic catgut. The muscularis and serosa are approximated and closed in one pass with 4-0 silk Lembert sutures.

6. The abdomen is irrigated with 2000 ml of sterile saline with an attempt to reach all areas.

7. A sump-style drain is placed intraperitoneally, and a Penrose drain or small Jackson-Pratt drain is placed suprapubically, exiting through separate stab wounds.

8. The abdomen is closed in layers in the conventional manner.

9. If a colostomy was performed, it is opened for fecal diversion, and the appropriate appliance is applied. Gauze and combine dressings are applied and secured with Montgomery straps.

BLADDER INTERVENTIONS

SUPRAPUBIC-TROCAR CYSTOSTOMY

Description. *Cystostomy* is creating an opening into the urinary bladder through a low abdominal incision or stab wound. When a drainage tube is inserted into the bladder through an abdominal incision, the procedure is a *cystostomy.* Trocar cystostomy requires puncturing and draining of the bladder with a needle or trocar and insertion of a catheter. This approach often accompanies other procedures, such as urethral suspensions and cryotherapy. Anesthesia may be general, regional, or local with sedation. Frequently the urologist will incorporate a flexible cystoscopy into the procedure.

Indications. Cystostomy may be indicated for temporary urinary diversion in cases of long-standing urethral obstruction or to protect a distal urethral repair during healing. Cystostomy may also be indicated for permanent urinary diversion as in cases of neurogenic bladder.

POSTOPERATIVE

Nursing Care and Discharge Planning for Repair of Vesical Fistulas

1. Depending on the involvement of the procedure, the patient may be discharged the same day or up to 4 days postoperatively.
2. Vaginal packing will be removed the first postoperative day.
3. Voiding trials begin at 2 weeks if healing is satisfactory. The suprapubic catheter is removed when urinary control returns. Frequency and urgency of urination is common for several months.
4. Sexual activity may resume after 6 weeks.
5. Abdominal drains are removed 1 to 4 weeks postoperatively, depending on the extent of involvement.
6. The patient will be receiving antibiotic therapy for 10 days to 3 months depending on the involvement and rate of recovery. If the fistula was extensive with abscess formation, a subcutaneous injection port may be inserted for systemic antibiotic therapy. Pain medication will vary depending on the involvement; PCA may be appropriate. A stool softener may be indicated.
7. A Foley catheter after vesicointestinal repair is removed after 5 to 7 days.
8. Postoperative urine cultures and serum electrolytes will be obtained as monitoring tools.
9. The patient should report any fever; unresolved pain; redness or heat at the incisional site; vaginal or abdominal wound discharge other than serous; anuresis, dysuria, vaginal urination; constipation or diarrhea; rash or urticaria; nausea or vomiting; intractable headache.
10. Strenuous activity should be avoided for 6 weeks. Other activity may resume as tolerated after 2 weeks.
11. Diet may slowly be resumed beginning with clear liquids and gradually advancing through long-term recovery protocol (liquid, bland, soft, etc.). Constipating and gassy foods should be avoided until fully recovered.
12. Fluid intake should be increased to 8 oz q2h for 2-3 weeks and maintained at 8 oz q4h until recovered. Fruit juices assist in maintaining potassium levels, but should be nonacidic and nongassy (apple juice).
13. Showers and baths are dependent on wound site and status according to physician's order.
14. Aspirin and other nonsteroidal antiinflammatory agents should be taken according to physician's order.

Perioperative risks. Concerns relative to cystostomy include obstruction of the catheter, urgency and pain caused by trigonal-catheter contact, inadvertent catheter dislodgment or removal, urinary infection, peritonitis, and persistent urinary site leak after catheter removal. The anesthetic risks previously discussed may all apply.

Equipment and instrumentation
Equipment
Electrosurgery unit
Suction unit
Instruments
Laparotomy instrument set
Trocar and cannula
Catheter stylet

Miscellaneous supplies

Foley catheters, #22 to 30 Fr with 5 cc balloon

Assorted Pezzer and Malecot catheters

Suprapubic catheter of choice

Urine drainage bag

Suture, 2-0 nylon on cuticular needle

Suture, 2-0 and 3-0 absorbable on CT-2 or SH-1 needle

Laparotomy pack

Sterile gowns

Sterile gloves

Drape towels, adherent

Sterile cloth towels

Suction tubing

Electrosurgery pencil with hand control

Radiopaque gauze sponges

Laparotomy sponges, small

Syringe, 10 ml, finger control

Hypodermic needle, #25 gauge, 1 1/4 inches

Gauze dressings

Local anesthetic of choice

Saline, 500 ml

Sterile water, 500 ml

Antiseptic prep solution

Absorbent prep drape

PREOPERATIVE

Nursing Care and Teaching Considerations for Cystostomy-Cystolithotomy

1. Review patient record for preoperative studies: urine culture, PT, PTT, CBC, serum and urine electrolytes, chest x-ray, ECG, cardiac enzymes, IVP, and cystogram.
2. Discuss planned procedure with patient, determine comprehension level, and explain as necessary.
3. Discuss postoperative expectations and restrictions.
4. Assess patient for medical and surgical history, allergies, range of motion and physical impairments, cardiovascular and pulmonary status, skin integrity, peripheral vascular circulation.
5. Check equipment and instrumentation for proper function and integrity. Ensure that appropriate catheters are available.
6. Check medications for dosage and expiration dates.
7. Position patient supine. Ensure that linen is free of wrinkles and body regions at risk for compromise are well padded.
8. Aseptically insert closed-system Foley catheter if indicated.
9. Prep and drape patient according to AORN standards and protect patient from pooling of solutions.
10. Document assessment findings and nursing interventions.

Procedural Steps

The patient is in the supine position. The patient is draped as described for routine suprapubic prostatectomy. When possible, a Foley catheter may be inserted into the urethra and the bladder distended with sterile saline or water at the outset for easy identification.

1. A short vertical, or Pfannenstiel, incision is made, the rectus fascia is exposed and transversely incised.
2. The rectus muscles are bluntly divided in the midline and retracted to reveal the prevesical fat. Minimal bladder surface is exposed by bluntly sliding the peritoneal fold upward.
3. Two stay sutures of 2-0 absorbable material are placed to the bladder wall, or the wall is grasped with Allis clamps. An incision is made between the sutures or clamps with the cutting current or knife blade.
4. The Allis clamps are positioned to grasp the full thickness of the bladder wall. Bleeding vessels in the bladder wall are clamped and ligated. The bladder contents are aspirated with a Poole suction.

CONSIDERATIONS The bladder opening may be extended if the bladder is to be explored for diverticula or calculi.

5. The catheter of choice is introduced into the bladder.
6. The incision is closed snugly about the catheter with 3-0 absorbable sutures to render the closure watertight about the cystostomy tube. A stab wound is made through the skin near the incision, and the catheter is brought out and connected to drainage.

CONSIDERATIONS If the cystostomy is for permanent diversion, the catheter may be sutured to the bladder wall with the 3-0 absorbable suture and to the rectus fascia with the 2-0 absorbable suture.

7. The muscle, fascia, subcutaneous tissue, and skin are closed with 2-0, 3-0, and 4-0 absorbable suture (or skin staples). The cystostomy tube is further secured to the skin with a 2-0 nonabsorbable suture to prevent it from being inadvertently dislodged from the bladder. A drain such as a Jackson-Pratt may be left in the prevesical space through a separate stab wound.
8. The wound is dressed.

CONSIDERATIONS If trocar cystostomy is the intent, the skin is nicked with a scalpel and the trocar is inserted into the bladder. The trocar obturator is withdrawn, and the bladder is drained through the trocar by suction. A catheter is passed through the trocar cannula into the bladder. The cannula is carefully withdrawn, and the catheter is sutured to the wound edges and the wound is dressed.

SUPRAPUBIC CYSTOLITHOTOMY

Description. Suprapubic cystolithotomy is the removal of calculi from the bladder. The surgical approach is similar to that described for subrapubic cystostomy. When the bladder is opened, calculi are identified and extracted. If indicated, bladder outlet obstruction may be repaired.

Indications. Calculi causing pain and obstruction of urinary flow that are too large to be safely removed endoscopically. Obstructions, such as prostatic enlargement or foreign bodies, are common causes of bladder calculi and may be corrected at the time of surgery.

Perioperative risks. The same risks apply as for cystostomy, with the patient at increased risk for infection because of urinary stasis from obstructing calculi.

Procedural Steps

The instrument setup used is as for cystostomy, plus Millin T-shaped stone forceps, Millin capsule forceps, Lewkowitz lithotomy forceps, Mason-Judd bladder retractors, long and short thyroid traction forceps, and retropubic needle holders or other long needle holders as desired.

1. Surgery proceeds as described in cystostomy steps 1 to 4.
5. The bladder is retracted open and manually explored.

STEP **5-1**

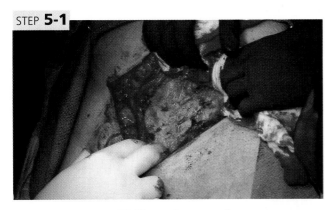

Bladder surface exposed.

STEP **5-2**

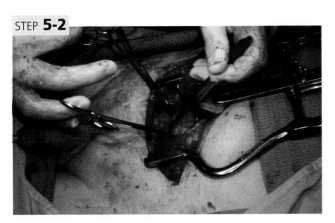

Bladder incised between Allis clamps.

STEP **5-3**

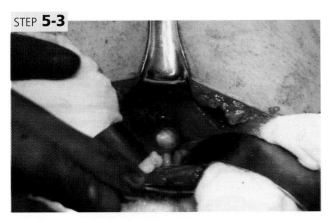

Bladder inspected, calculus revealed.

Calculi are grasped with the lithotomy instrumentation and removed.

STEP **5-4**

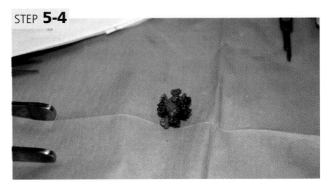

Bladder calculus.

6. Closure is the same as for cystostomy. A suprapubic catheter may be left in situ or the urethral Foley catheter placed preoperatively employed.

POSTOPERATIVE

Nursing Care and Discharge Planning for Cystostomy-Cystolithotomy

1. Monitor urinary pattern for signs of infection, retention, obstruction, calculus fragments, or bleeding.
2. Maintain closed drainage system, below bladder level.
3. Irrigate catheter as necessary to clear blood, fragments, or clots. Instruct patient in technique.
4. Provide appropriate antibiotic therapy to prevent infection. Reinforce need to take medication until gone.
5. Review pain medication prescribed; discuss restrictions and side effects.
6. Patient may be discharged the day of surgery. Activity may resume as tolerated, but strenuous endeavors should be avoided for approximately 2 to 4 weeks.
7. Review catheter and wound care.
8. Discuss reportable signs: fever, pain, urgency, distention, leaking around catheter, cloudy urine, warmth or redness at wound or drain site, anuria, and constipation.
9. Patient may resume diet as tolerated, increasing fluid intake to maintain good urinary flow.

CYSTECTOMY

Description. Cystectomy is the total excision of the urinary bladder and adjacent structures. Total cystectomy necessitates permanent urinary diversion into an ileal or colonic conduit. Conservative measures such as radiotherapy or chemotherapy may be used when the neoplasm is far advanced. In a male patient the prostate gland, seminal vesicles, and distal ureters are removed with the bladder and its peritoneal surface. In a female patient the bladder, urethra, distal ureters, uterus, cervix, and proximal third of the vagina are removed. Radical cystectomy with lymphadenectomy requires total excision of the urinary bladder and contiguous organs as well as pelvic lymph nodes (iliac and obturator). Urinary diversion is also performed in this slightly more extensive surgery.

Indications. Cystectomy is a surgical consideration when a vesical malignancy has not invaded the muscular wall of the entire bladder or when frequent recurrences of widespread papillary tumors do not respond to endoscopic or chemotherapeutic management. The patient should be medically able to withstand surgery with the expectation of reasonable longevity. Radical cystectomy with lymphadenectomy is indicated when larger tumors penetrate the full thickness of the bladder wall and invade the perivesical fat.

Perioperative risks. Intraoperatively it is imperative to maintain pulmonary and renal function, fluid and electrolyte balance, and the patient's body temperature. The patient is at risk for hemorrhage and shock with cystectomy.

Equipment and instrumentation

Equipment

Electrosurgery unit
Suction unit

PREOPERATIVE

Nursing Care and Teaching Considerations for Cystectomy

1. Incorporate nursing diagnoses.
2. Review patient record for reports of preoperative studies: serum electrolytes, cardiac enzymes, CBC, PT, PTT, serum chemistry survey, chest x-ray, ECG, pulmonary function tests, CT scan, bone scan, and MRI.
3. Discuss alternate methods of diversion with the patient. Assess comprehension that planned procedure may not be possible, necessitating an alternative route.
4. Ensure that patient had consultation with enterostomal therapist. Preoperatively an ileostomy bag should have been worn to determine the best placement.
5. Review patient records for indications of metastasis.
6. Interview patient regarding preoperative oncology consultation. Discuss the potential for chemotherapy or radiation therapy postoperatively.
7. Ascertain that mechanical and antimicrobial bowel preps were successfully performed.
8. Confirm that antibiotic therapy was instituted.
9. Assess the patient's nutritional level and evaluate the need for hyperalimentation perioperatively. Assess patient for skin integrity, range of motion, physical impairments, allergies, asthma, diabetes, cardiopulmonary status, peripheral vascular circulation.
10. Determine that blood is available (2 to 5 units). Patient may have autologous blood stored.
11. Ascertain that CVP and A-lines are in place or prepared for.
12. Check equipment, supplies, and instrumentation for proper function and integrity.
13. Check medications for dosages and expiration dates.
14. Assist surgeon and anesthetist to position patient. Utilize positioning pads where necessary. Ensure that monitoring lines and IV lines are unrestricted.
15. Apply patient dispersive pad and alternating compression stockings.
16. Aseptically insert closed-system Foley catheter.
17. Prep and drape patient according to AORN standards.
18. Document assessment findings and nursing care provided.

Alternating compression machine
Positioning pads
Instruments
Laparotomy instruments
Bladder instruments
Intestinal instruments
Clip appliers
Bookwalter retractor
Miscellaneous supplies
Laparotomy pack
Sterile gowns
Sterile gloves
Drape towels
Sterile cloth towels
Suction tubing
Electrosurgery pencil with hand control
Electrosurgery spatula tip, 6 inch
Hemoclips, a variety
Disposable staplers, TA, GIA, LDS
Stapler refills
Laparotomy sponges, small, large
Radiopaque gauze sponges
Kittner dissectors
Dressings
Montgomery straps
Double-J ureteral stents
Foley catheters, a variety
Ileostomy supplies
Red rubber catheters, a variety
Suture, 0, 2-0, 3-0 absorbable on CT-1 needle
Suture, 2-0, 3-0, 4-0 absorbable on SH-1 needle
Suture, 3-0, 4-0 silk on SH-1 needle
Ties, 0, 2-0, 3-0 long nonabsorbable and absorbable
Skin staples
Nylon, 2-0 on cuticular needle
Suture, 4-0 absorbable on PS-3 needle
Antiseptic prep solution
Absorbent prep drape

Procedural Steps

The patient is placed in the supine position with padding placed behind the knees and heels.

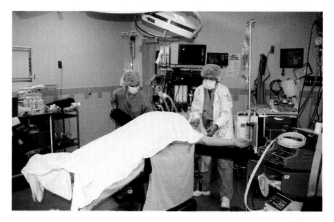

Patient in reverse Trendelenberg because of respiratory difficulties when flat.

The abdomen is widely draped to afford maximum access.

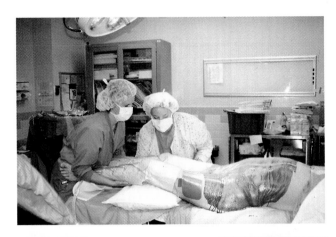

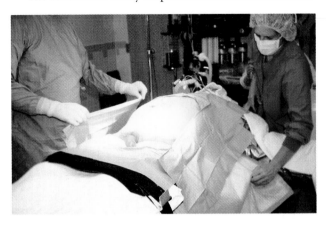

Instruments are as described for major abdominal procedures. For a male patient, if the prostate and seminal vesicles are to be removed, prostatectomy instruments should be added. For a female, instruments for vaginal and abdominal hysterectomy, as well as plastic surgery, should be added.

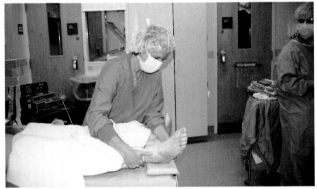

An abdominal shave and prep are carried out in a routine manner.

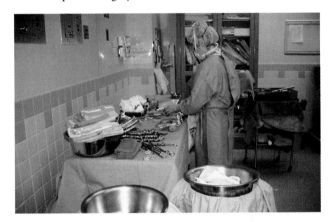

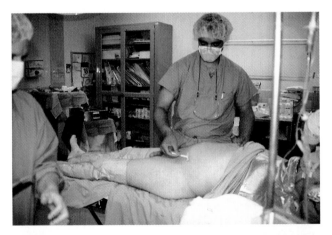

1. A midline incision from the epigastrium to the symphysis pubis, curving to the left of the umbilicus, is generally preferred.

2. The incision is deepened, the rectus muscles are retracted laterally, and the peritoneum is opened. At this point, long instruments are necessary.

3. In a male patient the bladder dome is lifted at its peritoneal surface. Dissection proceeds laterally on either side with ligation of the major vesical arteries.

STEP **3-1**

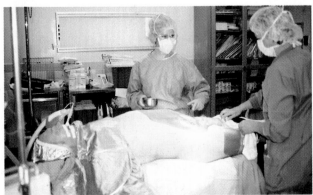

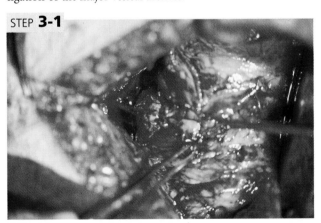

STEP **3-2**

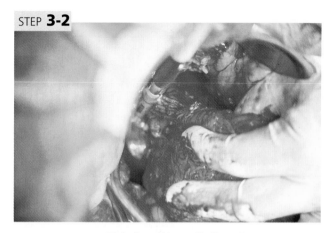

Vesical arteries are clip ligated.

The bladder is then retracted to expose the prostate and seminal vesicles, which are dissected free in continuity with the bladder. The dorsal vein is ligated with 0 silk ties or a vascular stapler.

STEP **3-3**

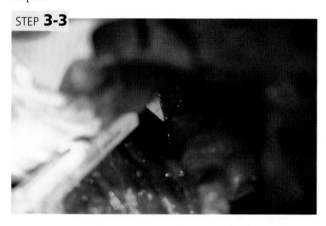

The vas deferens is divided, and the urethra is cut at the level of the pelvic diaphragm.

4. The surgical specimen consists of the bladder, distal ureters, prostate, seminal vesicles, and distal vas deferens and is removed en bloc.

STEP **4-1**

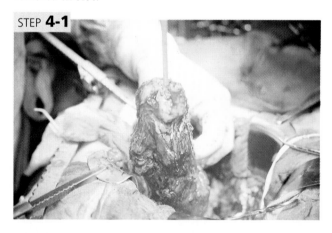

The urethra is ligated with absorbable suture.

5. Lap pads are placed in the denuded pelvis, and pressure is applied to reduce blood loss from oozing.

Nursing Care and Discharge Planning for Cystectomy

1. Patient must be observed for adequate pulmonary perfusion and oxygen supplied. Coughing, turning, and deep breathing are essential components of care.
2. Fluid and electrolyte levels must be monitored and replaced as necessary, especially sodium and potassium. If no alimentation occurs by 1 week, hyperalimentation may be necessary.
3. Catheters and stents should be inspected routinely for integrity and output.
4. The nasogastric tube should be connected to suction and seated so as not to stress the nares. Output should routinely be assessed and irrigations performed when indicated.
5. Alternating compression stockings remain until patient is ambulatory
6. Pain may be controlled with PCA, epidural catheter, or IM injection until alimentation begins. Oral medication is then instituted. Stool softeners should be provided once the intestinal tract is functioning.
7. Antibiotics are administered for approximately 5 days.
8. The patient will be discharged in 5 to 7 days.
9. Follow-up ureterograms and pouchograms are done 7 to 14 days postoperatively.

6. Urinary diversion by isolated ileal or colonic conduit may be performed. Direct anastomosis of the ureters to the colon may be performed by ureterosigmoidostomy.

7. The surgical approach for total cystectomy in the female patient is as described for the male patient, but the urethra is removed in continuity with the bladder and internal reproductive organs.

URINARY DIVERSIONS

Urinary diversions are required when cystectomy is performed. There are many possible approaches available to the practitioner. Those to be discussed include the classic and more common interventions seen. Preoperative nursing care and patient preparation will be the same no matter what diversion is chosen. Equipment and instrumentation is as described for cystectomy.

CUTANEOUS DIVERSION
Ileal Conduit

Description. The ileal conduit is the classic method by which the urine flow is diverted to an isolated loop of bowel. One end of the isolated loop is brought out through the skin so that the urine can be collected in a drainage bag, which is intermittently emptied. The selected site, usually in the right lower quadrant of the abdomen, above the belt line, is marked with a fine needle dipped in methylene blue to prevent erasure during skin preparation. The goal is to create a round, protruding stoma without wrinkles in the skin, to prevent urine leakage under the collecting device. Puckering around the stoma is minimized if a subcuticular technique is used when suturing the

Nursing Care and Teaching Considerations

Generic for Urinary Diversions

1. Incorporate nursing diagnoses.
2. Malnutrition and anemia need to be addressed before surgery. Hyperalimentation may be necessary perioperatively. Patient may have been on a clear liquid diet for 3 days preoperatively.
3. Review patient record for reports of preoperative studies: IVP, serum electrolytes, chest x-ray, bone scan, MRI, CT scan, CBC, PT, PTT, urine culture, urinalysis, ECG, serum chemistry survey (especially BUN, serum creatinine, alkaline phosphatase).
4. Determine if antibiotic therapy was successfully initiated.
5. Assess patient for allergies, skin integrity, diabetes, asthma, cardiopulmonary status, peripheral vascular circulation, range of motion, physical impairments (arthritis), presence of implants, nutritional status, previous radiation therapy,
6. Discuss perioperative course and determine comprehension and anxiety level: presence of stoma, need to wear appliance, nasogastric tube postoperatively, common stomal problems, positioning needs. Determine if enterostomal consult was accomplished.
7. Ascertain that preparations are made for CVP and A-line insertion. Determine if epidural catheter will be placed.
8. Check equipment, supplies, and instrumentation for function and integrity.
9. Check medications for dosages and expiration dates.
10. Position patient under guidance of surgeon and anesthetist. Ensure that IV lines are unrestricted and linen is smooth. Apply appropriate positioning devices.
11. Apply alternating compression stockings and patient dispersive pad.
12. Prep and drape patient according to AORN guidelines.
13. Document assessment findings and nursing interventions.

stoma in place. Cystectomy may be performed before or after this procedure, depending on the patient's condition and diagnosis. In some cases the surgeon may choose not to remove the bladder rather than to subject a debilitated patient to further surgery. In cases of bladder carcinoma, the surgeon may elect to treat the patient with radiation in an attempt to decrease the size of the tumor and "sterilize" the regional lymph nodes before performing a cystectomy.

Indications. The candidate for ileal diversion must have a retrievable ureter at least 1 cm in diameter with a thick, well-vascularized wall. The patient must be able to care for the appliance. Conditions amenable to diversion include neurogenic bladder, interstitial cystitis, and bladder carcinoma.

Perioperative risks. Surgical and anesthetic problems that have been encountered include anuria, intestinal or anastomotic obstruction, hyperchloremic acidosis, third-space losses, fluid and electrolyte imbalance, wound infection, wound dehis-

cence, anemia, paralytic ileus, intestinal fistula, ischemia and necrosis of the mesentery, urine leakage at the suture line, urinoma, redundant pouch requiring reoperation to shorten, stomal stenosis, stomal prolapse, peristomal dermatitis, hyperkeratosis, stomal scarring, stomal ischemia, parastomal hernia, calculus formation, and pyelonephritis.

Procedural Steps

The patient is placed in the supine position. A cystectomy and prostatectomy or hysterectomy are usually done at the time of surgery.

1. The bladder is decompressed with a catheter. The abdomen is entered through a midline abdominal incision. A self-retaining abdominal retractor is placed so that the viscera are excluded from the region of dissection.

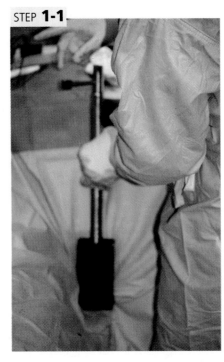

STEP **1-1**

Self-retaining retractor is attached to OR bed.

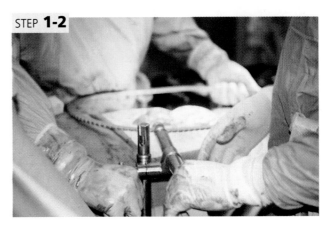

STEP **1-2**

Bookwalter being positioned.

2. The ureters are identified and mobilized by severing them 1 to 1½ inches from the bladder. A retroperitoneal tunnel is made so that the left ureter lies close to the right ureter.

3. The distal ileum and mesentery are inspected to identify the bowel's blood supply. A drain is passed through the mesentery, midway between the two main arterial arcades adjacent to the ileum at the proximal and distal ends of the selected segment. This segment usually comprises 15 to 20 cm of the terminal ileum, a few centimeters from the ileocecal valve.

4. Care is exercised to preserve the ileocecal artery and adequate circulation to the isolated ileal segment. The peritoneum is incised over the proposed line of division of the mesentery.

5. Intestinal clamps are placed across the ileum, and the bowel is divided flush with the clamps. The segment is opened and irrigated well with iodophor solution.

STEP 5-1

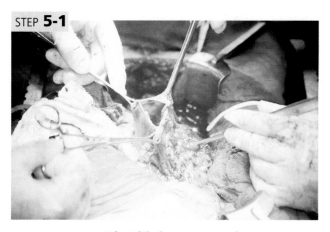

Selected ileal segment opened.

STEP 5-2

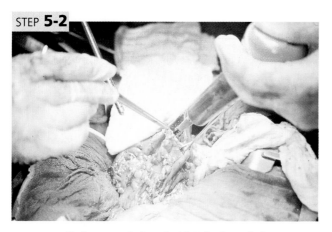

Ileal segment irrigated with Iodophor solution.

By gastrointestinal technique, the proximal end of the isolated ileal segment is closed first with a layer of absorbable sutures and then with a second layer of interrupted 3-0 or 4-0 silk sutures. The proximal and distal segments of ileum are reanastomosed end to end in two layers.

CONSIDERATIONS Staples may be used, and each staple oversewn with silk.

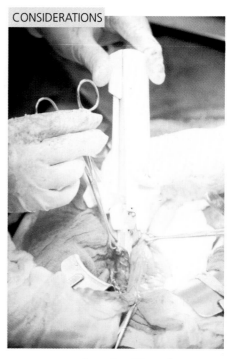

CONSIDERATIONS

Inserting GIA stapler.

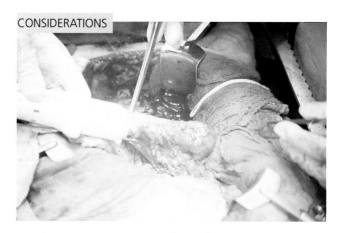

CONSIDERATIONS

Cross-stapling with GIA.

6. The mesenteric incision is closed with interrupted absorbable sutures.

7. The closed proximal end of the conduit segment is fixed to the posterior peritoneum. The ureters are implanted in the ileal segment with fine instruments and 4-0 absorbable ureteral sutures on atraumatic needles.

8. The peritoneum and muscle of the abdominal wall lateral to the original incision are separated by blunt dissection. The abdominal opening for the stoma is made.

9. The distal opening of the ileal conduit is then drawn through a fenestration in the muscle, fascia, and skin. The ileum is fixed to the fascia with quadrant sutures of 3-0 absorbable material. A rosebud stoma is constructed at the same time the ileum is sutured to the skin with subcuticular 4-0 absorbable suture.

10. Ureteral stents are usually left in the stoma, and a urinary collecting pouch is placed over the rosebud stoma to collect urine. The wound is drained with two Jackson-Pratt drains.

STEP **10-1**

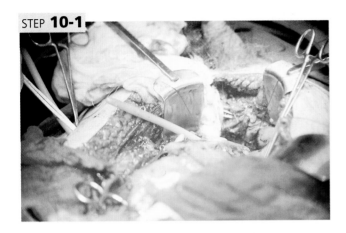

The abdominal incision is closed with 0 nonabsorbable suture. The skin is reapproximated with skin staples.

POSTOPERATIVE

Nursing Care and Discharge Planning for Ileal Conduit

1. Mannitol is administered to counter fluid volume shifts and prevent anuria.
2. Stomal stents and catheters are irrigated every 4 hours to prevent obstruction.
3. Ileostomy bag must be checked hourly and emptied routinely to prevent reflux and urinary backpressure leading to obstruction of urinary flow.
4. Hyperalimentation may be indicated if patient's nutritional level was not adequately corrected preoperatively.
5. Stoma should be routinely checked for leaks around appliance and appropriate stomal care provided. If leaks are severe, a blood-urea nitrogen (BUN) and loopogram may be indicated. It may be necessary to place a stomal catheter to low suction while healing takes place.
6. Stoma should be monitored for color and character of tissue, to determine vascularity and observe for ischemia or necrosis.
7. Nasogastric tube is maintained to suction to provide gastric decompression and assist in deterring ileus.
8. Antibiotic therapy is continued until tissues are well healed. Pain control may be provided with IV or epidural management. Stool softeners should be provided once patient is eating and peristalsis has returned.
9. Wound should be routinely checked, with dressings kept clean and dry.
10. Patient is discharged in 5 to 7 days.
11. Follow-up IVPs, CT scans, sonograms, loopograms, and BUN levels will be scheduled by the physician.

CONTINENT DIVERSION

Continent diversion requires a reservoir, an antireflux mechanism, and a catheterizable stoma that will not leak. Different parts of the bowel and the stomach have been used as continent reservoirs. The choice of the antireflux mechanism is dependent on the implantation site. The stoma does not require an appliance; therefore the site may be placed below the belt line or bikini line, making them catheterizable when the patient is sitting.

If the patient is dexterous and able to intubate the pouch and shows no psychologic or medical contraindications, he or she is a candidate. Contraindications include patients with insufficient bowel because of adhesions, previous resection, or disease (colitis); patients who have had radiation to the intestines; patients with limited life expectancy because of age, infirmity, or malignancy; and patients without the proper motivation to perform the care necessary.

Ileal Reservoir (Kock Pouch)

Description. A continent reservoir is constructed of ileum, without the use of the ileocecal region. Continence is achieved by the valve mechanism within the construction of the nipple valve attached to the skin. Instrumentation is discussed under cystectomy. Gastrointestinal staples may be used instead of or in addition to suture.

Perioperative risks. All the risks surrounding cystectomy apply. Additional problems encountered based on the nature of the diversion include efferent-valve malfunction, incontinence from ischemia, fistula formation, difficulty with catheterization, afferent-valve malfunction, urinary reflux, stenosis of stoma, urinary tract infection, calculus formation, inadequate pouch size, vitamin B_{12} deficiency, and hyperchloremic acidosis.

Procedural Steps

1. The mesentery is divided and suture or staple ligated along the avascular plane between the superior mesenteric artery and the ileocolic artery. The bowel is divided, and four segments are measured and marked with silk suture tags. These segments will serve as the efferent conduit, the pouch, and the afferent limb.

2. A portion of the proximal ileum is resected and discarded along with a wedge of mesentery. Suction is passed down the lumen to clear any fecal material or mucus. The proximal end is closed in an intestinal manner or stapled.

3. The segment to be employed is spread out in a U-shaped fashion. The sides are sewn together with 3-0 absorbable suture in a running fashion. The bowel is incised with electrocautery lateral to the suture into the two loops.

CONSIDERATIONS Gastrointestinal staples may be used to bring the sides together.

4. The medial edges are oversewn with 3-0 or 4-0 silk. The mesentery is cleared on the limb segments and the lumens are intussuscepted into the open pouch.

CONSIDERATIONS Marlex mesh is used to serve as a strut to prevent parastomal herniation and to fix the base of the efferent nipple to the abdominal wall, facilitating catheterization.

5. The TA or similar stapler is used to form each nipple and to attach the nipples to the back wall of the pouch..

6. An 8 Fr stenting catheter is placed inside the nipple of the efferent conduit to prevent making the collar too tight. The limbs are secured with 3-0 or 4-0 silk suture.

7. The pouch is closed in a gastrointestinal manner with sutures or staples.

8. The ureters are anastomosed, as described under ileal conduit, to the afferent limb.

9. A small stoma site is prepared as described under ileal conduit. A catheter of choice is placed in the stoma for post-operative care. Stents may be placed in the ureters for the immediate postoperative period. This will necessitate initial placement of an ileostomy appliance until all systems are functioning.

10. A drain is placed, exiting through a separate stab wound. Closure is in the standard manner for laparotomy. Retention sutures may be employed. Bulky absorbent dressings and Montgomery straps are applied.

Colonic Reservoir (Indiana Pouch)

Description. A continent reservoir is constructed of right colon, which may include the ileum and cecum, the ileal cecal

POSTOPERATIVE

Nursing Care and Discharge Planning for Continent Reservoir

1. Antibiotic therapy is continued until ureteral stents are removed at approximately 1 week.
2. Pain may be controlled with PCA, epidural injection, or IM injection. Oral medication is begun when alimentation resumes. Stool softeners should then be provided.
3. Hyperalimentation may be necessary if no alimentation occurs by 1 week. Nasogastric tube remains until alimentation begins.
4. Foley catheter is removed after 2 weeks. Cecostomy drain is removed in 3 weeks. Wound drains are removed in approximately 1 week. Ureteral stents are removed in 1 week.
5. Patient should be instructed to expect to need several trips to urinate at night in order to stay dry. The reservoir volume will increase over time. The patient must be taught stomal catheterization techniques.
6. Discuss the possibility of an artificial sphincter in the future.
7. Discuss the possibility of chemotherapy or radiation therapy.
8. Patient is discharged in 5 to 10 days.
9. Alternating compression stockings remain until fully ambulatory.
10. Follow-up studies will be done in 1 month to evaluate for hydronephrosis and reflux.
11. Wound and stomal care discussed under ileal conduit applies.

valve, and ascending colon. Intussusception of the ileocecal valve into the cecum and narrowing of the ileal segment attached to the skin allow for continence.

Perioperative risks. Risks surrounding cystectomy and the Kock pouch apply.

Procedural Steps

1. The large bowel is split down the antimesenteric border for approximately three fourths its length.
2. The U-shaped defect is closed in an intestinal manner.
3. The terminal ileum is sutured along it's length over a small red rubber catheter in an intestinal fashion.
4. The pouch is filled with 400 ml of saline, and a larger catheter is placed to determine catheterizability.
5. The ureters are tunneled into the cecum through its tenia. They are then tacked to the outer bowel wall, and the cecum is secured to the pelvic wall. Ureteral stents may be placed.
6. The pouch is secured to the abdominal wall. The stomal site is prepared as described in ileal conduit. A 22 Fr Malecot catheter is placed in the reservoir to drain the cecostomy, exiting through a separate stab wound.
7. All drains are brought to the outside through stab wounds. A wound drain may also be inserted.

BLADDER SUBSTITUTION

Description. Techniques to create a neobladder have utilized various segments of the intestinal tract. Some of the interventions developed include the following:

Right colocystoplasty. Depending on the extent of involvement, the right colon may be used to replace the bladder, the bladder and prostatic urethra, or the bladder and prostate with a direct enteric-to-proximal bulbar urethral anastomosis. This procedure has become more functionally effective with the use of intermittent self-catheterization and selective implantation of a prosthetic urinary sphincter.

Ileocecal bladder substitution. The ileum has been used as a reservoir to restore urinary continuity because it possesses a low intraluminal pressure. However, the short mesentery does not always permit the bowel to reach the urethra. The results with the current antireflux techniques are not consistently successful.

Sigmoidocystoplasty. Because of its ease of construction, bladder proximity, decreased obstruction from mucus, and large capacity, the sigmoid colon has been more appealing to many surgeons in their attempt to create a new bladder. More efficient emptying with a larger reservoir capacity seems to occur with a sigmoid replacement. Results yield higher intraluminal pressures, more effective urinary flow rates, and less nocturnal incontinence than with ileal segments.

Ileoascending bladder substitution. In an effort to improve the intestinal reservoir's capacity and antirefluxing effectiveness, the use of the ascending colon as a continent reservoir was introduced. This technique has several anatomic advantages over other methods of bladder replacement. The segment used can include the hepatic flexure and proximal transverse colon. A large-capacity reservoir is obtained, and colonic incision or tailoring is not required to achieve an appropriate shape. It easily reaches any site within the pelvis and can be anastomosed directly to the urethra without tension.

Indications. The ideal candidate for a bladder replacement after cystectomy for carcinoma is a patient with a normal urethra; a proximally located, well-differentiated bladder tumor, absence of carcinoma in situ; and proof, in the male patient, that the prostatic urethra is free of disease. High-dose radiation offers appreciable risks for postoperative complications and is contraindicated with enterourethral anastomosis.

Perioperative risks. There has been recurrence, renal damage, incontinence, and postoperative strictures and fistulas with ileocecal bladder substitution. Although most patients have attained daytime urinary control, 30% still have problems with enuresis. Deterioration of the upper urinary tract, as a result of infection and obstruction, has historically been a significant risk with this procedure. Because of this, ileocecal substitution is met with mixed reactions and recommendations. Other risks surrounding bladder replacement include hypokalemia, anemia, suture-line breakdown, fistula, and calculus formation.

Orthotopic Ileocolic Neobladder

Description. A bladder substitution utilizing the right colon and ileum is showing remarkable results in the last decade. The procedure relies on meticulous dissection of the prostatic apex with preservation of the urinary sphincter and neurovascular bundles as well as a watertight urethral anastomosis. Most patients have achieved a high degree of daytime continence and a minimum of nocturnal enuresis.

Indications. Considerations influencing patient selection include age, general health, and fitness for extensive, complicated surgery. Contraindications include previous radiation therapy, bowel disease (diverticulosis, Crohn's disease, colitis), and other major medical problems that might jeopardize the patient or procedure. Preoperative urethral biopsies are frequently performed to rule out tumor or cellular atypia in the urethra, which would prevent this particular intervention.

Perioperative risks. Risks include significant blood loss, pulmonary edema, pulmonary emboli, hypotension or hypertension, cardiac dysrhythmias, third-space losses, fluid and electrolyte imbalance, hypokalemia, hyperchloremic acidosis, and peripheral vascular compromise. Short-term complications encountered include bleeding, infection, urinary extravasation, bladder perforation, urethral stricture, fistula formation, urinoma, and small bowel obstruction.

Long-term problems that have occurred include chronic constipation or diarrhea, compromised enterohepatic circulation, vitamin B_{12} deficiency, and urinary incontinence in a small percentage of patients.

Procedural Steps

1. After cystoprostatectomy, the right colon is then reflected medially to the hepatic flexure. The distal ileum to be used in the neobladder is inspected.

CONSIDERATIONS The appendix may be used to catheterize the reservoir.

2. The small bowel is divided and laid in an S shape, and stay sutures of 2-0 or 3-0 absorbable material are placed.

3. The posterior walls are sewn from inside to outside with running 3-0 absorbable suture. A seromuscular wedge of the dependent cecum is excised, and the mucosa is everted with 4-0 absorbable sutures to form a bladder neck.

4. The left ureter is brought retroperitoneally under the sigmoid mesentery. A submucosal tunnel is created, and the ureters are reimplanted through the colonic wall. Anastomosis is done from the interior of the pouch. Anchor sutures of 3-0 or 4-0 silk are placed at the outer entry point. The wall of the colon is anchored to the psoas muscle with 3-0 or 4-0 silk to prevent migration of the neobladder.

POSTOPERATIVE

Nursing Care and Discharge Planning for Bladder Substitution

1. Hyperchloremic acidosis prevention requires close maintenance of the fluid and electrolyte balance and administration of hyperalimentation. Vitamin B_{12} levels should also be monitored.
2. Antibiotics are administered until the ureteral stents are removed, usually 7 to 10 days. An IVP is performed to assess the upper urinary tract before stent removal.
3. The suprapubic catheter and ureteral stents are irrigated twice daily to prevent mucous buildup. The suprapubic catheter is removed after 2 to 5 weeks.
4. The Foley catheter is irrigated twice daily to prevent mucous buildup. This is removed after 3 to 4 weeks. Urine output should be monitored for amount and character to assess for function and infection.
5. The patient may experience a bloating or "gassy" sensation as the bladder fills. The patient should void every 4 hours to develop a Valsalva maneuver and relax the perineal muscles to allow voiding. This will also prevent overdistention and potential perforation.
6. CVP and A-Lines are removed in approximately 1 week.
7. Pain may be controlled through PCA, IV, epidural or IM injection until the patient's alimentary function has returned. Orally administered pain medication may then be started. Stool softeners should be provided.
8. Alternating compression stockings remain until the patient is ambulating well.
9. The nasogastric tube is removed when bowel sounds are strong and alimentation has begun.
10. The patient is encouraged to ambulate early.
11. Coughing and deep breathing exercises are done daily to assist ventilatory process. IPPB may be indicated.
12. Dressings are kept clean and dry. Wound checks are made daily for signs of infection.
13. Patient is discharged in 5 to 14 days.
14. A pouchogram, cystogram, cystometrogram, or ureterogram may be done in 1 month to rule out hydronephrosis and establish continuity of the tract.
15. Patient should slowly resume dietary habits and activity. No strenuous activity for 6 weeks. If sexual activity is possible, it should be postponed for 4 to 6 weeks.

5. Ureteral stents are placed and brought out through the colonic segment through a separate abdominal stab wound. A catheter that serves as a suprapubic tube is placed.

6. Sutures of 2-0 absorbable material are placed around the urethral stump and tagged. A Foley catheter is inserted into the urethra in a retrograde manner. The urethra is anastomosed to the neobladder at the point of the new bladder neck.

7. The neobladder is closed in an intestinal fashion or with gastrointestinal staples in a side-to-side anastomosis.

8. Wound drains are placed to the outside. The bladder is filled to test for leaks.

9. The wound is closed in a conventional manner.

GLOSSARY

Colorometric test   Diagnostic test to evaluate for vesicovaginal fistula. Irrigation containing Methylene blue or Indiop carmine is instilled into the bladder, and discoloration of white gauze placed in the vagina indicates a positive test.

Connell   An inverting gastrointestinal stitch including all layers of the bowel.

Corpus   The main part of a structure or organ.

Lembert   An inverting gastrointestinal stitch where sutures are passed through the seromuscular layer, perpendicular to the axis of the bowel, excluding the inner bowel layer.

Nonseminomatous   Testicular germ cell tumor with low sensitivity to radiation therapy.

Orthotopic   Relating to the grafting of tissue in a natural position.

Preputial   Relating to being a prepuce, or foreskin.

Rami   A projecting part, elongated process; the upper branch of the pubis that extends from the pubic symphysis to the body of the pubis at the acetabulum and forms the cranial part of the obturator foramen; the thin lower branch of the pubis that extends from the pubic symphysis to unite with the ischium in forming the inferior rim of the obturator foramen.

Bibliography

1. American Urological Association, Allied: *Standards of urologic nursing practice*, Richmond, 1990, AUAA.
2. Association of Operating Room Nurses: *Quality improvement in perioperative nursing*, Denver, 1992, AORN.
3. Association of Operating Room Nurses: *Standards and recommended practices*, Denver, 1995, AORN.
4. Benumof JL, Saidman LJ: *Anesthesia and perioperative complications*, St. Louis, 1992, Mosby.
5. Brendler CM et al: *Controversies in prostate cancer: a series of debates*, Washington, 1995, AUAA.
6. Doughty DB: *Urinary and fecal incontinence: nursing management*, St. Louis, 1991, Mosby.
7. Droller MJ: *Surgical management of urologic disease: an anatomic approach*, St. Louis, 1992, Mosby.
8. Foster DC et al: *Urogynecology*, Baltimore, 1995, Johns Hopkins University.
9. Gershenson DM et al: *Operative gynecology*, Philadelphia, 1993, WB Saunders.
10. Gillenwater JT et al: *Adult and pediatric urology*, vols 1-3, St. Louis, 1996, Mosby.
11. Goldstein M: *Surgery of male infertility*, Philadelphia, 1995, WB Saunders.
12. Gray M: *Genitourinary disorders*, St. Louis, 1992, Mosby.
13. Hampton BG, Bryant RA: *Ostomies and continent diversions: nursing management*, St. Louis, 1992, Mosby.
14. Hinman F: *Atlas of urologic surgery*, Philadelphia, 1989, WB Saunders.
15. Leach GE: *Atlas of the urologic clinics of North America: vaginal surgery for the urologist*, 2:1, Philadelphia, 1994, WB Saunders.
16. Lepor H: *The urologic clinics of North America: advances in benign prostatic hyperplasia*, 22:2, Philadelphia, 1995, WB Saunders.
17. Lipshultz LI, Howards SS: *Infertility in the male*, ed 2, St. Louis, 1991, Mosby.
18. Litwack K: *Core curriculum for post anesthesia nursing practice*, ed 3, Philadelphia, 1995, WB Saunders.
19. Lytton B, et al: *Advances in urology*, vol 7, St. Louis, 1994, Mosby.
20. McGuire EJ et al: *Advances in urology*, vol 8, St. Louis, 1995, Mosby.
21. Meeker MH, Rothrock JC: *Alexander's care of the patient in surgery*, ed 10, St. Louis, 1995, Mosby.
22. Neih PT, Libertino JA: *Atlas of the urologic clinics of North America: use of intestine in urologic surgery*, 3:2, Philadelphia, 1995, WB Saunders.
23. Raz S: *Atlas of transvaginal surgery*, Philadelphia, 1992, WB Saunders.
24. Resnick MI, Novick AC: *Urology secrets*, St. Louis, 1995, Mosby.
25. Resnick MI, Kursh ED: *Current therapy in genitourinary surgery*, ed 2, St. Louis, 1992, Mosby.
26. Rothrock JC: *Perioperative nursing care planning*, ed 2, St. Louis, 1996, Mosby.
27. Seidman EJ, Hanno PM: *Current urologic therapy*, ed 3, Philadelphia, 1994, WB Saunders.
28. Smith AD: *Controversies in endourology*, Philadelphia, 1995, WB Saunders.
29. Tanagho EA, McAninch JW: *Smith's general urology*, ed 14, Norwalk, 1995, Appleton & Lange.
30. Vaiden RE et al: *Core curriculum for the RN first assistant*, Denver, 1990, AORN.
31. Walters MD, Karram MM: *Clinical urogynecology*, St. Louis, 1993, Mosby.
32. Whitehead ED, Nagler HM: *Management of impotence and infertility*, Philadelphia, 1994, Lippincott.

11

Open Interventions on the Upper Urinary Tract

The upper urinary tract includes the ureter, kidney, and adrenal gland. Procedures discussed will be those seen in everyday practice. Although an overview of kidney transplant will be presented, it is beyond the scope of this text to discuss recipient transplant and harvest from a living donor in detail. The settings that provide these services are limited to large institutions with dedicated transplant teams. The perioperative nurse on call is likely to become involved in kidney harvest from a cadaveric donor in almost any hospital setting, however, and this will be detailed.

The text and photographs in this chapter are intended to be generic for the specific interventions. Each is subject to alteration depending on the practice setting and the preference of the surgeon. Common surgical techniques and instrumentation are depicted and intended as an overview to enable the perioperative nurse to anticipate patient care needs. Instrumentation and actual equipment in practice will also vary according to physician preference and the procedural setting. It is important to focus on the principles involved in each procedure and consider the instrumentation as suggestions for the specialty of genitourinary surgery.

NURSING CARE

Urinary tract obstruction may develop as a result of stones, infections, tumors, congenital malformations, or previous operations on the urinary tract. Surgery is indicated to prevent renal obstruction and subsequent renal failure. Surgical approach in renal surgery is based on the patient's habitus, the need for exposure to a part or all of the kidney, and the surgical procedure to be performed. In the case of renal masses, attention is directed toward control of the vascular pedicle. For this reason patient position and surgical exposure are of prime consideration. The patient may be placed in the supine or supine-oblique position, modified Trendelenburg position, prone-oblique position, or the lateral position.

In routine renal surgery the patient is placed in the lateral position with the loin directly over the kidney rest. The operative flank is uppermost, with the patient's back brought to the edge of the operating room bed. The upper arm is supported on an overhead arm support, and the lower arm is extended gently or flexed at the elbow so that the hand rests on or under the head pillow. The lower axilla is supported with an axillary roll. The patient's legs are positioned by placing a pillow between them and flexing the lower leg at the knee. The upper leg remains extended. The kidney rest is then raised, and when

the desired bed flexion is achieved, 3-inch adhesive tape is used to stabilize the patient throughout surgery. A beanbag positioner is often employed to assist in stabilizing the patient in the lateral position.

The simple flank or transabdominal incision is most frequently used and may include removal of the eleventh or twelfth rib. The incision begins at the posterior axillary line and parallels the course of the twelfth rib. It extends forward and slightly downward between the iliac crest and the thorax. For the lumbar incision, the patient is placed in a supine or prone position with bolsters under the flank and lower thorax. This effectively places the flank in an oblique position, causing the abdominal viscera to fall away from the operative incision. This approach is used for renal neoplasms and affords an excellent approach to the renal pedicle. The thoracoabdominal exposure is employed primarily for large upper-pole renal neoplasms. The tenth and eleventh ribs are usually removed, and the chest cavity is opened, collapsing the lung. The leaves of the diaphragm are separated to expose the kidney. A large retractor, such as a Finochietto, and chest drains are required.

Precautions must be taken to ensure pulmonary excursion and prevent pressure injury, peripheral vascular compromise, and nerve damage. Alternating compression stockings should be utilized. General anesthesia, often augmented with an epidural catheter will be employed and a nasogastric tube may be placed.

Many of the patients will be elderly or compromised because of their disease condition. Both of these factors result in increased stress on the heart. When a patient suddenly develops hypotension and oliguria, and it is known that he or she has been well hydrated and the catheter is intact, a silent myocardial infarction must be addressed.

Hypothermia is useful in renal stone surgery as a means of prolonging the safe period of renal ischemia during extensive parenchymal manipulation. This method is also employed for surgery of the renal artery. A commercially synthesized ultrafiltrate of plasma is available as a sterile solution in liter bottles. If a slush machine is not available, slush may be formed by freezing or refrigerating 5 or 6 bottles for 4 hours. During the last 2 hours, the solution is shaken every 20 to 30 minutes to ensure that the ice forms into small, soft crystals. An 18 × 24-inch latex sheet with a center slit is draped around the kidney and secured close to the renal pedicle before the slush is employed.

Additional nursing diagnoses appropriate for interventions on the upper urinary tract may include the following:

Nursing Diagnosis	Perioperative Planning and Intervention
Hypothermia related to: Tissue exposure Room temperature	Provide warmed irrigations and intravenous solutions. Keep patient covered as much as possible; provide warm blankets. Adjust room temperature to afford comfort to patient as well as surgical team. Utilize warming blankets perioperatively as indicated.
Fluid volume excess related to fluid absorption	Document amount of irrigation employed. Observe and document cardiovascular status; note alterations. Observe and record respiratory status; note any changes. Observe for abdominal distention and discomfort; assess for rigidity. Note alterations in mental status. Insert Foley catheter. Administer diuretics as ordered. Postoperatively notify surgeon.
Urinary retention related to operative intervention	Assess abdomen for distention. Maintain patent, tension-free, and kink-free urinary catheter. Evaluate catheter position by determining length of catheter protruding from urethra; reposition catheter as necessary. If more than one half of a male patient's catheter is protruding, the tip may be in the prostatic urethra: Gently push catheter in toward bladder until urine flow appears and then gently pull back until slight resistance is met. Approximately two thirds should extend in the female patient. Determine status of gross sensory motor function, particularly after spinal anesthesia. Irrigate catheter as necessary; observe for clot formation; note amount and character of urinary output.
Fluid volume deficit related to: Blood loss Third-space losses Dehydration	Observe and document cardiovascular status; note alterations. Observe and record respiratory status; note any changes. Note alterations in mental status. Replace blood loss with packed cells, stored autologous blood, or plasma. Hydrate patient with intravenous (IV) electrolyte solutions. Monitor or insert central venous pressure (CVP) or arterial (A) line. Provide hyperalimentation.

The interventions involving the upper urinary tract will generally occur in an inpatient setting. Patient education must be individualized based on the data assessment and intervention. It is important to include significant others in the discharge planning and instruction. The pain encountered postoperatively will vary. Pain management and respiratory toilet techniques will assist the patient toward recovery. Local anesthetics may be instilled to provide comfort in the immediate postoperative period.

The operating lights, electrosurgical unit, and suction unit should be checked for proper function before the patient enters the room. Instrumentation should be inspected for damage, debris or corrosion, and proper action before use.

As perioperative patient care is implemented, the plan of care will be subject to adjustment on a continual basis based on data collected through the preoperative assessment and changing intraoperative circumstances. This ongoing evaluation and revision of care allows for an individualized approach. Once care has been implemented the postoperative assessment is completed. Often it will not be possible to accurately determine long-term outcomes. Immediate postoperative assessment allows for a baseline determination of the effect of the nursing interventions provided. Priority postoperative assessment data appropriate for the continual evaluation of nursing care includes but is not limited to:

- Awareness of reportable signs and symptoms of hemorrhage or infection
- Discussion of dressing, wound, and stomal care
- Discussion of probable postoperative pain
- Review of coughing and deep-breathing techniques to assist pulmonary exchange
- Awareness of need to ambulate as soon as possible to prevent stasis and pneumonia and assist peristalsis
- Awareness of diet or other restrictions related to the medication regimen
- Comprehension of the medication regimen ordered by the physician (aspirin and nonsteroidal antiinflammatory agents should not be used postoperatively unless cleared with the physician)
- Understanding the need for adequate fluid intake to accelerate healing and promote recovery from spinal anesthesia, if appropriate
- Review of drain care
- Review of catheter care

An overview of the care provided and the subsequent evaluation is recorded to provide for the continuity of care throughout the recovery period. This documentation should be individualized according to the procedure and the needs of the patient. Surgical settings differ, and perioperative documentation will have guidelines appropriate for the specific institution.

A summary of the intraoperative activities designed to achieve certain outcome criteria should be reported to the perianesthesia nurse. Information to be recorded and reported will vary according to the procedure performed. Reports may differ between surgical settings depending on the amount of preoperative instruction afforded the patient and services available to meet each patient's requirements. Priority information for the genitourinary patient may include the following:

- Wound status at the time of dressing application
- Patency of catheter or drains at discharge from the operating room
- Precautions pertinent to the patient's physical condition
- Amount of fluid loss and replacement
- Status of peripheral vascular circulation
- Skin integrity preoperatively and postoperatively
- Positions and devices employed for surgery
- Level of comprehension during preoperative instruction
- Information taught to the patient preoperatively and intraoperatively
- Untoward reactions encountered intraoperatively
- Nursing care provided

THE ROLE OF THE RN FIRST ASSISTANT

In addition to the aspects of perioperative assessment, planning, and intervention previously discussed, the RNFA can play a significant role with the family when a kidney harvest on a cadaveric donor is planned. The RNFA may serve as a liaison between the surgical team and the family along with the counselor from the transplant team. The RNFA, though not trained in grief counseling, has the background to explain appropriately what will occur during the surgical intervention. With perioperative background to draw on, the RNFA may console and gently support those left behind. Training in coping techniques and patient teaching may be adapted to this situation.

REMOVAL OF CALCULI

Equipment and instrumentation
Equipment
Electrosurgery unit
Alternating compression unit
Suction unit
Positioning devices
Fiberoptic light source
Instruments
Cystoscopy set
Laparotomy instrument set
Lewkowitz lithotomy forceps
Randall stone forceps, varied sizes
Silver probe, long
Bake's dilators
Long instruments
Deep retractors
Miscellaneous supplies
Laparotomy pack
Cystoscopy pack

PREOPERATIVE

Nursing Care and Teaching Considerations for Ureterolithotomy-Pyelolithotomy-Nephrolithotomy

1. Review IVP to determine patient position by location of calculus and appropriate patient position.
2. Review patient record for reports of preoperative studies: urine culture, prothrombin time (PT), partial thromboplastin time (PTT), complete blood count (CBC), cardiac enzymes, serum electrolytes, chest x-ray, electrocardiogram (ECG).
3. Assess patient for presence of infection, skin integrity, allergies, range of motion, physical impairments or limitations, previous surgery, medical history (diabetes), cardiovascular and pulmonary status, peripheral vascular circulation.
4. Interview patient for understanding of planned intervention. Establish comprehension and anxiety level. Review perioperative course.
5. Incorporate general nursing diagnoses.
6. Check equipment, instrumentation, and supplies for function and integrity. Supply appropriate positioning aids (lithotomy or frog-legged and supine-oblique or lateral).
7. Check medications for dosages and expiration dates.
8. Apply alternating compression stockings before induction of anesthesia. Aseptically insert closed-system Foley catheter after cystoscopy is completed while patient is still draped.
9. Position patient under guidance of surgeon and anesthetist. Ensure that linen is smooth and IV lines and catheter are unrestricted.
10. Prep and drape patient according to Association of Operating Room Nurses (AORN) standards.
11. Document assessment findings and nursing interventions.

Sterile gowns
Sterile gloves
Drape towels, 4
Sterile cloth towels
Vessel loops
Umbilical tape
Cystoscopy tubing
Electrosurgery pencil with hand control
Suction tubing
Electrosurgery spatula tip, 6 inch
Ureteral catheter, 5 Fr
Knife blades, #12, 10, and 15
Radiopaque gauze sponges
Kittner dissectors
Laparotomy sponges, small
Syringe, Asepto
Foley catheter, #14 or 16 Fr, 5 cc balloon
Urine drainage bag
Suture, 3-0 and 4-0 0n SH-1, UR and RB-1 needles
Suture, 2-0 and 3-0 on CT-1 needle
Suture, 4-0 on PS-3 needle
Skin staples

Sterile specimen container
Sterile saline, 1000 ml
Sterile water, 1000 ml
Sterile water, 3000 ml bag
Hypaque, 50% or other contrast material of choice
Syringe, 20 ml
Nephrostomy catheter
Penrose drain, $^1/_2$ inch
Jackson-Pratt drain
Jackson-Pratt reservoir
Ureteral stent
Gauze dressings
Antiseptic prep solution
Absorbent prep drape

URETEROLITHOTOMY

Description. The location of the calculus determines the surgical approach. A calculus high in the ureter requires a flank incision with possible removal of the twelfth rib; a more distal ureteral calculus requires a lower abdominal muscle-splitting incision.

A kidney, ureter, and bladder (KUB) x-ray film should be taken immediately before surgery to determine the exact location of the stone. The surgeon may also schedule a cystoscopic examination and attempt to remove the calculus endoscopically if the stone is in the most distal portion of the ureter.

Stones removed during surgery are usually subjected to chemical analysis. Stones obtained as surgical specimens should be submitted in a dry jar. Fixative agents such as formalin invalidate the results of the analysis.

Indications. Calculi in the renal pelvis may fall into the ureteropelvic junction and obstruct the flow of urine. However, calculi less than 1 cm in diameter may pass down the ureter and lodge at a more distal location, such as where the ureter crosses the iliac vessels or at the ureterovesical junction. A stone may remain in a renal calyx and continue to enlarge, eventually filling the entire renal collecting system (staghorn calculus). Hydroureteronephrosis, infection, and destruction of renal parenchyma frequently result from unrelieved obstruction.

Although the causes of many kidney stones are obscure, certain conditions such as obstruction, stasis, or imbalance of metabolism predispose their formation. Stones may form from various elements: calcium oxalate, calcium phosphate, magnesium ammonium phosphate, uric acid, calcium carbonate, or cystine.

Ureteral lithotomy is rarely performed because of the newer less invasive methods available. It is, however, important for the perioperative genitourinary nurse to have knowledge of this approach.

Perioperative risks. Risks related to ureterolithotomy include residual stone fragments, ureteral obstruction, injury to the ureteropelvic junction (UPJ) or ureterovesical junction (UVJ) injury, ureteral ischemia, ureteral colic, persistent drainage, ureteral stricture, bladder perforation, infection, adhesions, and urinoma. Anesthetic concerns include pulmonary edema, inadequate pulmonary excursion, pulmonary embolus, hypotension or hypertension, brachial or intercostal nerve injury, cardiac dysrhythmias, and compromised peripheral vascular circulation.

Procedural Steps

1. After cystoscopy with retrograde pyelograms an open-ended catheter is placed, if possible, and the Foley catheter is inserted. The patient is placed in supine-oblique or lateral position. Prepping and draping are performed in the usual manner.

2. The ureter is exposed extraperitoneally. The site of the calculus is located, and the ureter is freed a short distance distally and proximally.

CONSIDERATIONS With a lateral incision, it may be unnecessary to free the ureter. It may be stabilized around the calculus with vessel loops, umbilical tape, or Babcock clamps.

3. After exposure of the ureter, the calculus may be kept stationary with Babcock clamps or vessel loops applied above and below the calculus.

4. The incision in the ureter is made directly over the calculus. The calculus may then be easily removed with a Randall stone forceps.

5. A ureteral catheter is passed proximally and distally in the ureter as saline irrigation is instilled to check for ureteral patency and to dislodge any remaining fragments of calculus.

6. A double-J stent is passed into the ureter, and the ureter is closed with 4-0 absorbable sutures. A closed-system drain may be placed near the ureter and brought out through the wound or through a separate stab wound.

CONSIDERATIONS Stones should be placed in dry receptacles and sent to the chemistry laboratory for analysis.

7. The wound is closed in layers with 2-0 and 3-0 absorbable sutures. The skin is closed with a 4-0 subcuticular stitch or skin staples.

PYELOLITHOTOMY-NEPHROLITHOTOMY

Description. Pyelolithotomy. A lateral flank or posterior lumbar incision into the renal hilum, above the ureteropelvic junction, to remove a calculus located in the pelvis of the kidney. If the calculus is lodged at the UPJ, a dismembered pyelotomy and pyeloplasty may be considered. *Nephrolithotomy.* A lateral flank incision into the renal parenchyma to remove large or dense calculi.

Indications. Impacted large or complex calculi in the renal pelvis or body of the kidney causing recurrent infection, stasis, and obstruction. Open intervention is also indicated in patients with abnormal renal architecture, making a percutaneous approach difficult.

Perioperative risks. Problems that have been encountered with pyelolithotomy include damage to the ureteropelvic junction, bleeding, clot obstruction, prolonged drainage, and stricture. Risks inherent with nephrolithotomy include delayed intrapelvic hemorrhage, ischemic renal damage, renal artery injury, persistent infection, residual calculi, and pyelonephritis. Additionally, positional injury to the brachial plexus and damage to the intercostal nerve may occur. Anesthetic concerns include pulmonary atelectasis, phlebothrombosis, pulmonary embolus, pneumothorax, and hypertension.

Procedural Steps

1. Cystoscopy and retrograde pyelogram is performed. A ureteral catheter and Foley catheter are placed. The patient is placed in the lateral position and prepped and draped.

2. The renal pelvis is opened and the pelvic calculus gently removed.

3. The pelvis and collecting systems are thoroughly irrigated with saline using an Asepto syringe to dislodge the small remaining calculi and remove them from the kidney.

4. Nephrolithotomy or extended pyelolithotomy is employed when calculi are locked in the calyceal system and cannot be removed through a pyelotomy incision. In such cases the renal parenchyma above the calculus is incised and the calculus removed. In many instances such a situation is associated with a calyceal diverticulum.

5. After removal of the calculus, the collecting system is closed and the renal cortex reapproximated with deep hemostatic 2-0 absorbable sutures. A nephrostomy tube may be placed.

POSTOPERATIVE

Nursing Care and Discharge Planning for Ureterolithotomy-Pyelolithotomy-Nephrolithotomy

1. Intermittent positive-pressure breathing (IPPB) should be administered to the patient postoperatively until ambulating and exchanging well.
2. Early ambulation is encouraged.
3. Ureteral stents remain in situ for 10 days or until urinary drainage has spontaneously returned. The Foley catheter may be removed the first postoperative day. Intravenous pyelograms (IVPs) will be done before stent removal.
4. Antibiotic therapy should be continued according to the physician's order.
5. Urine should be monitored for signs of infection or obstruction. Cultures may be done a few days postoperatively.
6. Nephrostomy tubes remain in situ for 1 week.
7. Wound drains remain in place for 10 days, or until spontaneous urinary drainage has returned.
8. Pain may be controlled with epidural injection, patient-controlled analgesia (PCA), IV, intramuscular (IM), or oral therapy. Medications for ureteral colic or dysuria and stool softeners should be offered routinely.
9. Patient may be discharged about the fourth or fifth postoperative day (once the patient is eating, is afebrile, displays a clean wound, has begun having bowel movements, and may be controlled with oral pain medication).
10. Strenuous activity should be avoided for at least 1 month.
11. Diet may slowly be resumed as tolerated. Hydration is provided through IV therapy until appetite and tolerance return. Fluid intake should be increased to 8 oz q2h for 10 days once patient is able to eat and drink (half as fruit juice, half as water).

CONSIDERATIONS A nephroscope is sometimes used to localize and remove calyceal calculi. It is also useful for removal of residual fragments of staghorn calculi in the pelvic portion of the calyx.

6. An incision in the renal pelvis may be closed with 4-0 absorbable atraumatic sutures.

7. The renal fossa is drained with a Jackson-Pratt or similar closed drain and closed with 2-0 absorbable sutures. The wound and skin are closed with 3-0 and 4-0 absorbable suture or skin staples. All external drains are sutured in place with 3-0 nonabsorbable suture.

URETERAL RECONSTRUCTION

Description. Surgical excision of a section of ureter, generally involving the ureteropelvic or ureterovesical junction, and repairing the ureter and juncture to establish urinary drainage. The patient is in the supine or lateral position under general or regional anesthesia. An epidural catheter for anesthesia and postoperative pain management may be utilized. Alternating compression stockings are employed.

Indications. Reconstructive operations may be indicated because of a pathologic condition of the ureter that interferes with normal drainage. Conditions requiring ureteral reconstruction include stricture, trauma, low-grade ureteral tumor, and congenital ureterovesical reflux, as seen with ureterocele formation. Ureterocele is frequently associated with ureteral duplication, making identification of the functioning ureter critical.

Perioperative risks. Problems encountered during and after reconstructive procedures include hemorrhage, clot obstruction, acute pyelonephritis, urinary leakage, ureteral fibrosis, silent UPJ obstruction, suture granuloma, wound infection, incisional hernia, possible incontinence after ureterocele repair, and stent migration or calcification. Anesthetic risks are as mentioned with stone procedures.

Equipment and instrumentation
Equipment
Electrosurgery unit
Alternating compression unit
Suction unit
Positioning devices
Fiberoptic light source
Instruments
Cystoscopy set
Laparotomy instrument set
Long instruments
Deep retractors
Miscellaneous supplies
Laparotomy pack
Cystoscopy pack
Sterile gowns
Sterile gloves
Drape towels, 4
Sterile cloth towels
Vessel loops

Nursing Care and Teaching Considerations for Ureteral Reimplantation or Pyeloplasty

1. Review patient record for reports of preoperative studies: ultrasonograms, IVP, voiding cystogram, computed tomography (CT) scan, renal function parameters, PT, PTT, CBC, serum electrolytes, cardiac enzymes, urine cultures, chest x-ray, ECG. Urinary infection should be eradicated or controlled with antibiotics before intervention
2. Incorporate general nursing diagnoses.
3. Assess patient for allergies, skin condition, physical impairments, range of motion, presence of implants, peripheral vascular circulation, cardiopulmonary status, chronic disease condition (diabetes).
4. Interview patient and determine level of comprehension and anxiety regarding planned intervention. Discuss perioperative course.
5. Check equipment, instrumentation, and packaging for function and integrity. Check medications for dosage and expiration dates.
6. Provide appropriate positioning devices for positions planned (lithotomy or frog-legged and supine or lateral).
7. Apply alternating compression stockings.
8. Aseptically insert Foley catheter to closed drainage.
9. Position patient under guidance of surgeon and anesthetist. Ensure that IV lines and catheters are without constriction or tension. Determine that linen beneath patient is free of wrinkles.
10. Prep and drape patient according to AORN standards.
11. Document assessment findings and nursing interventions.

Umbilical tape
Cystoscopy tubing
Electrosurgery pencil with hand control
Suction tubing
Electrosurgery spatula tip, 6 inch
Ureteral catheter, 5 Fr
Knife blades, #12, 10, and 15
Radiopaque gauze sponges
Kittner dissectors
Laparotomy sponges, small
Syringe, Asepto
Foley catheter, #14 or 16 Fr, 5 cc balloon
Nephrostomy catheter of choice
Urine drainage bag
Suture, absorbable 3-0 and 4-0 on SH-1, UR and RB-1 needles
Suture, absorbable 2-0 and 3-0 on CT-1 needle
Suture, absorbable 4-0 on PS-3 needle
Skin staples
Sterile specimen container
Sterile saline, 1000 ml
Sterile water, 1000 ml

Sterile water, 3000 ml bag
Silicone tubing
Penrose drain, $^1/_2$ inch
Jackson-Pratt drain
Jackson-Pratt reservoir
Ureteral stent
Gauze dressings
Antiseptic prep solution
Absorbent prep drape

URETERAL REIMPLANTATION (UVJ REPAIR OR RECONSTRUCTION)

1. The patient is the supine position. The ureter is exposed through a transverse abdominal or Pfannenstiel incision.

CONSIDERATIONS Cystoscopy is generally performed first, and a ureteral catheter, passed retrograde, is used to identify and isolate the ureter.

2. The ureter is identified and the mucosa around the orifice dissected. The ureter is freed with long forceps and scissors outside the bladder.

STEP 2-1

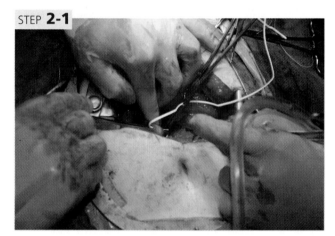

Placing vessel loop around ureter.

3. The bladder is opened, the ureteral orifice is located, and 4-0 traction sutures are placed.

STEP 3-1

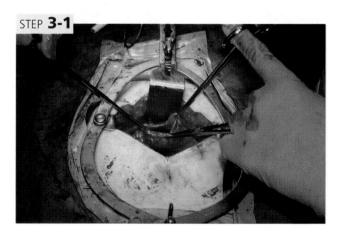

The bladder is incised.

STEP **3-2**

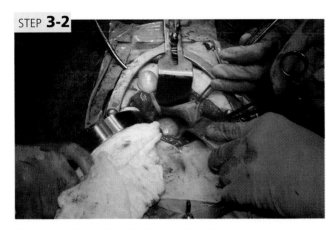

Ureterocele lying within bladder, to right of laparotomy sponge.

STEP **4-2**

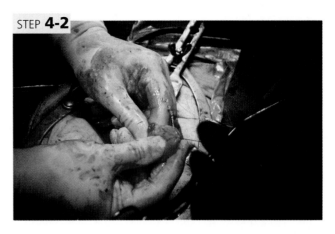

The ureterocele freed and outside the bladder; note urine exiting as (in upward stream) it is manipulated.

STEP **3-2**

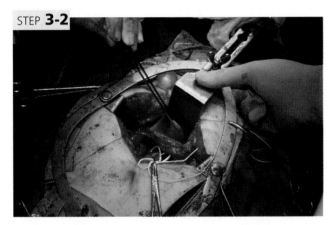

Traction suture placed on end of ureterocele.

4. The ureter is elevated with the traction sutures, freed from the mucosa and submucosa, and severed at the desired level.

STEP **4-3**

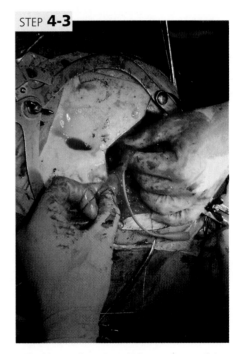

Red rubber catheter inserted to test ureteral patency.

STEP **4-1**

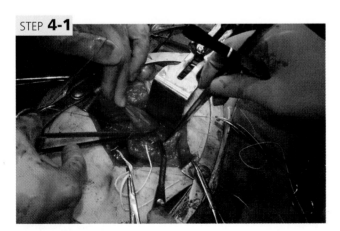

The ureterocele is dissected free of the bladder internal bladder wall.

STEP **4-4**

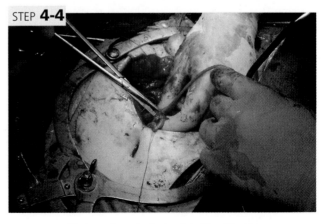

Ureterocele excised at point of healthy tissue.

STEP **4-5**

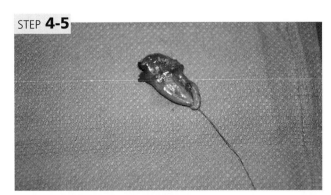

Excised ureterocele.

STEP **4-6**

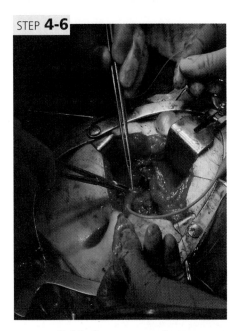

Fashioning new ureteral stoma.

5. The proximal stoma is transferred to the site of anastomosis.

STEP **5-1**

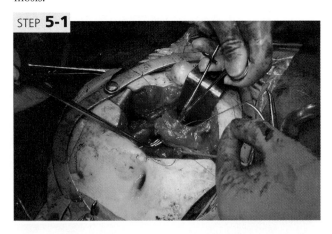

Passage is created with curved clamps, and the ureter is passed into the bladder.

STEP **5-2**

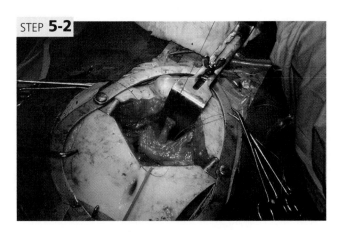

Refashioned ureteral stump.

The anastomosis is accomplished with fine dissection instruments and fine atraumatic sutures.

STEP **5-3**

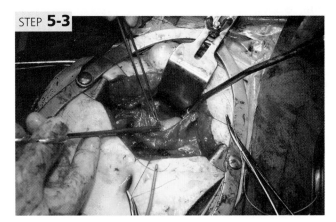

A mucosal pocket is created.

STEP **5-4**

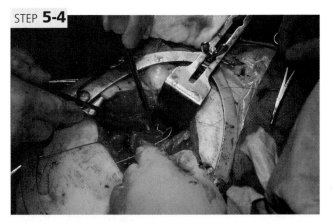

Ureter is anastomosed to the mucosal pocket.

6. A soft splinting stent is usually left in place until healing has taken place and free drainage is ensured.

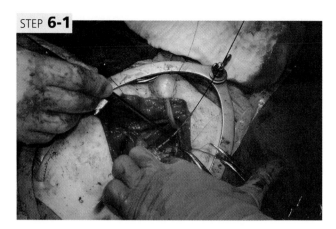

STEP **6-1**

Ureteral stent being placed.

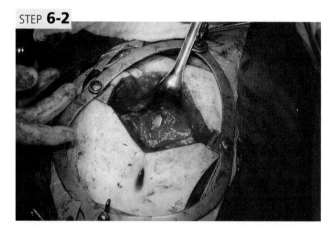

STEP **6-2**

Foley in bladder.

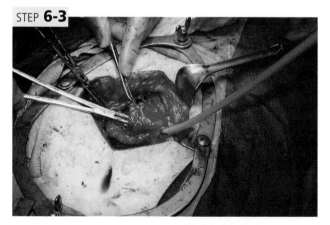

STEP **6-3**

Placing suprapubic catheter in bladder.

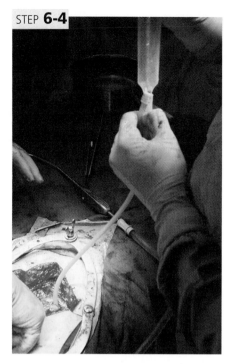

STEP **6-4**

Inflating bladder to test closure for leaks.

An extraperitoneal drain may be placed.

7. The wound is closed in layers and dressed in the routine manner.

DISMEMBERED PYELOPLASTY (UPJ REPAIR OR RECONSTRUCTION)8

1. The kidney and upper ureter are exposed through a supracostal flank incision.

2. Gerota's fascia is entered and the renal pelvis and ureter are freed while the kidney is rotated medially.

3. The ureter is freed and stabilized with a vessel loop below the level of the UPJ.

4. A 4-0 stay suture is placed in the tip of the ureter and the ureter is incised, trimmed, and shaped to the desired contour with fine forceps and scissors.

5. Anchoring sutures of 4-0 material are placed for traction during reconstruction of the renal pelvis. A diamond-shaped incision is made into the renal pelvis and the tissue removed.

CONSIDERATIONS The Foley Y-V-plasty technique may be followed. It converts a Y-shaped surgical incision of the renal pelvis into a V by drawing the apex of the arms of the Y to the foot of the Y with absorbable sutures.

6. Sutures are placed at each end of the refashioned renal pelvis, passed to the ureteral stoma and tagged. The pelvis is irrigated free of clots. The sutures are run in a continuous manner, creating the anastomosis.

7. A Silastic tubing may be used to stent the repaired pelvis until adequate healing has occurred. A nephrostomy tube is also placed within the pelvis to divert urine safely while the edema in the area of the plastic repair resolves.

8. Gerota's fascia is closed over the repair.

9. A drain is placed where the pelvis was reconstructed, and the surgical incision is closed in layers.

POSTOPERATIVE

Nursing Care and Discharge Planning for Ureteral Reimplantation or Pyeloplasty

1. Ureteral stent remains in place for 10 days. Spontaneous urinary drainage may not return for 10 days. IVPs will be done before stent removal.
2. Foley catheter may be removed the first or second postoperative day. A suprapubic catheter may be utilized instead of a urethral catheter.
3. Nephrostomy tubes are removed after 1 week.
4. Early ambulation is encouraged.
5. IPPB should be provided until patient is ambulating and exchanging well.
6. Pain may be controlled through epidural, PCA, IV, or IM therapy. Oral therapy begins once patient is tolerating food and liquid.
7. Antibiotics should be taken according to physician's direction until gone.
8. Patient should be hydrated with IV therapy until food and liquid tolerance is adequate for nutritional maintenance.
9. Urine is observed for volume and character to prevent obstruction and infection.
10. Patient may be discharged once bowels are functioning, diet is adequate, oral pain medication is tolerated, and there is no sign of fever or wound infection. Average is 5 days.
11. Postoperative IVP may be performed 3 or 4 days postoperatively.

KIDNEY REMOVAL

Equipment and instrumentation
Equipment
Electrosurgery unit
Alternating compression unit
Suction unit
Positioning devices
Instruments
Laparotomy instrument set
Long instruments
Vascular instruments
Deep retractors
Satinsky, Herrick, or Mayo pedicle clamps
Finochietto rib retractor, large

PREOPERATIVE

Nursing Care and Teaching Considerations for Kidney Removal

1. Review patient record for reports of any or all of the following preoperative studies: renal arteriography (possible with renal artery stenosis), CT scans and bone scans (for diagnosis of tumor), venogram (to rule out tumor extension to the renal vein), aortograms, inferior vena cavography, serum creatinine level and urograms of contralateral kidney (to assess function), lactate dehydrogenase (LDH) and liver enzymes (elevated with carcinoma). Other studies will include: PT, PTT, CBC, serum electrolytes, cardiac enzymes, urine culture, chest x-ray, ECG, IVP, magnetic resonance imaging, (MRI), pulmonary function profile, percutaneous renal biopsy.
2. Confirm that 2 to 4 units of blood has been prepared; patient may have autologous blood stored. IV crystalloids may have been initiated preoperatively.
3. Assess patient for comprehension and anxiety level regarding proposed procedure. Discuss perioperative course and common postoperative reactions.
4. Assess patient for allergies, range of motion, physical limitations, skin integrity, presence of other disease or infection, cardiopulmonary status. Infections of the urinary tract, teeth, or respiratory tract should have been treated. Antibiotics may have been administered preoperatively.
5. Check equipment, instrumentation, and sterile packaging for function and integrity.
6. Check medications for dosage and expiration dates.
7. Provide positioning devices appropriate for planned approach (bean bag, 3 inch tape, pillows, chest rolls, axillary rolls, Allen lateral armboard, kidney braces, pads for pressure sites).
8. Aseptically insert closed-system Foley catheter. Apply alternating compression stockings.
9. Slowly position patient under guidance of surgeon and anesthetist. Observe for signs of cardiovascular compromise and collapse. Provide padding to promote maximum pulmonary exchange. Ensure that all lines and drains are free of tension. Protect epidural catheter if in place.
10. If CVP or A-Line are not in place, be prepared to insert preoperatively. A nasogastric tube will be placed if the peritoneum is to be violated.
11. Prep and drape patient according to AORN standards.
12. Document assessment findings and nursing interventions.

Balfour, 2-inch and 2 $\frac{1}{2}$-inch blades
Matson costal periosteotome
Alexander costal periosteotome
Doyen rib raspatories, right and left
Bethune rib cutter
Double-action duckbill rongeur
Bailey rib approximater
Langenbeck periosteal elevator
Clip appliers

Miscellaneous supplies

Laparotomy pack
Sterile gowns
Sterile gloves
Drape towels, 4
Sterile cloth towels
Vessel loops
Umbilical tape
Electrosurgery pencil with hand control
Suction tubing
Electrosurgery spatula tip, 6 inch
Ureteral catheter, 5 Fr
Rubber catheter, 8 or 10 Fr
Knife blades, #10 and 15
Radiopaque gauze sponges
Kittner dissectors
Laparotomy sponges, small and large
Syringe, Asepto
Foley catheter, #14 or 16 Fr, 5 cc balloon
Urine drainage bag
Ligaclips, medium, medium-large, large
Suture, 0 and 2-0 nonabsorbable ties
Suture, absorbable 3-0 and 4-0 on SH-1, UR, and RB-1 needles
Suture, absorbable 2-0 and 3-0 on CT-1 needle
Suture, absorbable 4-0 on PS-3 needle
Skin staples
Sterile specimen container
Sterile saline, 1000 ml
Sterile water, 1000 ml
Penrose drain, ¹/₂ inch
Jackson-Pratt drain
Jackson-Pratt reservoir
Gauze dressings
Antiseptic prep solution
Absorbent prep drape

HEMINEPHRECTOMY

Description. Heminephrectomy is removal of a portion of the kidney. The patient will be in the lateral position under general anesthesia.

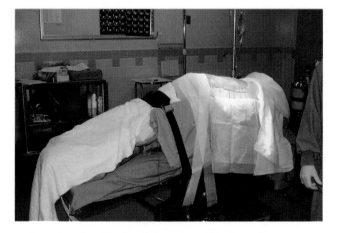

Posterior view of patient in lateral position for nephrectomy.

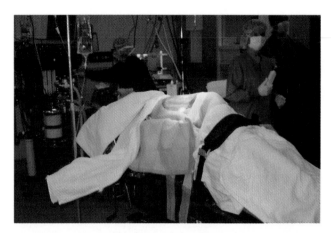

Anterior view of patient in lateral position for nephrectomy.

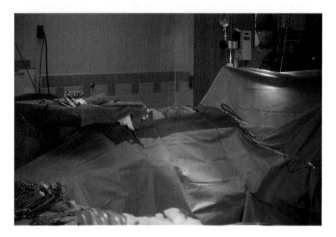

Patient draped for nephrectomy.

A Foley catheter is placed preoperatively.

Indications. Conditions involving the lower-pole or upper-pole of the kidney, such as calculus disease, trauma limited to one pole of a kidney, and localized carcinoma under certain circumstances. To preserve functioning renal parenchyma in the patient with a solitary kidney, patients with functional impairment of total renal function, and patients at higher risk for eventual renal failure (diabetes, hypertension, renal arterial disease).

Perioperative risks. Risks to follow may be applied to any of the nephrectomies to be discussed. These include delayed venous drainage; renal artery thrombosis; renal ischemia; damage to the intima; damage to and subsequent hemorrhage from the renal artery , aorta, or vena cava; renal insufficiency; distal ureteral obstruction; hydronephrosis; recurrence of carcinoma (9% to 17%); wound hemorrhage; ileus; fistula; infection; wound separation; and urinoma. Anesthetic risks include cardiovascular collapse from hyperextension, impaired vena caval return, acute cardiac decompensation on return to supine position, mediastinal flutter, pleura breach with a tear to the pleura or lung, lung collapse, pulmonary edema, pulmonary embolus, peripheral vascular compromise, intercostal nerve or brachial plexus damage, pneumothorax, phlebitis, deep vein thrombosis, atelectasis, hypotension or hypertension, and gastric regurgitation.

Procedural Steps

1. The kidney and its pedicle should be completely mobilized.

2. The main vessels may be temporarily occluded for only 20 to 30 minutes, after which progressive renal damage may occur. Local hypothermia may be indicated to prolong ischemic operating time.

CONSIDERATIONS Lasix or mannitol is given to promote diuresis before clamping of the renal artery.

3. The renal capsule is incised and stripped back.

STEP **3-1**

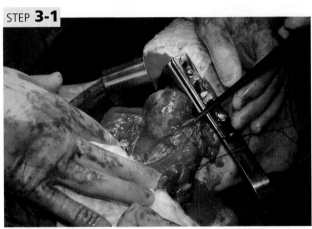

The renal capsule is incised; note tumor at proximal end.

A wedge of kidney tissue containing the diseased or damaged cortex is excised.

STEP **3-2**

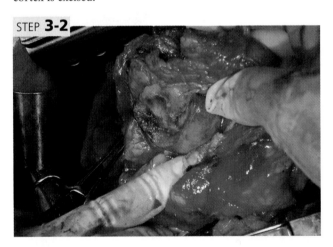

4. Interlobular fat or arcuate and interlobular arteries are clamped with Hopkins's clamps and suture ligated with 4-0 absorbable suture on urologic needles.

5. The open collecting system is reapproximated with a continuous 4-0 suture.

CONSIDERATIONS Ischemia resulting from the insult to the kidney often causes delayed venous drainage.

6. Perirenal fat is placed in the area in which tissue was excised, and the renal parenchyma is reapproximated with horizontal mattress sutures. If possible, the renal capsule is reapproximated with a continuous 2-0 suture.

NEPHRECTOMY

Description. Nephrectomy is the surgical removal of a kidney. The patient is in the lateral position under general anesthesia. An epidural catheter may be in place for postoperative pain management. A Foley catheter is placed preoperatively.

Indications. Nephrectomy is performed as a means of definitive therapy for many renal problems, such as congenital ureteropelvic junction obstruction with severe hydronephrosis, renal tumors, renal trauma, calculus disease with infection, cortical abscess, pyelonephrosis, and renovascular hypertension.

Perioperative risks. Risks are as for heminephrectomy.

Procedural Steps

1. The incision is carried through the skin, fat, and fascia.

STEP **1-1**

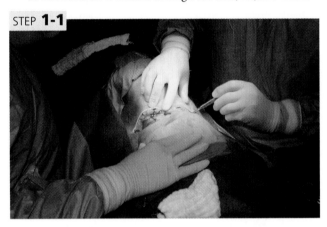

Bleeding vessels are clamped and ligated or fulgurated.

2. The external oblique, internal oblique, and transversalis muscles are sequentially exposed and incised in the direction of the initial skin incision.

STEP **2-1**

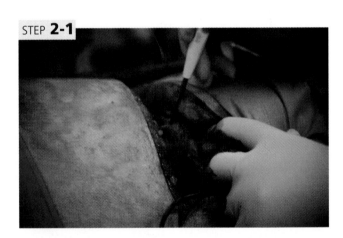

3. If necessary, a rib or ribs (eleventh or twelfth) may be resected to provide better access to the kidney. The periosteum is stripped with an Alexander costal periosteotome and Doyen rib raspatory.

CONSIDERATIONS A scalpel and heavy scissors may be used to cut through the lumbocostal ligaments. The rib is grasped with an Ochsner clamp and cut with rib shears, and the portion necessary to expose the kidney is removed.

4. Gerota's fascia is identified and incised with Metzenbaum scissors.

STEP **4-1**

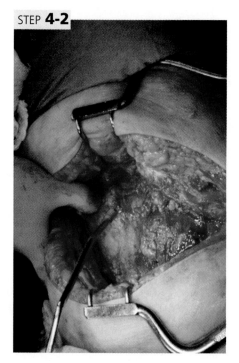

The incision is extended, and the kidney and perirenal fat are exposed by blunt and sharp dissection.

STEP **4-2**

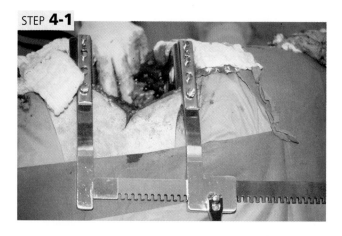

The kidney and renal fat are exposed by blunt dissection.

STEP **4-3**

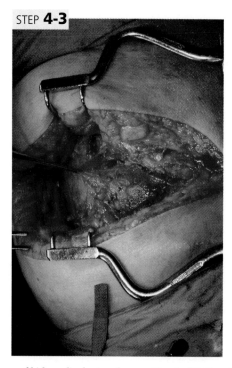

Exposure of kidney displaying abscess at level of Balfour blades.

STEP **4-4**

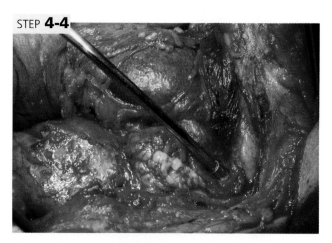

Close-up demonstrating kidney at far left, spleen behind suction, and diaphragm at level of suction tip.

STEP **4-5**

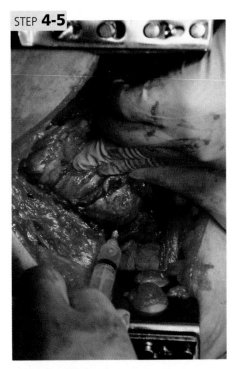

Aspiration of abscess for cytology and cultures.

STEP **4-6**

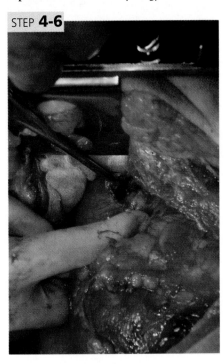

Opened abscessed cavity.

CONSIDERATIONS All perirenal fat that is removed during surgery may be saved in a small basin of normal saline. This may be used later as a bolster to stop bleeding.

5. The ureter is identified, separated from its adjacent structures, doubly clamped, divided, and ligated with absorbable 2-0 material.

6. The kidney pedicle containing the major blood vessels is isolated and doubly clamped; each vessel is triply ligated with nonabsorbable ties or hemoclips.

STEP **6-1**

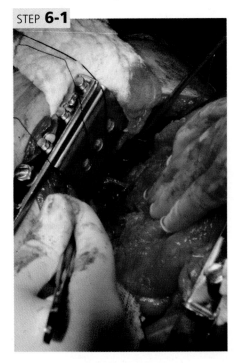

Renal artery isolated.

STEP **6-2**

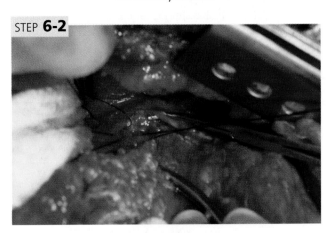

Suture ligatures being placed around renal vessels.

Each vessel is then severed. Two ligatures are left intact on the pedicle and the kidney is removed.

7. The renal fossa is explored for bleeding, and hemostasis is achieved. The fossa is irrigated with normal saline and suction. A drain is placed in the empty fossa and brought out through a separate stab incision in the skin.

8. The fascia and muscles are closed in layers with interrupted, absorbable sutures.

CONSIDERATIONS Retention sutures may be used in obese or chronically ill individuals in whom wound healing may be a problem.

9. The skin edges are approximated with interrupted sutures or with skin staples.

10. The drain is secured, and the wound is dressed.

NEPHROURETERECTOMY

Description. Nephroureterectomy is removal of a kidney and its entire ureter. The patient is in supine-oblique position under general anesthesia. An epidural catheter may have been placed preoperatively to allow postoperative pain management. The incision is extended anteriorly with the patient positioned and fully prepped and draped to access the flank and lower abdomen.

Indications. This procedure is indicated for collecting system tumors of the kidney and ureter.

Perioperative risks. Risks are as for heminephrectomy as well as the risk of urinary leak through the bladder incision.

Procedural Steps

1. The patient is placed in a supine-oblique position. The kidney and upper ureter are exposed, as described for nephrectomy. Simple nephrectomy is performed.

CONSIDERATIONS The kidney is placed in a plastic bag to prevent possible spillage of tumor cells. The ureter is not cut at this time but is mobilized as far distally as possible.

POSTOPERATIVE

Nursing Care and Discharge Planning for Kidney Removal

Postoperative care for the nephrectomy as well as adrenalectomy of the patient should be focused around the prevention of atelectasis, paralytic ileus, and wound infection.

1. Assist anesthetist and surgeon to return patient slowly to supine position. If large amounts of fluid were administered, acute cardiac decompensation may occur when patient is returned to supine position. The risk of cerebral vascular accident (CVA) or myocardial infarction (MI) is present, more so in the elderly. This may present immediately postoperatively or after discharge with typical anginal symptoms of MI or may be silent (hypotension, oliguria, and cardiac arrhythmia).

2. Patient should be assisted to cough and deep breathe. Provide pillow to splint flank. IPPB may be indicated.

3. Postoperative hypotension with fever and abdominal pain could indicate adrenal insufficiency. This occurs more often after radical or upper-pole heminephrectomy. Electrolytes and serum chemistry surveys should be drawn 1 day postoperatively and after discharge. Blood-urea-nitrogen (BUN), creatinine, and liver enzymes should be checked to diagnose early renal insufficiency.

4. An elevation of serum amylase with alkaline drainage or retroperitoneal fluid collection is suggestive of pancreatic injury. Hyperalimentation may be indicated. This is particularly true after left radical nephrectomy (the tail of the pancreas extends into the left renal space and is at more risk for injury, during left-sided interventions, than the pancreas itself when a right-sided procedure is performed). Injury is usually apparent intraoperatively, or immediately postoperatively. Injury to the right duodenum, during right nephrectomy, is generally immediately apparent.

5. Unremitting diarrhea may indicate vascular compromise to the descending colon after left nephrectomy. The risk is greater if a large lower-pole mass has been resected with injury to the adjacent inferior mesenteric artery.

6. Antibiotics (if indicated) and analgesics are administered intravenously until peristalsis returns. Pain management may also be accomplished with PCA or IM injections. Stool softeners should be provided upon return of peristalsis. Once alimentation occurs, oral medication is instituted. Patient should be instructed regarding the constipating effects of narcotics.

7. The wound drain remains for 5 to 10 days.

8. A chest tube may be in place if a thoracoabdominal approach was used. This is removed 1 or 2 days postoperatively.

9. The nasogastric tube, if used, remains until peristalsis returns, approximately 2 to 3 days.

10. CVP or A-lines remain until the patient is hemodynamically stable.

11. Alternating compression stockings remain until patient is ambulatory. Passive range of motion should be afforded until then.

12. The Foley catheter is removed in 3 to 5 days.

13. An IVP will be done 10 to 14 days after heminephrectomy to rule out distal obstruction and hydronephrosis.

14. Oral intake of fluid and food begins after peristalsis returns. Oral liquids are generally tolerated within 24 hours, and normal diet should resume soon after.

15. Early ambulation is encouraged. Normal activity may resume in 4 to 6 weeks. Strenuous activity (lifting more than 20 lb) should wait for 6 weeks. The patient may shower, climb stairs, and ride in a vehicle as tolerated.

16. Wound is assessed daily for signs of infection or separation. Instruct patient what to watch for. Wound dehiscence is uncommon, but subcutaneous herniation has been known to occur. Wound infection may occur, especially if the patient is diabetic with a history of pyelonephritis. The skin sutures should be removed, and the purulent material debrided. The incision is then packed with iodophor-soaked gauze that is changed daily.

17. If flank pain persists beyond the immediate postoperative period, the possibility of intercostal nerve root entrapment should be ruled out. If this has occurred, injection of a long-acting local anesthetic is often effective.

18. Patient may be discharged in 5 to 10 days. If the patient is young and in general good health and has a small wound, discharge could be the first postoperative day.

2. The operating room bed is adjusted so that surgery on the lower ureter may proceed. The lower genitourinary structures are identified and mobilized. The ureter and a small cuff of the bladder are removed in continuity, and the bladder is repaired with a single layer of 2-0 absorbable interrupted sutures.

3. The ureter and cuff of bladder are pulled superiorly into the flank incision, where the intact kidney and ureter may be removed from the surgical field.

4. A 14 or 16 Fr Foley catheter is left in the bladder, and drains are placed behind the bladder and in the empty renal fossa. The incision is closed in sequence in the usual manner.

RADICAL NEPHRECTOMY

Description. Radical nephrectomy is excision of kidney, perirenal fat, adrenal gland, Gerota's fascia, and contiguous periaortic lymph nodes. A lumbar, transthoracic, or transabdominal approach to the kidney is performed, depending on the size and location of the lesion. The transthoracic or transabdominal approach is preferred because the blood vessels of the kidney can be more easily reached and ligated before the tumor is mobilized, thus decreasing the possibility of tumor embolization into the bloodstream.

Indications. This procedure is performed for parenchymal renal neoplasms.

Perioperative risks. Risks are as for heminephrectomy as well as injury to the pancreas, spleen, or diaphragm and pleural effusion.

Procedural Steps

1. The procedure is as described for nephrectomy with the addition of adrenalectomy.

CONSIDERATIONS The renal pedicle is ligated before the kidney is mobilized, and Gerota's capsule is not incised but removed en bloc with the kidney.

2. Involved lymph nodes surrounding the renal pedicle are excised.

3. A chest tube is inserted if the transthoracic approach is used.

RENAL TRANSPLANTATION

Renal transplantation is the surgical placement of a donor kidney to alleviate the symptoms of end-stage renal disease. An allograft kidney is one obtained from a living related donor, a cadaveric donor, or a living unrelated donor. First attempted in the 1950s, an isograft is a kidney obtained from an identical twin.

Genitourinary surgeons are involved in the evaluation and management of patients who may undergo renal transplantation in several ways. The prevention, if possible, of renal failure caused by renal vascular or postrenal problems such as obstruction, before transplantation is necessary, is of primary consideration. The preoperative evaluation of the urinary tract in recipients and donors and the management of posttransplantation urologic disease and complications are additional roles the uro-

logic surgical team must fulfill. The transplantation procedure itself involves implantation of the ureter into the bladder, a bowel conduit, or neobladder and requires the urologic surgeon's contribution. Finally the evaluation and management of infertility and sexual dysfunction fall to the expertise of the urologist.

Candidates for transplantation must be able to withstand the operative procedure and be willing to accept the risks of surgery, rejection, and immunosuppression. Transplant recipients must be free of disseminated malignancy, extensive vascular disease, chronic infection unresponsive to treatment, tuberculosis, human immunodeficiency virus (HIV), hepatitis C, uncontrolled psychoses, ongoing substance abuse, active primary renal disease, chronic renal failure secondary to oxalosis, and medical noncompliance.

Urologic evaluation to rule out urinary tract infection, bladder dysfunction, and malignancy must be carried out. The minimal workup should include a urologic history, urinalysis, and a urine culture with a cytologic study. Patients with a history of voiding dysfunction should have a voiding cystogram, cystometrics with urethral pressure profile and external sphincter electromyelogram (EMG), and cystoscopy. Pretransplantation renal ultrasonography to rule out acquired renal cystic disease should be carried out in view of the increased incidence of malignant deterioration when this entity is present. A history of renal stone disease or infection requires radiographic visualization of the upper tracts, usually with retrograde pyelography.

Evaluation to rule out bladder scarring and noncompliance must be done well in advance of the transplant. Ureteral implantation into the native bladder is desirable whenever possible. When the patient has a urinary diversion, undiversion (ureteral reimplantation into the previously diverted urinary tract) may be indicated. The bladder may function only as a reservoir, requiring intermittent catheterization to be used. When the bladder capacity is compromised because of scarring, enterocystoplasty may be performed to provide increased compliance, capacity, and continence. Patients who have severe renal failure and require enterocystoplasty should learn to cycle their defunctionalized bladder with irrigation fluid to maintain compliance. Enterocystoplasty has resulted in poorly contractile bladders, requiring intermittent catheterization as well. Consideration should be given to using a portion of the stomach to augment these bladders because of its inherent ability to secrete acid and thereby decrease postaugmentation metabolic imbalance. Where the defunctionalized bladder (because of urinary diversion) has been subject to repeated infections (pyocystis) and the bladder cannot be rehabilitated, a cystectomy should be performed before the transplantation.

The need for recipient bilateral nephrectomy before transplantation has decreased in recent years, partially as a result of the improved ability to control metabolic problems (i.e., postnephrectomy anemia secondary to decreased erythropoitein production). Present indications for pretransplantation bilateral nephrectomy include renin-dependent hypertension unresponsive to medical treatment, renal failure caused by pyelonephritis with persistent bacteriuria, grade 3 to grade 4 reflux with or without bacteriuria, polycystic kidneys with significant infection or hemorrhage, heavy proteinuria producing severe nephrotic syndrome, renal malignancy, and kidneys diverted into conduits or cutaneous ureterostomies.

Nephroureterectomy should be performed where grade 3 to grade 4 reflux is present. When reflux is present, urine will drain antegrade into the bladder after voiding, predisposing the patient to urinary tract infection. Bladder function should be evaluated after nephrectomy, because of this risk.

The treatment of urethral problems such as urethral valves, strictures, and benign prostatism depends on urine production. Urethral valves can occur in the child or adult and should be resected. Benign prostatic hyperplasia (BPH) and stricture disease should generally be treated after the transplantation because of the tendency for recurrent stricture or bladder neck contracture to develop in the absence of urinary output. It may be preferable for the patient to have transurethral resection before renal transplantation, but the patient should then irrigate the bladder with antibiotic irrigation on a regular basis to avoid bladder neck scarring.

Additional problems affecting the urinary tract should be treated before renal transplantation allowing enough time for adequate wound healing before the patient is immunocompromised. These include undescended testicles, hydroceles, hernias, and hypospadias. Patients with chronic epididymitis should have either removal of the epididymis, or orchiectomy, to avoid sepsis and its associated morbidity.

The use of living donors, related or unrelated, provides for increased long-term success of the transplant. This is based not only on the relative absence of immunologic differences if the donor is related, but also on the availability of a donor before the recipient begins dialysis. Evaluation of the donor should be extensive because it may reveal undiagnosed medical problems in their early stages, representing one benefit the donor may receive. The presence of anatomic abnormalities in the donor kidney may not preclude the use of the kidney for transplantation. Such abnormalities include hypoplastic but otherwise normal kidneys, extrarenal pelvis, and congenital ureteropelvic obstruction. In addition to histocompatibility testing, the donor must also be evaluated for possible transmittable diseases, with testing that includes HIV, rapid plasma reagin, (RPR), cytomegalovirus (CMV), herpes, hepatitis C and B, and Epstein-Barr virus (EBV) titers. Females within childbearing age may be appropriate donors. The right kidney is generally chosen in this case, since it is more prone to hydronephrosis during pregnancy.

Renal transplantation is performed through an extraperitoneal right iliac fossa approach. The right iliac vein lies more anterior thus allowing for easier access. The left side is preserved for the possibility of second transplants. Careful ligation of lymphatics is performed to avoid postoperative lymphocele formation. Renal vein anastomosis is performed to the side of the external iliac vein, and the artery is anastomosed to the external iliac artery. In the case of multiple renal arteries, a Carrel patch may be anastomosed to the side of the external iliac artery. Heparinization is not required. Implantation of the ureter is performed by the extra or intravesical approach. Stenting the ureter is optional.

Complications attributable to urinary leak, ureteral stenosis, and UPJ obstruction average about 4%. Lymphatic fluid accumulations (lymphoceles) occur 1% to 18% of the time, and vascular complications (6% occurrence) may be attributable to venous or arterial kinking and venous or arterial torsion or stenosis. Late arterial stenosis may be attributed to rejection or may result from the technical intervention.

Renal biopsy is an important diagnostic step in confirming renal transplant rejection. Ninety percent of patients with an extreme elevation of serum creatinine, in the first month after transplantation, will demonstrate some evidence of rejection in the form of lymphocyte infiltration into the transplant biopsy specimens. Posttransplantation renal biopsy should be done if the serum creatinine has risen 20% above recent baseline levels, provided that renal ultrasonography has demonstrated a normal renal blood flow and no obstruction.

Demands for renal transplants continue to increase, with 10,000 performed annually: 25% from live donors and 75% from cadaveric donors. A backlog of over 10,000 organs per year exists. Length of hospitalization is generally 1 week, and 1-year cadaveric transplant survival averages 90%. Half of all kidney transplant recipients experience no rejection. The balance that do experience rejection respond to steroids or antihumoral therapy.

KIDNEY HARVEST (CADAVER DONOR)

Description. Kidney transplant entails transplantation of a living related or cadaveric donor kidney into the recipient's iliac fossa. The ideal cadaveric donor is young, free of infection and cancer, normotensive until a short time before death, and under hospital observation several hours before death. Permission to harvest the donor kidney must be obtained from the family and the medical examiner after brain death has been unequivocally established. Awareness of existing state legislation in this complex area is advisable. The donor is positioned supine and prepared for a xiphoid-to-pubis laparotomy.

Indications. A kidney transplantation is performed in an effort to restore renal function and thus maintain life in a patient who has end-stage renal disease. Preoperative management of the cadaver donor is vital to the success of the transplantation. As a result of the improvements in medical therapies, the only absolute contraindications for cadaveric donation are HIV and metastasis.

Perioperative risks. The risk involved in cadaver harvest revolves around the ability to maintain the patient on life support, with adequate ventilation and circulation for the organs. Kidney harvest is usually performed along with the harvest of several other organs. The aorta is cross clamped, and all organs are perfused with sterile iced saline. The heart, lungs, liver, and finally the kidneys are removed. Aseptic technique is critical to prevent organ contamination. Proper exposure is necessary to prevent damage to vessels integral to the transplant.

Equipment and instrumentation
Refer to nephrectomy, in addition to the following:
Bulldog clamps
Vascular clamps, angled, large
Deaver retractors, extra wide
Harrington retractors, small and large
Sternal saw or Lepshey knife and mallet
Centimeter ruler

Electrolyte solution (lactated Ringer's, Sachs, or Collins) cold in iced basin until needed

Intravenous extension tubes, sterile

Kidney basin with cold (4° C) intravenous saline solution (slush)

Stopcock, three-way

Needle catheter (Medicut), 18 gauge

Perfusion machine or kidney transplant equipment and ice

IV pole

Antiseptic prep solution

Absorbent prep drape

PREOPERATIVE

Nursing Care and Teaching Considerations for Kidney Harvest

1. Review donor's medical history for contraindications: chronic organ donor disease, ongoing systemic infection, intravenous drug abuse, malignancy, heart or lung disease, trauma to the donor organ, and HIV positivity.

2. Review donor's record for lab studies: blood typing, urinalysis, urine and blood cultures, BUN, serum creatinine, CBC, hepatitis B antigen evaluation, venereal disease, and HTLV-III, arterial blood gases, serum electrolytes, and liver enzymes.

3. Ascertain that the donor has been maintained on life-support systems: Organ perfusion, oxygenation, and hydration must be maintained. Arterial blood gases monitor ventilatory support. Dopamine may be administered if fluids alone are not able to maintain an adequate systolic blood pressure. Urine output is monitored, and antibiotics may be administered to combat and prevent infection.

4. After brain death has been established, the donor is taken to the surgical suite with respiratory and cardiac function mechanically maintained. Anticoagulant and alpha-adrenergic blocking agents are administered systemically during the procedure. Adequate renal perfusion and function are maintained with intravenous fluids and diuretics.

5. Family should be supported throughout to assist them in their decision and to cope with loss.

6. The patient is treated with respect, and attention is paid to maintaining body temperature, privacy, and aseptic technique.

7. Document nursing interventions.

Procedural Steps

1. A midline incision is made from the xiphoid process to the symphysis pubis with bilateral supraumbilical transverse extensions through the skin, subcutaneous layer, fascia, and muscle.

2. Hemostasis is obtained with clamps, ties, suture ligatures, and electrocoagulation.

3. The kidney, renal vessels, and ureter are carefully dissected with Metzenbaum scissors, DeBakey forceps, and Dean hemostatic forceps.

4. Heparin sodium, 15,000 units, is given intravenously 5 to 10 minutes before the renal vessels are clamped.

5. The usual method of resection is en bloc resection, which involves the removal of sections of the inferior vena cava and aorta with both kidneys in continuity. An incision is made along the route of the small bowel mesentery up to the esophageal hiatus. The entire gastrointestinal tract, spleen, and inferior portion of the pancreas are mobilized by dividing the celiac axis and the superior mesenteric artery, exposing the entire retroperitoneal region. The inferior vena cava and aorta are clamped below the renal vessels with vascular clamps, and the vessels are divided. Lumbar tributaries are secured with metal clips and are divided. The kidneys and ureters are freed from their surrounding soft tissues. The ureters are divided distally at the pelvic brim. The suprarenal aorta and inferior vena cava are clamped and divided at the level of the diaphragm, close to the bifurcation. The vessels and kidneys are severed from the surgical field, and the aorta and vena cava are ligated.

6. After removal of the kidneys, immediate perfusion with cold (4° C) electrolyte solution is carried out.

7. The kidneys are placed in a container of cold saline solution and surrounded by saline slush in an insulated carrier or placed on a hypothermic pulsatile perfusion machine for transport. A new preservative solution developed at the University of Wisconsin is being used in many institutions. It contains hydroxylethyl starch, providing a better metabolic substrate for organ metabolism. The cold ischemia time has been dramatically increased with this solution, allowing more time for transport.

8. While kidney perfusion is begun, the abdominal lymph nodes and spleen are removed for use in tissue typing.

9. The incision is closed with interrupted sutures.

10. Artificial life-support systems are terminated.

POSTOPERATIVE

Nursing Care and Discharge Planning for Kidney Harvest

1. Patient is prepared for transfer to the mortuary of choice according to institutional protocol.

2. Patient should be treated with respect throughout the perioperative course.

ADRENALECTOMY

Description. Adrenalectomy is partial or total excision of one or both adrenal glands.

Indications. Adrenalectomy may be performed for pheochromocytoma, Cushing's syndrome, hypersecretion of adrenocorticotropic hormone (ACTH) (70% of patients with Cushing's), primary tumor of the adrenal cortex, neuroblastoma, hyperaldosteronism, paraendocrine tumors, or secondary treatment of extra-adrenal tumors that depend on adrenal hormonal secretions, such as carcinoma of the prostate, lung, thymus, pituitary, and breast.

Perioperative risks. Risks surrounding adrenalectomy include liver damage, splenic damage, pancreatic damage, renal damage, wound hemorrhage, infection, retroperitoneal hemorrhage, hematoma, thrombophlebitis, portal vein injury, vena cava injury, hepatic vein injury, and subdiaphragmatic abscess. Anesthetic risks include cardiac dysrhythmias, hypertension, third-space losses (fluid-volume imbalance), hypovolemic and hyponatremic shock, dehydration, hypotension, renal shutdown, cerebral ischemia, hypoglycemia, hypokalemia or hyperkalemia, acidosis, inadequate pulmonary perfusion, pneumothorax, pulmonary edema, thrombosis and pulmonary embolus from venous stasis, and adrenal insufficiency.

Adrenal insufficiency may occur because of bilateral adrenalectomy for Cushing's syndrome, where treatment of the pituitary tumor responsible has not been effective, or after unilateral adrenalectomy, where the opposite adrenal has been suppressed or damaged. The postadrenalectomy or steroid-withdrawal syndrome may be gradual or abrupt in onset and includes symptoms of weakness, headache, fever, depression, nausea, vomiting, diarrhea, muscle aches, bone pain, loss of superficial skin layers, and hypotension. Patients who have had a total adrenalectomy will need lifelong replacement therapy including cortisone, and fluorohydrocortisone daily. Patients with a residual adrenal will have their replacement therapy tapered over 6 to 12 months.

Patients with Cushing's syndrome exist in a catabolic state with protein depletion and abnormalities of collagen synthesis. They are therefore prone to stress fractures, possibly related to positioning during surgery, abnormal wound healing, and ulceration of skin, with tearing of skin where tape is applied and development of stress ulceration prompting antacids, or histamine (H_2) blockade. Several studies have suggested a propensity to thromboembolism and deep venous thrombosis prompting the use of prophylactic measures such as low-dose heparin and antiembolism stockings in the appropriate setting.

Postoperative problems related to pheochromocytoma include hypertension and hypotension, hypoglycemia, and bronchospasm. Hypertension may present in the postoperative period if all tissues harboring pheochromocytoma have not been excised at the time of surgery. Dissection in the renal hilum may lead to injury to one of the renal arteries resulting in postoperative hypertension on a renovascular basis. Renal damage attributable to prolonged preoperative hypertension (as a result of elevated catacholamines) may lead to postoperative hypertension. Patients are treated with an alpha-adrenergic receptor blocking agent before surgery, usually phenoxybenzamine, which may contribute to hypotension in the early postoperative period. Third-space loss caused by extensive dissection may also be a contributing factor.

Patients with pheochromocytoma exhibit neurologic abnormalities on a long-term basis because of severe hypoglycemia caused by alteration of glucose metabolism. Patients may be more prone to bronchospasm postoperatively related to the decrease in catacholamines and their bronchodilatory effect.

Patients treated for aldosterone-producing adrenal adenoma with adrenalectomy may have alterations in electrolyte levels for 3 months and must be treated with appropriate steroid replacement (fluorohydrocortisone). Recovery of normal aldosterone levels may take as long as 12 months to develop but may be associated with moderate renal insufficiency.

PREOPERATIVE

Nursing Care and Teaching Considerations for Adrenalectomy

1. Patient may have been prepared for 2 days preoperatively with cortisone acetate, supplemented with IV administration immediately preoperatively and postoperatively if suffering from adrenal insufficiency (contraindicated with neuroblastoma and pheochromocytoma).

   Preoperative medical evaluation is appropriate focusing on the cardiovascular system because 40% of Cushing's syndrome deaths are attributable to cardiovascular disorders.
2. Review patient record for reports of CT scan, MRI, plasma catecholamines (epinephrine, norepinephrine, metanephrine, normetanephrine), PT, PTT, CBC, serum electrolytes, cardiac enzymes, chest x-ray, ECG, adrenal venogram.
3. Ensure that at least 2 units of blood are available. Check medications for dosage and expiration dates. Check equipment and instrumentation to assure proper function and freedom from debris.
4. CVP line will be in situ or inserted in the operating room after induction. A nasogastric will also be inserted.
5. Patient should be free of or under treatment for infection, hypokalemia, anemia.
6. Assess patient for allergies, diabetes, skin integrity, obesity, presence of implants, range of motion, physical impairments, and cardiopulmonary status.
7. Discuss perioperative course and postoperative reactions. Assess comprehension and anxiety level.
8. Aseptically insert closed-system Foley catheter. Apply alternating compression stockings and patient dispersive pad.
9. Position patient under guidance of surgeon and anesthetist. Provide appropriate positioning devices for approach chosen.
10. Ensure that IV and CVP lines and Foley catheter are free of constriction.
11. Prep and drape patient according to AORN standards.
12. Document assessment findings and nursing interventions.

Equipment and instrumentation
Refer to kidney removal

Procedural Steps

For unilateral adrenalectomy the patient may be placed in the lateral or supine position. When both glands may be explored, the supine or prone position is selected. The prone position is especially useful for debilitated patients with an advanced neoplasm.

Lateral Approach

1. A flank incision is performed as described for nephrectomy. The twelfth and sometimes the eleventh ribs are resected for optimum exposure of the upper pole of the kidney.

2. An opening is made through the transverse fascia with scissors. The pleura and diaphragm are protected with moist packs, and Gerota's capsule is incised to expose the kidney and adrenal gland.

3. The gland is identified and dissected free from the upper pole of the kidney by scissors and Babcock forceps. The blood supply of the gland is identified, clamped or clipped, and divided. Bleeding vessels are ligated.

4. To release the glands, the left adrenal vein, a branch of the left renal vein, is clamped and cut. The right adrenal vein, a tributary of the vena cava, is also divided. Fine vascular sutures may be required to repair inadvertent injury to the vena cava.

5. When hemostasis has been ensured, the wound is closed sequentially in layers: muscle, fascia, subcutaneous tissue, and skin.

Abdominal Approach

1. The abdominal wall is incised with an upper abdominal incision, and the peritoneal cavity is opened and explored. Bleeding vessels are clamped and ligated.

2. The abdominal wound is retracted, and the surrounding organs are protected with moist laparotomy packs.

3. The retroperitoneal area near the diaphragm is opened on the left side, exposing the renal fascia.

4. The renal fascia is opened to reveal the left kidney and adrenal gland.

5. The adrenal gland is freed from the kidney by sharp and blunt dissection. All bleeding vessels are clamped and ligated with no. 3-0 nonabsorbable sutures.

6. After hemostasis is achieved, the kidney is gently replaced in the renal fascia, which is closed with interrupted 2-0 absorbable sutures.

7. The peritoneum is closed over the left kidney and renal fascia.

8. The abdominal retractors are rearranged to give access to the peritoneum over the right kidney and adrenal gland. Care must be taken to prevent trauma to the liver.

9. The same procedure is repeated on the right side, taking care to clamp and ligate the short adrenal vein.

10. The abdomen is inspected for bleeding vessels, which are clamped and ligated.

11. The wound is closed as in a laparotomy.

Posterior Approach

1. The patient is placed in the prone position on chest rolls or a prone positioning device that has been adequately padded. (Refer to prone positioning, Chapter 5.)

2. The adrenal gland is approached at the level of the twelfth rib on the left and the eleventh rib on the right.

3. The kidney is retracted downward to expose the adrenal gland.

4. The apex and lateral margins of the gland are dissected free of surrounding tissue. Ligaclips are applied for hemostasis.

5. The adrenal vein is identified and doubly ligated with nonabsorbable ties and divided.

6. The wound is closed in a standard manner.

POSTOPERATIVE

Nursing Care and Discharge Planning for Adrenalectomy

1. Strict technique must be maintained during dressing changes and drain care. Patient is at increased risk for infection.
2. Narcotics must be used prudently. Decreased adrenal function exacerbates effect. Stool softeners should be provided.
3. Urine and serum electrolyte values should be drawn for the first week. Urine output is monitored. Inadequate tissue perfusion may cause decreased output requiring volume replacements. Increased diuresis results in sodium and potassium losses requiring volume replacements. Hyponatremia, hypokalemia, and hyperkalemia must be watched for (esp. with aldosteronism).
4. Blood pressure must be closely monitored. Persistent hypertension could indicate renal damage. Acute hypotension could be orthostatic hypotension or, if combined with other factors, indicative of an MI.
5. Blood glucose levels should be checked for the first 48 hours. Increased insulin secretion can lead to hypoglycemia (especially with pheochromocytoma and diabetes).
6. Patient should be assisted to cough and deep breathe. Provide pillow for splinting. IPPB may be indicated.
7. Foley catheter is removed 3 to 5 days postoperatively.
8. Steroids and catecholamines are indicated if the serum electrolyte, blood pressure, and pulse are indicative of adrenal insufficiency.
9. CVP and A-Lines are removed when the patient is hemodynamically stable.
10. Nasogastric suction is removed in 2 to 3 days, or when patient is eating.
11. Early ambulation is encouraged.
12. Diet should resume as soon as possible. Oral fluids are offered within 24 hours and normal diet resumes as soon as the patient tolerates it.
13. The patient may be discharged in 5 to 7 days.
14. Normal activity may resume in 4 to 6 weeks and strenuous activity in 6 weeks.

GLOSSARY

Carrel Anastomosis of a small, 4-6 sq cm section of aorta that includes multiple renal artery openings.

Cutaneous ureterostomy Diversion of the flow of urine from the kidney, through the ureter, away from the bladder, and onto the skin of the lower abdomen.

Foley Y-V pyeloureteroplasty Combined correction of a redundant renal pelvis and resection of a stenotic portion of the ureteropelvic junction.

Habitus Body build and constitution, especially as related to predisposition to disease.

Hilum The indented part of the kidney; a notch in or opening from a bodily part where blood vessels, nerves, or ducts leave and enter.

Nephrostomy Creation of an opening into the kidney to maintain temporary or permanent urinary drainage. A nephrostomy is used to correct an obstruction of the urinary tract and to conserve and permit physiologic functioning of renal tissue. It is also used to provide permanent urinary drainage when a ureter is obstructed or for temporary urinary drainage immediately after a plastic repair on the kidney or renal pelvis.

Nephrotomy Incision into the kidney, usually over a collecting system containing a calculus.

Oliguria Reduced excretion of urine.

Orthostatic hypotension Hypotension caused by erect posture.

Pyelolithotomy Removal of a calculus through an opening in the renal pelvis.

Pyeloplasty Revision or plastic reconstruction of the renal pelvis. Pyeloplasty is done to create a better anatomic relationship between the renal pelvis and the proximal portion of the ureter and to allow proper urinary drainage from the kidney to the bladder.

Pyelostomy An opening made in the renal pelvis for temporarily or permanently diverting the flow of urine.

Pyelotomy Incision into the renal pelvis used as an access to stones in the renal pelvis or collecting system.

Ureterectomy Complete removal of the ureter.

Ureteroenterostomy Diversion of the ureter into a segment of the ileum (ureteroileostomy), commonly referred to as "ileal urinary conduit," or into the sigmoid colon (ureterosigmoidostomy).

Ureterolithotomy Incision into the ureter and removal of an obstructing calculus.

Ureteroneocystostomy (ureterovesical anastomosis) Division of the distal ureter from the bladder and reimplantation of the ureter into the bladder with a submucosal tunnel.

Ureteroplasty Reconstruction of the ureter distal to the ureteropelvic junction.

Ureterotomy Result of utererotomy.

Ureterostomy Incision into the ureter for continued drainage from it into another body part.

Ureteroureterostomy Opening made by segmental resection of a diseased portion of the ureter and reconstruction in continuity of the two normal segments.

Bibliography

1. American Urological Association Allied: *Standards of urologic nursing practice*, Richmond, 1990, AUAA.
2. Association of Operating Room Nurses: *Quality improvement in perioperative nursing*, Denver, 1992, AORN.
3. Association of Operating Room Nurses: *Standards and recommended practices*, Denver, 1995, AORN.
4. Bennett AH: *Impotence*, Philadelphia, 1994, WB Saunders.
5. Benumof JL, Saidman LJ: *Anesthesia and perioperative complications*, St. Louis, 1992, Mosby.
6. Bia MJ et al: Evaluation of living donors, *Transplantation* 60(4): 322, 1995.
7. Busson M, et al: Analysis of cadaver donor criteria on the kidney transplant survival rate in 5129 transplantations, *J Urol* 154:356, 1995.
8. Drach GW: *Common problems in infections and stones*, St. Louis, 1992, Mosby.
9. Droller MJ: *Surgical management of urologic disease: an anatomic approach*, St. Louis, 1992, Mosby.
10. Flechner SM: Current status of renal transplantation: patient selection, results and immonosuppression In Novick A: *Urologic clinics of North America: renal vascular disease and transplantation*, 21(2):265, 1994.
11. Gillenwater JT et al: *Adult and pediatric urology*, vols 1-3, St. Louis, 1996, Mosby.
12. Gray M: *Genitourinary disorders*, St. Louis, 1992, Mosby.
13. Hinman F: *Atlas of urologic surgery*, Philadelphia, 1989, WB Saunders.
14. Litwack K: *Core curriculum for post anesthesia nursing practice*, ed 3, Philadelphia, 1995, WB Saunders.
15. Lytton B et al: *Advances in urology*, vol 7, St. Louis, 1994, Mosby.
16. McGuire EJ et al: *Advances in urology*, vol 8, St. Louis, 1995, Mosby.
17. Meeker MH, Rothrock JC: *Alexander's care of the patient in surgery*, ed 10, St. Louis, 1995, Mosby.
18. Normal DJ: Immunosuppression for renal transplantation: an overview, *New Developments in Transplantation Medicine* 1(2):13, 1994.
19. Resnick MI, Kursh ED: *Current therapy in genitourinary surgery*, ed 2, St. Louis, 1992, Mosby.
20. Resnick MI, Novick AC: *Urology secrets*, St. Louis, 1995, Mosby.
21. Rothrock JC: *Perioperative nursing care planning*, ed 2, St. Louis, 1996, Mosby.
22. Seidman EJ, Hanno PM: *Current urologic therapy*, ed 3, Philadelphia, 1994, WB Saunders.
23. Smith AD: *Controversies in endourology*, Philadelphia, 1995, WB Saunders.
24. Tanagho EA, McAninch JW: *Smith's general urology*, ed 14, Norwalk, 1995, Appleton & Lange.
25. Taylor RJ: Urological aspects of transplantation. In Vaughan ED: *Seminars in urology*, 7:2, Philadelphia, May 1994, WB Saunders.
26. Vaiden RE et al: *Core curriculum for the RN first assistant*, Denver, 1990, AORN.

12

Microscopic Interventions

Microsurgical instrumentation affords the genitourinary surgeon the opportunity to successfully manage small anatomic structures with minimal tissue trauma and accurate reconstruction. Additionally, refinements in microsurgical equipment have removed some of the earlier obstacles to successful surgical intervention. Optimal identification of minute structures in the male reproductive tract is achievable. As experience in the application of microscopic techniques increases, success rates for reconstructive procedures with a minimization of complications is improving.

All microsurgery requires the use of magnifying loupes or an operating microscope. Choice depends on the preference and training of each individual surgeon. Although loupes offer the surgeon more mobility intraoperatively, they are limited in providing high-power magnification and optimal lighting. Present-day operating microscopes offer a stereoscopic view, adequate illumination, and adjustable zoom focus. Specialists in urology began applying microscopic principles around 1964, beginning with extracorporeal renal vessel repair. Use of the microscope for genital reconstruction became popular in the 1970s through the efforts of Owen, Silber, and others.

Along with the equipment improvements, microscopic instrumentation and sutures have become more specific to urology. The need for precise grasping ability and atraumatic tissue manipulation, as well as length requirements, has led to new instrument development. Small structures in confined spaces that necessitate atraumatic manipulation and approximation have molded the creation of suturing material on specially designed needles.

Microscopic procedures in urology are considered outpatient procedures. The focus in patient education must be preparation for discharge shortly after the intervention. It is important to include significant others in the discharge planning and instruction. The pain encountered postoperatively will range from true discomfort to dull aching. Those that experience less discomfort are apt to discount the restrictions placed on their activity level. Delicate structures have been surgically manipulated, and it is important that all involved in the recovery period be aware of the need to curtail strenuous endeavors.

The patient will be in the supine position. It is easy to overlook the need to utilize certain comfort measures when he appears to be simply "lying down." Because these procedures can be lengthy, support should be provided beneath the knees and heels and under the sacral area. Additionally, any pressure points (back of head, scapula, elbows) should be adequately protected.

The anesthesia of choice for microscopic intervention may be general, spinal or epidural block, or local infiltration with sedation. The majority of the time monitored anesthesia care (local infiltration with sedation) is employed unless the length of procedure or the amount of dissection required necessitates another avenue. No matter what anesthetic is used, local anesthetic will likely be injected to control bleeding or to afford postoperative pain management.

Anesthetic complications to be alert for include allergic response to the local anesthetic (tinnitus, agitation, urticaria, itching, blurred vision, drowsiness, respiratory depression, cardiac dysrhythmias, and seizure activity), hypotension or hypertension, peripheral nerve damage, regurgitation of gastric contents, spinal headache, or excessive bleeding. The patient is instructed to refrain from taking aspirin and nonsteroidal anti-inflammatory agents for 10 days preoperatively. If this was not complied with, excessive bleeding could occur and the use of spinal anesthesia could be contraindicated.

There are many potential applications for genitourinary microsurgery. Some of these are hypospadias repair, penile revascularization, penile venous ligation, ureteral anastomosis, testis autotransplantation, microscopic varicocelectomy, vasotomy, epididymal sperm aspiration, autogenous or alloplastic spermatocele creation, vasovasostomy, and epididymovasostomy. The focus in this chapter is on those that have garnered the largest following at the time of this writing. Some of the procedures previously mentioned are currently seen only in large teaching or research hospitals. Additionally the perioperative genitourinary nurse may see variations in technique according to the individual surgeon's experience and preference.

The text and photographs to follow are intended to be generic for the specific microscopic interventions. Each is subject to alteration depending on the practice setting and the preference of the operating surgeon. Common surgical techniques and instrumentation are depicted and are intended as an overview to enable the perioperative genitourinary nurse to anticipate patient care needs. Instrumentation and actual equipment in practice will also vary according to physician preference, the procedural setting, and budgetary restrictions. It is important to focus on the principles of the microscopic interventions described and to consider the instrumentation as suggestions for the specialty of microurology.

NURSING CARE

Nursing diagnoses will have little variation for the microscopic techniques. Preoperative teaching and preparation and postoperative care and discharge planning will be identical for all vasectomy reversals, except for taking individual patient or procedure needs into account. General nursing diagnoses, preoperative planning, and perioperative interventions for a patient undergoing microscopic surgery might include:

Nursing Diagnosis	Perioperative Planning and Intervention
Risk for pain related to operative intervention	Review common postoperative course. Review pain-control regimen ordered by physician. Explain that medications should be taken regularly at first, before the onset of discomfort. Discuss other measures to decrease pain level: ice application, pressure dressings, scrotal support, minimized activity. Discuss restrictions that may be imposed by pain medication: alcohol, other analgesics to be avoided (aspirin), activity level.
Anxiety related to: Anticipated outcome Possible recurrence of presenting condition	Review purpose of planned procedure; ascertain comprehension level. Document expressions of anxiety by patient or significant others. Provide explanations and reassurance to the patient and significant others. Reinforce and review preoperative teaching; answer questions as necessary. Encourage participation in discharge planning; review discharge instructions. Keep significant others informed during intraoperative and postoperative phases. Verify understanding of reportable signs and symptoms. Allow significant others to spend time with patient preoperatively and postoperatively, if setting allows. Place follow-up call the day after surgery.
Risk for swelling related to: Fluid leakage Hematoma	Discuss possible complications and symptoms. Explain purpose and importance of ice application. Explain importance of minimizing activity for proper healing. Review activity regimen imposed.
Risk of infection related to: Operative intervention Medical status	Discuss signs and symptoms of infection. Review wound inspection and care and dressing care. Reinforce antibiotic therapy, if ordered, and importance of completing medication regimen (Antibiotic usage is patient dependent). Discuss precautions related to antibiotic if ordered (photosensitivity). Explain relation between adequate hydration and infection.
Risk for hemorrhage or hematocele related to: Vessel integrity Healing	Discuss signs and symptoms of bleeding. Reinforce importance of ice application. Review need to avoid aspirin and nonsteroidal medications for 10 days. Explain need for reduced activity level, review activity regimen. Discuss reasons for pressure dressings and scrotal support. Review bathing technique related to wound status: shower after 24 hours; do not scrub wound but gently cleanse and pat dry.

The perioperative genitourinary nurse caring for the patient undergoing microscopic intervention must also have a thorough working knowledge of the equipment and instrumentation to be used. It is essential to understand the various parts of the operating microscope and how to properly adjust it for maximum utilization. Spare bulbs and fuses should always be available. The proper position of the patient on the operating room bed in relation to the position of the microscope must be addressed. There must be enough clearance under the bed at the perineal level for the operating surgeon and assistant to sit comfortably. This may sometimes mean that the patient's buttock area will be in the cutout of the bed. To avoid physical strain for the patient, the cutout should be covered with a sturdy bed insert. Turning the pads on the bed so that the cutout in the pad is under the patient's neck is also advisable.

Instrumentation is extremely delicate and must be treated with care. Proper cleaning and maintenance is essential to keep the tools in good condition. Microscopic instruments should be cleaned throughout the procedure with a Merocel sponge moistened in sterile distilled water. Following the procedure the instruments should be immersed in warm distilled water with a mild instrument detergent and carefully scrubbed with a soft bristle brush. A minor soft-tissue instrument set should be available for opening and closure and in the event scrotal or inguinal exploration is necessary.

Microsutures are extremely expensive and should therefore be opened as they are needed. A minimum of two 10-0 and two 9-0 nylon sutures is generally required. Modified cutting, spatula, and lancet suture needles are necessary for vasal reconstruction. One of the most popular sutures presently available is a bicurved double-armed suture that is 2.5 cm in length.

Ideally, bipolar electrocoagulation using a fine-tipped jeweler's style forceps is employed for microscopic intervention. Less electric current is required, tissue damage is decreased, irrigation may be used during coagulation, and minimal coagulation of parent blood vessels results. If bipolar cautery is unavailable, a needle point on the monopolar electrocautery, which should be set at 25 W coagulation power or less, or a hand-held battery-operated ophthalmic cautery, may be used.

As perioperative care is implemented, the plan of care will be subject to change on a continual basis as a result of the data collected through the preoperative assessment and changing intraoperative circumstances. This ongoing evaluation and revision of care allows for an individualized approach. Once care has been implemented the postoperative assessment is completed. Often it will not be possible to properly determine long-term outcomes. Immediate postoperative assessment allows for a baseline determination of the effect of the nursing interventions provided. Priority postoperative assessment data appropriate for continual evaluation of nursing care for microscopic interventions might include:

- Understanding the importance of ice applied to the scrotum for 24 hours
- Awareness of reportable signs and symptoms of hemorrhage or infection
- Knowledge of the need to curtail strenuous activity (time frame varies according to intervention)
- Awareness of diet or other restrictions related to the medication regimen
- Comprehension of the medication regimen ordered by the physician (aspirin and nonsteroidal antiinflammatory agents should not be used for 10 days postoperatively)
- Understanding the need for adequate fluid intake to accelerate healing and promote recovery from spinal anesthesia, if appropriate
- Awareness of follow-up requirements—physician visit as scheduled, semen analysis in 3 and 6 months
- Readiness for discharge

An overview of the care provided and the subsequent evaluation are recorded to provide for the continuity of care throughout the recovery period. Documentation should be individualized according to the procedure and the specific patient needs. Surgical settings differ and perioperative documentation will have guidelines appropriate for the specific institution. A summary of the intraoperative activities designed to achieve certain outcome criteria should be reported to the perianesthesia nurse. Information to be recorded and reported will vary according to the procedure performed. Reports may differ between an outpatient and inpatient setting depending on the amount of preoperative instruction afforded the patient and services available to meet each patient's requirements.

Priority information for the genitourinary microsurgical patient may include:

- Precautions pertinent to the patient's preoperative and postoperative physical condition
- Wound status at the time of dressing application
- Status of peripheral circulation and skin integrity
- Positional devices employed
- Level of comprehension during preoperative instruction
- Information relayed to the patient preoperatively and intraoperatively
- Untoward reactions encountered intraoperatively
- Nursing care provided

The majority of the time, these procedures will be performed on an outpatient basis. The setting may be a free-standing facility or an outpatient hospital unit. It has been my experience that a free-standing facility offers more opportunity for perioperative contact with the patient. Many facilities perform the preoperative diagnostic laboratory studies and patient interview on the premises, increasing the ability to teach preoperatively. Additionally, more opportunity for postoperative reinforcement and the chance for direct patient follow-up care allows for greater continuity of care. Because free-standing facilities tend toward the smaller scale, communication between the perioperative, and perianesthesia care nurses is enhanced. The current trend toward cross-training affords all nursing personnel the opportunity to have a more comprehensive knowledge of the three aspects of perioperative patient care.

THE ROLE OF THE RN FIRST ASSISTANT IN MICROUROLOGY

During genitourinary microsurgery the RNFA functions in an expanded role, incorporating the perioperative nursing process while performing assistive behaviors. The need for an assistant, however, is surgeon and case specific in the field of microsurgery.

Preoperatively the RNFA frequently carries out the patient assessment and develops the individualized perioperative plan of nursing care. The RNFA can focus on specific patient needs such as positioning requirements, medication restrictions or allergies, and any unusual necessities discovered through the assessment data collected. If the RNFA is privately employed by the operating surgeon, this may have already been accomplished in the office setting and may then be communicated to the perioperative nursing team.

The RNFA is expected to understand the purpose of positioning techniques and should lead and teach the team when implementing this particular activity. For example, the knees, heels, and sacrum are supported with padding to alleviate low back strain, protect pressure points, and provide a comfortable intraoperative course. These procedures can be lengthy, and frequently the patient is sedated rather than under spinal or general anesthesia.

The RNFA is expected to understand and recognize the anatomy involved and the various surgical approaches and potential alterations. The team should be assisted in preparing for any given circumstance. For example, a vasovasostomy may turn into an epididymovasostomy, scrotal exploration, or inguinal exploration, because of vasal obstruction or uncontrolled bleeding. Identification of bleeding sites, aberrant and common vessels, and important reproductive structures is imperative for a good surgical outcome. Handling of tissue must be gentle and precise.

Intraoperatively the RNFA will lead the team in positioning and padding the patient, perform the skin shave and antiseptic prep, and assist with draping. During the operative intervention the RNFA will retract tissue, irrigate and sponge the operative site, stabilize vasal structures with tissue forceps, keep the field of vision clear, assist with evaluating the wound for hemostasis, identify bleeding sites, assist with electrocoagulation, irrigate the wound before closure, and suture and dress the wound. Additionally the RNFA will cleanse the patient of prep solution, evaluate skin integrity, and apply the scrotal support.

Postoperatively, the RNFA can evaluate patient outcomes based on the plan and implementation of nursing care. Patient

PREOPERATIVE

Nursing Care and Teaching Considerations for Vas Reversals or Sperm Retrieval

1. Incorporate all general nursing diagnoses and interventions for microurology.
2. Check microscope, overhead lights, operating room bed, and electrosurgery unit for proper function before patient's arrival.
3. Check all sterile supplies for package integrity. Check all medications for dose and expiration dates.
4. Check instrumentation for proper action and freedom from debris or damage.
5. Assess patient for comprehension of planned surgical intervention and anxiety level. Review as needed, including postoperative expectations and common sequelae.
6. Assess patient for skin integrity, peripheral circulation, presence of implants, low back syndrome, and general physical status.
7. Assess patient for allergies and medical condition. (asthma, obesity, past surgeries, etc.) Review pertinent laboratory reports (hemoglobin [Hgb], prothrombin time [PT], partial thromboplastin time [PTT], urine studies, fertility studies, etc.)
8. Document assessment findings.
9. Review postoperative expectations: ice application to scrotum for 24 hours, ambulation, avoidance of strenuous activity for 4 weeks, antibiotic (if indicated) and pain regimens, anticipated discharge from the facility, care of dressings, signs and symptoms to report, oral intake and diet, follow-up visit with physician, follow-up semen analysis at 3 and 6 months, resumption of sexual activity in 2 weeks.
10. Explain purpose of nursing interventions as they are implemented.
11. Establish range of motion of extremeties. Assess for low back stability.
12. Place patient in supine position with legs slightly separated and pad sacral area and under knees, heels, and other pressure sites. Be sure patient is well down on the bed to allow leg clearance for the surgeon.
13. If indicated, apply electrocautery dispersive pad to non-hairy, nonbony site away from any implants but as close to the operative site as feasible.
14. Reassess peripheral circulation after positioning. Ensure that IV lines are free of constriction.
15. Confirm that linen beneath patient is smooth.
16. Perform shave prep as described in procedural steps.
17. Aseptically prep and drap patient according to Association of Operating Room Nurses (AORN) standards and institutional guidelines. Protect patient from pooling of prep solution with absorbent towels; remove after prep.
18. Position microscope, video system, and electrosurgery unit to afford maximum utilization. Place two adjustable stools, one each side of surgical field.
19. Turn on electrical equipment. Microscope and video system will not be pulled into position immediately. They should be turned on when needed to conserve bulb usage.
20. Document nursing interventions.

---

instruction can be reinforced and other needs discovered intraoperatively may be addressed. The RNFA can also be assigned the follow-up call if appropriate. When privately employed, the RNFA has the opportunity to interact with the patient during the recovery process. Long-term outcomes may be evaluated and communicated to the perioperative nursing team. This will afford the team the chance to adjust future patient care based on the follow-up information acquired.

VASOVASOSTOMY

Description. Microscopic vasovasostomy is performed to reconnect previously severed ends of the vas deferens. The procedure may also be performed on men with a vas deferens that is partially obstructed as a result of inflammation or other causes. This is done with the aid of the operating microscope or magnifying loupes. Magnification is necessary because the lumen of the vas deferens is only 0.3 mm in diameter, and its accurate anastomosis to the opposite vas is the only way to assure technical success. This anastomosis is usually performed using a two-layer technique: 10-0 suture is placed in the inner layer of the vas and 9-0 suture is used to anastomose the outer muscular layer of the vas. Surgery time ranges from 2 to 4 hours.

Indications. Appropriate candidates for this procedure include men who have had a vasectomy within 5 years of the desired reversal. Longer intervals are associated with diminishing levels of success. Within the 5-year period success rates are in the range of 70%. Beyond 5 years the success rates average 50%.

Reanastomosis may often alleviate testicular pain, an occasional complication of vasectomy.

An effort should be extended to be certain that other factors that preclude a successful result have been eliminated. These include primary testicular failure as reflected by an elevated FSH (follicle-stimulating hormone) level, testicular atrophy, history of male infertility before the vasectomy, or infertility of the female partner. The method of previous vasectomy and its location may help in the planning of the vas reversal.

Performance of this procedure in an office setting under local anesthesia, with oral sedation, may be accomplished to help decrease the cost of the procedure for the patient (vasectomy reversal is not covered by many insurance carriers). In the operating room setting, anesthetic may be spinal, general, or local with sedation. The latter is the preferred choice, for it allows the patient to verbalize key sensations when they occur.

Perioperative risks. Inherent complications that can occur include hemorrhage, infection, inadvertent testicular artery injury, hematocele (collection of blood in the scrotum), postoperative occlusion of the anastomosis, untoward reaction to the local anesthetic, and granuloma formation.

Equipment and instrumentation

Equipment

Zoom microscope with foot pedals for focus, magnification, and position

Video camera system, microscope adaptable (optional)

Electrosurgery unit with bipolar capability

Bipolar micropoint forceps (jeweler's style)

Monopolar electrosurgery with spatula and needle-tipped pencil

Ophthalmic cautery

Adjustable stools, 2

Positioning pads

Head and neck supports

Safety strap

Absorbent towels for prep

Instrumentation

Minor soft-tissue instruments

Knife blade, #15 and #3 knife handle

Castroviejo or Barrraquer curved needle holder, nonlocking

Westcott scissors, sharp and blunt, 1 each *or*

Stevens tenotomy scissors, sharp and blunt, 1 each

Adventitial scissors

Microscissors (Vannas or choice), curved

Bishop-Harmon forceps, 2

McPherson forceps, 2

Castroviejo, 0.12 mm, fine-toothed forceps, 4

Tying forceps, straight or curved, 2

Jeweler's forceps, straight and J-shaped, #3 and #5, 2 each

Lacrimal probes, 0000-0

Vasectomy ring clamp, 1-2

Mosquito hemostats, curved Jacobson with fine, sharp point, 4

Gemini clamps, 2

Vasectomy Microspike approximater, vas-vas style

Micro bulldogs, 2

Microvessel clips and applier

Blunt irrigating cannula, no. 27

Miscellaneous supplies

Contrast material

Sterile tongue blade

Nylon, 10-0 on a microsurgery needle

Nylon, 8-0 or 9-0 on microsurgery needles

Suture, 3-0 absorbable on gastrointestinal needle

Suture, 4-0 absorbable on curved cutting needle

Antiseptic prep solution

Local anesthetic of choice

Saline, 0.9%, or balanced salt solution (BSS)

Small irrigation syringe

Tuberculin or insulin syringe

Syringe, 10 ml, with finger control

Hypodermic needles , #18 and #27 gauge, 1 $^1/_2$ inches

Jelco catheter, #24 or #26 gauge

Sterile glass slides, 4

Sterile applicators, or Weck-Cel spears, 12

Sterile gauze sponges

Scrotal support

Sterile basins

Gowns, 3

Gloves, 1 pair each

Drape towels, 5

Sterile towels, 4

Laparotomy pack *or*

Basic pack with fenestrated sheet *and*

Drape sheets, 2

Microscope drape

Procedural Steps

1. The patient is placed in the supine position with the legs slightly separated. A padded bolster should be placed under the patient's knees, heels, and sacrum to afford maximum comfort and relieve back strain. An absorbent towel is placed under the buttocks. A shave prep of the scrotum and application of an appropriate antiseptic solution is accomplished. The prep towel is then removed.

2. The entire perineum and suprapubic region should be prepped with the warmed antiseptic. Povodine-iodine (Iodophor) preparations may be chemically altered if placed in a solution warmer. The best method is to place the container in hot water for a short time or add warmed sterile water to the solution.

3. The perineal area is squared off with four towels and a laparotomy sheet or a small fenestrated sheet is placed. Additional drapes are placed over the legs and upper body if a small fenestrated drape is utilized. The patient's body should be draped completely.

CONSIDERATIONS When squaring off the perineum, the towels should surround the scrotum. It is advantageous if the penis lies cephalad securely under one of the towels. Some surgeons loosely tape the penis to the abdomen before prepping and draping. This will afford more working room for the surgeon and assistant.

4. After the vas deferens has been located by external manipulation, injection of local anesthetic may be performed.

STEP **4-1**

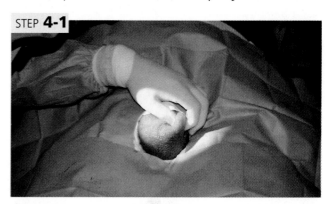

Injection is made into the scrotum and percutaneously into the vas.

STEP **4-2**

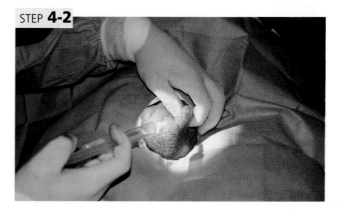

(The patient, if awake, may express the sensation of having a constricting sensation in his testicle.)

5. Bilateral vertical incisions, high on the scrotum, are made to expose each vas deferens.

STEP **5-1**

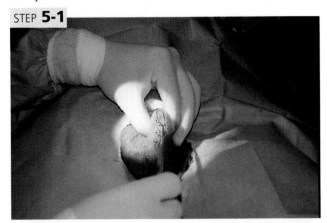

STEP **5-2**

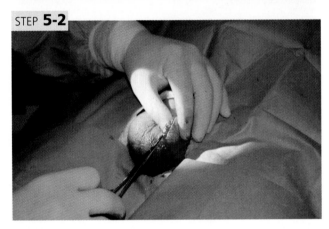

6. The testicle, epididymis, and vas are displaced from the scrotum if the ends of the previous vasectomy cannot be exteriorized. The site of the previous vasectomy is identified and the scarred area is resected.

STEP **6-1**

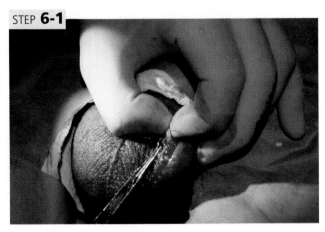

Identifying (isolating) vas.

STEP **6-2**

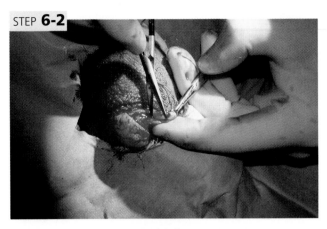

Freeing vas.

STEP **6-3**

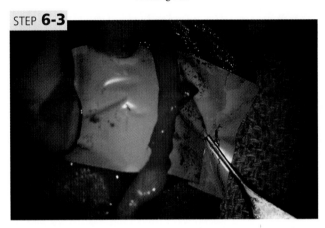

Locating previous vasectomy site.

The viable ends, with perivasal tissue intact, may be tacked to the incisional edge with a 4-0 absorbable suture. This may help ensure a tension-free anastomosis.

CONSIDERATIONS The vas may be reinjected with local anesthetic. The choice of anesthetic depends on surgeon preference. Two common choices are a 5 ml to 5 ml mixture of 0.5% plain bupivacaine Hcl (Marcaine) and 1% plain lidocaine, or 10 ml of 1% etidocaine Hcl (Duranest).

7. The proximal (testicular) end of the vas deferens is cut back until fluid is expressed.

STEP **7-1**

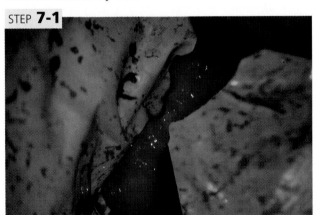

The testicular end of the vas is observed, and testicular fluid is collected onto a sterile glass slide. The color and consistency of the fluid is noted followed by observation under a laboratory microscope to determine the presence and motility of sperm.

CONSIDERATIONS Surgery continues even if results for sperm are negative unless an epididymal obstruction exists. The presence of copious, cloudy, or thin to creamy, yellow, water-soluble fluid usually indicates the presence of sperm cells. The presence of clear, watery fluid, or thick, white toothpaste-like fluid, or the absence of fluid are usually poor prognostic signs.

8. The distal (abdominal) end of the vas is placed on the sterile tongue blade and transected until a normal lumen is visible.

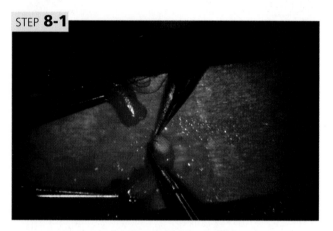

Vas placed on sterile tongue blade.

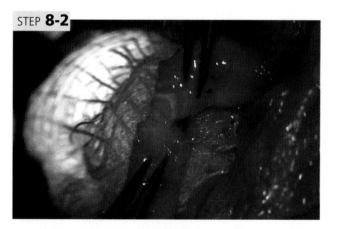

Viable vasal ends after dissection.

The distal and proximal lumens are then dilated with the tear duct probes or a microforceps.

STEP **8-3**

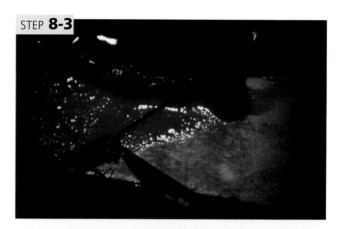

Dilating vasal ends with tear duct probe.

STEP **8-4**

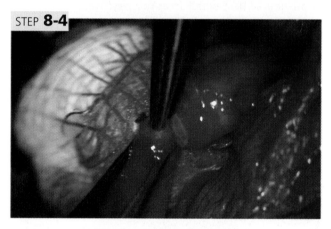

Dilating vasal ends with forcep.

Injection of sterile saline or balanced salt solution with a no. 27 blunt cannula or a Jelco catheter into the distal portion determines patency.

STEP **8-5**

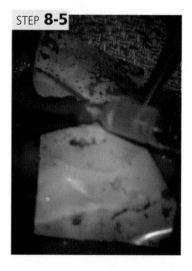

(The patient should express the feeling that he needs to urinate or ejaculate as the fluid enters the prostatic urethra.) Some surgeons choose to stain the vasal mucosa with methylene blue.

CONSIDERATIONS Excessive dissection may affect vasal vascularity and sympathetic nerve supply. Care must also be taken to avoid stripping the vas through excessive cauterization.

9. The two portions of the vas are secured in an approximater clip with background material or a sterile tongue blade placed underneath. Every effort is made to avoid significant tension and disturbance of the blood supply when the vas ends are positioned for the anastomosis. If the convoluted portion of the vas must be used, only a small section should be freed to maintain adequate blood supply.

CONSIDERATIONS The tissue should be periodically irrigated with sterile saline throughout the procedure. The heat from the microscope light tends to dry tissue rapidly. This may be accomplished with a small irrigation syringe of 0.9% saline or with the no. 27 blunt cannula on the balanced salt solution container. If applicators are used for sponging purposes, they should be slightly moistened and the cotton swirled tightly to a point. This will prevent clouding the field with flecks of the cotton. Weck-Cel spears are the preferred choice.

10. Two or three sutures of 9-0 nylon are placed in the outer layer without penetrating the lumen.

STEP **10-1**

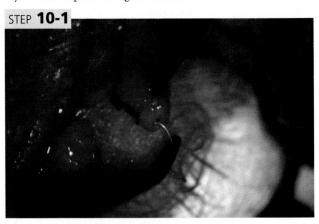

Placing first outer wall vasal stitch.

STEP **10-2**

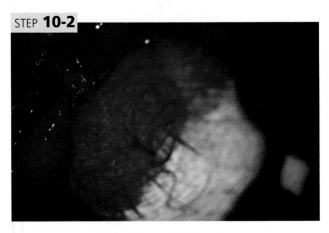

Back wall outer stitch in place.

11. Six sutures of 10-0 nylon are placed in the mucosa of the vas (inner layer).

STEP **11-1**

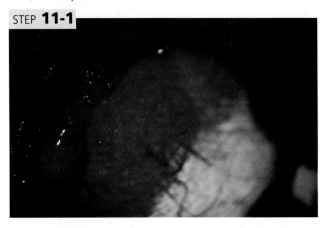

Placing inner top wall suture of 10-0 nylon.

STEP **11-2**

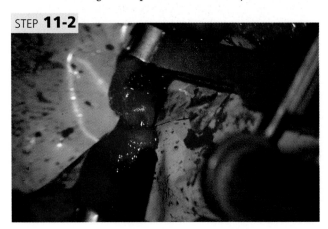

Partial closure of vasal ends.

The proximal end is sutured through the serosa to the mucosa and the distal end through the mucosa to the serosa. The approximater clamp allows the vas to be turned over so that the posterior wall can be visualized.

12. Nine sutures of 9-0 nylon are placed in the outer layer, without penetrating the lumen of the vas, to achieve a tight anastomosis.

STEP **12-1**

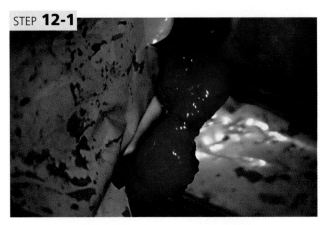

Completed inner layer of 10-0 nylon.

STEP **12-2**

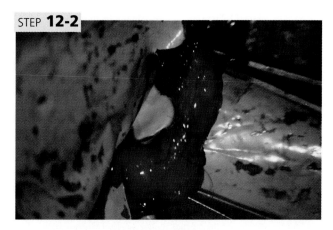

Completed anastomosis.

CONSIDERATIONS A single layer anastomosis of 9-0 nylon may also be performed depending on the situation and the surgeon's preference. The muscularis and mucosa are sutured in one pass with a triangular rather than a square suturing approach. A modification of this method places full-thickness sutures at 12, 3, 6, and 9 o'clock positions with intervening sutures in the muscularis only. Equal success has been reported with all three techniques though there may be greater risk of granuloma formation if the single-layer approach is not properly performed.

13. After hemostasis has been demonstrated, the scrotal incisions are closed in two layers with 3-0 and 4-0 absorbable sutures, in a running or interrupted fashion.

STEP **13-1**

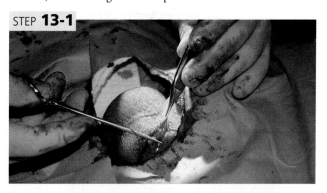

STEP **13-2**

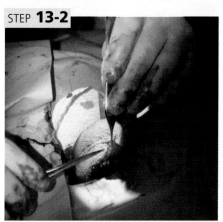

Gauze pressure dressings (fluffs) and a scrotal supporter or mesh underwear are applied.

EPIDIDYMOVASOSTOMY

Description. When there are not two viable segments of the vas deferens, a similar procedure, the epididymovasostomy, may be performed. Epididymovasostomy is a procedure in which the vas deferens is anastomosed to a tubule of the epididymis that has been demonstrated to contain fluid likely to harbor sperm cells. The epididymis is a wormlike structure closely attached to the testis and is made up of a convolution of tubules that carry sperm cells and testicular fluid from the testis to the vas deferens.

This procedure is performed by exposing the epididymis and incising the covering (peritoneum) over the epididymis to expose the underlying tubules. A tubule that appears distended with fluid is incised and anastomosed to the vas deferens. This is one of the most demanding procedures in microsurgery and may require over 5 hours for completion. Patency rates range from 60% to 85%, and pregnancy rates are from 35% to 56%. It can be as long as 1 year, however, before sperm cells appear in the semen analysis.

Indications. The epididymis is subject to the formation of obstructing scar tissue because of trauma and infection. Obstruction may occur after vasectomy, where a sperm granuloma has not relieved the obstructive effect of the vasectomy. If a vasectomy has been performed in a way that obstructs the vas, pressure may build up in the epididymis causing rupture of the epididymal tubules and obstruction at this site. Sperm granuloma formation occurs because of leakage of sperm cells and testicular fluid from the end of the transected vas and is named this because of its appearance under the microscope. The formation of a sperm granuloma relieves the pressure in the vas and epididymis thus preventing epididymal rupture. This formation prevents the most important cause of unsuccessful vas reversal. Obstruction of the epididymis may also be caused by congenital absence of the vas deferens.

An effort should be extended to be certain that other factors that preclude a successful result have been eliminated. These include primary testicular failure as reflected by an elevated FSH level, testicular atrophy, history of male infertility before the vasectomy, or infertility of the female partner. The method of previous vasectomy and its location may help in the planning of the vas reversal.

Perioperative risks. Inherent risks are the same as for vasovasostomy.

Equipment and instrumentation
Refer to vasovasostomy.
Vas to epididymis approximater clamp

Procedural Steps

The procedure begins as described for Vasovasostomy, steps 1 to 4.

5. Bilateral vertical incisions, high on the scrotum, are made to expose each vas deferens and epididymis.

STEP **5-1**

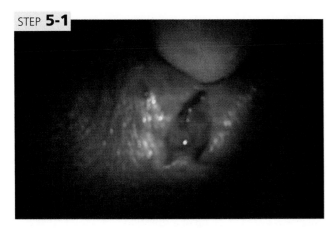

Incision begins.

6. The testicle, epididymis, and vas are displaced from the scrotum. The site of the previous vasectomy is identified, and the scarred area is resected.

STEP **6-1**

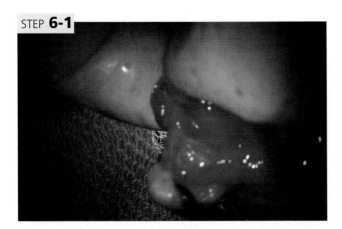

Exposing vas.

STEP **6-2**

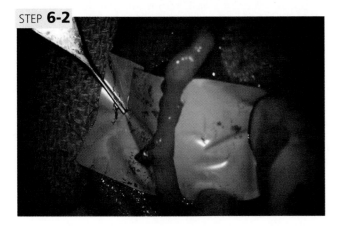

Vasectomy site exposed.

STEP **6-3**

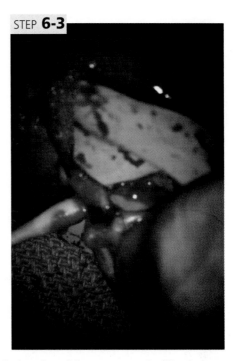

Occlusion of vas deferens apparent by dilated appearance.

The viable end, with perivasal tissue intact, may be tacked to the incisional edge with a 4-0 absorbable suture. This may help ensure a tension-free anastomosis.

7. The epididymis may be mobilized from the surface of the testicle just enough to allow a tension-free connection.

STEP **7-1**

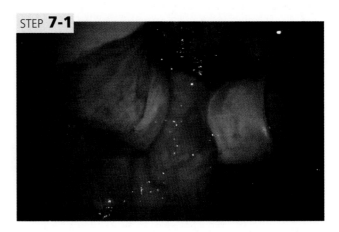

Exposing epididymis.

STEP **7-2**

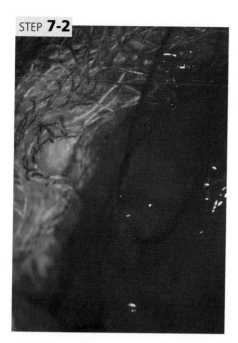

Mobilizing epididymis.

CONSIDERATIONS The vas may be reinjected with local anesthetic. The choice of anesthetic depends on surgeon preference. Two common choices are a 5 ml to 5 ml mixture of 0.5% plain bupivacaine and 1% plain lidocaine, or 10 ml of 1% etidocaine Hcl (Duranest).

8. The epididymis is incised until fluid is expressed.

STEP **8-1**

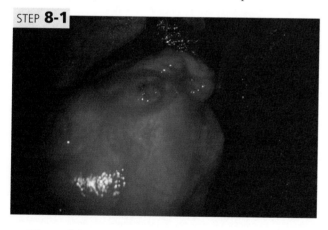

The epididymis is observed, and spermatic fluid is collected onto a sterile glass slide. The color and consistency of the fluid is noted followed by observation under a laboratory microscope to determine the presence and motility of sperm. The vasal segment may be irrigated with saline to determine patency.

STEP **8-2**

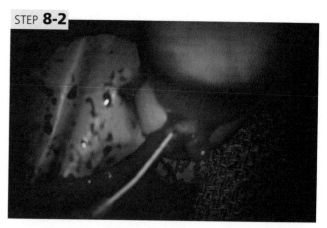

CONSIDERATIONS Irrigation of the epididymis should not be performed. The tubules are so delicate they could easily be blown out and consequently destroyed. Surgery continues even if results for sperm are negative unless an epididymal obstruction exists. The presence of copious, cloudy, or thin to creamy, yellow, water-soluble fluid usually indicates the presence of sperm cells. The presence of clear, watery fluid, or thick, white toothpaste-like fluid, or the absence of fluid are usually poor prognostic signs.

9. The vas segment and epididymis are secured in an approximater clip with background material or a sterile tongue blade placed underneath. Every effort is made to avoid significant tension and disturbance of the blood supply when the ends are positioned for the anastomosis.

CONSIDERATIONS The tissue should be periodically irrigated with sterile saline throughout the procedure. The heat from the microscope light tends to dry tissue rapidly. This may be accomplished with a small irrigation syringe of 0.9% saline or with the no. 27 blunt cannula on the balanced salt container. If applicators are used for sponging purposes, they should be slightly moistened and the cotton swirled tightly to a point. This will prevent clouding the field with flecks of the cotton. Weck-Cel spears are the preferred choice.

10. The mucosa of the epididymal tubule is anastomosed to the mucosal layer of the vas. The incised peritoneal covering is then anastomosed to the muscular layer of the vas.

11. Four to six sutures of 10-0 or 11-0 nylon are placed in the mucosa. The approximater clamp allows the vas to be turned over for visualization of the posterior wall.

12. A second layer of 9-0 or 10-0 nylon sutures are placed in the muscularis, without penetration of the lumen of the vas, to achieve a tight anastomosis.

CONSIDERATIONS Modifications may include a longitudinal versus a transverse incision of the epididymis, or the vas may be attached to the outer tunic of the epididymis in an end-to-side fashion.

The procedure concludes as described in Vasovasostomy, step 13.

POSTOPERATIVE

Nursing Care and Discharge Planning for Vas Reversals

1. Complete perioperative documentation including postoperative assessment.
2. Cleanse patient of prepping solution before dressing application. Assess skin integrity.
3. Evaluate status of peripheral vascular circulation.
4. Patient may resume diet as tolerated, starting with clear liquids.
5. Patient should drink 8 oz of liquid (half as water, half as fruit juice until eating normally) q2h for 48 hours to assist voiding process, offset infection, ensure hydration, accelerate healing, and promote recovery from spinal anesthesia, if employed.
6. Prescribed medications should be taken as directed. Aspirin and nonsteroidal antiinflammatory agents should be avoided until advised by physician to resume usage (10 days).
7. If antibiotics are ordered, they should be taken until gone. (Antibiotics are not routinely given either preoperatively or postoperatively; some situations may require their administration.)
8. Ice should be applied to scrotal region for 24 hours.
9. Patient may ambulate the same day of surgery. Effects of sedation or pain medication may result in dizziness. Caution should be emphasized.
10. Patient may resume sexual activity in 2 weeks if pain free.
11. Patient must avoid strenuous activity for 4 weeks. Scrotal support should be worn during this time.
12. Review symptoms of infection and hemorrhage (hematocele). These may include fever, warmth or redness at incisional site, swelling of scrotum, hematoma formation, and groin pain.
13. Review dressing care and bathing regime. Dressings should be kept dry and the inner layer removed as they become soiled. The patient may shower after 24 hours; wound should be cleansed gently with mild soap and patted dry. Dressings may be removed or decreased to only a light gauze covering after 24 hours.

EPIDYMAL SPERM ASPIRATION

Description. Aspiration of sperm from the epididymis is a procedure that is performed with an operating microscope to locate tubules that are distended with testicular fluid and sperm cells.

Microscopic epididymal sperm aspiration (MESA) requires the availability of an in vitro fertilization team, so that the aspirated sperm may be immediately processed and used for the selected in vitro technique or frozen for later use. The procedure must be timed according to the partner cycle of ovulation, if the in vitro technique is planned. Ova are aspirated as an office procedure just before MESA is performed.

Microscopic epididymal sperm aspiration should be performed using the micropipette technique. The tip of a 250- to 350-micrometer pipette is inserted into an epididymal tubule to retrieve sperm cells without contamination by red blood cells. After aspiration, the fluid is given to the in vitro fertilization team to process the sperm cells. Processing involves washing debris from the cells, retrieving the most active cells from the sample, and removing any red blood cells, if possible. This is critical, since red cells significantly interfere with sperm cell function.

After aspirating the sperm cells, the epididymal tubule is closed using microscopic technique. If adequate numbers of sperm cells can be obtained from one testis, the other side may be aspirated to add to the sperm bank if this is desirable. It may be necessary to aspirate sperm cells from the rete testis, tubules between the testicles and the epididymal head that carry cells to the head of the epididymis, if sperm cells are not found in tubules closer to the vas deferens.

Indications. The sperm cells retrieved may be used for intracytoplasmic injection into the partner's egg (ICSI), the most successful of the in vitro techniques available. This technique is not as dependent on the quality of the sperm as earlier techniques of in vitro fertilization (Fig. 12-1).

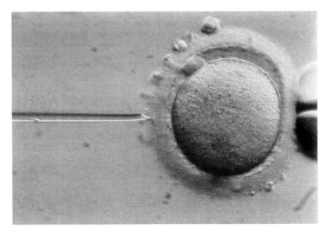

Fig. 12-1 Sperm in syringe (left) being transferred to egg in dish at right. Patient and wife had twins. *(Courtesy Main Line Reproductive Science Center, Wayne, Penn.)*

Using sperm cells from the epididymis and intracytoplasmic injection techniques, pregnancy rates may approach 50%. It may be possible to retrieve sperm cells by percutaneous aspiration of the testis, but the numbers of sperm cells retrieved by this technique are not as high as with MESA.

Perioperative risks. Possible complications include injury to the testicular artery with subsequent atrophy of the testis, bleeding with accumulation of blood in the scrotum (hematocele), granuloma formation, untoward response to the local anesthetic, and infection.

Equipment and instrumentation
Equipment
Refer to Vasovasostomy.
Instrumentation
As for vasovasostomy, excluding the following:
McPherson forceps
Lacrimal probes
Vasectomy ring clamp
Miscellaneous supplies
As for vasovasostomy, excluding the following:
Nylon 8-0 and 9-0 *and adding*
Methylene blue (optional)
Micropipettes, 4
Jelco catheter, 24 or 26 gauge, 12
Sterile basins

Procedural Steps

The procedure begins as described in Vasovasostomy, steps 1 to 3.

4. After injection of the local anesthetic into the scrotum, the larger of the two testes and its epididymis is exposed through a high vertical incision.

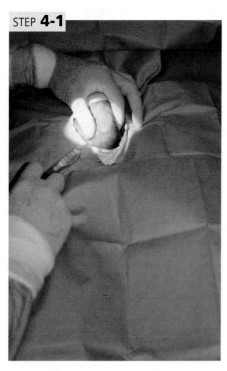

STEP **4-1**

Percutaneous local injection.

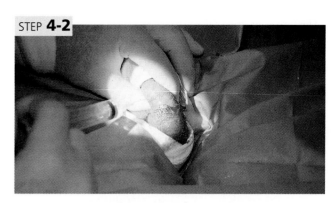

STEP **4-2**

Percutaneous local injection.

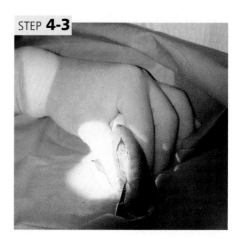

STEP **4-3**

Scrotal incision.

CONSIDERATIONS The larger testis will be the most likely to contain quality sperm cells. Choice of anesthetic depends on surgeon preference. Two common local anesthetic choices are a 5 ml to 5 ml mixture of 0.5% plain bupivacaine Hcl (Marcaine) and 1% plain lidocaine, or 10 ml of 1% etidocaine Hcl (Duranest).

5. The testicle and epididymis are displaced from the scrotum.

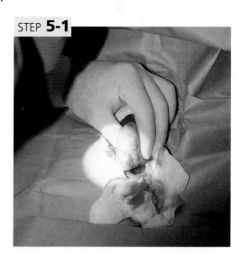

STEP **5-1**

The tunica covering the epididymis is incised after microscopic examination reveals a tubule or tubules that appear to contain testicular fluid and sperm cells.

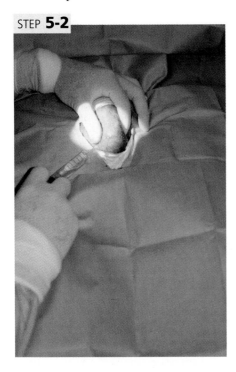

STEP 5-2

CONSIDERATIONS If necessary for pain control, the local anesthetic may be injected through the fascia of the spermatic cord once it has been properly exposed and visualized. The risk of testicular artery damage still exists, however.

6. The tubule is exposed by microdissection and associated bleeders are controlled because the epididymis is extremely vascular.

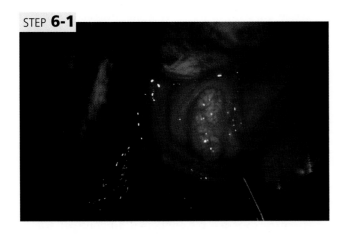

STEP 6-1

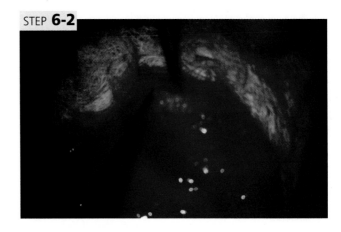

STEP 6-2

CONSIDERATIONS The tissue should be periodically irrigated with sterile saline throughout the procedure. The heat from the microscope light tends to dry tissue rapidly. This may be accomplished with a small irrigation syringe of 0.9% saline or with the no. 27 blunt cannula on the balanced salt container. If applicators are used for sponging purposes, they should be slightly moistened and the cotton swirled tightly to a point. This will prevent clouding the field with flecks of the cotton. Weck-Cel spears are the preferred choice.

7. A micropipette or #27 intercath on syringe containing sperm preservative is inserted into the tubule and fluid is collected for immediate delivery to the in vitro team.

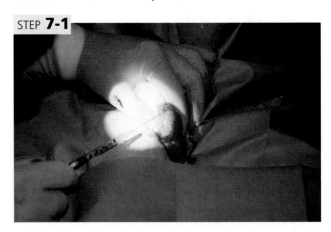

STEP 7-1

Spermatic fluid is aspirated.

8. The tubular incision is closed with interrupted 10-0 suture.

The procedure concludes as described for vasovasostomy, step 13.

CONSIDERATIONS Exploration and aspiration of the other side may be performed if adequate sperm cells have not been obtained from the first side.

POSTOPERATIVE

Nursing Care and Discharge Planning for Sperm Aspriation

1. Complete perioperative documentation including postoperative assessment.
2. Cleanse patient of prepping solution before dressing application. Assess skin integrity.
3. Evaluate status of peripheral vascular circulation.
4. Patient may resume diet as tolerated, starting with clear liquids.
5. Patient should drink 8 oz of water or juice every 2 hours for 48 hours to assist voiding process, offset infection, ensure hydration, accelerate healing, and promote recovery from spinal anesthesia, if employed.
6. Prescribed medications should be taken as directed. Aspirin and nonsteroidal antiinflammatory agents should be avoided until advised by physician to resume usage (10 days).
7. If antibiotics are ordered, they should be taken until gone. (Antibiotics are not routinely given either preoperatively or postoperatively; some situations may require their administration.)
8. Ice should be applied to scrotal region for 24 hours.
9. Patient should rest for 24 hours and may resume active ambulation the day after surgery.
10. Patient may resume sexual activity in 1 week if pain free.
11. Patient must avoid strenuous activity for 1 week. Scrotal support should be worn during this time.
12. Review symptoms of infection and hemorrhage (hematocele). These may include fever, warmth or redness at incisional site, swelling of scrotum, hematoma formation, and groin pain.
13. Review dressing care and bathing regimen. Patient may shower after 24 hours; wound should be cleansed gently with mild soap and patted dry. Dressings should be kept clean and dry and may be removed or decreased to a light gauze covering after 24 hours.

REVASCULARIZATION OF THE PENILE ARTERIES

The relationship of focal arterial occlusive disease to sexual dysfunction has led to efforts to rectify the resulting impotence. Investigational reconstructive surgery is taking place in patients who demonstrate correctable vascular disease in the large arteries. The most widely attempted repairs are end-to-end and end-to-side microscopic anastomosis of the distal inferior epigastric artery to the proximal deep dorsal artery near the pubic level, below the rectus muscle and Buck's fascia. Paramedian and infrapubic incisions are made, and the arteries are freed and tunneled. This procedure requires both a urologist and a vascular surgeon. Currently the success rate stands at 60% to 65%.

VARICOCELECTOMY

Description. Microscopic varicocelectomy uses the operating microscope to examine the contents of the spermatic cord before varicoceles are ligated. This provides for identification and preservation of the testicular artery, veins, and lymphatics before ligation of the varicocele. The procedure is carried out through a 1-inch incision at the top of the scrotum, under local anesthesia with intravenous sedation. The incidence of recurrent varicocele formation and hydrocele is less than 1%.

Indications. The presence of a varicocele, a dilated internal spermatic vein, located adjacent to the testis, is commonly associated with altered sperm cell function and appearance and male factor infertility. When varicoceles in this setting are ligated surgically, there is a high likelihood (70%) that semen quality will be improved, and fertility will result (48% during the first year after the procedure).

Perioperative risks. The likelihood of potential complications is small given the limited incision size and amount of dissection. Complications may include bleeding, hematocele, infection, ilioinguinal nerve injury, hydrocele, epididymitis, injury to the cord structures (vas, artery, lymphatics), adverse reaction to anesthetics or sedatives, and recurrence of the condition.

The conventional method of varicocele ligation in the retroperitoneum is associated with a 15% to 25% recurrence rate because of postoperative dilatation of branches not ligated during the procedure. In addition, ligation of the varicocele closer to the testis (in the inguinal canal) may be associated with the formation of a hydrocele (collection of watery fluid) around the testis in between 3% to 39% of cases.

Equipment and instrumentation
Refer to Vasovasostomy, adding the following:
Miscellaneous supplies
Suture, 5-0 absorbable on microsurgical needle
Suture, 4-0 absorbable on curved cutting needle
Papavarine HCl, 60 mg
Saline, 0.9%, 100 ml *or*
Lidocaine, 1% , 60 ml
Syringe, 3 ml
Penrose drain, 1/2 inch
Sterile basins

Procedural Steps

The procedure begins as described in Vasovastostomy, steps 1 to 3.

4. The spermatic cord is identified near the top of the scrotum.

CONSIDERATIONS This is a site where the cord is not surrounded by significant amounts of adipose tissue. The spermatic cord can easily be brought through a short (1-inch) incision in this location.

5. The incisional area is infiltrated with 1% lidocaine mixed with an equal volume of 1% etidocaine (Duranest) or 0.5% bupivacaine (Marcaine) with epinephrine.

6. A 1-inch incision is made and the spermatic cord is brought to the surface. Bleeders are controlled with bipolar electrocautery.

7. The spermatic cord is circled by a penrose drain and gently elevated through the incision. This allows for stabilization and control of the spermatic cord.

CONSIDERATIONS If necessary for pain control, the local anesthetic may be injected through the fascia of the spermatic cord once it has been properly exposed and visualized. The risk of testicular artery damage still exists, however.

8. A blunt-tipped needle is passed through the fascial layers of the cord, without piercing the vas, vessels, or lymphatics of the cord. The spermatic cord is infiltrated with a dilute solution of papaverine (1 ampule or 60 mg in 100 ml of 0.9% saline), and anesthetic solution.

POSTOPERATIVE

Nursing Care and Discharge Planning for Varicocelectomy

1. Complete perioperative documentation including postoperative assessment.
2. Cleanse patient of prepping solution before dressing application. Assess skin integrity.
3. Evaluate status of peripheral vascular circulation.
4. Patient may resume diet as tolerated, starting with clear liquids.
5. Patient should drink 8 oz of water or juice q2h for 48 hours to assist voiding process, offset infection, ensure hydration, accelerate healing, and promote recovery from spinal anesthesia, if employed.
6. Prescribed medications should be taken as directed. Aspirin and nonsteroidal antiinflammatory agents should be avoided until advised by physician to resume usage (10 days).
7. If antibiotics are ordered, they should be taken until gone. (Antibiotics are not routinely given either preoperatively or postoperatively; some situations may require their administration).
8. Ice should be applied to scrotal region for 24 hours.
9. Patient should rest for 24 hours and may resume active ambulation after that time.
10. Patient may resume sexual activity in 1 week if pain free.
11. Patient must avoid strenuous activity for 10 days. Scrotal support should be worn during this time.
12. Review symptoms of infection and hemorrhage (hematocele). These may include fever, warmth or redness at incisional site, swelling of scrotum, hematoma formation, and groin pain.
13. Review dressing care and bathing regimen. Patient may shower after 24 hours; wound should be cleansed gently with mild soap and patted dry. Dressings should be kept clean and dry and may be removed or decreased to a light gauze covering after 24 hours.

9. An incision is made under microscopic control, and dissection is carried out to identify the vas, testicular artery, and lymphatics, in addition to the associated veins.

10. The veins are carefully ligated and transected.

CONSIDERATIONS The tissue should be periodically irrigated with sterile saline throughout the procedure. The heat from the microscope light tends to dry tissue rapidly. This may be accomplished with a small irrigation syringe of 0.9% saline or with the #27 blunt cannula on the balanced salt container. If applicators are used for sponging purposes, they should be slightly moistened and the cotton swirled tightly to a point. This will prevent clouding the field with flecks of the cotton. Weck-Cel spears are the preferred choice.

11. The fascia of the spermatic cord is closed with absorbable 5-0 sutures. The cord is allowed to retract back into the depths of the wound after it has been determined that all veins have been ligated.

12. The incision is closed in a continuous, subcuticular fashion with 4-0 absorbable suture. Gauze dressings and a pressure dressing of gauze fluffs followed by a scrotal support are applied.

Bibliography

1. Association of Operating Room Nurses: *Quality improvement in perioperative nursing*, Denver, 1992, AORN.
2. Association of Operating Room Nurses: *Standards and recommended practices*, Denver, 1995, AORN.
3. American Urologic Association Allied: *Standards of urologic nursing practice*, Richmond, 1990, AUAA.
4. Benumof JL, Saidman LJ: *Anesthesia and perioperative complications*, St. Louis, 1992, Mosby.
5. Goldstein M: *Surgery of male infertility*, Philadelphia, 1995, WB Saunders.
6. Lipshultz LI et al: *Microsurgery,* Course Syllabus, Houston, 1995, AUA Surgical Learning Center.
7. Litwack K: *Core curriculum for post anesthesia nursing*, ed 3, Philadelphia, 1995, WB Saunders.
8. Meeker MR, Rothrock JC: *Alexander's care of the patient in surgery,* St. Louis, 1995, Mosby.
9. Resnick MI, Kursh ED: *Current therapy in genitourinary surgery*, ed 2, St. Louis, 1992, Mosby.
10. Tanagho EA, McAninch JW: *Smith's general urology*, ed 14, Norwalk, Conn, 1995, Appleton & Lange.
11. Tessier J et al: Principles of microsurgery. In Droller MJ:*Surgical management of urologic disease*, St. Louis, 1992, Mosby.
12. Vaiden RE et al: *Core curriculum for the RN first assistant*, Denver, 1990, AORN.
13. Whitehead ED, Nagler HM: *Management of impotence and infertility,* Philadelphia, 1994, JB Lippincott.

Advancements in Urology

Invasive Procedures

ULTRASOUND-ASSISTED INTERVENTIONS

The use of ultrasound by urologists has become an adjunct to surgical interventions as well a common office practice. There are several surgical interventions that are not possible without ultrasound imaging. These include:

- Imaging of the kidney for percutaneous access for renal biopsy or radiographic imaging when radiopaque contrast cannot be introduced into the collecting system.
- Transrectal imaging of the prostate in the treatment of carcinoma of the prostate. Two treatment options that may be used are percutaneous implantation of radioactive seeds (brachytherapy) or the placement of cryoprobes for cryoablation of the prostate.

The text and photographs to follow are intended to be generic for the specific interventions. Each is subject to alteration depending on the practice setting and the preference of the operating surgeon. Common surgical techniques and instrumentation are depicted and intended as an overview to enable the perioperative genitourinary nurse to anticipate patient care needs. Instrumentation and actual equipment in practice will also vary according to physician preference, the procedural setting, and budgetary restrictions. It is important to focus on the principles of the ultrasound interventions described and consider the instrumentation as suggestions for the specialty of genitourinary ultrasonography.

NURSING CARE

Nursing diagnoses will vary according to the extent and nature of the procedure performed and the patient's medical status. Nursing planning and care specific to each operative intervention are discussed under that procedure. General nursing diagnoses, preoperative planning, and perioperative interventions for a patient undergoing invasive ultrasound-assisted therapies might include:

NURSING DIAGNOSIS	PERIOPERATIVE PLANNING AND INTERVENTION
Risk for infection related to: Operative intervention Instrumentation Medical status	Obtain urine culture preoperatively; appropriately treat bacteriuria before procedure. Maintain aseptic environment and properly sterilize instrumentation. Insert catheter aseptically and maintain closed urinary drainage system. Use appropriate technique during surgical prep. Drape patient according to aseptic standards. Assess for signs of systemic infection and possible septic shock: fever, chills, rapid pulse, tachypnea, hypothermia, hypotension. Observe for signs of lower urinary tract infection: pyuria, dysuria, fever, lower back or abdominal pain without fever. Be alert to signs of wound infection: redness, edema, warmth, fever, exudate. Provide adequate hydration through IV solutions or fluid intake. Administer antibiotic therapies as ordered.
Risk for hemorrhage at wound site related to: Operative intervention	Discuss signs and symptoms of bleeding. Review need to avoid aspirin and nonsteroidal anti-inflammatory medications for 10 days. Explain need for reduced activity level, review activity regimen. Review bathing techniques related to wound status: shower after 24 hours; do not scrub wound but gently cleanse and pat dry.
Risk for hematuria related to: Operative intervention	Assess urinary output for signs of hematuria; report evidence of frank bleeding or clots. Provide adequate hydration through IV solutions or fluid intake.

NURSING DIAGNOSIS	PERIOPERATIVE PLANNING AND INTERVENTION
Risk for altered tissue perfusion related to: Operative intervention Positioning	Assess bilateral pedal and radial pulses perioperatively. Apply alternating compression stockings. Utilize and pad stirrups properly without compromise to neurovascular pressure sites (peroneal nerve, tibial nerve, popliteal space, calf area, Achilles tendon). Adjust position as necessary to maintain peripheral circulation. Avoid leaning against or on patient during operative intervention. Observe and document status of capillary refill and extremity temperature. Encourage early ambulation postoperatively.
Anxiety related to: Knowledge deficit Concern about outcome	Review purpose of planned procedure; ascertain level of comprehension. Document expressions of anxiety by the patient or family. Provide explanations and reassurance to the patient and family. Reinforce and review patient teaching; answer questions as necessary. Encourage participation in discharge planning; review discharge instructions. Keep family informed during intraoperative stage. Verify understanding of signs and symptoms to be reported. If patient-controlled analgesia (PCA) is to be utilized, confirm that contact has been established with home care provider. Visit patient, if hospitalized, or place follow-up call the day after surgery.
Risk for pain related to: Operative intervention Position Medical status	Discuss postoperative expectations. Review common postoperative course. Collaborate with health care team to plan pain control management. Have adequate assistance when moving patient. Assess and maintain comfort during positioning. Provide procedural and positional explanations. Review pain control regime ordered by physician. Explain that medication should be taken regularly at first, before onset of discomfort. Administer pain medication as ordered; explain side effects. If PCA is ordered, ensure patient's understanding of its use. Offer comfort measures to alleviate pain as appropriate (position, pillows, music). Discuss other measures to decrease pain level: ice application, pressure dressings, minimized activity, meditation, guided imagery. Assist patient to implement strategies to control pain through emotional and informational support. Discuss restrictions that may be imposed by pain medication: alcohol, other analgesics to be avoided (aspirin), activity level.
Altered pattern of urinary elimination related to: Instrumentation Operative intervention	Maintain patent, tension-free urinary catheter by securing to leg. Secure all connections. Keep collection device below bladder level. Ensure that tubing is free of constriction or kinks. Assess and document return flow of urine, include character and color. Observe for and document signs of dysuria. Irrigate catheter as indicated. Observe and document any abdominal distention. Maintain adequate hydration.
Fluid volume excess related to: Fluid absorption	Document amount of irrigation employed. Observe and document cardiovascular status; note alterations. Observe and record respiratory status; note any changes. Observe for abdominal distention and discomfort; assess for rigidity. Note alterations in mental status. Discontinue procedure as indicated and insert Foley catheter. Administer diuretics as ordered.

NURSING DIAGNOSIS	PERIOPERATIVE PLANNING AND INTERVENTION
Urinary retention related to: Operative intervention	Postoperatively notify surgeon. Assess abdomen for distention. Maintain patent, tension-free and kink-free urinary catheter. Evaluate catheter position by determining length of catheter protruding from urethra; reposition catheter as necessary. If more than one half of the catheter is protruding, the tip may be in the prostatic urethra: Gently push catheter in toward bladder until urine flow appears and then gently pull back until slight resistance is met. This should place it in the proper position. Approximately two thirds should be visible in the female patient. Determine status of gross sensory motor function, particularly after spinal anesthesia. Irrigate catheter as necessary; observe for clot formation; note amount and character of urinary output.
High risk for injury related to: Position	Correctly position patient in proper body alignment after adequate relaxation of leg and perineal muscles; avoid severe hip and arm flexion. Reduce pressure on sensitive neurovascular areas such as iliac crests, popliteal space, peroneal nerve, calf area, sacrum, shoulder, brachial plexus, and acromioclavicular region by padding as necessary. Assess character and presence of bilateral pedal and radial pulses perioperatively. Avoid pooling of prep solutions under buttocks, sacrum, or back. Avoid hairy areas or areas where prosthetic joint implants are in place when placing electrosurgery dispersive pad.

The perioperative genitourinary nurse caring for the patient undergoing invasive ultrasound-assisted procedures must also have a comprehensive working knowledge of the required equipment and instrumentation. It is essential to understand the operation of the operating bed, ultrasound machine, solution warming unit, pump irrigation system, cryotherapy unit, and other devices specific to the planned intervention.

Positioning the patient properly and safely on the operating room bed is essential. If the patient is to be in the prone or prone-oblique position, as with nephroscopy, the patient must be positioned with the area of interest accessible to C-arm imaging. This often requires imagination and unique utilization of the equipment at hand. For example, in most instances even a bed with C-arm capability is inadequate, in its normal position, for visualization of the flank area. The bed sections may need to be rearranged, meaning that the patient may be placed with his or her head at the actual foot. To do this, the head section must be attached to the foot end, and the bed turned around. When the patient is positioned, the flank should rest over what would normally be considered the break for the buttocks area. This also means that the pads for the bed must be rearranged, placing the longest pad under the patient's body with the cutout section at the patient's knee or head level. The shorter pad is placed over what is normally considered the chest section (Fig. 13-1). This is done to prevent pressure on the rib cage and iliac process. If the pads are placed such that there is a separation over the break in the table, they may shift and cause the flank to be pinched.

When invasive ultrasound-assisted interventions are performed, delicate endoscopy instrumentation will be employed. These instruments need to be handled with care to prevent fracture of the lens or fiberoptic components. Additionally a variety of ultrasound transducers may be used. They should be treated with respect to avoid damage to their internal mechanisms.

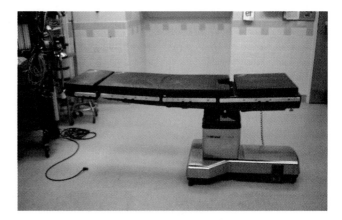

Fig. 13-1 Operating room bed rearranged for C-arm visualization of flank area.

As perioperative care is implemented, the plan of care will be subject to alteration and revision on an ongoing basis. All patient-centered activities must relate to the data collected during the preoperative assessment and to changing intraoperative circumstances. The perioperative genitourinary nurse should be cognizant of this possibility and be prepared to effectively adjust the plan of care. This ongoing adjustment allows for an individualized and patient-focused approach. Patient outcome is as dependent on the nursing interventions provided as it is on the expertise of the surgeon.

Once care has been implemented the postoperative assessment is completed. Often it will not be possible to properly determine long-term outcomes. Immediate postoperative assessment allows for a baseline determination of the effect of nursing care delivered. Priority postoperative assessment data appropriate for the continual evaluation of nursing care for invasive ultrasound-assisted interventions might include:

- Awareness of reportable signs and symptoms of infection or hemorrhage
- Knowledge of the need to curtail strenuous activity
- Cognizance of restrictions imposed by the medication regime
- Comprehension of the medication regime ordered by the physician (aspirin and nonsteroidal antiinflammatory agents should be avoided for 10 days)
- Understanding of the need for adequate fluid intake to accelerate healing, assist the voiding process, offset infection, and promote recovery from spinal anesthesia
- Review of follow-up requirements (postoperative physician visit, activity level, diet)
- Discussion of catheter care and wound care
- Readiness for discharge

An overview of the care provided and the subsequent evaluation is recorded to provide for the continuity of care throughout the recovery period. Documentation should be individualized according to the procedure and the specific patient needs. Surgical settings differ and perioperative documentation will have guidelines appropriate for the specific institution. A summary of the intraoperative activities designed to achieve certain outcome criteria should be reported to the perianesthesia care nurse. Information to be recorded and reported will vary according to the procedure performed. Reports may differ between an outpatient and inpatient setting depending on the amount of preoperative instruction afforded the patient and services available to meet each patient's requirements.

Priority information for the patient undergoing genitourinary ultrasonography may include the following:

- Precautions pertinent to the patient's preoperative and postoperative physical condition
- Wound status on discharge from the operating room
- Status of peripheral circulation and skin integrity
- Positions and positional devices employed
- Status of urinary output and catheter patency at discharge from the operating room
- Level of comprehension during preoperative instruction
- Presence of anxiety or fear during preoperative and intraoperative stages
- Information relayed to the patient preoperatively and intraoperatively
- Untoward reactions encountered intraoperatively
- Nursing care provided

ROLE OF RN FIRST ASSISTANT IN INVASIVE ULTRASONOGRAPHY

The RNFA may or may not play a role in invasive ultrasonography. If the RNFA is employed by the physician , his or her role will be much the same as with other interventions. The RNFA can be instrumental in preoperative teaching and postoperative follow-up care as well as a significant resource and liaison with the surgeon, patient, and office staff.

During the intraoperative stage the RNFA may be called on to operate the ultrasound equipment. There is little need for actual surgical assistance during the procedure. If the RNFA was involved with the preoperative planning, part of his or her role may be to attach any required ultrasonographic attachments onto the operating room bed. The RNFA may also lead the planning and implementation of patient care and patient positioning, apply the prep and drape the patient, insert the Foley catheter, and tend to the perineal and wound care. Dressings are not always indicated after these procedures.

PERCUTANEOUS NEPHROSCOPY WITH ULTRASONOGRAPHY

Description. Ultrasound imaging may be used to guide the injection of contrast material into the collecting system through a 22-gauge needle or to gain percutaneous access to the collecting system through an antegrade approach. The latter allows for insertion of a nephrostomy drainage tube or removal of an obstruction. Depth assessment is extremely precise as opposed to fluoroscopy, which requires compensation for image magnification. On the other hand, fluoroscopy affords a larger image.

Some disadvantages of ultrasound imaging are an obstructed renal pelvis that may be obscured by multiple renal cysts with hydronephrosis, calculi, and other factors such as obesity, overlying ribs, or colonic distention. It also may sometimes be difficult to visualize needle-tip placement in a minimally dilated renal pelvis.

The procedure may be performed under regional, general, or local anesthesia with monitored sedation. Depending on the patient's presenting complaint, any number of interventions may be accomplished using the ultrasound nephroscopically, with or without fluoroscopy. It is amenable to both an outpatient and an inpatient setting.

Indications. The patient may suffer from renal failure or have significant ureteral obstruction. In these cases intravenous and retrograde injection of contrast is either contraindicated because of further injury to the kidneys or not possible because of obstruction of the ureters. Other indications may include recurrent, febrile and afebrile, urinary tract infections; uremia with ureteral obstruction inaccessible through retrograde methods; pregnant women; obstructed transplanted kidneys; and congenital urinary system anomalies. Although generally contraindicated in the presence of urinary tract infection, toxic symptoms of pyonephrosis with urinary tract obstruction may be alleviated and allow for a specimen for culture to afford an appropriate treatment regimen. Additional indications for this antegrade approach are malrotation of the kidney, abnormal position of the kidney, horseshoe kidney, hypermobile kidney, and congenital ectopic kidney.

Intraoperatively ultrasound may be used to image the kidney to localize and extract calculi or to determine the extent of renal masses by examination or percutaneous biopsy for later excision. Frequently, nephroscopy is combined with nephrolithotomy or ureterolithotomy.

Patients should be typed and cross-matched or have 2 units of autologous blood stored preoperatively. Data indicate that percutaneous nephroscopy and nephrostomy has a transfusion rate of 10%. Additionally, a CT scan and x-ray film of the kidneys, ureter, and bladder (KUB) should be available.

Perioperative risks. Treatment is contraindicated in the presence of a urinary tract infection unless the condition cannot be assisted in any other manner. Complications associated with nephroscopy include hematuria, hemorrhage from the puncture site or kidney, violation of the pleura, injury to adjacent organs (bowel, spleen), ureteral penetration, and infection. Most vascular complications may be managed conservatively with bed rest, pressure dressings, transfusion, and clamping of the nephrostomy tube. Other vascular complications that have been documented include pseudoaneurysm, anterior venous fistula, and retroperitoneal hematoma that may require angioembolization or surgical repair. Anesthetic risks may include pneumothorax, hydrothorax, hemothorax, urothorax, pleural effusion, hypervolemia, hypothermia, hypotension, neurovascular injury, reaction to local anesthetics, and inadequate ventilation or respiratory depression resulting from the position or level of spinal anesthetic.

Equipment and instrumentation

Equipment

C-arm unit
C-arm-compatible operating room bed
Video unit with monitor, printer, VCR
Video camera
Camera cable
Electrosurgery unit
Electrohydraulic lithotrip for (EHL) unit
Fiberoptic light source
Fiberoptic light cable
Ultrasound machine
Positioning devices: pillows, rolls, pads, bolsters
Suction unit
X-ray aprons, thyroid collars, patient shield
Laser, if indicated
Laser goggles

Instrumentation

Ultrasound transducer, 3.5 MHz transabdominal
Nephroscope, flexible and rigid
Biopsy forceps, flexible and rigid
Stone baskets and graspers, variety
Amplatz dilators (or renal dilating system of choice)
Endopyelotomy instrumentation as indicated
Resectoscope as indicated

Miscellaneous supplies

Knife blade, #15
Knife handle, #3
Guidewire, 0.038 inch Bentson and J tipped
Mitty-Pollack needle, #22 gauge
Syringe, 50 to 60 ml
Control syringe, 10 ml
Hypodermic needle, #25, $1^1/4$ inches

PREOPERATIVE

Nursing Care and Teaching Considerations for Percutaneous Nephroscopy

1. Incorporate all general nursing diagnoses and interventions for invasive ultrasonography.
2. Check ultrasound, operating room bed, overhead lights, electrosurgery, video unit, fiberoptic light source, and suction unit for proper function before patient's arrival.
3. Check all sterile supplies for package integrity. Check all medications for dose and expiration dates.
4. Check instrumentation for proper action and freedom from debris or damage.
5. Patient is at higher risk for infection with nephroscopy. Ascertain that urine culture is negative or, if indicative of infection, the condition has been appropriately treated before surgery. Evaluate other pertinent radiologic and laboratory studies (prothrombin time [PT], partial thromboplastin time [PTT], hemoglobin [HgB], serum electrolytes).
6. Assess patient for comprehension of planned surgical intervention and anxiety level. Review as needed, including postoperative expectations and common sequelae.
7. Assess patient for skin integrity, peripheral vascular circulation, presence of implants, range of motion, and general physical status (allergies, limitation, past surgeries).
8. Review postoperative course: probable hematuria, possible renal or ureteral colic.
9. Document assessment findings.
10. Gather x-ray protection for personnel and patient.
11. Position video unit and C-arm monitor for optimal visualization.
12. Ensure that appropriate positioning aids are available (pillows, axillary roll, pads for bony prominences, chest rolls, etc.).
13. Rearrange operating room bed as previously discussed.
14. After the induction of anesthesia, if regional or general, insert Foley catheter aseptically to closed-system urinary drainage.
15. Under the guidance of the anesthetist, place patient in prone or prone-oblique position on the operating room bed, utilizing adequate assistance. Ensure that IV lines and foley catheter are free of constriction. Determine that adequate chest expansion is afforded.
16. Protect patient's thyroid and chest with leaded shield.
17. Prep and drape patient according to institutional and Association of Operating Room Nurses (AORN) guidelines. Provide appropriate protection from pooling of solutions with absorbent towels that are removed after prep.
18. Connect and turn on equipment (video system, fiberoptic light, electrosurgery unit, solution warmer, suction, ultrasound). Connect and open irrigant.
19. Patient is at higher risk for fluid-volume excess with nephroscopy because of large volumes of saline required when the tract is dilated and when calculi or tissue biopsies are retrieved. The patient should be carefully monitored for signs of fluid overload.
20. Document nursing interventions.

Open-ended catheter, 5 to 6 Fr
Ureteral balloon dilators
Amplatz coaxial dilators (or fascial dilators)
Leveen pressure syringe and gauge
Cobra catheter
Kaye tamponade balloon catheter
Nephrostomy tube
Endopyelotomy stent
EHL probe, 9 Fr
Bugbee fulgurator, 5 Fr
Electrosurgery fulgurating cable
Electrosurgery dispersive pad
Saline, 3000 ml bag or rigid container
Sorbitol or glycine, 3000 ml bag or rigid container
TUR irrigation tubing
Suction tubing
Sterile pack with draping system of choice (laparotomy
  pack)
Sterile gloves
Radiopaque contrast material
Local anesthetic of choice

Procedural Steps

1. A Foley catheter is aseptically inserted to closed drainage after induction of anesthesia (if regional or general is planned).

2. The patient is placed in prone or prone-oblique position on a table with C-arm capability. The side of interest is rotated up 30 to 45 degrees.

CONSIDERATIONS A rolled towel or similar positioning device may be employed under the midabdomen to reduce the spinal curvature, elevate the kidney, and decrease respiratory excursion of the kidney. Adjusting the operating room bed by "breaking" the foot section about 30 to 45 degrees ("break" as one would for lithotomy) may also accomplish the same purpose. It is important to elevate the chest adequately with chest rolls if the patient is prone. An axillary roll under the dependent side if prone-oblique position is used and under both axillae if prone position is used helps prevent brachial neurovascular damage.

3. Antiseptic prep is applied to the affected flank area, and the patient is draped. Local anesthetic may be instilled percutaneously.

4. A small incision is made at the desired puncture site. Insertion of a narrow 22-gauge trocar point needle with an outer sheath designed to accommodate an 0.038-inch guidewire through its outer sheath (Mitty-Pollack) may be used to achieve percutaneous access for calculus extraction. Access is attempted below the twelfth rib to avoid violation of the pleura or diaphragm.

CONSIDERATIONS Percutaneous access through the flank must avoid the pleural space and lung superiorly and the colon, liver, and spleen anteriorly. These structures are observed, and distances may be measured precisely, with ultrasound imaging and are thus avoided. The depth of the renal pelvis is localized with suspended respiration and the angle of entry determined by the angle of the transducer.

The avascular plane of Brodel, located 1 to 2 cm posterior to the lateral margin of the kidney, allows for a safe puncture lateral to the thick paraspinal muscles at a 20 to 30-degree angle in 70% of patients.

5. Access is accomplished and confirmed by observing a clear flow of urine from the needle hub with the stylet removed. A Bentson or small J-tipped guidewire is then introduced into the dilated calyx.

6. Sequential dilatation of the tract is performed with Amplatz dilators or a fascial balloon dilator.

7. An additional safety guidewire is introduced during dilatation.

8. The rigid nephroscope is introduced through the Amplatz sheath to visualize the collecting system. If the objective is only to place a nephrostomy tube for drainage, dilatation needs to be carried to just 8 to 10 Fr.

9. An open-ended ureteral catheter may be inserted through the nephroscope. Contrast material is infused through the catheter to visualize the collecting system.

CONSIDERATIONS Radiographic renal imaging better delineates the limits of the renal pelvis, and ultrasonography affords access to the renal pelvis

POSTOPERATIVE

Nursing Care and Discharge Planning for Percutaneous Nephroscopy

1. Complete perioperative documentation including postoperative assessment.
2. Cleanse patient of prepping solutions before dressing application. Assess skin condition.
3. Evaluate status of peripheral vascular circulation.
4. Assess urinary output and secure Foley catheter and nephrostomy drains.
5. Patient may resume diet postoperatively as tolerated, starting slowly with clear liquids.
6. Patient should drink 8 oz of water or juice every 2 hours for 48 hours to assist voiding process, offset infection, ensure hydration, and accelerate healing process.
7. Prescribed medications should be taken as directed, antibiotics until gone. Aspirin and nonsteroidal antiinflammatory agents should be avoided for 10 days unless advised by the surgeon as medically necessary.
8. Review symptoms of infection, hemorrhage, transient sensory nerve deficit, hematuria (fever, redness or warmth at puncture site, exudate, saturated dressings or oozing around nephrostomy disk, grossly red urine with or without clots).
9. Review dressing care and bathing regime. Patient may shower 24 hours postoperatively. Dressings should be kept clean and dry.
10. Review catheter and wound care.

for the injection of a contrast medium. Renal imaging may be accomplished to localize a renal mass or parenchyma for biopsy. In the latter case one must be aware of the likelihood of significant bleeding. This may result from a seemingly insignificant needle biopsy site in patients afflicted with a renal disease that requires biopsy for assessment.

10. If a calculus is seen and is small enough to be withdrawn it is done with a grasping forceps. If larger, it must be fragmented with ultrasonic, electrohydraulic, or laser lithotripsy. Every effort must be extended to render the kidney completely stone free.

11. If portions of the collecting system cannot be visualized through the rigid nephroscope, the flexible ureteroscope may be used through the Amplatz sheath.

12. If a lesion is found, it should be biopsied, if not done already, and treated by electrosurgical resection or laser fulguration.

13. The surgeon may perform an endopyelotomy by passing an endoscopic knife across the ureteropelvic junction (UPJ) and incising it longitudinally in the posterolateral position. This is followed by insertion of an endopyelotomy stent and nephrostomy tube.

14. After the procedure has been completed, the integrity of the collecting system and ureter should be documented with a nephrostogram before insertion of a nephrostomy tube.

TRANSRECTAL SEED IMPLANTATION WITH ULTRASONOGRAPHY

INTERSTITIAL RADIOTHERAPY AND BRACHYTHERAPY

Brachytherapy of the prostate gland is one procedure that validates the necessity of a collaborative, multidisciplinary approach to patient care. The radiation oncologist and medical physicist, in addition to the urologist, are integral to an optimum outcome from the initial planning stage throughout the postoperative surveillance. Additionally, radiology personnel, perioperative nursing staff, the anesthesia department, pharmacist, and laboratory technologists will be involved and are vital to patient care and teaching.

The facility that offers this treatment must be licensed for "Group 6" with the radioactive materials licensing department of their respective state.

Description. During percutaneous implantation of iodine-125 or palladium-103 seeds, the patient is positioned in the dorsal lithotomy position. The prostate is visualized with transrectal ultrasonic imaging, and the midportion of the prostate is located on a transverse image. This location becomes an index for positioning the axial ultrasound plane at the base of the prostate. The upper end of the needles used for implantation of seeds may then be positioned before the seeds are unloaded into the prostate. Approximately 2 to 3 hours should be allowed from start to completion. The procedure is amenable to outpatient management utilizing regional or general anesthesia.

Iodine seeds are commercially available in titanium-encased rods and may be obtained embedded in an absorbable suture. This allows them to remain positioned appropriately in relation to themselves and their location within the prostate. Additionally the risk of seed migration is minimized, and electrons are absorbed by the titanium wall.

Palladium seeds are plated onto a graphite pellet. The pellets are then loaded into titanium tubes with a lead marker. They are not presently available prethreaded.

The half-life of iodine (60 days) is longer than that of palladium (17 days) allowing the therapy to be delivered over the duration of tumor cell replication. The ability of tumor cells to multiply can therefore be altered. The rationale for using palladium is that the half-life of this isotope is shorter and affords a larger dose of radiation in a shorter time interval to more rapidly growing tumors: less than 12,000 cGy in 17 days versus 16,000 cGy in 60 days (1 cGY [centigray] = 1 RAD, or radiation absorbed dose).

Indications. Transrectal ultrasonography may be used for percutaneous implantation of radioactive seeds. This technique allows the delivery of significantly higher doses of radiotherapy to the prostate compared to external beam therapy, since the radius of penetration around each seed is only 5 mm and therefore spares adjacent organs. The typical radiation dose that can be delivered by external beam is approximately 6500 cGy. The dose that can be delivered with implantation of seeds is in the range of 12,000 to 16,000 cGy.

The patient will receive hormone therapy, to shrink the prostate gland, for 3 months before implantation. Patients with stage A or B prostate cancer are appropriate candidates. Selection is not influenced by a rise in the PSA, biopsy specimens indicative of further involvement, or age. Some patients will require radiation therapy before implantation. Preplanning is required to determine the dose of each seed, the spacing necessary between each seed, and the number of seeds required.

Six-year follow-up studies from multiple institutions indicate a disease-free interval and survival equivalent to the results of radical prostatectomy. If seed implantation is indicated as an adjunct to radiation therapy, it should be performed 3 to 4 weeks after the radiation treatment.

Perioperative risks. Intraoperatively there is the danger of implantation into the bladder; implantation too close to the urethra resulting in postoperative urethral stricture; implantation into the perineum if the needles are withdrawn too quickly; or implantation into the neurovascular bundle, since the anterior venous plexus is not distinguishable from the prostate on CT scan. There is also the chance of seed migration from seeds placed just outside the periphery of the gland and from the periprostatic plexus to the lung. Postoperative ecchymosis of the perineum is to be expected. Patients with a recent TURP (less than 60 days), a prostate gland measuring more than 60 cu cm, or a Gleason grade more than 6 should not be considered for this procedure. One alternative for the patient with a recent TURP is implantation concentrated in the periphery of the gland.

Few complications occur immediately postoperatively. Postoperative complications that may ensue in the first 12 months include acute cystitis, prostatitis, and urinary retention.

After 12 months, chronic prostatitis or cystitis; urethral stricture or contracture; stress, urge, or total incontinence; proctitis; and impotence have been documented. Some patients have required posttreatment TURP, bladder neck incision, suprapubic catheter insertion, or urethral dilatation to alleviate the above conditions. Less commonly, interventions such as laparotomy, colostomy, and urinary diversion have been necessary.

Anesthetic risks are the same as for any general or regional anesthesia. There appear to be no unusual anesthetic risks associated with brachytherapy of the prostate.

Equipment and instrumentation
Equipment
Ultrasound machine (Fig. 13-2)
C-arm monitor
Video monitor with VCR, printer
Stabilizing bar
Sledge
Stepping unit
Template
Shielding and loading apparatus (Fig. 13-3, *A*)
Shielding box (Fig. 13-3, *B*)
X-ray aprons and thyroid collars
X-ray shield for patient (thyroid and chest)
Video camera
Camera cable

Cystoscopy or electric bed (with C-arm fluoroscopy)
Allen stirrups
Armboards
Head and neck positioner
Alternating compression unit
Alternating compression stockings, thigh length
Electrosurgery unit
Electrosurgery dispersive pad

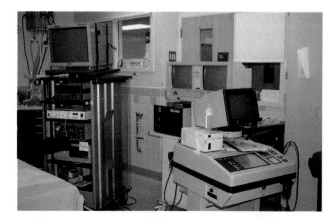

Fig. 13-2 Ultrasound, C-arm monitor, video monitor placed for optimal viewing.

PREOPERATIVE

Nursing Care and Teaching Considerations for Brachytherapy

1. Incorporate all general nursing diagnoses and interventions for invasive ultrasonography.
2. The patient should adhere to a clear liquid diet for 48 hours preoperatively and is NPO after the midnight before surgery.
3. A bowel prep or orally administered magnesium citrate is given the night before, and a Fleets enema is accomplished 2 hours preoperatively.
4. IV antibiotics are begun 1 hour preoperatively and continued orally for 8 days postoperatively.
5. Check ultrasound equipment, operating room bed, overhead lights, video unit, electrosurgery unit, fiberoptic light source, and alternating compression machine for proper function before patient's arrival.
6. Check all sterile supplies for package integrity. Check all medications for dose and expiration dates.
7. Check instrumentation for proper action and freedom from debris or damage.
8. Evaluate reports of pertinent preoperative studies (history and physical examination, chest x-ray films, PSA, prostate volume study, CT scans; PT, PTT, complete blood count [CBC], serum chemistry survey, and urinalysis).
9. Assess patient for comprehension of planned surgical intervention and anxiety level.
10. Review signs and symptoms to be reported (fever, excessive bleeding, unresolved pain, urinary retention).
11. Assess patient for skin integrity, peripheral vascular circulation, presence of implants, range of motion, and general physical status (allergies, limitations, past surgeries).
12. Review postoperative course: hematuria, ecchymosis of the perineum, Foley catheter for 24 to 48 hours, avoiding prolonged contact with pregnant women or allowing children to sit in the lap (2 months), antibiotics for 8 days, increased fluid intake (8 oz q2h), analgesia for pain.
13. Document assessment findings.
14. Gather x-ray protection for personnel and patient.
15. Ensure that Geiger counter and dosimeters are present.
16. Position ultrasound machine, video unit, and C-arm monitor for optimatl visualization.
17. Ensure that appropriate positioning aids are available (pillows, pads for bony prominences, etc.)
18. Rearrange operating room bed as previously discussed if electric bed is chosen over cystoscopy bed.
19. Under the guidance of the anesthetist, position patient in dorsal lithotomy on the operating room bed, utilizing adequate assistance. Ensure that IV lines are free of constriction.
20. Protect patient's thyroid and chest with leaded shield.
21. Prep and drape patient according to institutional and AORN guidelines. Provide appropriate protection from pooling of solutions with absorbent towels that are removed after prep.
22. Connect and turn on equipment (video system, fiberoptic light, ultrasound machine). Connect and open irrigant.
23. Document nursing interventions.

Geiger counter

Dosimeters (1 for each person in room)

Instrumentation

Cystoscopy setup (Fig. 13-4)

Transrectal radial transducer, variable frequency 6 to 10 MHz (probe)

Needles with stylet, 18 gauge, 21 cm, preloaded with seeds

Stabilizing needles, 2

Biopsy forceps

Strainer

Needle holder

Ruler

Scissors

Sponge stick

Thumb forceps, angled

Miscellaneous supplies

Electrosurgery pencil

Cystoscopy pack

Sterile towels

Cystoscopy tubing

Transducer cover

IV extension tubing

Stopcock

Syringe, 20 ml

Sterile solution basins

Sterile prep sponges

Sterile gloves, 1 pair each

Sterile radiation gloves, 2 pair

Povidone-iodine solution

Sterile water for irrigation, 3000 ml bag

Sterile water, less than 500 ml

Lubricating jelly (KY)

Absorbent towel for prep

Hypoallergenic tape, 3 inches and

Gauze *or*

Silk, 3-0 on curved cuticular needle

Procedural Steps

1. The patient is placed in the dorsal lithotomy position. He is prepped and draped as for cystoscopy.

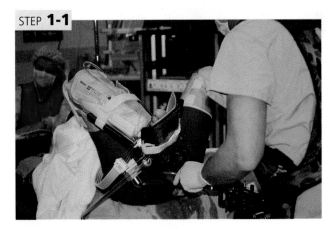

STEP **1-1**

Applying Iodophor prep.

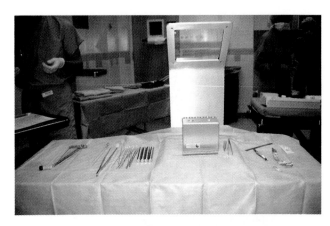

A

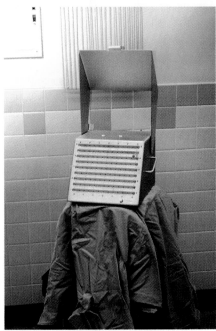

B

Fig. 13-3 **A,** Loading apparatus and table set-up for loading radioactive seeds. **B,** Shielding box.

CONSIDERATIONS The scrotum must be secured cephalad to allow a clear operating field. This may be accomplished with strips of 3-inch hypoallergenic tape placed in a sling (from one groin to the other over the posterior aspect of the scrotum) and crossover fashion (from the gluteal fold of one side to the opposite inguinal region). It is advisable to place gauze over the scrotum to protect the skin from shearing and tape burn. An alternative and perhaps better method is to place a traction stitch through the lateral edges of the scrotum and anchor it to the groin region.

2. At the initiation of the procedure a urethral catheter may be inserted to drain the bladder and refill it with 150 ml of sterile water. Contrast medium for fluoroscopy is then instilled to more clearly delineate the bladder neck.

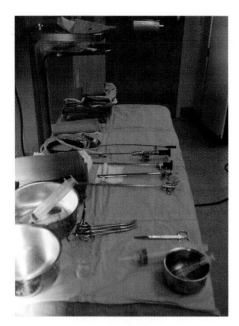

Fig. 13-4 Cystoscopy/seed implantation table set-up.

Alternatively a cystoscopy may be performed and the bladder drained. An open-ended ureteral catheter may be placed to instill contrast material and then removed. Ureteral catheters may also be placed if desirable.

STEP **2-1**

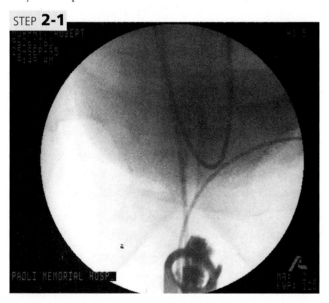

C-arm view of ureteral catheter in bladder and transducer in rectum.

These may remain in situ during the implantation.

CONSIDERATIONS The urethral catheter should be removed during implantation of seeds to avoid placement of seeds close to the urethra. The catheter causes the tissue surrounding the urethra to be compressed. If attempts are made to implant seeds into this compressed tissue, penetration of the catheter and urethra may easily occur.

Initially, C-arm fluoroscopy is utilized to judge the position of the needle at the base of the prostate referrable to the bladder. After several cases have been performed with fluoroscopy, it may be eliminated, and seeding may then be done with ultrasound imaging only.

3. Before seeding is begun, the ultrasound transducer must be positioned so that the posterior margin of the prostate is parallel to the axis of the ultrasound transducer.

STEP **3-1**

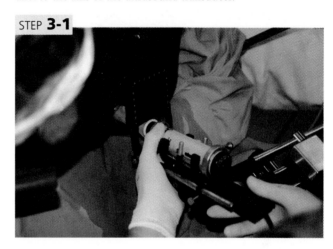

The direction of seed insertion and the transverse images of the prostate must have a similar appearance to those on the preoperative volume study. The volume study and implant worksheet are utilized for continual verification of coordinates. The probe must be securely anchored so that the seeding procedure may be completed without alteration in the position of the prostate relative to the needles used to implant seeds. A stabilizer bar is attached to the operating room bed. This secures the "stepping unit," which allows a 5 mm incremental forward and backward motion of the transducer. The "sledge," which holds the transducer, is attached to the stepping unit.

STEP **3-2**

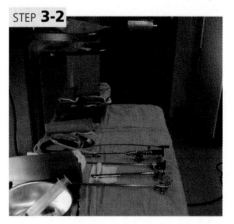

CONSIDERATIONS The transducer (probe) should be covered with a sterile "condom" (balloon transducer or probe cover). This is then filled with 15 ml of sterile water to remove any artifact. Filling the condom with too much fluid will change the configuration of the prostate and alter the anatomic presentation. The transducer will be aimed with the tip toward the floor at a 20-degree angle. The posterior wall of the prostate must be far enough away from the probe so that the posterior row of seeds lies just inside the posterior capsule.

4. Seeds are implanted by means of loaded needles placed in the prostate according to the template plan obtained from the radiotherapist.

STEP 4-1

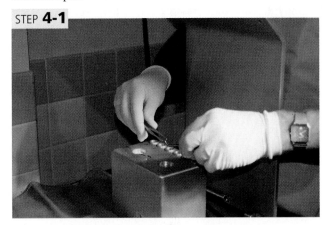

Loading iodine-125 seeds onto absorbable suture.

STEP 4-2

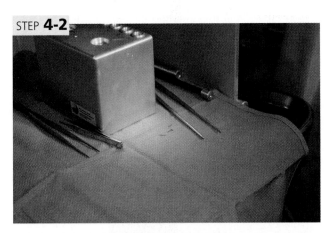

Seeds after loading onto suture.

STEP 4-3

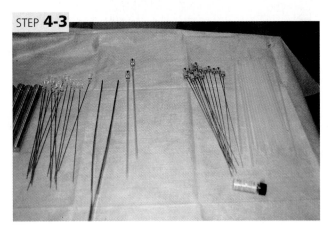

Needles used for seed implantation.

STEP 4-4

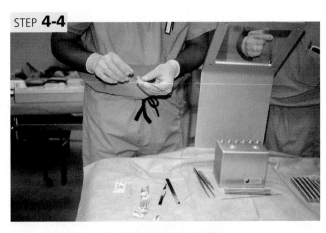

Loading seeds into needles.

STEP 4-5

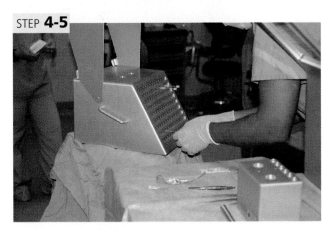

Placing needles in numbered shielding box.

For appropriate positioning of the needles a template with labeled grid is attached to the transducer so that needle placement matches the grid locations on the plan.

CONSIDERATIONS The template plan is obtained preoperatively by utilization of the ultrasound and the transducer anchoring equipment to measure and map the appropriate seed sites within the prostate. This may be accomplished in the surgeon's office, radiology department, or oncology clinic.

CONSIDERATIONS

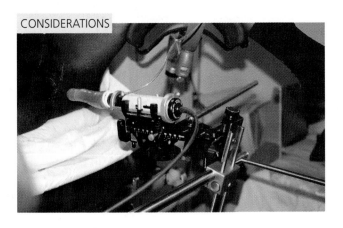

The grid is labeled alphabetically *Aa, Bb, Cc,* etc. The center of the prostate correlates with *D* on the grid. It is best to place the center seeds slightly off center to avoid the urethra. The volume of the apex of the gland is drawn somewhat larger on the plan.

STEP **4-6**

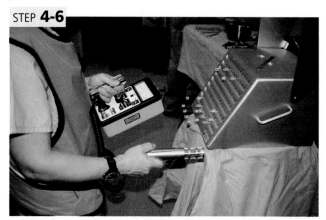

Throughout the procedure, random room checks with the Geiger counter will be performed to determine radiation levels.

All personnel will be scanned before leaving the room at the end of the procedure.

5. Stabilization of the prostate may be achieved with stabilization needles that are placed lateral to the center into the right and left lobes of the prostate and moved once the anterior seeds are in place. Another method is to use a Foley catheter as a tractor for implantation of the periphery and until implantation near the urethra occurs. The best method may be to overcompensate for the rotation of the prostate by angling or turning the needle slightly opposite to the direction desired.

6. The most anterior seeds are placed first.

STEP **6-1**

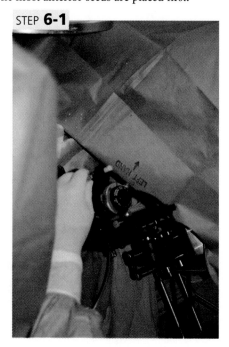

Placing first anterior needle.

STEP **6-2**

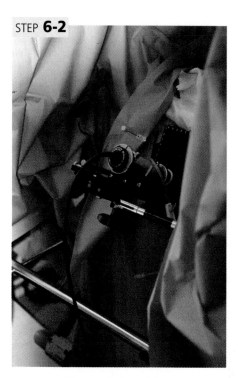

First needle in position.

This is so that imaging of the anterior portion of the gland is not obscured by the ultrasonic shadows created by seeds placed posteriorly.

STEP **6-3**

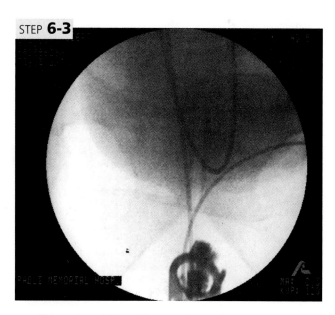

C-arm view of first seed row in place and second row in position on needle.

If single seeds are used, the bevel of the needle should be sealed with bone wax to keep the seed in place until implantation. If strands are utilized, Anusol HC (hydrocortisone) is used to seal the bevel before implantation. Strands should be cut cleanly with electrocautery to seal the ends and prevent fraying. Frayed ends may be split further when the stylet is inserted into the needle and adversely affect seed placement. Contrary to normal needle insertion with the bevel up, these needles are placed into the prostate with the solid, or back side, up.

CONSIDERATIONS Every effort is extended to avoid implanting seeds into the bladder or too close to the urethra to avoid the necrosis that causes significant postoperative irritative symptoms. The preoperative implantation plan should take into consideration the position of the urethra in the prostate so that it can be avoided during seed implantation. The bladder neck and rectum must be avoided during implantation to prevent urethrorectal fistula formation, irradiation of the bladder, and scarring at the bladder neck level.

When placing the anterior seeds the needle may become lodged in the pubic bone. The needle tip is visualized as a bright echo, and the angle may be altered to compensate for the bone. Alternatively the placement of the anterior seeds may be postponed until the end when the template may be dropped down, the probe positioned parallel to the pubic arch, and the needles inserted past the anterior portion into the prostate.

7. During implantation, measurements can be taken from the hub of the needles to the template to check the location of the needle tips, since this distance should not change, and such measurements assure positioning of the first seeds at the base of the prostate. The distance, in centimeters, from the needle hub to the needle trocar is equal to the number of seeds in each needle.

STEP **7-1**

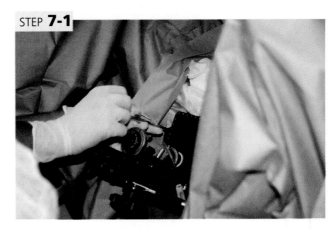

Measuring needle depth.

POSTOPERATIVE

Nursing Care and Discharge Planning for Brachytherapy

1. After recovery from anesthesia, the patient may be discharged with prescriptions for oral analgesics and antibiotics as warranted. A skin rash or other side effect should be reported to the surgeon (nausea, diarrhea, constipation, itching).
2. A #16 or 18 Fr, 5 cc Foley catheter will be in place for 24 to 48 hours.
3. Patients should be warned of the possibility of slight bleeding beneath the scrotum (ecchymosis), hematuria for 24 hours, and bruising between the legs. Bloody urine or clots after 24 hours should be reported to the surgeon.
4. Later side effects include frequent urination, dysuria, burning, urgency, and decreased stream that may continue for 1 to 4 months.
5. Heavy lifting or strenuous activity should be avoided for 2 days.
6. Diet may return to normal as tolerated. The patient should increase fluid intake to 8 oz of water or juice every 2 hours for at least 2 days.
7. Fever should be reported to the surgeon.
8. Hormone therapy is discontinued after implantation to allow tumor cells to replicate during the half-life of the chosen seeds.
9. Radiation concerns dictate avoiding prolonged close contact with pregnant females. Maintaining a distance of 6 feet is considered aedequate for their safety.
10. Children should not sit in the patient's lap for the first 2 months after the implantation.
11. Patients should be instructed that objects they touch are not radioactive and that bodily wastes are not radioactive.
12. Sexual intercourse may resume 2 weeks after the implant. A condom must be used for 2 months, however. Ejaculate may be discolored a brownish black initially.
13. Urine should be strained, since seeds will occasionally be passed through the urine. If passed seeds can be retrieved, they should be placed into the provided container with a tweezers and returned to the cancer facility.
14. Follow-up CT scan is done 2 days postoperatively to determine the exact position of the seeds within the prostate and to determine that all areas of the prostate are being treated optimally. Occasionally it may be necessary to administer additional external beam radiation therapy or to implant additional seeds.
15. Follow-up visits with the oncologist and surgeon will be scheduled every 3 to 6 months for 5 years. Transrectal ultrasound exam, PSA levels, and other exams will be performed periodically during these visits.
16. Biopsies of the prostate are done yearly for 2 years. If biopsy results return positive after 18 months, there is probably still viable tumor present.

CONSIDERATIONS The needle is inserted beyond the desired site and then retracted. The bladder wall can generally be felt with the needle tip, and insertion should just enter the wall but not pass through it. The first seed will then determine where the remainder will lie because the seeds will fall into a plane that follows the first seed in a specific needle. The target volume is greater than the actual volume of the prostate so that the capsular edge of the prostate and just beyond are also subjected to seed penetration. These peripherally placed seeds have a higher energy and may also have a greater tendency for migration because the tissue is not dense enough to hold the seed in place. The base of the prostate is also slightly overimplanted.

8. Cystoscopy should be carried out at the end of the treatment so that seeds protruding into the urethra or left in the bladder may be removed.

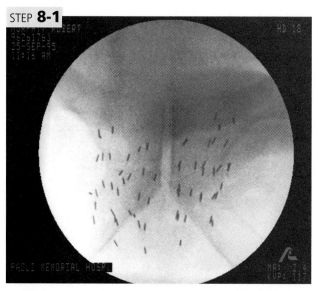

STEP 8-1

C-arm view of completed seed placement.

Bleeding from percutaneous sites is brief, but perineal echymosis should be expected. Patients are generally able to void 24 to 48 hours after implantation.

TRANSRECTAL CRYOSURGICAL ABLATION WITH ULTRASONOGRAPHY

Description. Transrectal ultrasound may be used to image the prostate for cryosurgical ablation. During this procedure five 3 mm probes are inserted percutaneously into the prostate. Liquid nitrogen is then circulated through the probes to freeze the gland. This causes cell destruction and cell membrane rupture during thawing. Long-term results for this procedure are not available so far, but 5-year statistics indicate equivalent results compared to surgery. Of 382 patients treated, 80% had negative prostate biopsy results, and 50% had PSA levels less than 1 ng/ml. The 1-year continence rates are over 99%, making this an attractive alternative to conventional therapy. Definitive results regarding postcryosurgical erectile dysfunction are still not available, but may be a significant consideration for the sexually active patient since the recovery rate is anticipated to range between 30% and 50%.

During cryosurgery, a suprapubic catheter is inserted, since the swelling that occurs in the prostate interferes with voiding. The suprapubic catheter allows urinary drainage and trials of voiding, until the swelling has subsided enough to allow micturition to occur (approximately 14 days).

The freezing process may be extended beyond the prostatic capsule, potentially eradicating extracapsular extension. The purpose is to eradicate locally recurrent cancer and effect a cure. The procedure may kill diverse populations of cancer cells, including chemoresistant and androgen-resistant forms.

Indications. A feasible, less-invasive option for patients suffering from prostate cancer. One of the advantages is that all the therapeutic options are still open to the patient, including repeat cryosurgery, radiation therapy, hormone therapy, observation, or surgery. Recurrence of an elevated PSA and positive biopsy results after cryosurgery prompt additional therapy. A prior TURP may increase the difficulty but is not a contraindication. Patients with extensive local tumor that does not allow for adequate visualization of disease extension or that poses increased risk to ureters, bladder, or rectum if fully encompassed by freezing may not be candidates for cryoablation.

Perioperative risks. Complications that have been documented include urethrorectal and urethrocutaneous fistula, urethral necrosis, ureteral obstruction, retention caused by sloughing of prostate tissue, transient renal failure, incontinence caused by freezing of the external sphincter, impotence (incidence lower than that with other approaches), sepsis, hemorrhage (rare), the usual anesthetic risks associated with regional or general anesthesia, myoglobinuria, and hemoglobinuria.

Equipment and instrumentation
Refer to cystoscopy setup in addition to the following:
Equipment
Cryotherapy delivery system (Fig. 13-5)
Liquid nitrogen (Fig. 13-6)
Solution warming unit
Pump irrigation system
Ultrasound machine
Alternating compression machine
Alternating compression stockings, thigh length
Allen stirrups
Instrumentation
Cystoscopy setup
Knife handle, #3
Needle holder
Scissors
Adson tissue forceps
Cryosurgical probes, 5, and tubing
Ultrasound radial transducer, 6 to 10 MHz (Fig. 13-7)

Bookwalter retractor
Miscellaneous supplies
Knife blade, #11
Silk, 3-0 on cutting needle
Chromic, 3-0 on cutting needle

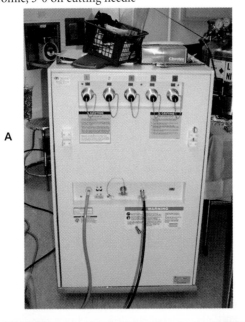

A

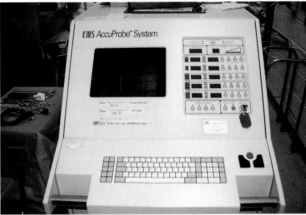

B

Fig. 13-5 A, Cryotherapy delivery system.
B, Cryotherapy unit control panel.

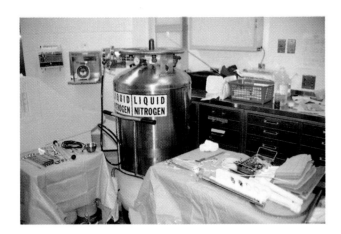

Fig. 13-6 Liquid nitrogen.

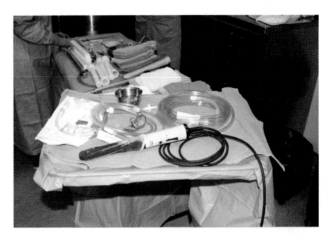

Fig. 13-7 Transrectal ultrasound transducer and tubings.

Procedural Steps

1. The patient is positioned in the dorsal lithotomy position (low or exaggerated by surgeon preference).

CONSIDERATIONS The procedure averages about 2 hours. Alternating compression stockings and Allen boot stirrups, or well-padded candy-cane stirrups, are employed.

2. The perineum is shaved, prepped with a provodine-iodine (Iodophor) solution, and draped as for cystoscopy.

STEP **2-1**

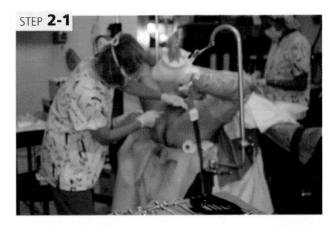

STEP **2-2**

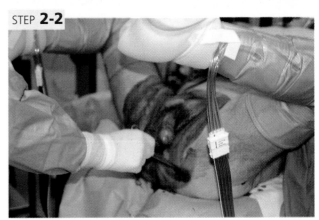

PREOPERATIVE

Nursing Care and Teaching Considerations for Cryotherapy

1. Incorporate all general nursing diagnoses for ultrasonography
2. Prophylactic antibiotics are administered preoperatively and continued intraoperatively and for 1 to 5 days postoperatively.
3. It is preferable if the patient adheres to a liquid diet for 24 hours before surgery. He is NPO after midnight the night before surgery.
4. A Fleets enema is given the night before surgery.
5. Preoperative work-up includes CBC, PT, PTT, chest x-ray, CT scans of the pelvis and abdomen, and bone scans.
6. Check ultrasound machine, operating room bed, overhead lights, video unit, fiberoptic light source, and alternating compression machine for proper function before patient's arrival.
7. Check all sterile supplies for package integrity. Check all medications for dose and expiration dates.
8. Check instrumentation for proper action and freedom from debris or damage.
9. Check function of cryotherapy delivery system and ensure that adequate liquid nitrogen and five cryoprobes are available.
10. Assess patient for comprehension of planned surgical intervention and anxiety level.
11. Review signs and symptoms to be reported (fever, excessive bleeding, unresolved pain, urinary retention).
12. Assess patient for skin integrity, peripheral vascular circulation, presence of implants, range of motion, and general physical status (allergies, limitations, past surgeries).
13. Review postoperative course: hematuria, ecchymosis of the perineum, suprapubic catheter possible for 7 to 14 days, antibiotics for 2 to 5 days, increased fluid intake (8 oz q2h), analgesia for pain.
14. Document assessment findings.
15. Position ultrasound machine for optimal visualization.
16. Ensure that appropriate positioning aids are available (pads for bony prominences etc.)
17. Under the guidance of the anesthetist, position patient in dorsal lithotomy on the operating room bed, utilizing adequate assistance. Ensure that IV lines are free of constriction.
18. Prep and drap patient according to institutional and AORN guidelines. Provide appropriate protection from pooling of solutions with absorbent towels that are removed after prep.
19. Connect and turn on equipment (solution warming unit, irrigation pump, fiberoptic light, ultrasound machine). Connect and open irrigant.
20. Document nursing interventions.

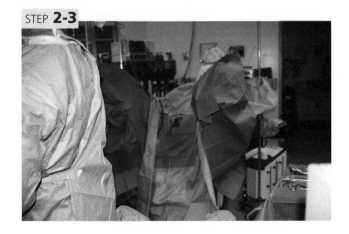

STEP **2-3**

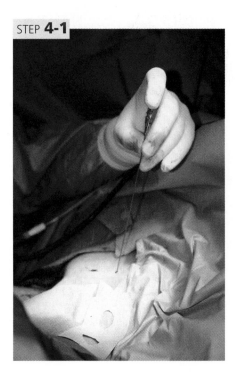

STEP **4-1**

3. A cystoscopic examination is carried out to assess the external sphincter, prostatic urethra, bladder neck, and bladder (trigone in particular).

CONSIDERATIONS The bladder is filled with sterile irrigant to facilitate percutaneous insertion of a Cope suprapubic catheter.

4. An 18-gauge needle with trocar is inserted suprapubically into the bladder.

The trocar is removed to allow passage of the 0.038 inch guidewire through the needle.

STEP **4-2**

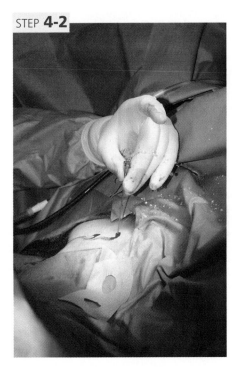

Suprapubic needle following withdrawal of trocar.

STEP **4-3**

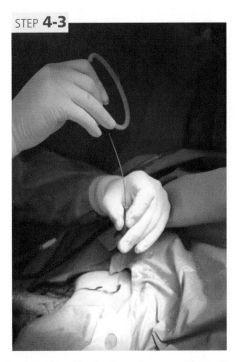

Passing .038 guidewire through suprapubic needle.

STEP **4-4**

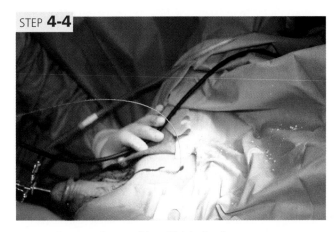

Suprapubic guidewire in place.

The tract is then progressively dilated with #6 to 12 Fr fascial dilators.

STEP **4-5**

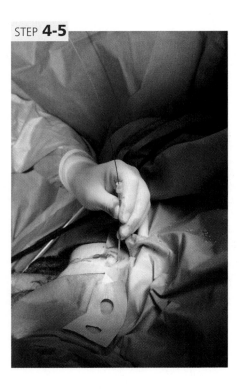

The catheter is placed in the bladder dome to reduce bladder spasms and is connected to drainage.

STEP **4-6**

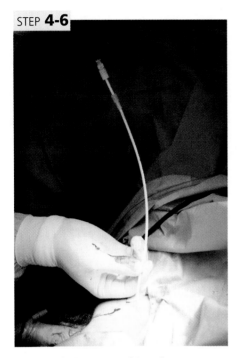

Placing suprapubic catheter.

STEP **4-7**

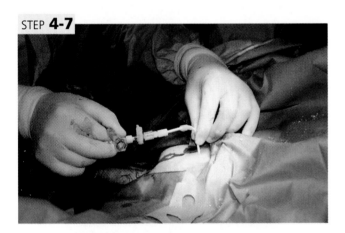

Attaching suprapubic catheter to drainage.

5. A trocar with cannula is inserted into the bladder through a 1 cm suprapubic incision placed between the pubis and the suprapubic catheter.

STEP **5-1**

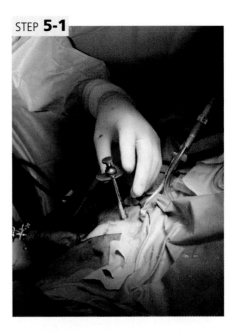

Cystoscopic evaluation is performed to assess puncture site and bladder integrity.

STEP **5-2**

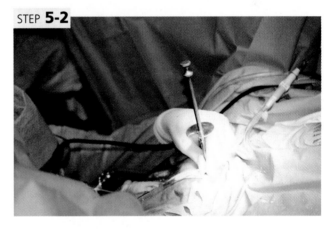

6. As the trocar is removed, irrigation tubing is passed through the cannula into the bladder and out the urethra under cystoscopic guidance.

STEP **6-1**

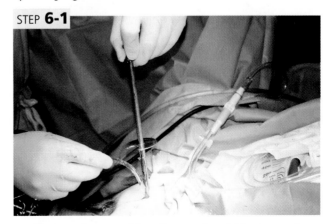

The trocar is removed from the cannula as tubing is passed.

STEP **6-2**

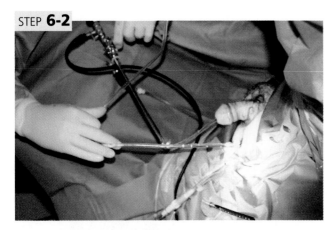

The tubing is grasped and pulled out through the urethra.

This tubing is attached to sterile water irrigant that is circulated through a solution warmer and irrigation pump system to raise the urethral temperature during the freezing process.

STEP **6-3**

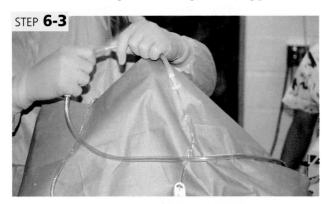

The tubing is attached to warmed sterile water.

STEP **6-4**

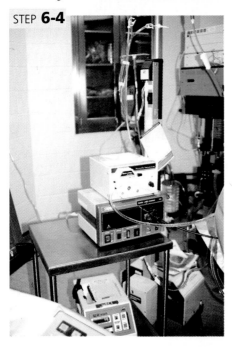

Irrigation, pump, warming unit, and TED sequential unit.

7. The scrotum is tethered to the lower outer abdominal wall using a 3-0 silk stay suture.

STEP **7-1**

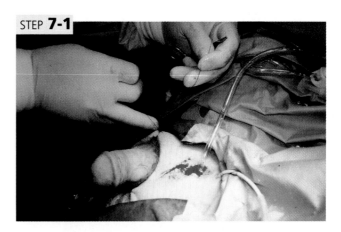

8. A Bookwalter retractor is attached to the operating room table with the oval ring extending over the patient's genitalia.

9. Transrectal ultrasonography is carried out, and the volume of the prostate is calculated. The anatomy of the bladder neck, trigone, seminal vesicles, and urogenital diaphragm are noted.

STEP **9-1**

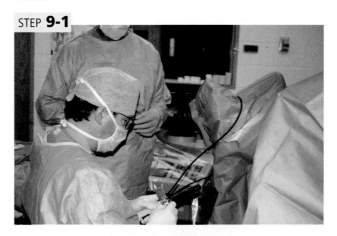

Attaching needle guide to transducer.

STEP **9-2**

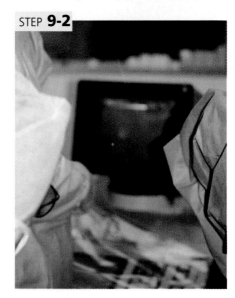

Surgeon observing ultrasound monitor during transrectal exam.

10. Five 18-gauge needles with trocar obturators are inserted into the prostate at the 10, 2, 4, 6, and 8 o'clock positions with their tips placed within 5 mm of the upper extent (base) of the prostate.

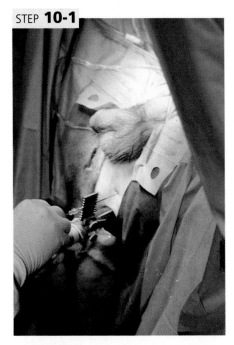

STEP **10-1**

Placing first trocar needle in perineum.

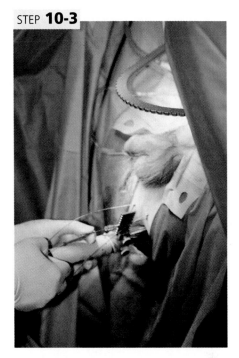

STEP **10-3**

Passing second guidewire into perineum.

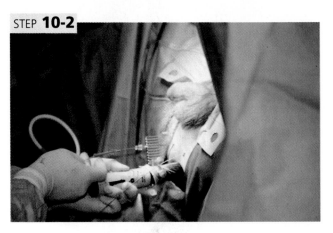

STEP **10-2**

Passing first guidewire through first needle tract.

As each needle is inserted, the trocars are removed and 0.038 J-tipped guidewires are inserted.

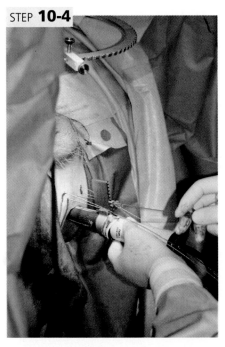

STEP **10-4**

Placing fifth trocar needle in perineum.

11. Once all wires are in place, fascial sleeved dilators are used to create tracts into the prostate. A stab wound may be necessary initially to allow entrance of the dilators.

STEP **11-1**

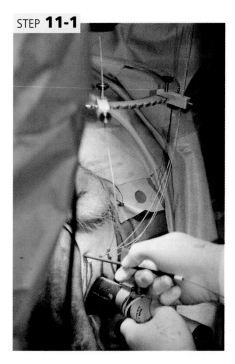

Dilating first tract in perineum.

STEP **11-2**

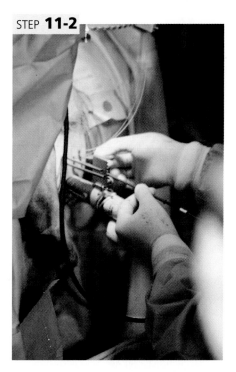

Stabwound incision to allow insertion of fascial dilator.

The dilators are removed, leaving the sleeves in situ for placement of the cryoprobes. Each sleeve is irrigated with saline to confirm their position before placement of the cryoprobes.

STEP **11-3**

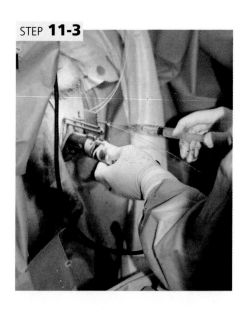

12. The cryoprobes are inserted and the cryotechnician is instructed to "stick all probes." This will adhere the probes to the prostate so that they will be stabilized.

STEP **12-1**

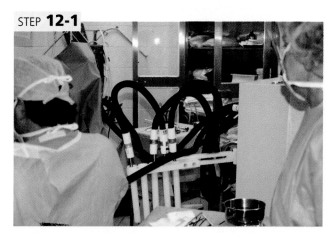

Cryoprobes extending from cryotherapy machine, first probe being positioned.

Elastic straps should be used to support the probes, attaching them to the ring of the retractor.

CONSIDERATIONS The freezing process is begun at the anterior aspect of the gland so that the border of the freeze zone may be observed on the ultrasound monitor progressing posteriorly. Care is taken to avoid freezing the rectal wall and bladder neck and below the pelvic floor. The exact temperature of the peripheral freeze is not really known. Some surgeons place thermocouples into the prostate to determine this.

CONSIDERATIONS

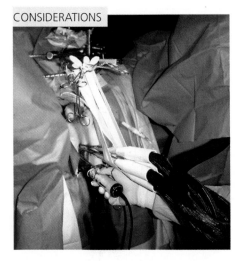

Cryoprobes held in place with elastic straps.

13. Freezing is begun through the anterior probes, followed by complete freezing to the prostate-rectal border. The freeze temperature is −180° C.

13. Ultrasonographic examination is performed on the apex of the gland to assess for residual unfrozen tissue. The probes are thawed and withdrawn 1 to 2 cm. When the probes have been repositioned, this remaining apical tissue should be frozen.

14. After all tissue has been frozen, the procedure is terminated by removing the cryoprobes once they have been "unstuck" (thawed).

15. The warming tubing is removed, and its insertion site and all cryoprobe sites are closed with a 3-0 absorbable suture on a cuticular needle.

16. A #18 Fr, 5 cc Foley catheter is inserted and connected to straight drainage if the urine is bloody. The catheter may be removed the following morning.

Patients treated with cryosurgery are generally admitted to the hospital, and discharged the following morning unless bleeding, fever, or anesthetic complications prevent their discharge.

Noninvasive Procedures

FLUOROSCOPE-ASSISTED INTERVENTIONS

In 1963 the physicists of Dornier Systems Ltd. and Friedrich Shafen discovered that shock waves could travel through body tissue and fragment calculus material without loss of energy. In 1980, Chaussy and associates treated the first patient and in 1982 reported their first series of 72 treated patients. Presently over 80% of urinary tract calculi may be treated with shock-wave lithotripsy, avoiding transurethral or percutaneous instrumentation. Several modifications of the original Dornier extracorporeal shock-wave lithotriptor (ESWL) have been developed and are commercially available.

POSTOPERATIVE

Nursing Care and Discharge Planning for Cryotherapy

1. Most patients are discharged on the first or second postoperative day.
2. Gross hematuria, bladder spasms, and perineal ecchymosis are common sequelae in the first 24 hours postoperatively.
3. Enforced diuresis with IV fluids, diuretics, and liquids as tolerated will help avoid clot formation and retention.
4. Rectal suppositories should be avoided; instead bladder spasms are treated with oral medication.
5. Oral analgesics will be prescribed for pain management. Oral antibiotics are ordered for 1 to 5 days postoperatively.
6. Warm sitz baths and a soft cushions or "hemorrhoid ring" often decrease the patient's perineal discomfort.
7. Care and maintenance of the suprapubic catheter are an important focus for teaching. Spontaneous voiding usually returns in 7 to 14 days. The patient should be instructed to monitor postvoid residual volume. Once this is below a range of 50 to 60 ml on a consistent basis the catheter may be removed.
8. Postoperative follow-up care will include serial PSA levels, digital rectal exams, and transrectal ultrasound evaluations every 3 months postoperatively and postcryotherapy prostate biopsies after 6 months and then yearly.
9. Document nursing interventions and teaching.

All lithotriptors have an energy source, a focusing device, a coupling medium (water), and a stone-localization device (fluoroscopy, ultrasound). High-energy shock waves are generated in air or water by the abrupt release of energy into a small space. When the shock wave meets a boundary between substances of different densities, the stress level between the substances at this interface may overcome the tensile strength of the calculus. As the shock wave penetrates through the stone, a part of the wave is reflected creating a stress on the calculus that results in fragmentation. Repeated shocks ultimately may decrease the size of the calculus to fragments smaller than 2 mm.

The original spark-gap extracorporeal shock-wave lithotriptor (Dornier Human Model-3, or HM3) offered a spark-plug energy source, an ellipsoid reflective focusing surface, water-bath coupling device, and fluoroscopy with two image intensifiers for stone localization. An extremely cumbersome unit, it required a large area for installation. Patient positioning was often difficult, and the physiologic effects of near–total body immersion produced anesthetic difficulties. Additionally it required regional or general anesthesia and was limited to this single function. Although no longer in production, it is still found in many institutions. A modified version offers anesthesia-free treatment but is less powerful.

Second-generation units (Dornier HM4, MFL5000, MPL9000) use water-filled bags, fluoroscopy or ultrasonography, and a dry bed. The HM4 and MPL9000 allow for multidisciplinary use, whereas the MFL5000 (Fig. 13-8) allows for transurethral endoscopic interventions and multidisciplinary lithotripsy. The power of the generator being used determines the need for some method of intraoperative pain management.

Third-generation units (Dornier MFL5000U, MPL9000X) offer a combination of fluoroscopy and ultrasonography, which may be used simultaneously, an electromagnetic shock wave source, and, depending on the power of the generator, anesthesia-free intervention. Electromagnetically induced unfocused shock-wave impulses with an acoustic lens are combined with a tube of degassed water for focusing and inclination of the shock wave and a water cushion for acoustic coupling .

The most recent lithotriptor uses shock waves that are generated from rapid expansion of ceramic elements excited by a high-voltage pulse. This is the piezoelectric crystal shock-wave generation method with monitoring by real-time ultrasonography. It is the only device that is truly pain free because of the lower output frequency employed. No patient analgesia is necessary, the noise level is decreased, the radiation exposure is eliminated, precise localization of radiolucent calculi (important where uric acid stones are prevalent) is possible, no cardiac effects result from treatment, the incidence of *steinstrasse* is decreased, and fewer side effects occur because of the small focal area. On the other hand, therapy generally takes longer, may carry a higher repeat-treatment rate, success with ureteral calculi is minimal, obesity interferes with stone localization, and larger stones are not so readily treated.

With the investigation of the shock-wave method of noninvasive urinary stone treatment, further developments and refinements will be forthcoming. Lithotriptors throughout the country will vary considerably because of the rapid advancements being made. Lithotriptors, other than the water-immersion units, have become multifunctional. Although the newer lithotriptors are less expensive than earlier versions, hospitals and treatment centers that invested in first- and second-generation equipment may be reluctant to purchase these newer-generation units when faced with current economic restraints. Thorough evaluation to determine whether the unit in place has paid for itself, has outlived its usefulness, or carries significant trade-in value will affect whether it is feasible and cost effective to convert systems presently in place.

Two types of lithotriptors are commonly used presently, one requiring water immersion and one utilizing membrane-enclosed water cushions. Although the same precautions and potential sequelae apply no matter which method is employed, it has been shown that water-bath treatments pose the higher risk. The ESWL suite, or mobile trailer, houses all the equipment needed to perform the procedure.

NURSING CARE

Perioperative nursing assessment must include a review of the patient's cardiac and respiratory status, bleeding profiles, presence of infection, a negative pregnancy test for females where applicable, and baseline vital signs. It is also important to ensure that the patient has complied with preoperative restrictions, in particular avoidance of aspirin and nonsteroidal antiinflammatory agents for 5 to 10 days preoperatively.

Nursing diagnoses for patients undergoing ESWL therapy will be the same no matter what type of unit is to be employed. The major difference between the two approaches lies in the degree of risk. Common nursing diagnoses for the ESWL patient include:

NURSING DIAGNOSIS	PERIOPERATIVE PLANNING AND INTERVENTION
Risk for infection related to: Ureteral stent Medical status	Confirm that urine culture is negative for bacteria. Maintain aseptic environment and properly sterilize instrumentation before stent insertion. Use appropriate technique during surgical prep before stent insertion. Drape patient according to aseptic technique before stent insertion. Observe for indications of fever, dysuria, or pyuria. Provide adequate hydration through IV solutions or fluid intake. Administer antibiotic therapies as ordered.
Risk for pain related to: Operative intervention Ureteral stent Passage of fragments Passage of clots	Review common postoperative course. Review pain control regime ordered by physician. Explain that analgesics should be taken regularly at first, before the onset of discomfort. Discuss other measures to decrease pain level: relaxation therapy, guided imagery, minimize activity. Discuss restrictions that may be imposed by pain medication: alcohol, other analgesics to be avoided (aspirin), activity level.
Anxiety related to: Anticipated outcome Knowledge deficit Possible recurrence of presenting condition	Review purpose of planned procedure; ascertain comprehension level. Document expressions of anxiety by patient or significant others. Provide explanations and reassurance to the patient and significant others. Reinforce or review preoperative teaching, answer questions as necessary. Discuss process of shock-wave therapy and why bruising and hematuria may occur. Encourage participation in discharge planning; review discharge instructions. Keep significant others informed during intraoperative and postoperative phases. Verify understanding of reportable signs and symptoms. Allow significant others to spend time with patient preoperatively and postoperatively if setting allows. Place follow-up call the day after surgery.

NURSING DIAGNOSIS	PERIOPERATIVE PLANNING AND INTERVENTION
Altered pattern of urinary elimination related to: Instrumentation Presence of ureteral stent Passage of fragments or clots	Assess and document return flow of urine, include character and color. Observe for and document signs of renal or ureteral colic and dysuria. Observe and document any abdominal distention. Observe for hematuria. Maintain adequate hydration.
Risk for injury related to: Position in hydraulic sling Shock-wave therapy	Correctly position patient in proper body alignment in hydraulic sling (if applicable) after adequate relaxation: 1. Protect ECG leads, IV site, epidural catheter with adhesive transparent waterproof coverings. 2. Ensure adequate personnel to safely transfer patient to and from sling. 3. Ensure that patient's back from the scapula level up is supported by foam backrest. 4. Support patient's head in horseshoe headrest. 5. Secure patient with safety straps across upper chest, thighs, ankles, and diagonally across abdomen. 6. Assess for and relieve pressure on sensitive neurovascular areas. 7. Avoid undue stretch on muscles, ligaments, and joints. 8. Position arms across chest or on padded armrests when sling is raised and lowered. If patient is supine or prone, provide padding under knees or chest, axillae, and ankles. Assess character and presence of bilateral pedal and radial pulses perioperatively. Explain that some bruising may occur over focal shock-wave sites. With water bath unit, facial bruising, though not common, has occurred.

The perioperative genitourinary nurse caring for the patient undergoing ESWL must also have a comprehensive working knowledge of the equipment. It is important to understand the operation of the operating bed, the hydraulic sling, and the ESWL unit.

Positioning the patient properly and safely on the operating room bed or in the hydraulic sling is essential. It is critical to an optimal outcome that the patient be aligned for maximum contact between the working head of the ESWL unit and the calculus. This is aided by the presence of the stent and the use of C-arm fluoroscopy. If the calculus is located near the pelvic bone, the patient may be placed prone on the bed or gantry (sling) so that the shock wave may be directed at the sacroiliac notch. Another method is to elevate the buttock and flank area with a foam wedge approximately 30 degrees off the bed and angle the working head to align with the target site.

As perioperative care is implemented, the plan of care will be subject to alteration and revision on an ongoing basis. All patient-centered activities must relate to the data collected during the preoperative assessment and to changing intraoperative circumstances. The perioperative genitourinary nurse should be cognizant of this possibility and be prepared to effectively adjust the plan of care. This ongoing adjustment allows for an individualized and patient-focused approach.

Once care has been implemented the postoperative assessment is completed. Often it will not be possible to determine long-term outcomes properly. Immediate postoperative assessment allows for a baseline determination of the effect of nursing care delivered. Priority postoperative assessment data appropriate for the continual evaluation of nursing care for ESWL might include the following:

- Awareness of reportable signs and symptoms of infection or hemorrhage

- Knowledge of the need to curtail strenuous activity
- Cognizance of restrictions imposed by the medication regime
- Comprehension of the medication regime ordered by the physician (aspirin and nonsteroidal antiinflammatory agents should be avoided for 10 days unless otherwise directed)
- Understanding of the need for adequate fluid intake to accelerate healing, assist the voiding process, offset infection, and promote recovery from spinal anesthesia
- Review of follow-up requirements (postoperative physician visit, activity level, diet)
- Discussion of ureteral catheter care
- Readiness for discharge

An overview of the care provided and the subsequent evaluation is recorded to provide for the continuity of care throughout the recovery period. Documentation should be individualized according to the ESWL approach and specific patient needs. Surgical settings differ, and perioperative documentation will have guidelines appropriate for the specific institution. A summary of the intraoperative activities designed to achieve certain outcome criteria should be reported to the postanesthesia care nurse.

Priority information for the ESWL patient may include the following:

- Precautions pertinent to the patient's preoperative and postoperative physical condition
- Status of peripheral circulation and skin integrity
- Positions and positional devices employed
- Status of urinary output and ureteral catheter patency at discharge from the ESWL suite
- Fluid replacement
- Level of comprehension during preoperative instruction
- Presence of anxiety or fear during preoperative and intraoperative stages

- Information relayed to the patient preoperatively and intra-operatively
- Untoward reactions encountered intraoperatively
- Nursing care provided

ESWL (EXTRACORPOREAL SHOCK WAVE LITHOTRIPSY)

Description. Calculi that are treated with shock-wave lithotripsy are fragmented by the energy focused on the stone with the lithotriptor. Shock waves reverberate inside the calculus causing fragmentation, initially at the front and back of the shock-wave path, with ultimate complete or partial destruction of the calculus. The amount of destruction is dependent on the number and energy of the shock waves delivered and the hardness of the stone. This technique is effective, since shock waves can be transmitted and focused through tissue without loss of energy.

Shock waves may range from 500 to 2000 impulses and are administered over a time period that can vary from 30 minutes to 2 hours. A loud reverberating popping sound occurs each time a wave pulse is activated. It is advisable that ear plugs be worn by all.

The requirement for anesthesia is determined by the power of the shock wave, the area of shock-wave entry at the skin level, and the size of the shock-wave focal point. The summation of shock waves used during the procedure can cause pain at the skin level.

Typically, general, spinal, or local anesthesia is used with the first-generation lithotriptors, such as the HM-3. Later versions have been developed to allow for lithotripsy with only intravenous sedation, oral sedation, or a transcutaneous electrical nerve stimulator (TENS unit).

In the era of open intervention for stone disease, urologists were reluctant to offer surgical intervention because of the 20% risk of prolonged wound discomfort, cost of hospitalization, lengthy recovery, and potential morbidity. It is believed that approximately 60% of patients were treated too late to avoid significant, disease-related, preoperative, and postoperative complications. Urologists have become more aggressive with the advent of the less-invasive ESWL, and patients are being treated earlier, thus avoiding the significant sequelae previously encountered.

Indications. Radiographic demonstration of a calculus or calculi in a ureteral tract that will allow passage of fragments. The need for ancillary procedures such as ureteral stenting (stones greater than 1.5 cm) or percutaneous nephrostomy (staghorn calculi, where a large volume of stone fragments will cause obstruction or where percutaneous stone extraction is contemplated for the complex calculi in a "full kidney") must be evaluated. The incidence of renal infection as a result of stone disease rises relative to the length of time the calculus has been present and the increase in the size of the calculus during that time. A calculus that has existed for 2 years carries an infection rate of 58% and a growth rate of 26%. After 5 years these rates convert to 70% and 39%, respectively. At 10 years, they rise dra-

matically to 83% and 78%. Additionally, 26% of patients are asymptomatic at 2 years. At 5 years, 17% remain asymptomatic, and after 10 years, only 11% are without symptoms. In the first 5 years, 80% of patients require treatment.

It is important to assess for and eliminate urinary tract infection, determine renal function, and review the results of coagulation studies. The patient must be informed of alternative therapies and potential complications, including the potential necessity of repeat treatments or auxiliary procedures to remove fragments.

Stone-free rates after lithotripsy depend on the location, size, and composition of calculi. Generally, stone-free rates range from 80% to 90% for renal and upper ureteral calculi, and 70% for lower ureteral calculi. Calcium oxalate monohydrate and cystine calculi are difficult to fragment relative to stones of other composition such as calcium oxalate dihydrate. Stones greater than 1.5 cm may require more than one treatment to render the kidney stone free in 90% of afflicted patients. Stones larger than this may require additional procedures such as percutaneous or ureteroscopic approaches to achieve complete elimination of calculus material. Patients with stones greater than 1.5 cm, or who require hospitalization because of renal colic, are more likely to benefit from the placement of a ureteral stent before the procedure.

Contraindications include pregnancy, coagulopathy, distal obstruction, and uncontrolled infection with urosepsis. Partial loss of parenchyma is not considered a contraindication to ESWL.

Perioperative risks. The overall mortality for ESWL is 0.02%. Iliac artery and vein thrombosis have been reported with lithotripsy for ureteral stones, and shielding of lungs is necessary in infants and children to prevent pulmonary damage. Renal artery aneurysm rupture has not been reported so far.

Patients presenting with a large obstructing stone (greater than 3 cm) may have a diminished effect from treatment because of the lack of available expansion space in the kidney. A large calculus may cause particle shielding or not allow room in the kidney for the full impact of cavitation, resulting in less effective fragmentation of the stone. The accumulation of these stone fragments (*steinstrasse* or "street of stones") in the ureter occurs in less than 5% of lithotripsy cases and is located in the upper ureter 18% and the lower ureter 75% of the time. Intervention for *steinstrasse* is required in 35% of this 5% because of a solitary kidney, pain, total obstruction, or a 3 cm length of ureter full of fragments. Varying degrees of success have been realized with the use of adjunctive therapies to assist propulsion of fragments. Attempts include hydration, diuretics, and prostaglandin inhibitors to augment peristaltic waves while allowing ureteral dilatation and aiding stone passage.

A staghorn calculus is a complex branching calculus carrying a high morbidity and involving most of the renal pelvis and at least two major calyces. These tend to cause increased system dilatation resulting in an adverse effect on the post-treatment stone-free rate. If the renal system is "overdilated," the propulsion of fragments is less effective because they settle into the dilated sections and are distanced from the peristaltic action that aids expulsion. If the stone burden created by a staghorn calculus exceeds a surface area of 500 mm, or if a large calculus exists (greater than 3 cm), it may best be treated with anatrophic nephrolithotomy or percutaneous nephrostolithotomy.

The use of a stent prior to ESWL is dependent on the patient and the character of the calculus or calculi. It should also be determined that the urine culture is negative. Studies show that complication rates decrease if a stent is utilized with a stone greater than 1.5 cm. A stent placed before ESWL generally allows the patient a shortened hospital stay or treatment as an outpatient, tends to decrease the need for ancillary interventions, reduces overall complications, and assists in proper positioning for ESWL by delineating the ureteral anatomy and the precise stone location. On the other hand, those patients who tend to readily form stones may demonstrate calcification of the ureteral stent in a relatively short period of time. Other problems related to ureteral stents have been flank discomfort, hematuria, nausea, vomiting, frequency, urgency, dysuria, bladder spasms, renal colic, or ureteral colic, perforation, urinoma, suture irritation of the urethra, vesicoureteral reflux, fragmentation, incontinence, stent migration, premature stent removal, obstruction, and sepsis. Some of these events may be avoided by proper selection of stent material, diameter, and length; by accurate placement; and by removing the tether at the urethral end. Without a stent the risk of silent renal obstruction resulting in loss of kidney function, obstruction of the ureter, nephritis, and sepsis is increased.

Gross hematuria is seen almost universally, resolves in 12 to 48 hours, and is believed to be attributable to parenchymal edema, which spontaneously heals within 1 week. Subcapsular or perirenal hematoma caused by perinephric fluid collections are seen in 15% to 30% of cases. The incidence appears to be higher in the hypertensive patient. Subcapsular hematoma may resolve in 6 weeks or require 6 months, whereas perirenal hematoma will usually be relieved in a matter of days. Calcification, scarring, loss of nephrons, and dilated veins have been demonstrated in treated animal studies. Less than 1% of patients have demonstrated cardiac dysrhythmias, myocardial infarction, pulmonary contusion, pancreatitis, or splenic rupture One study shows an increase in hypertension from 3% to 8%, but this is not confirmed by other studies. Renal colic has been exhibited in less than 25% of patients, obstructive pyelonephritis in 2% to 6%, and sepsis in 0.5%. Impairment of renal function may be seen in patients with solitary kidneys. The majority of lithotripsy patients will demonstrate little or no long-term morbidity.

Complications related to shock-wave lithotripsy result from the cavitation effects of treatment and are proportional to the number of shocks. Whole blood exposed to shock waves demonstrates breakdown of red blood cell membranes and the release of free hemoglobin into solutions. The ability of the kidney's tubular cells to survive shock waves is related to the number of shock waves to which the kidney is exposed and not the energy level. Bone-growth abnormalities have been demonstrated in rats exposed to shock-wave lithotripsy, with shortened extremities in 17% of treated animals. Additionally, injury to the lung has been demonstrated in laboratory animals as exhibited by the expectoration of blood. No apparent injury to the heart muscle or spinal cord has been shown.

Instrumentation/equipment. If a stent is to be inserted immediately before the procedure, the patient will be taken to the operating room. A cystoscopy, retrograde pyelogram, and stent insertion setup should be prepared and all the associated nursing guidelines followed (refer to Chapter 7). If the stent is already in place or one will not be used, the patient is taken to the ESWL suite for the intervention. The equipment is stationary, and the unit is stocked with appropriate positioning and protective devices (Fig. 13-8).

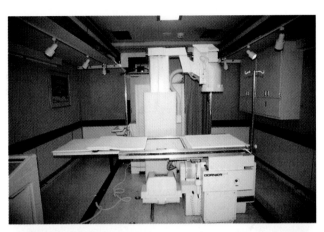

A

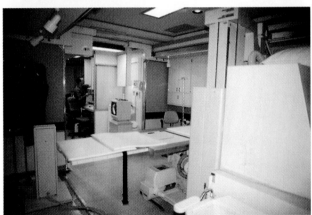

B

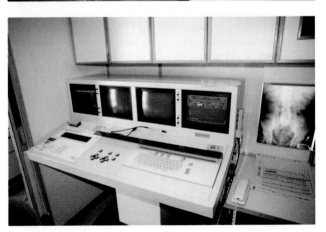

C

FIG. 13-8 **A,** ESWL trailer set-up with Dornier MFL 5000. **B,** ESWL trailer set-up. **C,** Monitors for ESWL.

Nursing Care and Teaching Considerations for ESWL

1. Incorporate all general nursing diagnosis and interventions for ESWL.
2. Check ESWL unit and operating room bed or hydraulic sling for proper function before patient's arrival.
3. Check all medications for dose and outdates.
4. Patient is at risk for infection with ESWL. Ascertain that urine culture is negative or, if indicative of infection, the condition has been appropriately treated before surgery. Evaluate reports of other pertinent preoperative studies (PT, PTT, Hgb, serum electrolytes, chest x-ray, ECG, IVPs).
5. Assess patient for comprehension of planned surgical intervention and anxiety level. Review as needed, including postoperative expectations and common sequelae.
6. Assess patient for skin integrity, peripheral vascular circulation, presence of implants, range of motion, and general physical status (allergies, limitations, past surgeries).
7. Review postoperative course: probable hematuria, renal or ureteral colic, flank pain, possible bruising.
8. Document assessment findings.
9. Gather x-ray protection and ear plugs for personal and patient.
10. Ensure that appropriate positioning aids are available (pillows, axillary rolls, pads for bony prominences, waterproof tape, etc.).
11. Under the guidance of the anesthetist, position patient on the operating room bed or into hydraulic sling, utilizing adequate assistance. Ensure that IV lines are free of constriction. Ensure that IV site, ECG leads, and epidural catheter are protected if water-bath unit is employed.
12. Protect patient's thyroid and chest with leaded shield.
13. Apply petrolatum to affected flank to prevent air bubbles.
14. Connect and turn on equipment.
15. Document nursing interventions.

Procedural Steps

1. Position the patient in the shock-wave path on the lithotriptor using the localization system of the machine (usually fluoroscopy, possibly ultrasonography).

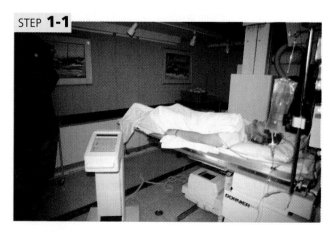

STEP **1-1**

Patient positioned for ESWL utilizing Dornier MFL5000.

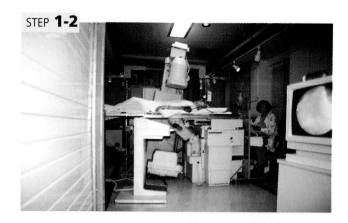

STEP **1-2**

Establishing shock wave path for fragmentation process.

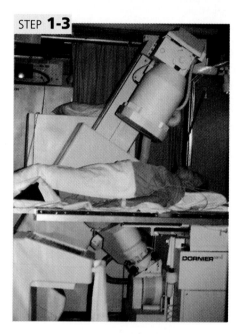

STEP **1-3**

Lithotriptor in shock wave path position.

2. Select an energy level and number of shocks appropriate for the position, size, and composition of the stone, and the habitus of the patient.

3. Monitor the destruction of the stone with the imaging system during the procedure.

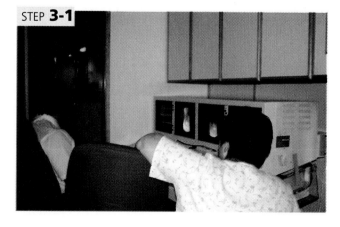

STEP **3-1**

POSTOPERATIVE

Nursing Care and Discharge Planning for ESWL

1. Complete perioperative documentation including postoperative assessment.
2. Cleanse patient of petrolatum. Assess skin condition.
3. Evaluate status of peripheral vascular circulation.
4. Assess urinary output and patency of ureteral catheter. If a tethered catheter is in place, ensure that the suture is secured without tension.
5. Patient may resume diet as tolerated postoperatively, starting slowly with clear liquids.
6. Patient should drink 8 oz of water or juice every 2 hours for 48 hours to assist voiding process, offset infection, ensure hydration, and accelerate healing process.
7. Patient should avoid strenuous activity for at least 2 days postoperatively.
8. Prescribed medications should be taken as directed, antibiotics until gone. Aspirin and nonsteroidal antiinflammatory agents should be avoided for 10 days unless advised by the surgeon as medically necessary.
9. Review symptoms of infection (fever, pyuria, dysuria), hemorrhage, transient sensory nerve deficit, hematuria, ecchymosis or petechiae (redness, warmth or bruising of face or at shock-wave entry and exit sites), grossly red urine with or without clots.
10. Review ureteral catheter care. If infection or extreme discomfort occurs, stent may need to be removed to be eliminated as the possible causative agent.
11. Discuss possibility of renal or ureteral colic until majority of fragments have passed, clots have cleared, or stent is removed.
12. Urine should be strained for fragments; particles should be taken to physician on first postoperative visit to be sent for qualitative analysis.
13. KUB will be performed on first postoperative visit even in absence of symptoms of obstruction. These may be repeated as indicated for 2 to 4 weeks.
14. If the patient has a history of previous stones, a 24-hour urine collection will be performed once postoperative IVUs indicate the patient is stone free. This allows assessment of the patient's metabolic status for future stone-forming potential (elevated uric acid, calcium, oxalates, subnormal excretion of citrates). An appropriate stone-risk diet may be prescribed after review of the urine study.
15. Document nursing interventions and teaching.

4. Provide patient with appropriate prescriptions for analgesics, antibiotics, and postoperative instructions before discharge.

Bibliography

1. Association of Operating Room Nurses: *Quality improvement in perioperative nursing.* Denver, 1992, AORN.
2. Association of Operating Room Nurses, Inc.: *Standards and recommended practices,* Denver, 1995, AORN.
3. American Urologic Association Allied, Inc: *Standards of urologic nursing practice,* Richmond, 1990, AUAA.
4. Babian RJ, Chodak GW: Is cryosurgery effective in treating prostate cancer. From Course Syllabus: *Controversies in prostate cancer,* Washington, DC, 1995, AUA.
5. Benumof JL, Saidman LJ: *Anesthesia and perioperative complications,* St. Louis, 1992, Mosby.
6. Blasko et al: *Ultrasonically guided* ^{125}I /^{103}Pd /^{192}Ir *implantation for the treatment of prostate cancer,* Seattle, 1995, Pacific NW Cancer Foundation.
7. Brundage DJ: *Renal disorders,* St. Louis, 1992, Mosby.
8. Chaussy C et al: *Extracorporeal shock wave lithotripsy,* Munich, 1982, Karger Verlag.
9. Clayman RV et al: A comparison of in vitro cellular effects of shock waves generated by electrohydraulic, electromagnetic, and piezoelectric sources, *J Urol* 141:228A, 1989.
10. Delius M: This month in investigative urology: effect of extracorporeal shock waves on the kidney, *J Urol* 140:390, 1988.
11. Desmet W et al: Iliac vein thrombosis after extracorporeal shock wave lithotripsy *N Engl J Med* 321:907, 1989.
12. Droller MJ: *Surgical management of urologic disease,* St. Louis, 1992, Mosby.
13. Dyer RB et al: Magnetic resonance imaging evaluation of immediate and intermediate changes in kidneys treated with extracorporeal shock wave lithotripsy, *J Lithotripsy Stone Dis* 2:302, 1990.
14. Elbers J et al: The effects of shock wave lithotripsy on urease positive calculogenic bacteria. In Lingeman JE, Newman DM, eds: *Shock wave lithotripsy,* New York, 1988, Plenum Press.
15. Fedullo LM et al: The development of steinstrasse after ESWL: frequency, natural history, and radiologic management, *AJR* 151:1145, 1988.
16. Fegan JE, Preminger GM: Extracorporeal shock wave lithotripsy. In *High Tech Urology,* Philadelphia, 1992, WB Saunders.
17. Fine J et al: Effect of medical management and residual fragments on recurrent stone formation following shock wave lithotripsy, *J Urology* 153:27, 1995.
18. Fischer N et al: Cavitation effects: possible cause of tissue injury during extracorporeal shock wave lithotripsy, *J Endourol* 2:215, 1988.
19. Grimm PD et al: Ultrasound-guided transperineal implantation of iodine-125 and palladium- 103 for the treatment of early stage prostate cancer, *Atlas Urol Clinics No Am* 2:2, 1994.
20. Jaegar P et al: Morphologic changes in canine kidneys following extracorporeal shock wave treatment, *J Endourol* 2:205, 1988.
21. Keeler L et al: Extracorporeal shock wave lithotripsy for lower ureteral calculi: treatment of choice, *J Endourol* 4:71, 1990.
22. Kirby RS, Christmas TJ: *Benign prostatic hyperplasia,* London, 1993, Gower.
23. Kroovand RL: Extracorporeal shock wave lithotripsy in the pediatric stone patient: problems and results, *Probl Urol* 1 (4)682, 1987.
24. Lepor H: *Urologic clinics of North America: advances in benign prostatic hypertrophy,* Philadelphia, 22:2, WB Saunders, May, 1995.
25. Lepor H, Lawson RK: *Prostate diseases,* Philadelphia, 1993, WB Saunders.
26. Litwack K: *Core curriculum for post anesthesia nursing,* ed 3, Philadelphia, 1995, WB Saunders.
27. McAteer JA et al: Cell culture and in vitro systems to assess the bioeffects of ESWL, *J Urol* 141:228A, 1989.
28. Meeker MR, Rothrock JC: *Alexander's care of the patient in surgeryy,* St. Louis, 1995, Mosby.
29. Moran ME et al: Effects of high energy shock waves on chick embryo development, *J Urol* 143:167A, 1990.
30. Randazzo RF et al: The in vitro and in vivo effects of extracorporeal shock waves on malignant cells, *Urol Res* 16 (6)419, 1988.

31. Resnick MI, Kursh ED: *Current therapy in genitourinary surgery,* ed 2, St. Louis, 1992, Mosby.

32. Rothrock JC: *Perioperative nursing care planning,* St. Louis, ed 2, 1996, Mosby.

33. Rubin JI et al: Kidney changes after extracorporeal shock wave lithotripsy CT evaluation, *Radiology,* 162:21, 1987.

34. Smith AD: *Controversies in endourology,* Philadelphia, 1995, WB Saunders.

35. Smith JA: *High tech urology,* Philadelphia, 1992, WB Saunders.

36. Tanagho EA, McAninch JW: *Smith's general urology,* ed 14, Norwalk, 1995, Appleton & Lange.

37. Vaiden RE et al: *Core curriculum for the RN first assistant,* Denver, 1990, AORN.

38. Walsh PC et al: *Campbell's urology,* ed 6, Philadelphia, 1992, WB Saunders.

39. Yeaman LD et al: Effect of shock waves on structure and growth of the immature rat epiphysis, *J Urol* 141, 670, 1989.

Index